McGRAW-HILL SERIES IN WATER RESOURCES AND ENVIRONMENTAL ENGINEERING

Ven Te Chow, Rolf Eliassen, and Ray K. Linsley, Consulting Editors

CHANLETT: Environmental Protection

GRAF: Hydraulics of Sediment Transport

HALL AND DRACUP: Water Resources Systems Engineering

JAMES AND LEE: Economics of Water Resources Planning

LINSLEY AND FRANZINI: Water Resources Engineering

METCALF AND EDDY, INC: Wastewater Engineering: Collection, Treatment, Disposal

WALTON: Groundwater Resource Evaluation

WIENER: The Role of Water in Development: An Analysis of Principles of Comprehensive Planning

ENVIRONMENTAL
PROTECTION

**McGRAW-HILL
BOOK COMPANY**

New York
St. Louis
San Francisco
Düsseldorf
Johannesburg
Kuala Lumpur
London
Mexico
Montreal
New Delhi
Panama
Rio de Janeiro
Singapore
Sydney
Toronto

EMIL T. CHANLETT

*Professor of Sanitary Engineering
Department of Environmental Sciences and Engineering
School of Public Health
University of North Carolina, Chapel Hill*

Environmental Protection

This book was set in Times New Roman.
The editors were B. J. Clark and Michael Gardner;
the cover was designed by Anthony J. Paccione;
and the production supervisor was Ted Agrillo.
The drawings were done by Oxford Illustrators Limited.

Library of Congress Cataloging in Publication Data

Chanlett, Emil T
   Environmental protection.

   (Water resources and environmental engineering series)
   1. Environmental engineering. I. Title. [DNLM: 1. Air pollution—Prevention & control.
2. Environmental health. 3. Sanitation. 4. Water pollution—Prevention & control. WA 670
C459e 1973]
TD145.C45   614.7   72-8118
ISBN 0-07-010520-0

**ENVIRONMENTAL
PROTECTION**

456789—MAMM—7654

To
ELISKA LOWBEEROVA CHANLETT
and
DANIEL ALEXANDER OKUN

CONTENTS

Foreword   xi

Preface   xiii

1 The Quality Factors for Environmental Protection   1

Population Trends and Resource Use   1
The First Level—Health Effects   6
The Second Level—Comfort, Convenience, Efficiency, and Esthetics   11
The Third Level—The Effects on the Balance of Ecosystems and
 Natural Resources   14
The Quality of the Environment and Resource Management   17
Ecology and Ecosystems   23
Meteorology   27

**2 Some Principles of Epidemiology and of the Sciences Which
 Underlie Environmental Protection**   36

Epidemiology   37
The Fate of Our Pathogens   45

The Mass of the Dose 55
A Mathematical Expression That Predicts Several Environmental
  Phenomena 58
Electromagnetic Energy and Its Spectrum 60

3 Man's Use of Water Resources **64**

The Need 64
The Quantities 65
The Qualities for Drinking and Domestic Use 75
The Sources and Their Use 89
Attaining and Maintaining Quality for Domestic Use 101
Water for Recreation 117
Water for Agriculture 127
Water for Industry 131
Possible Changes and Developments 132
An Appraisal of Man's Management of Water 134

4 Disposal of Excreta and Wastewaters **139**

The Need 139
Dilution and Pollution 142
Sewage Treatment and Process Choices 150
Industrial Wastewaters 167
The Disposal of Human Excreta without Sewers 178
Possible Changes and Developments in Managing Human Excreta 186
An Appraisal of Man's Management of His Own Excreta and
  Wastewaters 191

5 Our Air Environment **196**

Encounters with Contaminated and Polluted Air 196
Toxic Gases, Vapors, Dusts, and Fumes Producing Occupational Diseases 200
Our Community Air 223
Changes and Developments 271
Appraisal 274

6 Solid Wastes Management **277**

The Solid Wastes Issues 277
Phases and Choices 288
An Agricultural Waste—Animal Manure 305
Improvements and Developments 309
An Appraisal 311

7   Vector Control   **314**

The Rationale of Control   316
A Classification of Control Methods   317
Insecticides   320
Vectors and Hosts, and the Mechanisms of Transmission   327
Malaria Eradication—A Global Campaign   336
Rodent Action and Man's Counteraction   340
Schistosomiasis   349
Changes and Developments in Controlling Animal Vectors   353
An Appraisal of Man's Control of Insects and Rodents   355

8   Food Protection from Source to Use   **359**

Compatibilities and Contrasts between Cultural Patterns and Food
   Protection Goals   359
Three Primary Targets of Food Protection   360
Achieving Food Protection in Growing, Processing, Storing,
   Transporting, and Retailing   384
Achieving Food Protection in Final Preparation and Serving   400
Washing and Sanitizing Food-processing Equipment and Food-
   handling Utensils   405
Tests and Inspections for Food Protection   409
Changes and Developments to Come   411
An Appraisal of Food Protection   413

9   Ionizing Radiation and Its Control   **418**

The Origin of Ionizing Radiations   420
The Emissions   427
Units and Measurements   430
Biological Damage from the Ionization of Tissue   436
Limits on Exposure and on Dose for Voluntary and Official Groups   445
Radiation Protection—Principles and Techniques   451
Instrumental Measurement   459
Changes and Developments   464
Appraisal   469

**10   Electromagnetic Energy in the Range of Ultraviolet, Visible
      Light, Laser, the Radio Frequencies, and Microwave**   **473**

Ultraviolet   475
The Visible Range   478
Laser, Coherent Light   491

The Radio Frequencies and Microwave   498
Possible Changes and Developments in the Use of Certain Segments
    of the Electromagnetic Energy Spectrum   504
An Appraisal of Man's Management of Certain Segments of the
    Electromagnetic Energy Spectrum   506

11   The Energies of Heat and Sound   **509**
Heat and Man   509
Sound, the Unwanted Form—Noise   523
Changes and Developments   544
Appraisal   547

Name Index   **555**
Subject Index   **559**

A characteristic which has set people apart from other species has been their ability to control many aspects of their environment. Throughout recorded history man has continually struggled to manage his natural environment in order to improve his health and well-being. The sanitary code of Moses in the Old Testament, which is as sound today as it was when written, gave direction to man's efforts, but it was not until the "sanitary awakening" following the industrial and scientific revolutions that major environmental control progress was made. In recent years environmental sanitation in many parts of the world has led to large reductions or virtual elimination of diseases spread via the environment, such as the insect-, rodent-, water- and food-borne infections. Not long ago these diseases were at the top of the list of causes of death and morbidity.

Continuous environmental vigilance is necessary to keep these weeds in the garden of humanity from increasing to the proportions which still exist among a large part of the earth's population. Man's successes in the control of environmental-borne diseases have not reduced the need for ever-increased efforts of effective management of the total environment. The population explosion, an affluent society with desires for a vast array of products, increased radiations, the automobile, greater energy use, increased food production needs, and other developments have created strains on parts of the ecological systems.   Perhaps never in history has man demonstrated such great concern for his total environment as in now being witnessed in many parts of the earth, particularly in those areas which have benefited most from man's environmental control efforts toward more effective uses of human, material, and natural resources.

This text is appropriately man- and health-oriented in its approach to environmental protection.   It recognizes man's place and role in the ecological system and encompasses most aspects of environmental control and protection.   Emphasis is placed on the "why" and sufficient treatment of the "what" and "how to" of the following areas: effects on man's health, effects on ecosystems, and effects on comfort, convenience, and esthetics.

The sections of each chapter dealing with Changes and Developments and An Appraisal of management and protection efforts further illustrate man's position in the system and aid the student in the evaluation of progress as well as environmental-control needs.

I used a draft of this book three times for a rather broad one-quarter course on environmental control that met four times per week and was taken by groups of undergraduate students, very heterogeneous as to educational background, including fine arts, education, social science, science, and engineering.   I found the text to be very satisfactory for most of the students.   Those who had taken college-level biology, chemistry, and physics were able to pursue the text material quite thoroughly.   Those whose education in science was very limited, while unable to understand the organic chemistry of pesticides, the detailed biology of certain diseases, or the activated sludge process, did obtain a grasp of the "whys" of environmental control, together with extensive improvement in their overall scientific understanding of concepts that enabled them to analyze more logically environmental information and at least, relate their thinking to scientific principles.   On the whole these students of diverse basic educational backgrounds found the text stimulating and interesting.   The text material is well organized and cohesive, and the ideas are clearly presented.

This text will be a useful reference for the professional who seeks answers to the "whys" of environmental problems.   However, its greatest value should be for the education of the student entering the health, environment, and associated fields, and to those people who, as concerned citizens, wish to acquire a better basic understanding of environmental problems.

HAROLD B. GOTAAS
Walter P. Murphy Professor
The Technological Institute
Northwestern University
Evanston, Illinois

PREFACE

Environmental protection is man-centered. This book states the rationale for the management of our water resources, of our excreta and wastewaters, of our air environment, of our solid wastes, of commensal insects and rodents, of our food, and of exacerbations of physical energy to prevent the impairment of health, to promote our efficiency and comfort, and to safeguard the balances in natural ecosystems. The principles of environmental protection are emphasized. The objectives of design and practice are given without detailing design or practice methods. The consequences of mismanagement of the major environmental components are examined at three levels: effects on health; effects on comfort, convenience, efficiency, and esthetics; and effects on the balances of ecosystems and of renewable resources. The first chapter develops and illustrates these three levels of man's concern for the earth's environmental quality and the interrelations among these. The driving forces of the " P game " are identified. These are the exponential growth of people, production, power, places, and pollutants. The impact of this growth on the water, air, and land cycles of nature are cited.

These three cycles offer one unifying theme for teaching environmental protection. The topical Chapters 3 through 8 are arranged in the order of water, air, and land. The book is fitted to such an approach with the added selective use of the material on the physical energies in the last three chapters, which cover ionizing radiations, electromagnetic energies, heat, and sound.

Chapter 2 provides an introduction to epidemiology, the study of the environmental and social factors that determine man's health, the fate of biological pathogens in the free environment, and the importance of the mass of the dose in disease processes. Although directed to biological agents in Chapter 2, these matters are equally applicable to chemical and physical agents. These applications are made in the chapters on air, food, vector control, and radiations. Two phenomena that are encountered again and again in environmental protection are examined briefly in Chapter 2. These are the mathematical expression for first-order, or monomolecular, reactions and the electromagnetic energy spectrum. These two common denominators require enough development to impress students of environmental protection with the unity of the processes of nature, which we so readily tend to isolate into specialized studies and exclusive domains.

Chapter 2 provides a base for a second approach to teaching environmental protection. That is the identification and grouping of biological, chemical, and physical agents. The separation of biological and chemical agents in the topics covered in Chapters 3 through 8 would be too disjointing, if followed rigorously. The biological and chemical agents are dealt with jointly under the environmental media of water, wastewater, solid wastes, and food. Except for treating radioactivity in water and food under those subjects, the physical energies stand apart in Chapters 9 to 11.

Each of the nine topical chapters conclude with sections on Changes and Developments and an Appraisal of our management and protection efforts. The views are mine and reflect over 30 years of professional practice in the wide span of environmental protection. There is certain to be disagreement with these views from other professional practitioners. There is the risk that time will speedily make the comments outdated. These have been retained because trial use of draft copies of the text by students at Northwestern University has shown them to stimulate student interest and to provoke lively discussion.

The book is written with the anticipation that its users will have an understanding of chemistry, biology, physics, and mathematics to the extent of basic principles and recallable familiarity with terminology and symbols. New or unusual units are identified and explained. This holds particularly for the treatment of the physical energies. The choice of English and metric units has been a compromise. Design and performance data on water, wastewater, airflow, and solid wastes are in English units. Chemical concentrations and physical energy values are in metric units. Temperatures are given in both the Fahrenheit and Celsius scales. The transition from English to metric units is welcomed with a reluctance to abandon precipitously the familiar design and performance landmarks in English units.

The perplexing issues of chemical toxicants and pollutants in environmental media are met in the context of the media and of their use. Therefore, information and comment on low-level concentration of organics in water, of pesticides and weedicides, and of food additives are found in the chapters on water, air, vector control, and food protection. The discussion on rationale of ionizing radiation and limits on exposure and dose contributes to an understanding of the difficulties that are met in decisions on low-level exposures from any environmental contaminants for long time spans. This handling of the issues deprives the reader of a handy compend on the subject. It does provide the information for formulating an understanding and obliges recognition of the use setting in which the choices must be made. A reasoned position on pesticide residues and on food additives requires knowledge of the beneficial uses of these materials.

The book is offered to meet the needs of a one-semester course in environmental protection. It is likely that only a graduate group of students from the several specialties, seeking a broadening of their information on all aspects of the environment, will undertake cover to cover use of the book. For other groups selective use is recommended. Some groups will find that a single reading of the chapters on vector control and food protection suffices without elaboration in classroom work. This may hold for engineering students. Other groups may find the discussion of industrial wastewaters, agricultural wastes, coherent light, and heat can be managed as reading assignments without classroom treatment. This may hold for sanitarians, although that professional group rarely finds itself with an excess of knowledge for the variety of questions addressed to it by the people it serves. The book is fitted to college groups at the undergraduate level who seek an understanding of environmental issues or an introduction to the field with thought of specialization in it by further professional preparation. The first group is usually from very mixed backgrounds ranging from the natural sciences to the fine arts. The task rests with the instructor to delineate the depth and detail of the subject matter which such students are expected to master both from the instructor's material and from any book. For the latter group, a sampling of scientific detail in the form of chemical reactions, organic structural formulas, physics and mathematical equations, and biological classifications and behavior is given to convince such students that environmental protection depends upon the sciences which they have sought to master and that it is a field of applied sciences in which they can test their mettle to solve scientific and social problems.

The book is directed to the question "Why?" rather than to "What?" or "How to?" The data in tables and graphs, in many instances from original sources, are designed to answer "Why?" The answers are not always complete and are sometimes controversial. The text is addressed to the tables and graphs and avoids repetition in words of the data set forth in the tables and graphs. This makes the projection of the illustrative material from the book during classroom use an effective teaching method. It also provides for assignments requiring analysis of tabular and graphic data as an adjunct to learning by active cerebral engagement with the material in the book. A source of visual aids and a problem manual for teachers are planned.

I would not have had the audacity to undertake writing this book without the strong and active support of my Department Head, Dr. Daniel A. Okun, and my wife, Eliska Lowbeerova Chanlett. The help of those who did technical review of chapters and sections of subject matter for which they are recognized authorities gives me confidence in the scientific accuracy, subject always to more recent findings, and courage to face the discovery of errors which likely persist. Colleagues of my own department who did technical reviews are Morris A. Shiffman on epidemiology and food protection; Charles O'Melia on water resources; Richard Cole on excreta and wastewater; James C. Lamb on industrial, recreational, and agricultural water and wastewater; Arthur C. Stern on the air environment; Newton Underwood on the ionizing and nonionizing radiations; and Robert Harris on heat and sound. Dr. George Kupchik of Hunter College reviewed the chapter on solid wastes. The quality of the chapter on vector control owes much to generous assistance of the scientific staff of the Vector Biology and Control and Malaria Eradication groups of the World Health Organization through interviews, the provision of data, and a painstaking review of the draft text. A particular debt is owed to Roy J. Fritz and N. G. Gratz for reviewing the chapter material on insects, rodents, and control measures; to James Haworth on malaria eradication; and to F. S. Barbosa on schistosomiasis.

My appreciation goes to Miss Gill Ryan of Coventry, England, and Mrs. Pat McCotter of Trenton, North Carolina, for suffering through the task of transcribing the first two-thirds of hand copy to a draft typing. The demanding work of completing the draft and preparing the manuscript was skillfully executed by Mrs. Pat Blunden of Chapel Hill, North Carolina. The many individuals and organizations which have graciously permitted use of previously published material are cited in source references and are here additionally thanked for sharing their work to enrich this book.

EMIL T. CHANLETT

THE QUALITY FACTORS FOR ENVIRONMENTAL PROTECTION

POPULATION TRENDS AND RESOURCE USE

The quality of our environment is determined by the intricate processes of mankind's making a living and enjoying life. In that process water, food, land, and air are used in man's activities. The changes that man produces during this use affect his health, his comfort, his esthetic senses, his efficiency, and his capacity to attain a satisfactory social adjustment. There are individually perceptible benefits or detriments. Additionally his use of the four essentials for life affects the dynamics of all plant and animal life on earth, by altering the ecological balances. Finally, his methods of using land, water, and air particularly as waste disposal sinks have impaired their quality so that these are no longer usable in some instances for his own needs and purposes. The assessment of ecological changes and of the beneficial use of our land, water, and air resources requires collective wisdom. The rapid increase in the world's population and the accelerating rate of use of all natural resources are making the consequences of misuse more drastic, more widespread, and more readily evident to large numbers of people. The response is political action to control gross abuses.

Figure 1-1 graphs the world's population and its rate of growth. Table 1-1

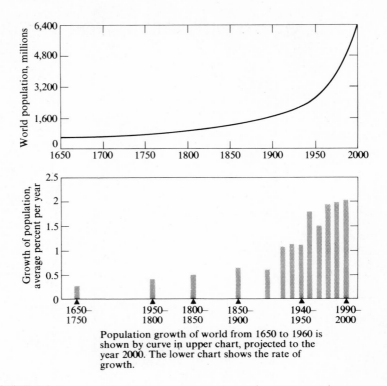

Population growth of world from 1650 to 1960 is shown by curve in upper chart, projected to the year 2000. The lower chart shows the rate of growth.

FIGURE 1-1
The world's population. [*Source:* "*Population*," authors Kingsley and Davis, (Copyright © 1963, *Scientific American, Inc.*) All rights reserved.]

presents the numbers by selected years and by major regions. If resource use remained at a constant per capita rate, a doubling of resultant waste production by the year 2000 would be formidable enough. However, the technological escalation of production makes a rising per capita rate of use the usual pattern. Figure 1-2 states the case for iron ore output for the world, the United States, and other countries. Petroleum use in the world is rising at about 8 percent per year. Table 1-2 projects the natural resource use of 1960 to the requirements of the year 2000. It is the stated goal of governments and of international organizations to achieve a continued increase in the standard of living for all people. Confronting the aspirations of the rest of the world to attain the level of United States consumption throws all the estimates on known reserves into the columns "ridiculous" and "absurd." The Ehrlichs sum it up this way (Ref. 1-1, pp. 61–62): "To raise all of the 3.6 billion people of the world

Table 1-1   ESTIMATED POPULATIONS OF THE WORLD AND ITS MAJOR REGIONS, IN MILLIONS, IN 1900, 1950, 1960, AND 2000, WITH COMPARISONS OF INCREASES FROM 1900 TO 1950 AND FROM 1950 TO 2000 NUMERICALLY AND AS A RATIO

| Area | Estimated population, millions | | | Projected population, millions, year 2000 | Increase, millions | | Ratio of increase, 1950-2000 to 1900-1950 |
	1900	1950	1960		1900-1950	1950-2000	
World	1,550	2,518	2,995	6,907	968	4,389	4.6
Africa	120	209	254	663	89	454	5.1
North America	81	168	199	326	87	158	1.7
Latin America	63	163	206	651	100	488	4.9
Asia	857	1,389	1,679	4,250	532	2,861	5.4
Europe, including U.S.S.R.	423	576	641	987	153	411	2.7
Oceania	6	13	17	30	7	17	2.4

Table 1-2   PROJECTIONS FROM 1960 TO 2000 OF NATURAL RESOURCE UTILIZATION BY THE UNITED STATES*

Resource	Unit of measure	1960 use	2000 requirement
Cropland, including pasture	10^6 acres	447	476
Timber	10^9 ft³	11	47
Freshwater withdrawal	10^9 gpd	84	149
Oil	10^9 barrels	3.2	10.0
Natural gas	10^{12} ft³	13.3	34.9
Coal	10^6 short tons	436	718
Nuclear power	10^9 kWh	...	2,400
Iron ore	10^6 short tons	131	341
Primary aluminum	10^6 short tons	2.1	13.3
Primary copper	10^6 short tons	1.7	4.5

* These projections are based on a population increase from 180 million in 1960 to 330 million in 2000, and an increase in gross national product value from $503 billion in 1960 to $2,200 billion in the year 2000.

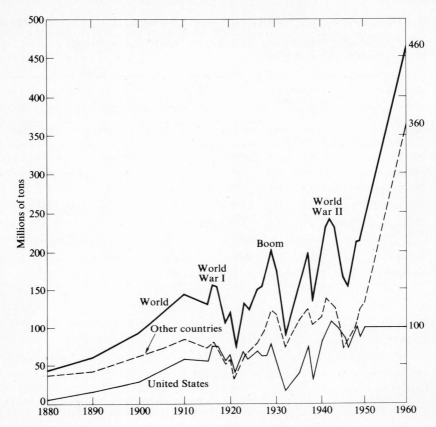

FIGURE 1-2
Iron ore—output of the world and of the United States, 1880 to 1960. (*Source:
W. S. Woytinsky and E. S. Woytinsky, "World Population and Production,"
p. 785, The Twentieth Century Fund, N.Y., 1953, with 1960 data supplemented.*)

to the American standard would require ... the extraction of some 75 times as much
iron as is now extracted annually, 100 times as much copper, 200 times as much lead,
75 times as much zinc, and 250 times as much tin."

To meet that long step forward solely from the known reserves, only the iron
reserves would meet the need. All others are far exceeded. Note that this extrapolation was solely for the 3.6 billion already on board and that it makes no provision for
increased per capita consumption by the present "haves." It only provides for bringing the present "have nots" to the level of the haves. It is conjecture, but it does
underscore the finite size of nonrenewable mineral resources, as we now can get at
them technologically and economically. These are the constraints which will make
recycling a much more attractive engineering feat than it has been.

Table 1-3 shows the tempo of growth of urban populations in the United States and in two developing countries, India and Pakistan. In such countries the shift is taking place more rapidly and in the face both of more limited financial capacity and of less technical experience for providing the services of water supply, sewerage, solid-waste collection and disposal, and control of air pollution and food hygiene. The impact of the shift from rural to urban areas on sanitary services is both quantitative and qualitative. The number of new users outstrips existing capacities. In case of failure, the results hit a target of concentrated susceptibles. An example is the Delhi, India, outbreak of infectious hepatitis in which the contamination of the public water supply by the virus of that disease from sewage produced an estimated 29,300 cases over a period of 3 months in 1955 to 1956.

Urban concentrations intensify the deficiencies of housing, transport capacity, and food storage and distribution. The deficiencies magnify crowding, noise, insect and rodent populations, air pollutants, and street filth. These factors are detrimental to health and well-being with identifiable roles in the etiology and epidemiology of disease and impairment. The effects of urbanization on privacy, on the privilege of space, on the experience of family and near-neighbor interaction, on the ease of access for recreation and for leisurely pursuits, and on a man's identification with a community are ill-defined. The shape and condition of the physical environment influence these matters. Thus, these are the responsibility and concern of engineers, sanitarians, planners, health officers, and sociologists. Social mechanisms in the public and private sectors to bring an interdisciplinary capability to confront these issues have been mustered to a limited degree to define the problems. The achievement of solutions is your task.

Our knowledge of the identification of the quality of the physical environment with effects is quite precise in terms of the cause of disease and physiological

Table 1-3 THE TEMPO OF GROWTH OF URBAN POPULATION IN INDIA, PAKISTAN, AND THE UNITED STATES, IN MILLIONS OF PEOPLE

	India		Pakistan		United States
1901–1911	0.4		8.5	1900–1910	39.3
1911–1921	8.3		16.1	1910–1920	29.0
1921–1931	19.1		32.1	1920–1930	27.3
1931–1941	32.0		44.1	1930–1940	7.9
1941–1951	41.4		41.9	1940–1950	19.5
1951–1961	26.4 (urban redefined) 34.0 (urban as defined in 1951)		56.4	1950–1960	10.9 (estimated)

impairments.   These will be previewed as first-level effects.   The effects upon comfort, convenience, esthetic senses, and efficiency are less well defined although more readily noticed and accepted as fact by people.   Thus colored, turbid water is rejected by all of us despite bacteriological tests which certify that it is free of intestinal bacteria common in man.   Such effects will be previewed as second level.   Beyond these concerns for the effects on man are the effects on the planet he dominates.   Those of us who operate from the limited point of view of health effects, or who may be interested in the positive influences of the second-level effects must also recognize the overlap effects on the ecological balances in the plant and animal kingdoms and the condition and very existence of all natural resources.

Man's technological management of energy for his sole benefit has been developing for a scant 200 years.   The sequence has been thermal, electrical, and nuclear energy development and utilization.   In the process, the first century was marked by an unbridled exploitation of human resources for individual profit.   The second century has been marked by an unbridled exploitation of natural resources with a shift from individual to corporate profit.   The use of natural resources is rapidly becoming subject to governmental controls which are increasingly restrictive on the range of individual or corporate decision on their use.   The human equation is simple.   When too many people became the victims of the 14-hour day, of child labor, and of the neglect of the hazards of work, the collective social conscience demanded and brought changes, at least in the democracies of Great Britain and the United States.   We are now at the stage in which too many people feel the effects of polluted water, polluted air, and despoiled land to let the dancers go on without paying the piper his due.

THE FIRST LEVEL—HEALTH EFFECTS

Infectious Diseases and Our Environment

The health effects of deficiencies or excesses in the environment have been characterized by the identification of specific causes and effects.   The most spectacular achievement of the biological sciences in the last 100 years has been the identification of pathogenic organisms.   The speedy application of this knowledge through the organization of public health and public works agencies has enormously lightened the burden of infectious diseases on man.   Figure 1-3 shows the record of mortality rates from typhoid fever in Chicago from 1860 to 1942.   Figure 1-4 shows the record of murine typhus fever cases in the United States and 10 southern states from 1932 to 1957 and the effects of control measures.

Appendix 1 is a roll call of infectious diseases by an environmental agent or by a vector which is dependent on environmental conditions sometimes created by man and

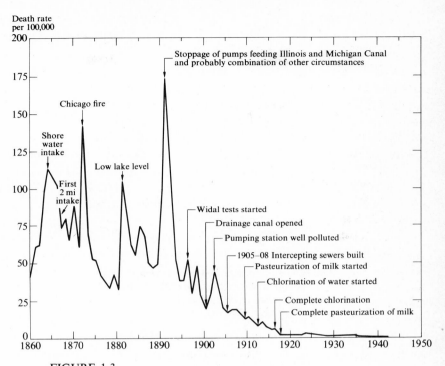

FIGURE 1-3
Death rates from typhoid fever per 100,000 total population, city of Chicago from 1860 to 1942. (*Source: L. L. Dublin, A. J. Lotka, and M. Spiegelmann, "Length of Life," fig. 21, p. 159, The Ronald Press, New York,* © 1949.)

always controllable to an effective degree by him.   The repetitions and duplications appear in any schematic arrangement of diseases, agents, and environmental factors, as human feces is the most frequent means of exit of pathogens.   Milton J. Rosenau's "short circuit" from the anus of one man to the mouth of another is not always short and not often directly evident.   The intermediate routes include hands, water, soil, food, insects, and rodents.   The role of air as an environmental transmitter of pathogenic organisms remains dubious and undetermined with the exceptions of such rare diseases as psittacosis, "parrot fever," and in the hospital environment.

Toxic Chemicals in Air, Food, and Water

Toxic chemicals have reached man by air, skin contact and absorption, food, and water throughout recorded medical history.   The association of cause and effect for lead is attributed to Hippocrates about 400 B.C.   Georgius Agricola in the sixteenth century

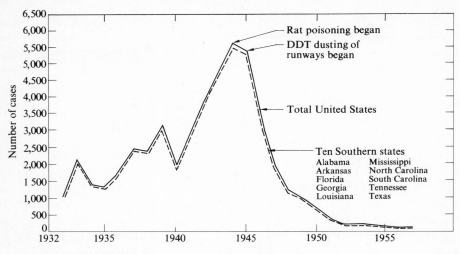

FIGURE 1-4
Annual number of reported murine typhus fever cases in the United States and in 10 southern states, 1932 to 1957. [*Source: G. J. Love and W. W. Smith,* "*Murine Typhus Investigations in Southwestern Georgia,*" *Public Health Rep.* (*U.S.*) 75, 1960, p. 430, *Fig.* 1.]

and Bernardino Ramazzini in the seventeenth century knew enough about the occupational occurrence of certain diseases and substances encountered to write books on occupational diseases.   Ever since, the list of toxicants has grown longer.

The indictment of occupational toxicants is firmer than that for biological agents as it is quantitative with remarkable accuracy.   This holds particularly for substances at the extremes of exposure times.   Long-term epidemiological studies have established the concentrations in air of lead, mercury, free silica, and manganese which will produce disease after years of occupational exposure.   Substances producing transient effects such as narcosis from the gases and vapors of aliphatic hydrocarbons and brass founder's ague from zinc oxide fumes are similarly well documented in terms of concentration in air, time of exposure, and physiological effects.

The quantitative validity of hazardous concentrations of toxic substances in foods is less certain.   The population at risk varies from fragile infants to physiologically impaired old people.   Intakes of food types are variable.   Therefore reassuring margins of safety are applied in interpreting toxicological evidence from experimental animal feeding.   The indictment is reinforced from time to time by recurrence of poisonings.   Examples are cadmium poisoning when cadmium-plated ice-cube trays were used to prepare a frozen dessert of citrus fruit concentrates and when acute methemoglobinemia overcame 11 aged patrons of a Chatham Square (N.Y.) café, whose oatmeal was salted with sodium nitrite in place of sodium chloride (Ref. 1-2).

There are limits on the concentrations of additives for coloring, preserving, and flavoring foods. The limits are particularly restrictive for substances suspected of being carcinogenic. A more recent concern has been residuals from farm use of antibiotics in poultry feeding and treating mastitis in milk cows, and use of a variety of chemicals as pesticides and herbicides. The difficult technical and political decisions that must be made are exemplified by the cranberry crisis of 1959, when residuals of aminotrazole (ATZ), a recognized carcinogen, were found in extensive samples of fresh and canned cranberries already on the store shelves for the Thanksgiving and Christmas dinners of millions of American families. The intricacies of the case are concisely presented in Brown (Ref. 1-3, p. 100). Consumer reaction was well measured by Thanksgiving sales 70 percent below normal and Christmas sales 50 percent of the usual.

Permissible concentrations for seven toxic chemicals in sources of drinking water are given in both Drinking Water Standards of the Public Health Service and in International Standards for Drinking Water of the World Health Organization. The numerical values are conservative to provide a safety factor. For chemicals such as lead, arsenic and cadmium, which are stored in the body, allowance is made for the possible intake from sources other than water. Recorded injury from toxic substances in drinking water in this century are limited to nitrates and fluorides. Each of these have unique actions and targets. Excesses of nitrates in water used in babies' formulas in the first few months of life are reduced to nitrites in the digestive tract and produce methemoglobinemia. Fortunately the frightening blue appearance produces action, usually hospitalization. Off the high-nitrate water, the baby's blood is restored to its normal hemoglobin-carrying capacity of oxygen. The fascinating discovery of the relation of fluorides and tooth quality extends over 50 years. The establishment of a minimum concentration in drinking water for the formation of decay-resistant teeth and a maximum to prevent tooth mottling and staining rests on sound epidemiological studies. Four million Americans on naturally occurring fluoride in their drinking water provided the epidemiological evidence.

The fact that airborne contaminants in community air could be more than a nuisance was forceably demonstrated in the United States at Donora, Pennsylvania, over a weekend in October 1948. When 10 percent of a community's population feel sufficient respiratory distress to seek medical aid, a health crisis exists. The Donora investigation did not produce a neat, clear-cut cause and effect explanation. It did introduce a team of industrial hygiene experts of the Public Health Service to the complexity of community air pollution. At least three environmental factors make the conditions differ from occupational exposure to single toxic substances. Localized meteorological patterns determine dilution. The types of sources determine the components and concentration of the mixture of contaminants which must be inhaled. The makeup of the mix, humidity, and sunlight influences the interactions of the contaminants and the resultant products and conditions.

Rachel Carson's *Silent Spring* provoked more public consternation and scientific response than the Donora air pollution episode, because it dramatized the presence and the effects of the residues of synthetic organic pesticides in the general environment.   The behavior of these residues in gaining global distribution and in entering the food chain is underlined by DDT in the fatty tissue of penguins in Antarctica. Man is able to store as much as 270 milligrams of DDT per kilogram of fat for a period up to 18 months without apparent ill effects.   These storage levels resulted from intakes of 35 mg/day, which makes it evident that DDT is of a very low order of toxicity. The issues at stake are two.   DDT and analogous chlorinated hydrocarbons do not decompose readily in the free environment.   Global distribution has resulted.   These compounds are now in the metabolic pathways of animals and plants.   There is no certain answer to whether there will be perceptible effects over long periods of time. Increasing concentration in the food chain has occurred.   Used to control Dutch elm disease, DDT was ingested by earthworms from the fallen leaves and accumulated in the worms.   Robins fed on the worms and died.   It was the silencing of the robins which aroused Rachel Carson.   Another example of DDT accumulations through food chain or food web is shown later in Fig. 1-9.

The release of long-lived radioactive isotopes into the environment raises similar questions.   Once freed to water or air, the radioactive atoms behave chemically as the stable element with the same number of protons.   What are the consequences of incorporating even extremely low concentrations of radioactive elements in the cycle of life?   To date the management of radioactive wastes has been most conservative. In view of our ignorance of long-term effects, this has been a prudent policy.   The facts remain that ^{90}Sr is now in our bone structure, that ^{85}Kr appears as a contaminant in all concentrates of krypton, and that ^{14}C has increased beyond that from the natural cosmic actions in the earth's atmosphere.

Health Effects of Uncontrolled Physical Energy

The sources of exposure to uncontrolled physical energy result largely from man's manipulation of heat, mechanical power, electricity, and nuclear phenomena.   All these are encountered in natural occurrences such as climatic extremes, earthquakes, lightning, and electromagnetic radiations from the sun and stars.   The list of discrete agents is lengthening either through their application or as unwanted by-products. These include vibration, sound in various forms, ultraviolet and infrared light, microwave, and coherent light beams.   With the exceptions of badly managed mechanical power, ranging from a mishandled power saw to an automobile, which produces hundreds of thousands of permanent disabilities and thousands of deaths each year, the fatal consequences of excessive exposure to physical energy are relatively few.

Physiological effects of the widespread exposures to heat and noise are either not permanent or not severe impairments.

This enumeration of environmental factors which produce direct effects on physiological functions is not all inclusive. For example, allergic substances in air and soil distress thousands of people. Poisonous insects and reptiles cause injury to a few and outright fear in many. An American regards his car affectionately, despite the collective toll of 60,000 deaths per year in vehicle accidents. He regards rattlers and copperheads with abject horror and rushes for the hoe, although deaths from snake bites average less than 20 per year in the United States.

THE SECOND LEVEL—COMFORT, CONVENIENCE, EFFICIENCY, AND ESTHETICS

The distinction between health effects measured by changes in physiological function and the effects of human sensitivity and desire for an environment which is pleasing, comfortable, and convenient is not merely an academic matter. The economists increasingly insist upon justifying expenditures on a cost-benefit basis and upon establishing priorities of action in accord with the return on investment. These require that the characteristics of a problem and the results of its solution be distinguishable. Such a necessity is evident if the costs and benefits of managing the pollution of a stream have to be weighed. The sanitarian rarely thinks in such terms in a systematic way in recommending food sanitation actions, although he makes such judgments in emphasizing one recommendation over another. The air pollution control officer confronts a difficult mixture of causes and effects in which physiological impairments are harder to identify and measure than the assaults on the senses of sight and smell.

Three Senses—Sight, Smell, and Taste

Everyone, by the senses of sight, smell, and taste, makes a measure of the quality of the environment around him, of the liquids and solids offered and of the air breathed. Individual expectations, acceptances, and tolerances are a product of cultural and social conditioning with wide variations in which educational and economic levels have a strong influence. Water and food are judged by their appearance, their taste, and their odor. Air is judged by its freedom from dust and odor. All of our surroundings are judged by the absence of litter and filth. These qualities are not satisfactorily or easily stated in quantitative terms. A few exceptions are the turbidity and color of water, sediment in milk, and particulates in air.   In these instances the standards are arbit-rary, but measurements can be replicated and comparisons made.   For the remainder, descriptive terms and subjective evaluation must be used.   Efforts to define tastes and odors hold particular interest as many people are quite sensitive to them, especially when there are changes and first encounters.

Heat, Noise, and Light

Extremes of physiological strain of thermal stress are largely occupational exposures. The desire to enjoy thermal comfort is universal.   Man has devoted a lot of effort to beat the heat and to keep out the cold in the process of civilizing himself.   Ingenious architectural forms and judicious use of structural materials are examples of such efforts. Mechanical heating and cooling systems with year-around thermostatic and humidity controls have made thermal control possible for increasingly large volumes of space. The Houston Astrodome is a case in point.   The standards of thermal comfort rest on a subjective response.   The widely used effective-temperature charts are derived from the responses of trained subjects to many combinations of dry-bulb and wet-bulb temperatures, of humidity, and of air movement.   The patterns of these variables are compatible with the body's physiological responses to temperature changes and the heat transfer mechanisms of conduction, convection, radiation, and evaporation.

As with heat, functional effects of high noise levels have been observed in noisy work places.   The effects are temporary or permanent hearing losses, usually in the high-frequency ranges.   Studies of an African tribe unaccustomed to civilized noise hint at cardiovascular responses.   One useful definition of noise is "unwanted sound." Our urbanized, mechanized way of life has produced an increasing number of sources of unwanted sound.   Our desire for quiet is subjective and dependent on our own activity and location at the time.   The shattering racket of a high-powered outboard motor boat on a lake at dawn produces a completely different reaction than the same noise multiplied many times during that afternoon's boat races or water-skiing exhibi-tion.   Noise control is a comfort expectation that the people will increasingly demand of those who shape and control the environment.

Visible light is a short segment of the electromagnetic energy spectrum.   In variable intensity, quality, and quantity, it is with man always.   Yet precise evidence of detrimental effects of a permanent nature on the eyes is not at hand.   There is ample evidence on the relations of lighting and the capacity to do a visual task.   These needs have been best defined for work places.   Esthetics and comfort enter into the design and use of any environment in which lighting is controlled.   Interior decorators use lighting to create a desired "atmosphere."   Illumination qualities which can be managed are intensity, contrast, color, and glare.

Structural Characteristics, and Ease, and Efficiency

In going down a flight of steps a variation in riser height as little as one inch will be sensed.   This is a minute example of our response to dimensions, or at least to dimensional changes.   Differences in floor hardness among terrazo, cork, and carpeted surfaces are sensed.   These examples must have extensions to the whole range of things which surround us and which we use.   Furniture, bathroom equipment, tools, machines, household appliances, vehicles of all sorts, sports and recreation equipment all have characteristics which affect the ease of use.   Layouts of shops, offices, kitchens influence efficiency.   The absence of positive influences is expressed in accidents.   The presence is expressed in, "It's a joy to have."

Ergonomics treats all these effects and influences in the working environment. The goal of ergonomics is the optimal use of energy—human, mechanical, thermal, electrical, and nuclear.   That goal is the endpoint of the interaction of the human being, the device in use, and the surroundings.   On the human side all possible physiological and psychological elements are considered.   Anthropometric, sensory response, and work capacity factors are considered.   The optimum match between these and the device is sought.   In the device are such things as its dimensions; the shape, color, and position of controls and indicators; its speed and speed changes; and its output of noise, vibration, heat, and airborne wastes.   In practice the problem may range from optimum dimensions of a work table to the most efficient layout of the control console of a nuclear reactor.   For the surroundings there is the search for the optima of thermal comfort, air quality, acoustic characteristics, illumination, and color combinations.   Additionally there may be such items as durability, maintenance ease, skid properties of surfaces, fire retardation, and planning for escape and evacuation.

There have been limited achievements of these goals in work places.   Many of the human factors have been difficult to define.   After definition, the transformation of the device and surroundings to fit the human need confronts a variety of compromises.   The system of man, machine, and work place must still be a combination which produces quality goods at a marketable price.   The most severe test of ergonomics is the effect on the cost per unit produced.

The development of commercial aircraft is an example of the extensive application of these ideas.   In commercial flying the stakes are high.   These are the safety of passengers, crew, and craft; the comfort, feeding, and entertainment of passengers; and the work efficiency of the crew.   These must be met in the face of such hostile environmental factors as noise, vibration, use of inflammable liquids, external temperature extremes, air pressure changes, directional and velocity changes, and the maintenance of a self-contained water, waste, and air system.   The crew must manage the integrated equipment aboard for propulsion and control, for maintaining the internal environment, for navigation, and for communication.   All this must be provided for within constraints of space and weight. The final combination must be operationally safe and economically profitable. A successful commercial plane affords a case study of environmental control.[1]

Ergonomics of the work place and the environmental factors of aircraft design and operation demonstrate the scope of the task which must be taken on in planning and managing the environment to achieve the best human physiological and psychological responses. The objective must be more than preventing negative responses of disease, impairment, discomfort, and annoyance. It must be to produce and enhance the sense of well-being. It must be to provide an environment which will facilitate the processes by which people attain fully their potential of social and personal adjustment.

There are large gaps in how to plan an environment to meet the whole spectrum of human needs. Although public health people have done relatively little to fill these gaps, it has not been for the lack of vision and guidance of a few public health leaders. A notable example is the breadth of C. E. A. Winslow's *Basic Principles of Healthful Housing* in 1939. He grouped 30 principles as fundamental needs for the control of contagious diseases, for the prevention of accidents, for physiological comfort, and for psychological benefit. For a sizable portion of the slum people of the cities of America the rudimentary needs for the control of contagious diseases as delineated by Winslow have not been met. The fitting of the jigsaw puzzle of human needs and natural and social resources is an exciting prospect which gives meaning to all professional efforts.

THE THIRD LEVEL—THE EFFECTS ON THE BALANCE OF ECOSYSTEMS AND NATURAL RESOURCES

The activities of those engaged in environmental control to achieve health benefits have had direct effects on the ecological balances of plant and animal life. The effects have been both beneficial and detrimental. The involved professional groups in the United States of America, placed in chronological order of their development, are sanitary engineers, sanitarians, industrial hygienists, air pollution managers, and health physicists. Each of these groups are in varying degrees responsible for the disposal of liquid, airborne, and solid wastes. The disposal methods in use are affecting our water, air, land, and subterranean resources. Therefore, these professional groups must harmonize their methods and operations with the efforts to protect plant and animal wildlife and to conserve our natural resources.

[1] Ross McFarland, "Human Factors in Air Transport," McGraw-Hill, New York, 1946.

Safeguarding the Ecological Balances

The efforts at liquid waste control have been favorable for fish and plant life with one exception. The primary effort has been to reduce the solids and putrescible organic load on receiving waters. According as this conserves the dissolved oxygen reserves in the water, fish and plant life are not cut short. The exception has been the increase in the enrichment of receiving waters in phosphates and inorganic nitrogen by sewage effluents. In its usual cycle the treatment of liquid wastes accelerates the formation of the oxidized states of phosphorous and nitrogen. More significantly, phosphate-base detergents and fertilized-field runoff have increased the concentration of phosphates in sewage. These enrichments have increased the production of some algae which appear in vast numbers as a " bloom," to the detriment of the usual balance. This has occurred in Lake Washington, Seattle, and in lakes in Wisconsin.

Insect control has produced some surprising results, in which the method used to suppress one species favors the reproduction of another. An enthusiastic mayor of an Amazon River town ordered the cutting of all shade cover on wet lands around the town to reduce production of a biting pest mosquito. The deterrent to the pest breeding favored the breeding of a malaria vector which required sunlit waters. In another instance the release of high-salinity ocean water to a freshwater swamp prevented the breeding of a malaria vector but resulted in a profusive emergence of a brackish-water pest mosquito. The fly *Musca domestica* jolted the status of DDT as a miracle insecticide. A few common houseflies had the genetic endowment to metabolize DDT before the toxicant acted on its nervous system. These survived to produce generations with the same unique characteristic. They absorbed DDT with impunity.

Shifts in existing ecological balances have been caused by the pesticide residuals. Residuals of DDT in the Miramichi River, New Brunswick, Canada, nearly eliminated a year's production of young salmon in 1954 and 1956. The DDT did not directly affect the salmon. The stream insects, their food supply, were killed and failed to return for 2 years. At Clear Lake, California, DDD, an analog of DDT, moved through the food chain from the lake water with a concentration of 0.02 ppm by weight to plankton with 5 ppm to fish with fat containing from hundreds to thousands of ppm. Grebes that fed on the fish died. For a detailed tracing of DDT through the food web of an estuarian life regime, see Fig. 1-9.

Fortunately no such dramatic effects on existing ecology have been caused by the discharge of radioactive wastes to the general environment. Painstaking investigations have been and continue to be carried out to plot the course of such contaminants. Such sensitive indices as the egg fertilization of salmon spawning in the Columbia River, which receives low-level wastes from the nuclear plants at Hanford, Washington, have not shown observable changes. The presence of long-lived radioactive chemicals in plant and animal tissue is, of course, recognized. The long-range consequences of this new factor in the cellular environment cannot be predicted. That makes mandatory a continued conservative management of such wastes. As the number of sources of these wastes increases, further restrictions on discharges to the free environment will be in order.

The discharge of carbon dioxide, CO_2, and sulfur dioxide, SO_2, from the burning of fossil fuels may be producing worldwide climatic effects. There is evidence that the effect of SO_2 may offset the CO_2 effect. CO_2 is being added to the earth's atmosphere at the rate of 6 billion tons/year. By the year 2000 the concentration of CO_2 in our air will increase from about 300 ppm by volume to 375 ppm, a 25 percent increase. CO_2 is a strong absorber and back radiator of infrared radiation. The increased CO_2 in the air is estimated to be capable of causing rises of from 1 to 7°F in the average temperature near the earth's surface, depending upon water-vapor behavior. SO_2 in the air has a hygroscopic action and increases haze. As water vapor absorbs infrared radiation, the increased haze will offset the CO_2 "greenhouse" action. Scientists studying these phenomena must work with rather fragmentary data gathered in a period which is infinitesimal compared with the earth's balancing processes for handling CO_2 by plant use, by ocean solution, and by mineral combination, over hundreds of thousands of years. The predictions of these changes are as yet uncertain. It is clear that man's recent and accelerating use of fossil fuels is having geophysical consequences. Even our management of stack gases for the immediate reduction of localized air pollution may influence these consequences.

The Effects of Waste Disposal Methods on the Future Uses of Natural Resources

The impairment of our water and air resources by the unrestricted disposal of wastes by dilution is already evident to a severe degree in heavily urbanized and industrialized areas. The unrestricted dumping of tailings and strippings from open-pit mining has left ugly scars of land areas, unfit for other uses. To permit these resources to be used to such a degree is a broader license than organized society can afford to issue. Selfish use in the short run must yield to selfish requirements over a somewhat longer run.

The use of subterranean space for waste disposal has been successful for oil brine wastes, and to a limited extent for sewage in combination with groundwater recharge. Seepage pits for the disposal of intermediate-level radioactive wastes use the absorptive capacities of the substrata. The burial of solid wastes contaminated with radioactivity is a long-term commitment of land use. The economic pressures for the immediate utilization of such sites seldom permit detailed consideration of the future requirements for the same site. In the short history of sanitary landfill for the disposal of municipal refuse, there have been examples of choice of sites which a few years later were regretted. The minimum obligations to those to come are careful mapping, recording, and marking of such sites, an inventory of types and quantities of wastes, and a surveillance of the fate of the wastes.

THE QUALITY OF THE ENVIRONMENT AND RESOURCE MANAGEMENT

From 1962 to 1967 five major committees of experts and of citizens of high reputation reported on the deterioration of the environment of the United States. The reports have become identified by the names of the chairmen. These are the Paul M. Gross report to the Surgeon General of the Public Health Service in 1962, the John W. Tukey report to the President's Scientific Advisory Committee in 1965, the Athelstan Spilhaus report to the National Research Council and National Academy of Sciences, in 1966, and the Ron M. Linton report to the Secretary of the Department of Health, Education and Welfare in 1967 (Refs. 1-4 to 1–7).

Amid the wealth of data and penetrating analyses that these reports present, six needs stand out.

1 The need to apply fully the existing technology of environmental control.
2 The need to involve a wider range of scientific and managerial skills in waste and pollution issues.
3 The need to intensify and to extend the collection and analysis of baseline and surveillance data on pollutants and their effects.
4 The need for investigation and research on the long-term effects of low concentration of contaminants, acting singly and collectively on ecosystems.
5 The need to deal with wastes and residues as part of the cycle of resource use for which producer and consumer must accept responsibilities and costs.
6 The need to fit governmental jurisdictions and administrative mechanisms for environmental control to the area and scope of the problems and their solutions.

The concern expressed by the organizations requesting these reports results from the pressures of our technological escalation, our population escalation, and our urban concentration. These are not peculiar to the United States. Technological growth is shared very unevenly in other nations. While Japan, Germany, and the U.S.S.R. are moving rapidly in this, most nations of Asia, Africa, and Latin America have the benefits and the problems of technological change only in a few urban centers or in areas rich in minerals or oil.

Table 1-1 on world and regional population shows absolute increases estimated for the years 1950 to 2000 from two to five times those for the years 1900 to 1950.

The increase for Asia will equal the total population of the world in 1958.   The pressures of such increases on the quality of our environment as set forth in this chapter are frightening.   There are indications that the major portion of that pressure will be exerted in towns and cities with the worldwide phenomenon of migration from rural to urban living continuing.

The committee reports spell out the urgency of the situation in the United States.   In many large cities of the world the need is greater, as the rudimentary services of water supply and sewerage have not been met.   Before the plans to meet these needs can be realized, a new wave of migration and births in excess of deaths produces more areas within those cities without water and sewer service.   Such has been the case in Sao Paulo, Lima, Bombay, Calcutta, Guatemala City, and Bangkok.   The concentrations of people in these cities are producing waterborne and airborne wastes which are overwhelming the dilution capacity of adjacent water and of the local air envelope, two resources regarded as natural and inexhaustible.   The tasks are enormous and the time finite.

The P Game and the Systems of Water, Air, and Land

We are in the "P game," the exponential rises of people, production, power, places, and pollution.   These must be fitted to the natural systems of our water, air, and land. The P game has some staggering stakes.   Edwin Dale of the *New York Times* has strikingly capsuled the exponential growth of the United States economy with $100 billion growth in the 13 years from 1944 to 1957 and a projection of a $500 billion growth in the 13 years from 1969 to 1981 (Ref. 1-8).   All the values of goods and services produced are in constant-value dollars.   The growths in three 13-year periods are:

    1944–1957 $100 billion
    1957–1969 $300 billion
    1969–1981 $500 billion

Dale states (Ref. 1-8, p. 28):

> That is the law of compound interest.   These are not numbers; they are tin cans and smoke and auto exhaust.   There is no visible escape from it.   Applying the same percentage growth to a larger base every year, we have reached the point where our growth in one year is half the total output of Canada, fully adjusting for inflation. Another dizzying and rather horrifying way of putting it is that the real output of goods and services in the United States has grown as much since 1950 as it grew in the entire period from the landing of the Pilgrims in 1620 up to 1950.

Electrical power use in the United States is at 1.5 billion kWh and rising at 7 percent a year.   We now require a generating capacity of about 1 kW per capita.

To produce that power each year we burn 300 million tons of coal, 9 billion gallons of oil and 3 trillion cubic feet of gas.   The hydro-generated electricity is small.   Nuclear-reactor-generated electricity is still small, but rising rapidly.

The number of places is important, as decisions on environmental quality are determined by governmental response.   In the United States, the 50 states; 3,000 counties; 18,000 villages, towns, and cities; and 40,000 special districts, townships, and local authorities can rarely be ignored, bypassed, or circumvented.   Each has a bit of sovereignty, zealously exercised as it sees its interest and its good.

The number of pollutants can be enumerated by a look at you.   How much mess do you make each day?   You put out 5 pounds of solid wastes each day.   This is food waste, paper, bottles, cans, plastics, and just trash.   You use and dirty 50 gallons of water a day, bathing, hand washing, and toilet flushing.   Your sewered waste requires about 0.2 pound of dissolved oxygen per day.   That sounds modest enough, but nature has squeezed us badly on that item.   Oxygen is not very soluble in water. Natural water that has 80 pounds of dissolved oxygen in a million gallons is very well oxygenated.   Streams that have already received a load of wastes may not have enough to keep trout and bass alive.   These fish require about 40 pounds in a million gallons.   Your daily waste load requires all the oxygen that is in 5,000 gal of water that has just enough dissolved oxygen in it to keep trout and bass alive.

You do most of your dirtying of air when driving a car.   A car that runs 10,000 mi/year, the United States' average, dumps $3\frac{1}{2}$ pounds of carbon monoxide per car per day, $\frac{3}{4}$ pound of particulates out the tail pipe, and $1\frac{1}{2}$ pounds of unburnt hydrocarbons per day.   That's a "fifth" size of whiskey bottle full of gasoline.   Your share of all the mess discharged from all sources into the air is 4 lb/day.   Of this, 60 percent is from motor vehicles, 30 percent from electricity generation and manufacturing, and 10 percent from space heating and solid-wastes burning.

Manufacturing and agricultural liquid and solid wastes have not been assigned to you.   That would bring your per capita water use to 2,100 gallons per day (gpd). That is 9 tons.   The solid wastes from animal and food production makes the Augean stables that Hercules flushed out a modest accumulation.   It is a matter of about 2 billion tons/year, or 55 lb/(capita)(day).

These prodigious quantities of wastes must find a place in the cycles of our water, air, and land systems with or without some degree of treatment or preparation for assimilation.   The determinants of the assimilative capacity of water, air, and land are natural constraints of any geographical area.   Local meteorology limits the amount of wastes which can be diluted and carried away by the air.   The local streamflow, rainfall, and runoff limit and determine the amount of wastes that can be discharged into creeks, streams, rivers, and lakes.   The local soil characteristics determine land disposal of wastes, use of groundwater, and application of groundwater recharge for wastewater reclamation.   The local topography sets the risks of floods, erosion,

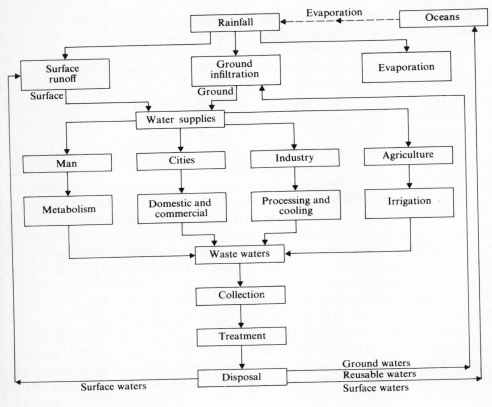

FIGURE 1-5
The environmental system of water. [*Source: Rolf Eliassen, Stanford University.*]

and use for solid waste burial.   The extent of natural constraints must be known for the prudent use of these resources.

The best-developed and most widely used method of fitting a waste load to the natural constraint of an environmental receptor is the use of the Phelps-Streeter[1] formulas for predicting the extent of dissolved-oxygen use in a stream by the bio-oxidizable wastes discharged into the stream.   The method provides a means of predicting the biochemical oxidation demand, BOD, that one can impose on a stream and still maintain in the water a dissolved-oxygen concentration needed for aerobic stabilization or for a desired species of fish.   It provides the means for the rational and prudent use of the assimilative capacity of the stream with the benefit of establishing

[1] H. W. Streeter and E. B. Phelps, Pub. Health Bull. 146, U.S. Pub. Health Service, Washington, D.C., 1925.

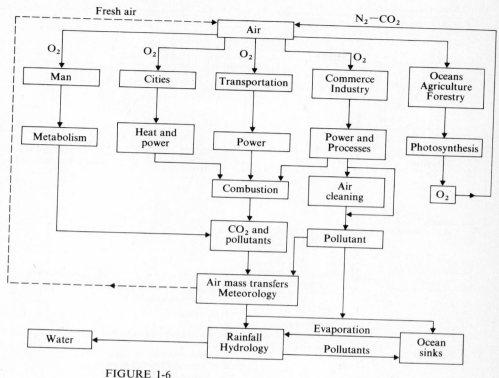

FIGURE 1-6
The environmental system of air. [*Source: Rolf Eliassen, Stanford University.*]

a well-nourished variety of aquatic plant and animal life, of stabilizing the organic oxidizable wastes of man and some of his production activities, and of utilizing a water resource without deteriorating its quality for other beneficial uses.   Similarly, methods are now in use for predicting the behavior of pollutants discharged into the air. There are equations for the diffusion of stack plumes under certain meteorological conditions.   There are mathematical models for estimating the ambient air concentrations of pollutants for known or assumed emission rates from particular process and materials sources of pollution.

One route that must be followed to protect our environment is to expand and improve the techniques for keeping our waste discharge loads within the assimilative capacity of the environment. Such methods require detailed and correct knowledge of the behavior of the biological, chemical, and physical cycles in water, in the air, in the soil, and on the land. All these are interacting, while the separations are in the mind of man as he tries to comprehend these and to manage them. In the real world of nature there is no consciousness that the path of carbon dioxide from the air to

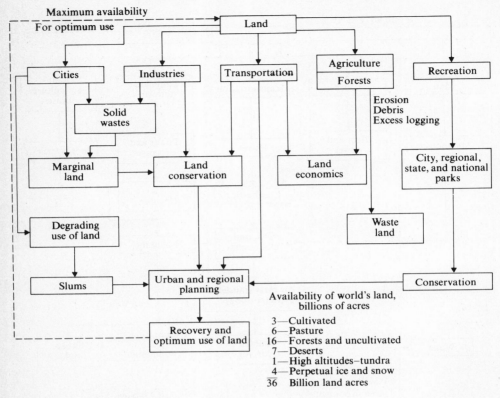

FIGURE 1-7
The environmental system of land.   [*Source: Rolf Eliassen, Stanford University.*]

dissolution in the ocean water to the deposition of calcium carbonate in coral is a pass from air to water to land, and that there are physical processes of solution and subsidence, chemical processes of conversion to bicarbonates and carbonates, and biological processes as aquatic living forms utilize the chemical constituents in their metabolisms.

Whatever detail of environmental action and response is under study, it is useful to be aware of the framework of systems and of cycles in which it functions.   Dr. Rolf Eliassen of Stanford University develops environmental protection from the three environmental systems, water, air, and land.   The components of these three systems are shown in Figs. 1-5 to 1-7.   The water system functions by the natural hydrological cycle with the assistance or interference of man-made means.   The hydrological cycle describes the path of water from cloud precipitation to runoff and percolation on the ground to evaporation from water, ground, and plant surfaces to return to vapor in

air, ready again for cloud formation.   There are well-described cycles of the key elements of animal and plant life.   These are the carbon, nitrogen, and phosphorous
cycles.   Another major cycle included in the air environment system is the heat-
transfer cycle among land, water, air, and outer space that produces the air movements
on earth which we recognize as weather.   How these systems and cycles affect living
things, their functions, their structure, and their organization is the concern of ecology.

ECOLOGY AND ECOSYSTEMS

Some of the man-produced biological, chemical, and physical agents are also part of
the natural scheme of biological, chemical, and physical actions.   Some of these
actions have been exacerbated by man's modification of the natural environment.   A
large number of chemical and physical agents have been added by man in his mastery
of energy sources in the last 200 years.   Until the steam engine, man had very slight
multiplication of his muscle power.   His power supplements were windmills, sails,
water wheels, and draught animals.   The energy explosion, since James Watt improved
the crude steam-powered British mine pumps, has been thermal, electrical, internal
combustion of petroleum products, and nuclear.   Every use of this fantastic energy
potential produces wastes—solid, liquid, or gaseous.   On dumping, these end some-·
where on the land, in the water, or in the air.   This energy waste by man changes the
constituent energy in the environment and must to some degree influence the energy
transfer processes which determine the structure and function of everything in that
environment.   How much?   Favorably for what constituents?   Unfavorably for
what constituents?   These are ecological questions.

   In applying his new-found energy, man dumps the parts he has not learned how
to use or does not consider worth recovering.   He also uses that new energy to make
major alterations in the environment: land cultivation on a grand scale; surface runoff
control by dams, canals, and drainage; extraction of mineral and petroleum products;
city and road building; removal of forests and grasslands; and now he is starting on the
oceans, outer space, and the forces that determine weather.   To the present, these
actions have been scarcely questioned except, "Will it make money for me if I use
money (mine or somebody else's) to make the changes?"   Two immediate cases in
the United States have been the development of the supersonic transport, SST, airplane, and the construction of the crude-oil pipeline across the Alaskan tundra to get
the North Slope oil to market at the lowest cost and presumably maximum profit.
The only real "environmental crisis" is how public opinion and public policy will
evolve answers to such propositions.   In the past, the questions were not even asked
in public.   The environmental alterations change the energy transfer processes as

much as the waste energy dumps do, and raise the same questions.   The rational answers require ecological expertise.   The actual answers come from some peculiar consensus of our value system expressed through the network of social and political processes and actions.

The definition of ecology is in the Greek words *ekos*, "the house," and *logos*, "knowledge of."   It is knowing what makes our dwelling place function.   The tough questions are whose dwelling places and for what fitness of function.   Man appears to be the only species significantly able to call the shots.   The dilemma he is recognizing is that calling the shots solely for his immediate aggrandizement is changing the energy transfer system drastically and perhaps so rapidly that the present generation of decision makers does not want to live long enough to see the consequences of their choices.

Eugene Odum succinctly and brilliantly explains ecology as the study of structure and function of nature in "Relationships between Structure and Functions in Ecosystems."[1]   The very good collection of papers edited by Edward J. Kormondy (Ref. 1-9) includes Odum's article.   Scientists, usually biologists and now some chemists and others, study the structure of an energy community.   It may be small and self-contained as a pool of water in a rocky outcrop on a mountain top.   It may be large as an inland lake.   It may be a watershed of a square mile or two.   Sticking with structure, the data are on species, numbers, distribution in space and seasons, life history, nutrients, light, and heat.   They give essentially a quantitative description of a stationary mode, although cycles are observed.   Function of the energy community engages the dynamics of biological energy flows, rates of reproduction, respiration, death and transfiguration; of chemical energy transformation, the cycles of nitrogenous, carbohydrate, mineral, and fatty compounds, and the role of enzymes; and of the regulatory interactions among the biological, chemical, and physical actors in the play called life.   The dynamics of such interrelated patterns of materials, energy, and living things, both sustaining the patterns and being sustained by these, is an ecosystem.   Odum therefore prefers to define ecology as "the study of the structure and function of ecosystems."

Figure 1-8 is a modification of Van Dyne's diagram (Ref. 1-10, p. 329).   The modification is that Van Dyne's network of interrelated arrows among man, climate, soils, plants, and animals is overlaid on the three intersecting circles of land, water, and air.   Van Dyne very purposefully puts man down twice.   Once it is as a component among animals.   The second time it is as the manipulator.   Indeed, in his own terms man does not question that he is master.   A number of religious, philosophical, and mythological themes assure man that he is master and that all around him is his to manipulate.   Ecology is beginning to examine the complexities of these systems and

[1] *Jap. J. Ecol.*, **13**:108 (1962).

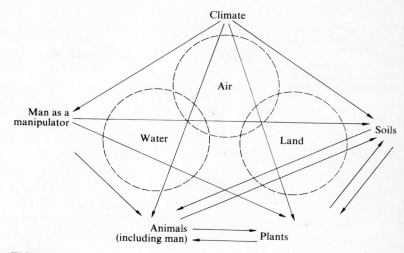

FIGURE 1-8
Understanding ecosystems requires understanding interactions among several
components. [*Modified from G. M. Van Dyne* (*Ref.* 1-10, *p.* 329).]

to venture a few predictions.   As a result of the energy explosion and all that has come
with it, the manipulator's influence on the ecosystem or on many interacting ecosystems has been accelerated and intensified at an increasing rate.   Whatever man
identifies as his own environment, external and internal, shares in these formidable
changes.   This has produced reactions of curiosity, concern, and alarm.   It has produced three hypotheses with variants.   These are:

1 The impacts of technology, urbanization, and population density are outstripping
    man's biological capacity to adapt.   The impairments can appear in time scales
    varying from an individual's lifetime, to a generation or two, to an evolutionary
    span of time.
2 The impacts of technology, urbanization, and population density are so violent
    that the stability of the present ecosystem is being changed so rapidly as to
    threaten the collapse of the earth's life support system.
3 The impacts of technology, urbanization, and population density require the
    maximum utilization of the assimilative capacity of the physical environment
    for the support of the human race.   This can be done by applying present knowl-
    edge fully and effectively through existing social and political mechanisms be-
    fore catastrophe.

Ecology and ecosystems underscore the fact that man is not in this game of life,
the energy transfer system, by himself or for himself.   Man-centered environmental

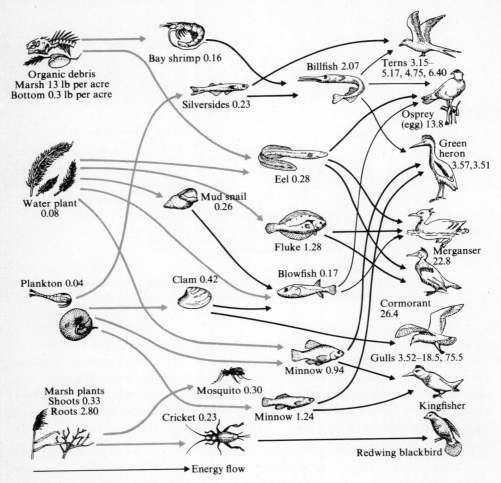

FIGURE 1-9
Portions of a food web in a Long Island estuary, showing the concentrations of DDT in milligrams per kilogram in each organism in the ascending energy regime. [*Source: From "Toxic Substances in Ecological Cycles," G. M. Woodwell. Copyright © 1967 by Scientific American Inc. All rights reserved.*]

protection deals with the health and comfort consequences of ill-managed or non-managed biological, chemical, and physical agents moving cyclically or haphazardly in our land, air, and water spheres.   The forces which influence man also influence other living things and the nonliving processes that support life.   For the most part the effects stated in this book on ecological balances are incomplete, for our knowledge of these is rudimentary.   In isolated cases the data are substantial, although limited to the specific conditions of the ecosystem and characteristics studied. An example is the behavior of DDT in the food web embracing dead forms, plant life, plankton, crustacea, insects, fish, and birds, in a Long Island estuary. This study by George M. Woodwell, Charles F. Wurster, and Peter A. Isaacson is summarized in Fig. 1-9.

METEOROLOGY

Meteorology is the study of the changes of a number of physical parameters in the atmosphere. These include temperature, pressure, water content and state, and radiant flux. These elements and their variations produce horizontal and vertical circulation, cloudiness, and precipitation Their behavior has a marked, even decisive, effect on the wastes we attempt to discharge into the air. The weather elements determine dispersion. Without horizontal or vertical air movement, dispersion is nil except from very high stacks with high discharge velocities and temperatures. Solar radiation affects the reactions of pollutants in the air. Pollutants provide condensation nucleii for water vapor, which produces haze and cloudiness that in turn obscures sunshine. These perceived weather characteristics have more effect on, and meaning for, people than the ritual recital of technical weather observations.

Figure 1-10 diagrams one scheme of zone names for the earth's envelope and physical data on each zone, in the case of distance and temperature in three scales. The zonal divisions of Fig. 1-10 are by temperature gradients. The speed-of-sound trace parallels the temperature values, as sound propagates in air in accord with air temperature. Sound moves faster in warm air. At the top of the figure, the thermosphere extends from an altitude of 85 km, about 50 mi, to 500 km, 300 mi, beyond the scale of our figure. The high and rising temperatures in the thermosphere are due to the absorption of solar radiation by the sparse population of molecular and atomic oxygen, atomic nitrogen, and at still higher altitudes, hydrogen and helium. Satellite-gathered data reveal that above 250 to 400 km, 150 to 240 mi, temperatures are quite constant and fantastically high in the few molecules and atoms present. The average is 1500 K in the isothermal region, with peaks of 2000 K corresponding to solar activity peaks. The molecular species present absorb solar radiation to a frequency of 1×10^{15} Hz, a wavelength of 200 nm. The subsequent dissociation and ionization is exothermic with the release of heat. The solar radiation absorbed is in the very short or "extreme" ultraviolet range. The units used are frequency in hertz (Hz), or cycles per second, and wavelength in nanometers (nm). One nanometer is one-billionth of a meter, 1×10^{-9} m, and is the same as one millimicron.

The next zone of particular meteorological interest, which has affected life on earth since its inception, is the ozonosphere. In this space, from 10 to 50 km (6 to

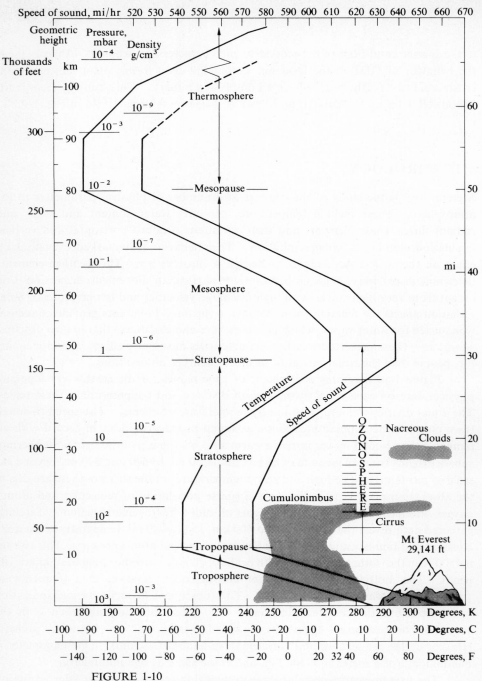

FIGURE 1-10
The zones of our atmosphere to an altitude of 120 km. (*Source: U.S. Navy Weather Research Facility, the Navy, Washington, D.C.*)

30 mi), ozone absorbs ultraviolet in the frequencies from 1.5×10^{15} to 1.0×10^{15} Hz, 200- to 290-nm wavelength. This absorption maintains the heat balance of the atmosphere and particularly of the zone in which we usually move, the troposphere. The major part of the action is at about 50 km (30 mi) and accounts for the temperature rise in the stratosphere, which coincides with the ozonosphere in altitude. The absorption of ultraviolet in the ozonosphere produces the temperature gradient of the stratosphere. The reactions among oxygen species and ultraviolet are regenerative.

$$O_2 + hv \rightarrow O + O$$
$$O_2 + O + M \rightarrow O_3 + M$$
$$O_3 + hv \rightarrow O_2 + O$$
$$O_3 + O \rightarrow O_2 + O_2$$

The hv, a Planck quantum, is the ultraviolet energy. The M is a third partici- pant such as nitrogen to accept the excess energy of the O_2, O combination. The third reaction is the primary source of heat released as the O_3 decomposes. The ozone concentrations in the ozonosphere are many times those of highs in the troposphere. The maximum concentration is about 10 ppm in the altitudes of 25 to 30 km (15 to 20 mi). The reported concentrations in the troposphere reach only 0.04 ppm. The relation of particular gaseous concentrations in the stratosphere to the behavior and fate of pollutants emitted on earth is not certain. There may be a migration and transformation of carbon monoxide from the troposphere to the stratosphere. In 1961, C. Junge, a leader in atmospheric chemistry, discovered a sulfate aerosol layer at an altitude of 20 km (12 mi). The particles were less than 1 μm in diameter and were largely ammonium sulfate. Their origin is likely sulfur dioxide, perhaps from our pollutants. The zonal scheme of Fig. 1-10 is not the only one in use. A simpler division from earth out to the domain of astronauts and cosmonauts is troposphere, stratosphere, ionosphere, embracing the meso- and thermosphere of Fig. 1-10, and exosphere for all space beyond 1,000 km (600 mi) from the earth.

The troposphere is labeled by the Greek word *tropos*, which means "turning." The gaseous content of this zone is constantly turning in turbulence and mixing. Its behavior makes our weather with its swirling air masses, endlessly shifting cloud for- mations, relentless movements of cold and warm fronts, and dynamic creation of high- and low-pressure areas. We see and feel the results of these actions as clear, cloudy, rainy, or windy days; as fog, rain, sleet, snow, or hail; as lightning; as tornados, cyclones, hurricanes, or typhoons. The energy source for all these manifestations is the sun. Its heating of the land and water on the earth's surface and of the air about it produces a vast heat engine or thermodynamic transfer system.

The troposphere is a uniform gaseous mixture with a height of 18 km (11 mi) at the equator and 11 km (5 mi) at the poles. On a clean, dry basis, nitrogen and oxygen make up 99.032 percent of the mixture by volume. Adding argon at 0.934 percent and carbon dioxide at 0.031 percent brings the account to 99.997 percent.   That leaves 0.003 percent for numerous other elements.   This account does not provide for our addition of contaminants and pollutants.   Nor does it provide for a most important and variable component, water vapor.   A global average estimate of water-vapor content in air at any time is 3 percent.   The water vapor and carbon dioxide in the air provide the greenhouse roof of the earth.   These constituents of our air absorb some of the sun's incoming radiation, and more importantly, absorb the reradiation from the earth's surface.   Water vapor strongly absorbs two ranges of the earth's back radiation.

Carbon dioxide fills in much of the absorption gap between the two absorption ranges of water vapor.   On the average the water vapor absorbs six times as much radiation as all the gases, including carbon dioxide.   Without this conservation of the earth's heat by the water vapor and carbon dioxide, the climate of this planet and things on it would be different.

Of the sun's radiant energy striking the planet and its air envelope, 42 percent is reflected back to space, 43 percent is absorbed on the land and water surfaces, and 15 percent is absorbed by the atmosphere.   The earth's surface and atmospheric heating is uneven, with the equator a peak high and the poles the lows.   This initiates the basic wind pattern as the hot equatorial air rises and moves toward the poles and the cold polar air moves toward the equator in lower strata.   Even without the effect of the earth's rotation, the pattern is not simply that of up from the equator and pole-ward with a cold stream moving below from the poles to the equator.   Cooling of the hot equatorial air and mixing at 30° latitude produces the first mixing region and deviation.   The second is at 60° latitude, another mixing zone as the remaining, cooling equatorial air makes its further descent and encounter with the cold polar air. Figure 1-11 is a schematic of the events for the Northern Hemisphere.

The effect of the earth's rotation must now be added.   It is that of trying to draw a straight chalk line from the center to the edge of a rotating phonograph record. The trace is a curving path.   The effect of the earth's rotation on wind direction and velocity is described as the Coriolis effect, named after the nineteenth-century French physicist who described it.   The Coriolis force is at right angles to the wind direction. Therefore, in the Northern Hemisphere a wind from the equator to the pole, a south wind, tends to be pushed in an eastward direction, making the movement a southwest wind.   Remember that winds are directionally identified by the direction from which they are coming.   The directional patterns are reversed in the Southern Hemisphere. The combination of mixing at the 60 and 30° latitudes, of the Coriolis effect, and of the null movements at encounter zones at the 30° points and the equator produce circulation patterns that have become part of our literature and culture.   In the Northern Hemisphere, these are the calms, the doldrums at the equator, and the horse latitudes at 30° north.   The winds are the trades from the northeast from the horse latitudes to

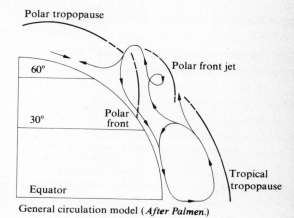

Polar tropopause

60°

30°

Polar front jet

Polar
front

Equator

Tropical
tropopause

General circulation model (*After Palmen.*)

FIGURE 1-11
A schematic of air movement from the equator to the North Pole under thermal forces. (*Source: U.S. Public Health Serv. RATSEC Training Handout PA-ME*-31, *5a*.12.62, *p.* 2.)

the doldrums, the prevailing westerlies from the horse latitudes to 60° north latitude, and north of that line the less well known but bitterly felt polar easterlies from the northeast. The last penetrate the great central plain of Canada and the United States in the winter months and battle it out with the prevailing westerlies in a series of cold and warm fronts to the discomfort and dismay of the inhabitants.

The general wind patterns of the world are established by the thermal upthrust of the hot equatorial air. Additionally, there is local air movement initiated by localized heating and cooling of sizable air masses. These movements are of great importance in moving pollutants away from our cities. In their absence stagnations and inversions result in disagreeable and decidedly unhealthy air for breathing. Figure 1-10 diagrams the troposphere with a temperature gradient from 15°C (59°F) at sea level to −55°C (about −70°F) at an altitude of 10,000 m (32,500 ft). These changes are about 6.5°C/1,000 m (or 3.5°F/1,000 ft). The gradient, a decrease in temperature with altitude, holds for large quiet air masses. It is called the *normal environmental lapse rate*. The term is neatly in accord with the dictionary definition of lapse, "to fall away by degrees." In the lower troposphere, a zone from the surface to an altitude of about 2,000 m (6,500 ft), the temperature varies considerably from the normal environmental lapse rate dependent on the character of the underlying surface and the rate of radiation from it.

In instances in which the temperature increases with altitude, that is, the change is inverted from the normal decrease, the condition is termed an *inversion*. An inversion may begin at ground level and extend upward, a ground inversion. Such a condition occurs at night when the ground cools rapidly and lowers the temperature of the air near the ground below that of the air above it. See line *c* in Fig. 1-12. This condition limits vertical movement, which depends on the buoyancy of warm air in a

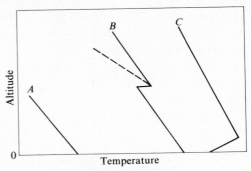

FIGURE 1-12
Examples of commonly occurring environmental lapse rates. (*Source: Class notes of Prof. H. B. Gotaas, Northwestern University, on meteorology and climatology, p. 05.013.*)

A   Normal environmental lapse rate.
B   Thermal inversion.
C   Ground inversion.

larger cooler parcel of surrounding air.   Alternately, the inversion condition may occur in a layer of air at some altitude above the ground.   See line *b* in Fig. 1-12. This thermal inversion layer is a barrier to upward movement.   In effect it is a lid. In conjunction with local topography, as in the case of the Los Angeles basin, an upper-air thermal inversion can create a stagnated air mass just as a cover does over a pot of boiling soup.   The thermal inversion layer can be formed above valleys at night as the cool denser air slides down the hillsides into the valley while a warm layer remains above the ridge tops.   The meteorologists describe the condition of no vertical motion of air as *stable equilibrium*, and those in which there is vertical movement as *instability*.   The thermal inversion is one set of conditions resulting in stability.   To understand and to predict other cases of stability and instability, it is necessary to examine the behavior of parcels of air moving in a large air mass at temperatures different from one another.

A parcel of warm air, say over a city, surrounded by a large mass of cooler air moves upward.   It starts at ground pressure of, say, 1,000 mbar (760 mm of mercury or 14.7 psi).   As the pressure around decreases with altitude, the warm air parcel expands.   As it expands it cools.   There is no outside source of heat to provide the energy for the expansion.   The air parcel provides that energy from its own heat which results in its cooling.   The process is called *adiabatic*, meaning that there is no loss or gain of heat to the parcel to or from outside sources.   Conversely, a parcel of air forced down into higher pressures will be compressed and become warmer.   The increased temperature is due to confining the gas molecules to a lesser volume.   The rate of cooling of a parcel of dry air on ascent, or of cooling on descent is a constant with altitude change. It is 1°C/100 m (or 5.5°F/1,000 ft).   This is the dry adiabatic-process lapse rate.   It states the temperature change of a parcel of air rising or falling. In air in which there is no motion, the temperature change with altitude is in accord with the normal environmental lapse rate.   The adiabatic lapse rate is a special and constant case of the lapse rate of air in vertical motion.   This special parcel is moving in a large mass of surrounding air that is essentially stationary.   Therefore, the surrounding air is changing in temperature in accord with the normal environmental lapse rate.   The relation between the adiabatic lapse rate of an air mass and the environmental lapse rate determines conditions of vertical equilibrium.

The thermal conditions in the surrounding air, defined by the environmental lapse rate, and in a particular parcel of air, defined by the adiabatic process rate, determine whether there will be vertical movement of the air parcel.   When the environmental lapse rate is less than the adiabatic lapse rate, there will be no vertical movement.   The condition is described as stable.   When the environmental lapse rate is greater than the adiabatic-process lapse rate, there will be motion.   The condition is described as unstable.   This is so because the parcel of air moving upward cools at the adiabatic-process lapse rate.   However, it will still be warmer than the surrounding air mass which is dropping in temperature at the environmental lapse rate.   As the surrounding air continues to be cooler than the air parcel, vertical motion continues.   For the dispersal of ground-level pollutants to the upper altitudes, unstable conditions are desirable as there is vertical movement of the polluted air parcels. Figure 1-13 illustrates a parcel of dry air, warmed to 26.5°C (80°F) that starts moving upward in the surrounding 21°C (70°F) air at the dry adiabatic-process rate of 5.5°F/1,000 ft (1°C/100 m).   At 2,000 ft the parcel is at a temperature of 69°F (20.5°C). The surrounding air drops in temperature at the normal environmental lapse rate of 3.5°F/1,000 ft (6.5°C/1,000 m).   It is 63°F (17°C) at 2,000 ft.   The air parcel at 69°F (21°C) is still warmer than the surrounding air.   It will continue to rise.   The behavior and predictions become more intricate as water-vapor content is taken into account as the latent heat changes of water condensing or evaporating affect the temperature of an air parcel.   For saturated air the adiabatic-process rate is lower than that of dry air because of the release of latent heat as water vapor condenses.

All of us are more aware of the more forceful horizontal air movements, the winds.   Four characteristics of winds affect the behavior of air pollutants and their effects on us.   Wind direction determines whether the pollutants are carried to sensitive receptors—man, other animals, plants, and susceptible property.   Wind speed determines the travel time to such receptors.   It also provides dilution as a higher-speed wind will spread out the pollutant load from a constant emission source into longer air paths and larger air volumes.   Dilution of air pollutants from a constant source is directly proportional to wind speed.   Winds are rarely constant for prolonged periods.   There are variations in direction and velocity.   These changes contribute to the distribution of pollutants by diffusion due to the eddy motions of wind variations.   Even low levels of wind variation produce diffusion in the order of one thousand times the diffusion caused by molecular motion.   Winds in their

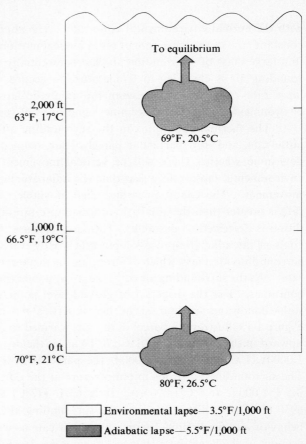

To equilibrium

2,000 ft
63°F, 17°C

69°F, 20.5°C

1,000 ft
66.5°F, 19°C

0 ft
70°F, 21°C

80°F, 26.5°C

☐ Environmental lapse—3.5°F/1,000 ft

▨ Adiabatic lapse—5.5°F/1,000 ft

FIGURE 1-13
Environmental lapse rate exceeds adiabatic process rate, which causes air parcel to rise.

encounter with changes in topography and surface characteristics and with natural and man-made structures produce turbulence. This is generally beneficial in distributing air pollutants. The exceptions are eddies and backwinds around or between large buildings and occasionally natural formations which may trap and concentrate pollutants or carry these to ground levels.

REFERENCES

1-1 EHRLICH, PAUL R., and ANNE H. EHRLICH: "Population, Resources, Environment," W. H. Freeman and Company, San Francisco, 1970.

1-2 ROUECHÉ, BERTON: "Eleven Blue Men," Medallion Books, Berkeley Publishing Corporation, New York, 1955.

1-3 ROBERT M. BROWN (ed.): "The Dynamic Spectrum, Man, Health, and Environment," *Natl. Sanit. Found., Monogr.* 5, Ann Arbor, Mich., 1966, p. 100.

1-4 Report of the Committee on Environmental Health Problems to the Surgeon General, *U.S. Public Health Serv. Publ.* 908, 1962.

1-5 Environmental Pollution Panel, President's Science Advisory Committee: Restoring the Quality of Our Environment, The White House, November 1965.

1-6 Waste Management and Control, *NAS-NRC, Publ.* 1400, 1966.

1-7 The Task Force on Environmental Health and Related Problems: A Strategy for a Livable Environment, *U.S. Public Health Serv. Rep.*, June 1967.

1-8 DALE, EDWIN: The Economics of Pollution, *The New York Times Mag.*, Apr. 19, 1970.

1-9 KORMONDY, EDWARD J. (ed.): "Readings in Ecology," Prentice-Hall, Inc., Englewood Cliffs, N.J., 1965.

1-10 VAN DYNE, GEORGE M.: "The Ecosystem Concept in Natural Resource Management," Academic Press, Inc., New York, 1969.

2

SOME PRINCIPLES OF EPIDEMIOLOGY AND OF THE SCIENCES WHICH UNDERLIE ENVIRONMENTAL PROTECTION

The applications of biology, chemistry, physics, mathematics, and the engineering sciences will be evident in the chapters which follow. Less evident will be the need for a comprehension of human values and behavior, of political processes, of economics, and of administrative methods. Some supportive review of all these matters will be needed from time to time. Three matters are selected for review or introduction in some detail. These are the nature of epidemiology, the fate of pathogens in the free environment, and the mass of the dose of injurious agents. Brief comment is made on the first-order equation of the law of mass action and on the electromagnetic spectrum. These are unifying concepts which recur in several processes of environmental changes and manifestations. At a few points in this book, an understanding of the rudiments of fluid mechanics will be useful but not a necessity. The three fundamental equations describing fluid flow and its energy states are the equation of continuity, Bernoulli's theorem, and frictional requirements. As each reader's need for such understanding varies greatly, even brief comment on fluid flow is not undertaken.

EPIDEMIOLOGY

For the century from 1850 to 1950, epidemiology was the unchallenged source for the rationale of preventive medicine and environmental sanitation. This was the century of triumphs of Western white man over communicable diseases in his cities, his military forces, and more slowly among his farming people. He took his public health methods with his trade and his colonization. He got a boost in microbiology and immunology from the speedily developed skills of the Japanese. The key to grasping what epidemiology is about is to examine the three Greek words that form it: *epi*, over; *demos*, the people; *logos*, knowledge. "Knowledge of what is over the people" cannot stand by itself. In the phrase "epidemiology of disease," epidemiology does make sense. The epidemiologist literally looks at the dead, dying, ailing, and escapees as a collective and asks, "What has come over you people?" To answer a devastating respiratory epidemic that swept Europe in 1743, the Italians said it was *l'influénza*, the French *la grippe*, and the English that it came from the mainland and quite properly should carry an Italian or French name. Two centuries earlier, John Caius had described it as "the Sweat" (Ref. 2-1, p. 21). The question, "What has come over you people?" demanded an answer when large numbers of people in a community concurrently had the same symptoms and were subject to common events. Thus, the circumstances provided a basis for a detectivelike sorting of the evidence, making the question more frequently answerable in the face of an outbreak or epidemic of a single disease. Epidemiology is not and never has been limited to epidemics or to communicable diseases. Diabetes has an epidemiology as do distinct types of cardiovascular disorders and the nutritional diseases, scurvy, beriberi, and pellagra, resulting from specific vitamin shortages. The objective of epidemiology is to find the factors that influence and cause the occurrence of disease among people as a collective in order to provide a rationale for control and prevention. At a minimum, some sign of public action by way of investigation and information has allayed panic and delayed a wholesale exodus from the cities. Panic and flight happened in the Middle Ages when rat-borne plague appeared. R. Pollitzer tells of the rich and knowledgeable packing up and taking off when considerable increases in the number of dead rats were noted. They had their cue from existing epidemiology or folklore and had no intention of becoming added statistics of the new epidemic. Their discretion exceeded their valor and well it might as the hypothesis of flea-borne plague was still in doubt in the early 1900s.

Three classics of nineteenth-century epidemiology of communicable diseases are still in print. These are Peter Ludwig Panum, 1847, on measles in the Faroe Islands; John Snow, 1849, on the mode of communication of cholera on Broad Street, Golden Square, and adjoining streets of London; and William Budd, 1873, on typhoid fever outbreaks that he had analyzed in 1853 and 1866 in Wales and England. These are most accessible and somewhat abbreviated in Roueché's collection of epidemiological studies (Ref. 2-1).   Roueché includes a 1552 account of "The Sweat or Sweating Sickness" by the English physician, John Caius.   It was an epidemic disease that rolled across England in five waves from 1485 to 1551, and is believed to have been a virulent influenza.   The spread in time and cause extends to "Glue-Sniffing in Children," Helen H. Glaser and Oliver N. Massengale, 1962, of the University of Colorado Medical School.   In between in the time span is Matthew Carey's account of Philadelphia's enduring 11,000 cases, with 4,000 deaths, of yellow fever among its 50,000 people from July 26 to October 26, 1793.   Who fled, who stayed, and what they did is a remorseful reminder of the fragility of the social structure under assault. Some samplings from the three classics show what epidemiologists seek.   Panum, a young Danish medical graduate, was sent to the Faroe Islands in 1846 in the middle of a measles outbreak.   There had been no measles on the island since 1781, 65 years before.   From April to mid-September, 6,000 of the 7,782 islanders had full-blown measles, with about 100 deaths.   Panum saw about 1,000 of the cases and made four observations:

1   The incubation period, the time from exposure to the definite symptom of a rash, was 14 days.
2   The time of highest risk of transmission was during the rash.
3   Transmission had to be by person-to-person contact and possibly contaminated clothing, and not by miasmas.
4   Those who had had the measles in 1781 did not get it again.

Snow's dramatic account which cites the Broad Street pump as the mode of transmission, with the Broad Street brewery workers as a control group because of the proprietor's daily allotment of malt liquor, closes with these words:

> Each epidemic of cholera in London has borne a strict relation to the nature of the water supply of its different districts, being modified only by poverty and the crowding and want of cleanliness which always attend it.

This exemplifies the environmental control product of epidemiology, the mode of transmission.   With that known, control can be planned.   Note Snow's perception that susceptibility or the ability to cope with the waterborne infection is modified among the poor, the crowded, and the dirty.   The number of such miserable collections of humanity, with burdens also of poor nutrition and ignorance, are increasing. Every urban center and a fair share of rural areas have poor people, poor not only in worldly goods but in ability and incentive.   The education and training of these unfortunates to the maxima of their potentials is the only change worth seeking which will have lasting benefits.   Table 2-1 presents data assembled by Snow on three separate water services for London in the 1840s.

Roueché's selection, "Typhoid Fever: Its Nature, Mode of Spreading, and

Prevention," covers two of the outbreaks William Budd had studied.   Here are Budd's words on the hotel outbreak following Cowbridge Race Week, Cowbridge, Wales, November 1853 (Ref. 2-1, p. 83):

> From this and other considerations I was led to infer that drinking water was the most probable vehicle of it.
>   A visit to the courtyard of the hotel left in my mind no doubt that this was the true view of the case.   The cesspool and drain, which I was informed had received the bulk of the diarrhoeal discharges from the fever patient, was at the time of the outbreak so near to the well, that under the conditions of soil and locality, percolation from one to the other was inevitable.

Such an observation, even to the selection of words, would well serve a sanitarian's or sanitary engineer's report today, over 100 years later.   Budd's studies included a rural outbreak of typhoid fever in Kingswood, England, in 1866.   The conditions are sketched in Fig. 2-1.   Of the upstream and downstream clusters, Budd wrote (Ref. 2-1, p. 87):

> The little stream, laden with the fever-poison cast off by the intestinal disease of the man who had been stricken with the same fever some weeks before, was the only bond between them.

During a field visit to Kingswood, a gentleman stated to Budd:

> The only wonder is that all these poor people have not died of fever long ago.   For any time these last six years, but in the summer especially, to anyone coming down this lane, the stink had been enough to knock a man down. ...   [Budd stated that] it was down the stream that the seeds of the plague flowed.
>   Higher up, the stream was common sewage only; lower down, it was sewage plus the specific excreta of the fever patient.
>   Hence the cardinal difference in the fate of those who were exposed to its emanations in the two situations.   The only inference that it seems possible to draw from these facts is, that while sewage charged with the specific fever-poison is all-potent in breeding fever, sewage not so charged has no power to breed it at all.

Table 2-1   DATA OF JOHN SNOW ON CHOLERA AMONG THREE WATER SERVICES IN LONDON

Water service and source	No. of houses served	Dead from cholera	Deaths in each 10,000 houses
Southwark and Vauxhall Co's.: From polluted part of Thames River	40,046	1,263	315
Lambeth Co. From upstream intake " quite free from sewage of London "	26,107	98	37
Rest of London	256,423	1,422	59

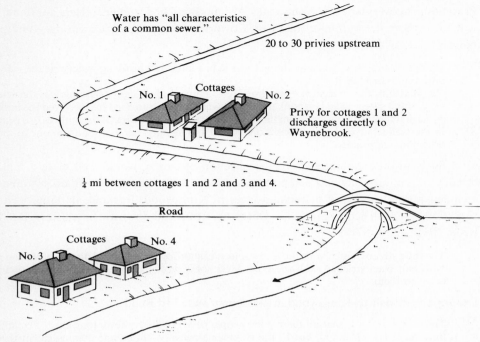

The events:

1. Father of family in cottage 1 returns from St. Philip's slum of Bristol with typhoid fever. His family is well. He has "profuse diarrhea;" for two weeks his excreta discharge to Waynebrook.

2. At end of 4th week, several persons in cottages 1, 2, 3, and 4 are attacked by the fever. There had been no contact between those in cottages 1 and 2 and those in cottages 3 and 4.

3. There were no cases upstream of cottages 1 and 2 despite the condition: "the stink has been enough to knock a man down."

FIGURE 2-1
Sketch of housing clusters along Waynebrook, Kingswood, England, and the occurrence of typhoid fever in 1866.

In this Budd was singling out the mode of transmission and stating that there was an etiological agent that had to be present.   Identification of the etiological agent is a most powerful tool in combating disease and managing the environment, for that singles out the cause, be it disease, disablement, discomfort, or distraction.   The studies of Panum, Snow, and Budd were made before the pathogenicity of bacteria was recognized.   Samples and references to many epidemiological studies of varying types are in this book as these are the fabric of the rationale of environmental control of the hazards to man and the risks he chooses to accept for real or fancied benefits of

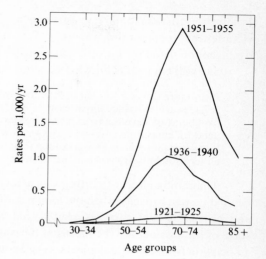

FIGURE 2-2
Death rates for cancer of the lung and pleura in England and Wales in 5-year age groups in three time intervals, 1921 to 1925, 1936 to 1940, and 1951 to 1955. [*Source: Sartwell (Ref.* 2-2, *p.* 15).]

technology, growth, and the increase and concentration of his numbers.   Examples in this book which do not concern either epidemics or infectious diseases are the fluoride-caries relation, ionizing radiation effects, noise effects, the accident syndrome, the significance of DDT residues in human fat, such information as is available about microwave effects on man, and occupational disease studies which successfully defined safe working levels in the workroom air for toxic dusts, gases, and vapors.

For a formal introduction to epidemiology and public health statistics read the first three chapters of Sartwell (Ref. 2-2).   The basic methods of epidemiology, experimental controlled observations, and uncontrolled observations are stated and illustrated.   The changing patterns of disease and causes of death are emphasized under dynamics and distribution.   For example, in 1920 coronary artery disease was not even among the 189 causes of death in the classification list used in the United States.   In 1930, it was charged with 1 percent of all deaths in the United States, and by 1959 with 17 percent of deaths.   Sartwell cautions that the bulk of the increase reflects advances in medical knowledge and changes in terminology of disease diagnosis.   Figure 2-2, from Sartwell, shows the change in death rates from lung cancer in England and Wales in 5-year age groups plotted for three different time periods.   Such displays raise three questions:

1 Is the change a real shift in the natural occurrence of disease among like groups of susceptibles?
2 Is it a shift in the number of susceptibles making up the cohort identified by age and geography?
3 Can the cause of the change be identified?

Finding the answers to these questions is much more difficult than the epidemiological victories that required the mustering of circumstantial evidence to fix a specific causative agent or mode of transmission of a specific communicable disease.

Sartwell comments on what he terms "temporal associations" (Ref. 2-2, p. 16):

> Even more difficult to deal with is the situation where prolonged exposure to an agent is necessary to induce the disease.   With certain carcinogens employed in industry the likelihood of developing cancer increases with duration of exposure.   Since the frequency of cancer increases with age anyhow, and since individual susceptibility varies so that some individuals, however long their exposure, do not get the disease, it is not easy either to demonstrate the association or to put it in quantitative terms.

These difficulties of sorting out associations from cause and effect are simply beyond human capacity when the total mix of environmental contaminants, pollutants, and physical energy excesses are charged with impairing human behavior.   At no stage of the sort-out are the means of measurement sufficiently sensitive to distinguish association from cause and effect.   The September 1968 issue of the *American Journal of Public Health*[1] contains the papers of a symposium on epidemiology and the environment.   Specific examples of the confrontation with real data are given both on individual physiological function variables in diurnal, seasonal, and annual cycles and on the short- and long-cyclical jumps and jogs of specific diseases in large populations such as all of New York City.   Among a group of young men under standard metabolic conditions, Frederick Sargent found physiochemical properties of the blood to vary among individuals by 10 percent for nonprotein nitrogen, 20 percent for cholinesterase, and 42 percent for alkaline phosphatase.   E. J. Cassel and his colleagues examined mortality data and rises in sulfur dioxide and particulates in air in New York City.   As the length of time span of their observations was expanded from 2 months to 1 year to 3 years, "it became clear that elevated air pollution levels were not necessarily associated with increased mortality."   Robert E. Carroll, reporting during the symposium on the epidemiology of New Orleans asthma, stated:

> The nature of the allergen that causes New Orleans' periodic episodes of asthma attacks remains an enigma.   Very sophisticated air sampling for a number of years has failed to produce any consistent findings.   Prior hypotheses, implicating burning dumps or dust from a grain elevator, no longer seem tenable.

The examples produce some sobering thoughts which are wholly absent from the glib words of politicians and, unfortunately, of some professional practitioners who have espoused the dirty environment as a worthy mate to give purpose to their lives.

Most of us will profit by reading Chaps. 2 and 3 of Ref. 2-2.   In these, Paul Densen lucidly and concisely deals with "Statistical Reasoning and the Health of the Population."   Morbidity and mortality rates and ratios in common use and "bench

---

[1] *Am. J. Public Health*, **58**:1638–1683 (1968).

marks" on these are given. The difference between *incidence* and *prevalence* is clarified once again. Incidence is a rate which must be on a time base. Prevalence is a ratio of the number of people afflicted to the total number of exposed population, however you choose to define "exposed." Two quotes from Densen give the flavor of his thinking.

> The study of man and his responses to his total environment, particularly as they are related to the phenomena of health and disease, is essentially the study of variation. The statistical method is a powerful tool for the investigation of this variation. ...
> (Ref. 2-2, p. 43)
> Apart from the acute respiratory diseases and accidents, the major threats to the health of the population are the chronic diseases—heart disease, stroke, cancer, arthritis, mental disease, and others. These are all diseases for which knowledge of the etiology and natural history is still far from complete. As has been pointed out by Stewart (1960), the goal of the attack on these diseases is prevention of disability. Until more is learned about how to prevent the diseases themselves, this must be the goal of preventive medicine—a goal which, at the present time, can only be achieved through the development of adequate methods of medical care.
> (Ref. 2-2, p. 73)

That statement is not hopeful for prevention and does not consider that possible causes of the chronic diseases cited are factors in our physical environment. The possibility of such environmental causes rests on fragmentary information such as less cardiovascular disease in hard-water areas, more cardiovascular disease where trace metals such as vanadium are in the water, and the violent responses to impact noise that were shown in the cardiovascular system of a South Sahara tribe adapted to a nearly noiseless surrounding. There is presently expansive conjecture on chemical contaminants' being carcinogens. There are several organics which produce cancers in mice after sizable doses and exposures. Some of these are human carcinogens in occupational exposures and among heavy users of smoked foods. Some specific substances are asbestos fibers, radon-gas-decay daughters, and alpha-benzopyrenes. Conjecture is unlimited when additive, potentiating, and synergistic actions among two or more compounds is presupposed on a "what if?" basis. "What if you ingest this one, inhale that one, and absorb the other one?" The dilemmas of toxicology and radiation biological effects are cited in the chapters on water, food, and radiations.

Figure 2-3 is a model that is helpful and likely oversimplified. Shown as a teeter-totter, the model is dynamic, seeking to keep within a range of teeter to totter that is accepted as functionally healthy. Biochemistry and molecular physiology emphasizes that the interaction between host and disturbing agent or agents is at particular cell locations. Therefore, all forces and factors outside of that interaction locus are the entire external environment. That must include the nutritional and emotional levels and the homeostasis of the susceptible man. This is environment in its universal sense as indeed there is a localized biochemical environment within the cell, determining the behavior of particular molecules, atoms, and orbital electrons at

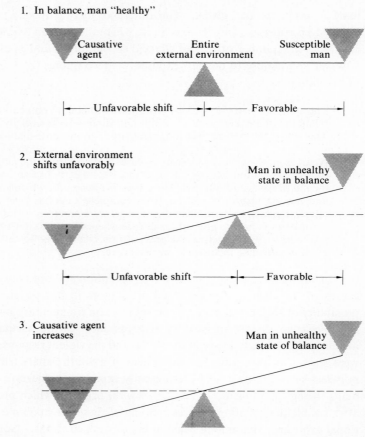

FIGURE 2-3
A diagrammatic balance among the susceptible man, the causative agent, and the man's entire external environment.

that locus of interaction. Our ignorance of these matters is vast, and for all but a few specific agents that ignorance is total. A few mechanisms are known, at least in part, such as CO and hemoglobin, alpha-particle energy transfer in human tissue, microwave and laser energy effects on specific cells in the human eye, ^{90}Sr deposition in the bone, DDT and DDE storage in fatty tissue, and the specificity of some viruses to cell reactions.

All this goes on in a living system which has survived by adaptation. Darwin set down the broad principles based on his observations of gross anatomical differences within a species and among the species. More recent eloquent words on the subject

of man's staking his survival on his ability to adapt come from René Dubos in h
books, *Man Adapting*[1] and *So Human an Animal*[2]. Man's cohabiting species, plant
and animal, are included in the stakes. In the earth's long process of survival and
adaptation many species have gone to fossils. Man is different from those which got
the extinction ticket, because he appears to have the power and resources of choice.
The growing mess of dirty water, air, food, and land are his own doings, which can be
controlled. Dubos is convinced that the natural process of adaptation is too slow to
counterbalance the deleterious environment which man is shaping about himself at an
accelerating rate. Therefore, human behavior must change to delay or postpone for
a man's lifetime immediate self-gratifications, primarily of material goods and excessive childbearing, to bring man into a more promising balance with earth. This is
not for the earth's sake, but for man's own survival as something resembling an intel-
ligent being privileged to develop his potentials freely and to use his endowments, vast
or modest, in harmony with life about him. The test rests upon the total intelligence
resources of the species. Epidemiology must be applied at every hopeful point,
including the epidemiology of human behavior, which is a product of mental health.
Control technology, which is the contents of this book, is important. It is only a
tool. Its use rests on the value system of each of us and of our collectives of family,
neighborhood, town, state, nation, and world. The humanities are the nurture of our
values. The scientist, technologist, manager, and political leader without that nurture
are menaces to our survival.

THE FATE OF OUR PATHOGENS

Survival Factors

The pathogens of man are most comfortable in our bodies, which offer a remarkably
constant environment of pH, temperature, nutrients, and biochemical support. Of
course, these are not symbiotic. The pathogens are "imperfect" parasites as their
presence wrecks the equilibrium of our body's biochemical and biophysical environment, makes us sick, and produces the state we call disease. Our excretions become
disorderly, our temperature increases, our nutrient system bobbles about, our blood
composition changes; we are sick, acutely or chronically. During the process, the
organisms leave our bodies as adult, larva, cyst, or egg forms. Usually the departure
is in coughs, sneezes, nasal drip, and spit from the lungs, throat, nose, and mouth; in
our urine and feces; from our blood by blood-sucking insects; and from surface

---

[1] Yale University Press, New Haven, 1965.
[2] Charles Scribner's Sons, N.Y., 1968.

tact transport by flies as in trachoma and yaws.   How do these
_arture?   What is their fate in the free environment?   These
have a very rough time outside our bodies.   It is not rough enough
in" entirely.   Even with man-assisted controls, pathogens survive their
rious voyage from man to man.   Events in 1970 reminded us of man's shortsighted management of his environment, including a typhoid fever outbreak on the
Pacific and Orient ship *Oronsay*, cholera in the Crimea and Caucasus regions of the
U.S.S.R., which spread to West Africa, and viral meningitis in the South Bronx section
of New York City.   Myriads of pathogens start the new generation in man's tissues.
Some specific information on the numbers in man's feces are in the chapter on wastes,
in man's food in the food protection chapter, and among the animals in the vector
chapter.   With such fantastic numbers starting the migration, a few make it.   The
cruel demanding selection by survival earns enough successes against formidable environmental and biological odds to keep the pathogens among us.   Several malariolo-
gists, observing the perilous journey of the plasmodia, have noted that there ought not
to be any malaria.   The odds are very much against making it through the cycle.   In
malaria and in our man–external environment–man cycles of communicable diseases,
the survivors overcome physical, biological, and chemical adversity in the free environment.

Table 2-2 does not contain any surprises when the elemental processes of life are

Table 2-2   FAVORABLE AND UNFAVORABLE ENVIRONMENTAL
FACTORS FOR THE SURVIVAL OF THE PATHOGENS OF
MAN IN THE FREE ENVIRONMENT

Favorable	Unfavorable	Comments on survival
Moisture	Drying	Drying is the most adverse condition.
Low temperatures	High temperatures	Pathogens survive freezing; 60°C kills in 1 min or less; 100°C is a certain killer.
pH range, 5–9	pH below 5 and above 9	Specific organisms have a narrower favorable range than 5–9; none are acidophils of alkalophils.
Shade	Sunlight	The UV of sunlight and drying are killers.
Freshwater	Saline water	Survival in freshwater is much longer than seawater.
Clean water	Polluted water	Competitive forms of life in polluted waters kill pathogens.
Sterile soil	Natural soil	Competitive forms of life in natural soil kill pathogens.

in mind.   Pathogen survival from feces at low temperatures, including freezing, is well documented in frozen meats and natural ice on contaminated lakes and ponds. Of course, there is no multiplication at low temperatures as life processes are quite dormant.   The presence of other organisms in natural soil and in polluted waters is unfavorable for pathogens.   Those of human origin are victimized by protozoa, bacteriophages, viruses, and antibiotics.   The certain effects that drying and heating have on microorganisms have been applied for millenia by man to control food spoilage during storage until the next harvest.   An unrecognized benefit was killing pathogens on the foods being preserved.

The Survival of Pathogenic Bacteria from Feces

Since their identification in feces less than 100 years ago, numerous studies have been made on the survival of pathogenic bacteria from feces in the environment, in privies, in septic tanks, and during the unit processes of sewage treatment.   The information is most extensive for *Salmonella typhosa* and *Vibrio cholera*.   Table 2-3 shows that their

Table 2-3   SURVIVAL DATA ON TWO INTESTINAL PATHOGENIC BACTERIA IN THE FREE ENVIRONMENT

Survival time	*Salmonella typhosa*	*Vibrio cholera*
1 In feces	Min., 8 days Max., 5 months General, 30 days	7–14 days unless frozen, then survives winter-long freezing
2 In water	Sterile, 15–25 days Tap, 4–7 days Raw river, 1–4 days Drainage canal, 2 days	1–5 days 1–2 days 2–3 days Rivers of India, $\frac{1}{2}$–$1\frac{1}{2}$ days
3 On foods	Vegetables and fruits: Min., 15 days Max., 40 days General, 20 days	On meat 7–14 days On fish 3–4 days ambient temperature On fish 10–12 days in ice box Raw milk 1–1.5 days at 22–25°C
4 On natural soil	Min., 1 day Max., 2 years in moist frozen General, under 100 days	Moist tropical, 7 days Russian winter, 4 months Dry brick dust, 3 days max.
5 With heating	In milk at 80°C, 2 s In milk at 62°C, 36–42 s In milk at 60°C, 76–82 s	In water at 100°C, 0 In water at 80°C, 5 min In water at 56°C, 30 min In water at 40°C, 3 days

survival times must be estimated in days at ambient temperatures. The patterns indicated in Table 2-2 are followed. *V. cholera* is less resistant than *S. typhosa* under the conditions listed except for its longer survival on heating in a liquid. *V. cholera* lasts 1 hour in sour milk and only 5 min in the Indian curd milk called *dahi*. The resistance through freezing winters requires discarding the widely held notion that cold kills.

Survival data on other pathogenic bacteria are plentiful on specific conditions such as recovery from tomatoes; rate of death in sludge digestors; survival on coins, paper money, and telephone handsets. A comprehensive analysis can be made on the survival of *Mycobacterium tuberculosis*, both hominis and bovis, in the free environment. These are tough organisms with high resistance to heat and drying. Aside from bovis transmission in milk, environmental transmission of tuberculosis is not supported by the epidemiological patterns.

The Survival of *Entamoebia histolytica*

Waterborne outbreaks of amoebic dysentery have been very rare. The world's first large recorded one was in Chicago in 1933. There have been no more than a half-dozen waterborne outbreaks in the world since then. From 1930 to 1962 there have been 28 other outbreaks in mental hospitals, Indian reservations, United States colleges, and rural families. Yet there is much information on *E. histolytica* survival, as it forms resistant cysts. The cysts persist in water, on soil, on food, and through conventional chlorination of water. For field-troop protection, during World War II, the U.S. Army supported investigations on cyst survival and kill to get water-hygiene methods for field water points and for individual canteens. *E. histolytica* cysts differ markedly both in survival time for relatively small temperature increases

Table 2-4 SURVIVAL OF THE AMOEBOID AND CYSTIC FORMS OF *Entamoeba histolytica*

Survival	Time and conditions
1 In water, amoeboid-form cysts	3 days at room temperature 5 weeks at 37°C 153 days at 12–22°C 37 days at room temperature "Few" days at 37°C 90 days at 0°C with $\frac{1}{3}$ reduction for each 10°C increase
2 In soil, cysts	6–8 days in moist soil at 24–34°C
3 In water treatment, cysts	99.99% removal by coagulation and rapid sand filtration
4 Drying and heating, cysts	5 min at 65°C 10 min at room temperature "Few" minutes at room temperature on human hands

and in their requirement for increased chlorine residuals with water temperature increases.   Conflicts appear between reports of the early 1920s and recent work, due to changed techniques for isolating, identifying, and counting the organisms.   Experiments done with cysts from cultures rather than with cysts of human intestinal origin show the cultured cysts to withstand higher combinations of chlorine concentrations and exposure times than freshly excreted cysts.   Finally, the apparent wide variations in survival data must be viewed in the probability span of all biological responses. Disease and its environmental control is a biological game of chance played with the best judgment of the odds and not with the expectation of winning 100 percent of the chances or 100 percent of the time.

Table 2-4 shows that *E. histolytica* cysts are more resistant than *S. typhosa* and *V. cholera* in the free environment, and most markedly, 10 times more for survival times in water.   More dramatically, the cysts have survived from 10 min to 48 hours in chlorine concentrations in water up to 500 mg/l.   The World War II studies of S. L. Chang and Gordon Fair led to the decision to develop and use iodine compounds for cyst kill in field water supplies where sand filtration could not be used.   For satisfactory kill by chlorine, 30-min contact at pH of 6 to 7 with superchlorination doses was needed.   Temperature increases of 10°C required 40 percent increases in chlorine residuals.   A doubling of cyst population required a 30 percent increase in chlorine dose.   Such conditions are too demanding for routine field use.   These data do bear out the resistance of the cysts to chlorine in water.   This is remarkable for any microorganism and particularly so for an intestinal pathogen, even if it is a protozoan.

The Survival of Hookworm and Roundworm

These intestinal parasitic helminths seem remote from our urbanized life.   Their continued presence among some 2 billion of us is documented in the chapter on wastes. That signals our lack of determination to apply the rudiments of preventive medicine and environmental sanitation, the hygienic disposal of feces, to the billions of people in millions of rural villages.

Table 2-5 shows that the survival ranges in time of the two most damaging helminths is a matter of weeks, indeed months, for not unusual ambient temperatures. Survival at low temperatures is again characteristic, as for those pathogens in Tables 2-3 and 2-4.   The only naturally protective condition is sun-drying.   With 5 days survival for hookworm eggs and 20 days for the roundworm, dependence on that protection is too slow to prevent recycling and added infections.   The egg ladened feces must not be discharged by man, woman, or child on the ground surface.   If some form of water-carried sewage disposal cannot be devised, the infectious feces must be dropped in pits.   Ample data are extant on helminth survival in the unit processes of sewage treatment.   There is very substantial removal by primary settling.   That places such helminths as hookworm, roundworm, whipworm, and the tapeworms in the sludge.   Survivals in sludge digestors from 2 to 6 months have been observed. Flash heat drying is required for the kill.   The only secondary bio-oxidation process that can do a consistent 99 percent removal is intermittent sand filtration.   The chlorination levels used in sewage treatment leave the excreted forms of helminths unscathed.

A Look at Human Viruses in the Free Environment

Our knowledge of human viruses and human viral diseases is a peculiar patchwork of prevention by immunization, as for smallpox and rabies (after exposure for man); prevention by vector control before the virus was known, as in the case of yellow fever and dengue; isolation from the free environment without substantial evidence of environmental transmission, as for poliomyelitis; and concern for an epidemic risk of environmental transmission of a virus that has not been cultured, as in the case of infectious hepatitis.   For the last virus, the Australia antigen found in the serum of Australian aborigines and isolated in 1969 from one-third of over 200 hepatitis patients is a long step toward tissue culture and immunization development.   Further, the cultured hepatitis virus will be studied to find feasible environmental controls.

Table 2-5   SURVIVAL DATA ON TWO INTESTINAL HELMINTHS, HOOKWORM AND ROUNDWORM, *Ascaris lumbricoides*

Survival	Hookworm	Roundworm
1 In feces	8–12 weeks at spring temp. 4–6 weeks at summer temp. 1–2 days with lime addition	Composting ends eggs. Eggs last 6 months in pits.
2 On soil	6–12 weeks max. 3 weeks at 35°C 9 weeks at 27°C 10–12 weeks at 15°C 1 week at 0°C 5 days in direct sun	5–6 months in winter. 3 weeks in moist soils resulted in 50% of eggs embryonating in sun and in 90% making it in shade; 20 days kills in sunned sand.
3 Temperature	Hatching: 20–35°C favorable 40°C max. 8–10°C min.

Survival of eggs: above 60°C, killed 50-60°C, 1–5 min 40–50°C, "few" min | Hatching: 27–30°C favorable with relative humidity of 75–80%; embryonated after 40 days at −2 to −17°C

Survival of developed embryos: 12 to 18°C, 30 days −6 to −17°C, 10 days −6 to −17°C, killed in 20 days |

A major triumph of molecular biology is recognition of animal viruses as one of the two nucleic acids, ribonucleic acid, RNA, or deoxyribonucleic acid, DNA. These bits of genetic material have an extracellular state as submicroscopic particles surrounded by a protein. Some of these virus particles, or virions, have a passage in the free environment in one of three ways. The viruses of German measles, measles, mumps, smallpox, chicken pox, and influenza have a droplet-airborne passage. The viruses of yellow fever, dengue, some hemorrhagic fevers, several encephalitides, and less certain disease entities are grouped as arthropod-borne animal viruses. There are about 150 such viruses with varying chemical properties. The grouping is based on their propagative cycle among the vertebrates: man, other mammals, birds, and certain reptiles and amphibians. The arthropod vectors are mosquitos, sand flies, midges, ticks, and mites. The third passage which is most puzzling and threatening is the exit of certain viruses from man's intestine with his feces. Solely on that behavior, the poliomyelitis viruses, infectious hepatitis virus, enterocytopathogenic human orphan (ECHO), and the Coxsackie viruses are called *enteroviruses.* Coxsackie is a geographical tribute to the New York State town where a new virus was isolated. Viral classification on biochemical characteristics is already in use among microbiologists. The crude grouping used here is justifiable by its provision of some handhold to public health and environmental protection practitioners to identify these virus appearances in the free environment.

The fascination of the enigmas of human viral diseases is found in what we do know about epidemiological and environmental behavior of the entero viruses. These viruses survive in the free environment. Mack, Mallman, et al.,[1] made 118 isolations of Polio types I and III, Coxsackie and ECHO, from 1,403 at-plant raw sewage samples. These included 88 recoveries from the East Lansing, Michigan, plant, which receives residential sewage, and 30 from the Lansing plant which receives a substantial load of industrial wastewater. The point is the survival in sewage of these specialized forms of life which require host cells for replication. For all its complexities and for all its intense study, the epidemiology of poliomyelitis and its paralytic manifestations has not supported waterborne transmission of the disease.

Transmission of Viruses by the Water Route [Ref. 2-3] reports the papers and discussion of a symposium on the issue held December 6–8, 1965, at the Robert A. Taft Sanitary Engineering Center, Cincinnati, Ohio. The observations which follow are my summary of the salient presentations by an international group who have studied the matter in laboratory and field work and who have reflected on the epidemiological and sanitary evidence of the realities and risks of human virus transmission through the environment to produce disease.

---

[1] *Sewage Works J.,* **30**:957 (1958).

1   The enteroviruses which can be isolated and cultured—polio, Coxsackie, ECHO —are readily found in sewage and survive conventional treatment. Settling reduces recoveries by 3 to 12 percent. The unit process of "activated sludge" reduces the recoveries by 75 to 90 percent. Bizarrely, the reoviruses, probably from animals, are recovered with 20 percent more successes after activated-sludge treatment of the sewage than in the raw sewage entering the plant.

2   Conventional water-treatment processes cannot be relied upon to remove enteroviruses. Flocculation and settling removes Coxsackie A-2 very well, A-1 partially. But these processes have slight effect on polio and apparently also slight effect on the infectious hepatitis virus. Free available chlorine at 1 mg/l for 30 min does inactivate enteroviruses not shielded in particulates.[1]

3   Enteroviruses survive in natural waters about 2 months in temperate zone winters and about 1 month in temperate zone summers. Coxsackie B-3 is the toughest, Polio I is the frailest, ECHO 6 is in between these in survival time. Survival is even longer in raw sewage and very heavily polluted waters. The most extensive data result from the work of T. G. Metcalf and W. C. Stiles in estuarine waters of New Hampshire.

4   Shellfish transmit infectious hepatitis to man by storing and, under most conditions, concentrating the virus in their diverticulum and drainable fluids. Shellfish transmission accounts for about 1 percent of reported infectious hepatitis in the United States. Such transmission was first verified in Sweden in 1955 in an outbreak of 630 cases. In the United States 84 cases appeared on the Gulf Coast and 485 in New Jersey and the Northeast in 1961. Two further outbreaks occurred in 1964 with 193 cases in south New Jersey and Philadelphia and 123 cases in Connecticut. Virus accumulation in shellfish is rapid, within 2 to 4 hours during active feeding. Survival in dry stored shell stock at 5°C is long, up to 1 month. Depuration, self-cleansing, is thorough during active feeding in clean waters for 2 to 4 days. The risk of infectious hepatitis in eating raw shellfish taken from United States Gulf Coast and Atlantic Coast waters is greatest from midsummer to late fall and rises as pollution increases, even when indexed by coliform tests. The two 1961 infectious hepatitis outbreaks were caused by shellfish "bootlegged" from "closed" waters. Shellfish sanitation officials had found high coliform densities in the growing waters and in accord with U.S. Public Health Service Shellfish Sanitation procedures had prohibited harvesting shellfish. Improved methods of depuration are being developed at the U.S. Food and Drug Administration Northeast Shellfish Sanitation Research Center, Narragansett, Rhode Island.

---

[1] N. A. Clarke and S. L. Chang, *JAWWA*, **5 1**:1299 (1959).

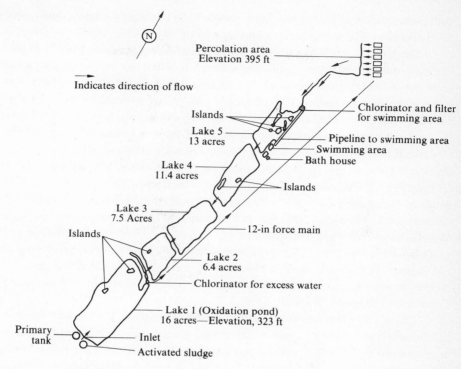

FIGURE 2-4
Diagrammatic map of Santee project reclaiming Santee town wastewater for recreational uses of boating, fishing, and swimming. [*Source*: *Berg* (*Ref.* 2-4, *p.* 402).]

The Santee Project reclaims the wastewater from a southern California community of 12,000 people for recreational use in a series of five lakes.   Figure 2-4 is the diagrammatic map and requires careful attention to the arrows to grasp the flow pattern.   Top-quality water for swimming in a part of lake 5 has been through the activated-sludge process, an oxidation pond in lake 1, chlorination at the end of lake 1, a pass through a natural percolation bed, flocculation, diatomaceous earth filtration, and a final chlorination before it is piped to the swimming area.   The second filtration removes iron and manganese picked up in the natural percolation bed.   No virus recoveries have been made on water going through all these steps.   None were recovered from experimental additions of attenuated Polio III virus after a 200-ft pass along the percolation bed.   No viruses were recovered from the recreational lake samples over a 33-month period.   The project has been in development and study since 1962 with joint participation of health and water people from the federal, state, county, and town governments. There has been swimming use of lake 5 since 1965.

There is a compelling necessity for information on the behavior of viruses in the free environment, most evidently for water. It is not an overwhelming menace of waterborne viral diseases presently. Infectious hepatitis, of which the least is known, is the only viral disease epidemiologically recognized as waterborne. To 1965, the world provided 50 alleged outbreaks of waterborne infectious hepatitis. J. W. Mosely, reviewing the epidemiological consequences of human viruses in water at the 1965 Cincinnati symposium, judged 30 of these to provide adequate data for such a classification. Even accepting all 50 as validly waterborne, the total cases are about 35,000. Of these, 28,475 cases are ascribed to the Delhi disaster of 1955 to 1956, noted in some detail in the chapter on water. The next 12 outbreaks, ranked by number of cases, account for 4,758 cases. That leaves less than 2,000 cases attributed to 37 outbreaks. Mosely uncovered eight outbreaks of poliomyelitis considered waterborne in the 40 years from 1913 to 1953. Six were in Sweden from 1913 to 1949, producing at most 336 cases. The seventh was in Huskerville, a residential subdivision near Lincoln, Nebraska, with 45 cases, 17 paralytic, in 1952. The eighth was in Edmonton, Alberta, Canada, in 1953 with 75 cases.

The urgency remains as the concentration of people in urban and suburban areas throughout the world imposes water reuse, planned or unplanned, and a quality deterioration that is subtle rather than overt. Three questions are posed concerning the removal of viruses, of traces of organic chemicals potentially carcinogenic or mutagenic, and of traces of heavy metals, recognized as toxic in the occupational setting, in wastewaters, and in polluted natural waters, surface and ground:

1 Are present water-treatment processes sufficient to remove these contaminants?
2 Are present sewage-treatment processes reducing these consistently?
3 Can wastewaters be reclaimed with probability statistics reasonably established on the risks of such contaminants passing through?

A few answers and some suggestions are in later chapters. Grueling work in laboratories, in pilot plants such as the Advanced Waste Treatment Research Program at Lebanon, Ohio (started by the U.S. Public Health Service and continued by the Environmental Protection Agency of the United States), and in controlled field applications such as the Santee Project will produce the material for the professional judgments that must be made in day-to-day decisions that commit private and public capital. Such decisions are the crucial ones which shape our environment and knowingly or unknowingly set its quality.

THE MASS OF THE DOSE

The mass of the dose needed for an assaulter to produce human damage is another component in the relationship of the susceptible human, the environmental conditions, and the assaulter, whether of a biological, chemical, or physical form.   How much can a man take?   Some kind of answer must be given for all exposures, with the hope of protecting a very large percentage of all of us, say at least 95 percent and, it is hoped, 99 percent.   Who from what?   The ground crewman at jet airports against noise; the traffic cop at a downtown intersection against vehicle exhaust, heat or cold, and noise; the ghetto kid who eats flaking paint against lead; the nuclear physicist against ionizing radiation; the sandwich-vending-machine customer against microwaves from the microwave oven; the rice-paddy worker against malaria; somebody somewhere against each and all of the environmental conditions offered for study in this book and several surfacing during its preparation.   A few questions, facts, and dilemmas are widely applicable.

On the Exposure

1 Is it short and occasional as a burst of radiation from an x-ray machine?
2 Is it continuous with a well-defined intake of the carrier but with variable concentration of the pollutants as in urban community air for one who works and lives in the city?
3 Is the intake variable but the concentration of the suspected agent constant as with brominated vegetable oil, BVO, in fruit flavored soft drinks?
4 Is it a matter of chance that is approximately predictable as a bite on an airport transient by a female anopheline in an area of low endemicity of malaria?
5 Is it an exposure to a material present widely in the environment, reaching everyone all the time and in everyone's body as with lead present in variable, usually very low, concentration in our food, air, water, and even skin contact surfaces?

On the Exposed

1 Does the exposed man, woman, or child know there is a risk?   Contrast the skilled crop-dusting pilot applying parathion with the youngster who's "paw" mobilizes him to harvest tobacco on which in 1970 he is using parathion for the first year and thinks it is not different from the DDT he has used for 25 years.
2 Is the exposed person acceptably healthy, or is there an overt or subtle somatic, genetic, or emotional factor influencing the body's processes for coping with the intake?   Those affected by such factors range from the normal young in rapid growth to the underfed, the alcoholic, the cardiorespiratory cripple, the drug

victim, or the patient in therapy. An example of the last, a bit exotic, is the cardiac recovery patient who has a battery-powered pulse generator about the size of a small matchbox fastened to his chest. The pulse normalizes the heartbeat signal. It is a "heart pacemaker." In a microwave field such as that produced by ground radar control systems for airport landing and takeoff control, the heart pacemaker signal is seriously disturbed and cannot provide support for its patient. The answer is not to ban radar, not to prohibit such people from entering microwave fields. The answer is to shield the pacemaker circuit so that the microwave energy cannot penetrate it.

3 Do the exposed enjoy their right to environmental and medical surveillance to verify that exposure is not greater than professionals judge to be an acceptable risk for the benefits gained from the exposure? Such surveillance is provided to a limited degree. The job is being done for not more than 25 percent of United States workers who are in exposures for which there is enough knowledge to provide protection. The job is being done well for U.S. Atomic Energy Commission's controlled nuclear materials and installations, and it is being done to the full extent of agreed-upon knowledge of risks and of controls. For all of us in the United States there is a variable effectiveness of control, from good for biological contaminants in our water and milk, to negligible for noise in our communities, homes, and most work places. The basis for control varies from sound scientific reasoning to emotional irrationality. The national chemophobia is offered as an example of the latter—quite peculiar among a people who each year consume $15 billion worth of ethyl alcohol, who burn $10 billion worth of tobacco, who dally with marijuana in increasing numbers and support a gangster-managed international trade in hard drugs, and who accept 60,000 street and road killings for the convenience of unprecedented automobility with the added fillips of alcohol, speed, and more acceleration power than brake power.

On the Quantities for Injurious Dose or Exposure

1 The most is known on the physical-energy doses, or exposure, which will produce injury in man and in a number of animals and plants. These energies include ionizing radiation, nonionizing radiation, temperature extremes, noise, and vibration. Most of these can be measured precisely to very low levels with ready discrimination in such things as wavelength (or frequency), energy, and power. Usable thresholds can be set for single exposures and for continued lower levels for occupational exposures. Acceptable exposures for humans for a lifetime or for generations at very low levels in fractionated doses and irregular periods are prudent, practical professional guesses.

2 A substantial and reliable collection of data exists for some 400 toxic chemicals

used, generated, or produced in manufacturing operations.   This is the contribution of industrial hygiene and occupational medicine.   It developed from and for adults sufficiently healthy to make it to the time clock each day and to the pay window each week.   Caution, reticence, and in some instances prohibition, is dictated before extrapolating these data to all manner of beings, media, and conditions.   Beyond the industrial poisons, information becomes fragmentary, with pharmacology a major source of identification of toxic compounds.   Large doses of notorious substances are well known.   Then there is the trail-off to guesses for toxicants for which the identity is obscure, the time of exposure long, and the dose tiny.

3   Surprisingly little is known on the quantity of a biological agent needed to produce injurious infection.   How many typhoid bacteria must be in a glass of water to produce a human case?   How many *Clostridium perfrigens* in your lunch will give you a food infection?   Nobody knows.   For medical and environmental control of the bacterial pathogens, such information has not been needed.   The goal has been "wipe 'em out."   The widespread occurrence of salmonella in a variety of foods is necessitating serious consideration of bacteriological standards which permit a limited number of salmonella to be present. For the helminths—ascaris and hookworm—a patient prognosis can be made from egg counts per gram of feces.   Rarely can the goal of helminth control by medical and environmental methods be eradication.   The goal is to eliminate worms to a low level of infestation and keep it there.   There have been studies on the ratio of coliform bacteria to typhoid fever bacteria in feces and in sewage just as there are now estimates of enteroviruses in water.   In the study of fecal bacterial travel in the Ohio River from Cincinnati to Louisville, the investigators C. C. Ruchoft, E. B. Phelps, and Wade Hampton Frost interpreted their data on the assumption that the ingestion of one *Salmonella typhosa* would produce typhoid fever.   Their goal was to get at coliform survival numbers and travel time and the required dilution and treatment.   It is doubtful that any of the three distinguished sanitary scientists would not have risked ingesting one *S. typhosa*.   Virologists looking at viral concentrations in water are being asked to relate these to risk of infection.   S. A. Plotkin and M. Katz have offered the contention "that one infective dose of tissue culture is sufficient to infect man if it is placed in contact with susceptible cells" (Ref. 2-3, p. 163).

On Potentiation and Synergism

All the facts and conjectures on the mass of the dose make up a sea of uncertainty. The question, "What if there is potentiation?" produces a whirlpool of doubt. "What if there is synergism?" produces a tidal wave of terror.   These are devastating questions for those trying to arrive at workable values for acceptable exposures or intakes for a specific assaulter.   To potentiate is to make powerful and to intensify. The concurrent presence of a second agent makes a first one more intense in its effect without the second one's having a defined toxic effect in itself.   Synergism is the joint action of agents, usually two, which by their complementary functions produce an effect quite apart from what either can produce singly.   Relatively little is known of these formidable threats to dealing with environmental contaminants and pollutants. The number of identified, recognized instances have been limited.   For human responses to toxic chemicals, concurrent physiological stresses of fatigue, sleeplessness, temperature extremes, and poor feeding are more certain contributors to intensified effects than identified synergistic or potentiating chemicals from the environment.

A MATHEMATICAL EXPRESSION THAT PREDICTS SEVERAL ENVIRONMENTAL PHENOMENA

There is a mathematical equation which is useful for predicting a number of phenomena that add to or subtract from environmental quality.   It is quite familiar in one form or another to chemists, physicists, some biologists, demographers, and all mathematicians and statisticians.   It is also a constant tool of bankers and loan sharks as in one form it is the compound interest rule.   It is a unifying common statement useful in the study of environmental quality issues.   It provides a link among the rates of microorganism growth and death; rates of solubility and precipitation; rates of stabilization of sewage and stream degradation with respect to dissolved oxygen content; rates of radioactive decay; rates of attenuation and transmission of forms of electromagnetic energy such as gamma and x-rays, visible light, and infrared; and rates of heat transfer.   The equation will be used in several places in this book in varying degrees of detail.   To the chemists it is identified as the monomolecular law of mass action and by some as a first-order reaction.   To mathematicians it is a form of $y = e^{ax}$ function in which a "constant" e is raised to a variable power x.

In words, the monomolecular reaction law states that the amount of material disappearing as in radioactive decay, or appearing as in the growth of bacteria, in a unit of time—say an hour, day, or year—is a fixed percentage of the amount present at the beginning of that unit of time and of each thereafter.

The compounding of interest on $1,000 for 50 years at 5 percent interest is helpful to emphasize the effect of the law.   The $1,000 at 5 percent interest compounded annually for 50 years produces $11,467.40.   If not compounded, the interest yield is $50 per year, or $2,500, for the 50 years.   The original investment then has a worth of $1,000 in principle and has $2,500 in interest for a total of $3,500.   Compounding gained $7,967.40.

In the application to human population growth, an increase of 2.5 percent/year produces a doubling in a little less than 30 years. Thus, a country with 100 million people in 1970, increasing at 2.5 percent a year, must organize its existence for 200 million in year 1999. If the population growth were not compounded, but a simple additive of 2.5 million/year, the 30-year increment would be $30 \times (2.5$ million), or 75 million. The compounding produces an added 25 million for which resources and facilities must be organized. This difference appears modest, but in dealing with people, it is translated into housing, schools, roads, fuel, power, health services, food supply, and wastes management.

The arithmetic and calculus development of the equations for first-order, or monomolecular, reactions are given with singular clarity and in step-by-step detail in Ref. 2-4, pp. 85–89 and 126–139. Two useful expressions of these equations are the logarithmic form and the exponential form. For decreasing concentration

$$k = \frac{2.303}{t} \log \frac{c_0}{c}$$

This states that the reaction velocity constant k can be computed if the concentration c_0 is known at time zero, the reaction is allowed to run for time t, and the concentration c is observed at the end of time t.

The exponential form appears more formidable and requires the use of e^x and e^{-x} tables, or slide rules with such scales.

Then

$$c = c_0 e^{kt}$$

is for phenomena in which the concentration is increasing, as in bacterial growth;

$$c = c_0 e^{-kt}$$

is for phenomena in which the concentration is decreasing, as in the use of dissolved oxygen in a stream.

Data following these equations plot on semilogarithmic graph paper as a straight line, and on arithmetic paper as exponential curves.

Some users of this book will do some practice problems, learning or relearning the use of e^x tables. All will encounter the expression with different symbols in place of c, c_0, and k. In place of c, there are n for number of atoms, nuclei, or curies; I for intensity, L for biochemical oxygen demand (BOD) as it expresses load on the stream. In place of k, the radioactive decay constants for each radionuclide are given by the Greek letter λ, lambda. Occasionally the variable power is not time; therefore t is not used. For example, $p = p_0 e^{-kh}$ describes the decrease in atmospheric pressure p with an increase in altitude h. When units change and vary in usage along with symbols, a cool head and hand are needed to come through unscarred arithmetically. Despite the initial complexity and the continued pitfalls of arithmetic mistakes, these expressions are most useful and knit together many environmental phenomena already well-known and likely some that need to be known.

ELECTROMAGNETIC ENERGY AND ITS SPECTRUM

Figure 2-5 in a unifying sweep displays the work of Isaac Newton and Christiaan Huygens on visible light in the late 1600s, of William Herschel on infrared in 1800, of J. W. Ritter on ultraviolet in 1801, of James Clerk Maxwell on the relation of electricity and magnetism set forth in his six differential equations in 1860, of Heinrich Rudolf Hertz on radio waves in 1888, of Willhelm Konrad Röntgen on x-rays in 1895, of Ernest Rutherford on alpha and beta emissions in 1911 to 1914, and then into the last 60 years with the avalanche of theory and application.   That avalanche has put bits and pieces of electromagnetic energy into household use in every corner of the world.   The examples UHF, VHF, M band, 48 meter band, UV, TV, radar, microwave oven, infrared, x-ray, citizen's band, and ac electricity are used and talked of from the towering urban apartments of the sophisticated and the rich to the humble huts of the Guatemalan highlands and Thailand plains, where the transistor radio converts electromagnetic energy to words and music on battery power.

Electromagnetic energy is a package of electricity and magnetism traveling at the speed of light at a discrete frequency and wavelength, and carrying a discrete amount of energy.   These discrete characteristics are defined by:

1   Frequency × wavelength = speed of light.
2   Energy of each package = Planck's constant × frequency.

The range of frequency and hence of wavelength is so great that no single unit of length is satisfactory for practical exchange and daily use in the variety of applications of electromagnetic energy.   Figure 2-5 carries frequency in hertz (Hz), which is identical with cycles per second, and wavelength in centimeters despite the cumbersome exponents.   With these units, *1* and *2* above become:

1   The number of Hz × wavelength in cm = 3×10^{10} cm/s.
2   Energy in erg = 6.62×10^{-27} erg $\cdot$ s × the number of Hz.

This is good, usable physics.   It does not however help many to shape a picture of electromagnetic energy.   Figure 2-6 does that at a slight risk of oversimplification bothersome to physicists and electrical engineers.

In Fig. 2-6 it all starts with electrons, from the local radio station's transmitter, racing up the antenna lead at a speed close to that of light.   They dash along our

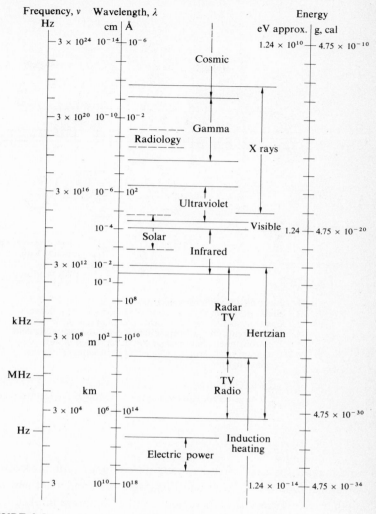

FIGURE 2-5

The electromagnetic spectrum.   [*Source*:   *B. G. Ferris* (1960), *Electromagnetic Radiation, N. Eng. J. Med.*, **275**:1100 (*Nov.* 7, 1966).]

exaggerated antenna.   As they do they generate a magnetic field.   That is the wonder of it all.   Our electrons reach the end of the antenna.   They cannot get off.   They race to the other end.   This action creates an electromagnetic field in the surrounding space. The electromagnetic field is propagated at the speed of light.   Enormous pulsations of the electric and magnetic fields, like a giant football inflating and deflating, build up on our antenna along its long axis.   Suddenly a combination package of electricity

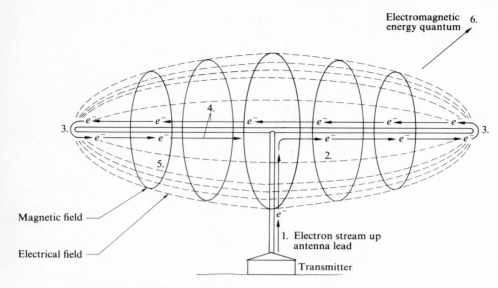

1. Electron stream moves up antenna lead.
2. Electron stream moves to end of antenna. Cannot leave.
3. Electron stream moves to other end of antenna.
4. Electron movement along antenna generates magnetic field.
5. Electromagnetic field propagates at the speed of light.
6. Quantum of electromagnetic energy "broadcasts" at the speed of light.

FIGURE 2-6
The generation of electromagnetic energy along an exaggerated radio broadcasting antenna.

and magnetism tears off at the speed of light to give you the latest information on what breakfast food to eat, what hair dressing to use, and what new misery man has thrust upon man. Planck says there goes another quantum in obedience to my law and my constant. You have not had to wait very long for the advice you asked for by switching on your receiver. It all happens at the speed of light, 3×10^{10} cm/s, 300,000 km/s, or 186,000 mi/s. That is $7\frac{1}{2}$ trips around the world at the equator in 1 s.

The units used to describe electromagnetic energy are a great headache to those who deal with its many varieties from the short-wavelength, high-frequency gamma rays to the long-wavelength, low-frequency microwaves. Those concerned with these energies and their effects on man or other living things have to deal with the entire range. The radioman stays in his bit of the range and talks about "long wave" and "short wave." In the whole spectrum, both are very long, say from 10^6 cm (1,000 m) to 10^2 cm (1 m). The TV man talks about VHF (very high frequency) and UHF (ultra high frequency).   Both are low frequencies in hertz, or cycles per second, in the whole spectrum.   Furthermore, the TV man has been of no help at all by switching from wavelength to frequency in his designation of the pieces of electromagnetic energy he uses.   Appendix 2 puts together the fundamental characteristics of the electromagnetic energy spectrum and the terms used by the day-by-day practitioners.   It provides a pad of sorts for the morass of units and terms and a "bench mark" from which to view the startling scene.   Indeed, the first public message on the telegraph in 1844 from Baltimore to Washington, D.C., 44 mi, was well chosen from the Old Testament, Book of Numbers, "What hath God wrought?"   Even less answerable is, "What is man doing with the electromagnetic energy spectrum?"

The concern of this book is that he does not wreck himself and other living things in the course of using it for better or for worse.   The particular issues on electromagnetic-energy "risks in use" are in chapters on the management of physical energy released in the environment and, as appropriate, in the chapters on water and food.   The electromagnetic energy spectrum unifies the conception of all that.   It is not only unified in nature, it is all part of a whole.   Man fractionated it as he came to know it bit by bit.   Maxwell, a bare 100 years ago, suspected that his electromagnetic equations would also apply to visible light, ultraviolet, and infrared.   X-ray was 35 years away, and gamma 50 years away from identification, so Maxwell had no clues from these exhibitions of electromagnetic energy.   But in less than 100 years from 1860, it would all be common stuff for all of us.   The responsibility of the professional practitioners of the subjects in this book is to see that these energies do not warm up the wrong things in the wrong places at the wrong times.

REFERENCES

2-1   ROUECHÉ, BERTON: "Curiosities of Medicine," Medallion Books, Berkeley Publishing Corporation, New York, 1963.

2-2   SARTWELL, PHILIP E. (ed.): "Maxcy-Rosenau Preventive Medicine and Hygiene," 9th ed., Appleton Century Crofts, New York, 1965.

2-3   BERG, GERALD (ed.): "Transmission of Viruses by the Water Route," Interscience Publishers, John Wiley & Sons, Inc., New York, 1967.

2-4   DANIELS, FARRINGTON: "Mathematical Preparation for Physical Chemistry," McGraw-Hill Book Company, New York, 1928.

3

MAN'S USE OF WATER RESOURCES

THE NEED

A brief exposure to a water shortage at home or a short stay in an area where water is in short supply is a stern reminder of our dependence on water for survival and for the enjoyment of a high standard of life. A United States suburbanite in the face of a water shortage first sacrifices the sparkling appearance of his car, then the lawn and shrubs, then a high level of bodily and domestic cleanliness. His fellow man in water-scarce areas or water-scarce seasons has not reached the point where such sacrifices can be exacted from him. First, he must fit his food growing to his water supply, then water for his animals, then whatever can be spared for bodily and domestic cleanliness. What cannot be spared is shared. A marvel of water conservation and use is the village water hole, "the tank," in central India during the dry season. Maximum beneficial use has a full dimension. The quality requirement is that it feels wet. The quantity requirement is met by whatever is there. These are acceptances of compelling necessities, not a lack of joy for clean and abundant water. The management of the village water hole can be improved with hygienic gains in the process. The management of the water resources of all communities can be improved. The gains in that task in the western countries in the last 100 years were made with strong incentives for waterborne disease control. The incentives and the practices are now being extended throughout the developing world. At the same time, the squeeze of easily accessible sources and of rising demands, sometimes for competing uses, is pushing the development of the political art and of the applied science of water resource management to the position of a specialty in its own right with sophisticated skills for analyzing the maximum beneficial use at minimum cost. Water is a renewable resource. That renewal is accomplished by natural and man-managed processes. Man is at his best when he aids and abets natural processes in such ways as by control of runoff and evaporation through reforestation and cover crops, by storage, by groundwater recharge, and by fitting his use to the yields which can be replenished naturally. The paradox of the world's water resources is that while it is generously abundant in its totality, man has not reached the point of social and technological development either to live where the water is or to bring the water easily to the places where he is.

THE QUANTITIES

Of an approximated 40 million cubic miles of water on and in earth, not more than 0.5 percent is readily accessible for man's use. Of the total, 97 percent is in the oceans and salty seas; $2\frac{1}{4}$ percent is in snow and ice, with some usable on melting. Of the 3 percent of the total rated as fresh, some is frozen and much is in ground strata over 2,500 ft below the surface. Only one-tenth of the total freshwater is estimated to be in groundwater strata less than 2,500 ft below the surface. Of that source, a safe withdrawal, which would not deplete or deteriorate it by saline water intrusion, is placed at 0.5×10^{10} million gal/year. Rain and snowfalls recycle 12×10^{10} million gal/year, but three-fourths of this falls on the saline oceans and seas. Thus, 3×10^{10} million gal/year precipitates on land. This is distributed as rather rapid evaporation and plant transpiration to the atmosphere, percolation to replenish the groundwater, and runoff to streams, lakes, and man-made impoundments. The runoff to man's most accessible sources is about 1×10^{10} Mgal/year. Such global estimates indicate the limit of readily available fresh water, which is about 1.5×10^{10} Mgal/year. That is the sum of runoff and safe groundwater withdrawals.

The necessity of rational management to meet rising usage by more people, more manufacturing, more irrigation, and more recreation becomes more evident when the questions of where it is and where it is needed are joined. Across the world one-third of the land areas is well watered, and two-thirds arid to semiarid. The same fractions can be applied to the United States from east to west excepting the western slopes of the Sierra Nevada mountains and the northwest corner of the country, which records our highest annual average rainfall. On a still smaller geographical scale, but hardly insignificant, California illustrates the urgency of managing the distribution of water between where it is and where it is needed. Irrigation needs of the central valley south of Sacramento and manufacturing and population needs of the Los Angeles basin require managing water distribution to the users from the whole length of the Sierra slopes down the valley, as well as across the southern desert from the Colorado River.

Water uses present startling paradoxes as so much is wholly out of managed decisions. Figure 3-1 requires careful study and the application of two water resources terms. *Beneficial use* of water is its utilization for production, for physiological requirements, for pleasure, and for property protection and survival. This means use, with varying scales of planning and management, for manufacturing and processing, for food production on land and in water, for domestic and public needs, for recreation, and for flood control. Other beneficial uses are for hydro-power production, navigation, and waste transportation. Such uses along with recreational use and commercial fishing in fresh waters do not require the water to be withdrawn from the stream. Thus 22 percent of the total precipitation which reaches streams is used beneficially without being withdrawn. Note that only 7.5 percent of the total precipitation is withdrawn for irrigation, industry, and municipal supply. Adding the last percentages to the 39 percent of natural precipitation which waters farm crops, pastures, forests, and browse vegetation, makes up the 68 percent of annual precipitation that is in beneficial use. The remaining 32 percent passes through the hydrologic cycle without beneficial use as that percentage of precipitation falls on non-economic vegetation. Each beneficial use has some minimum quality requirements. But the term *beneficial use* does not carry any connotation of maintaining that quality during and after that use. On the contrary, in most uses the quality is deteriorated. Since that limits the water's next use, water resource management must deal with quantity and quality.

The second term, *consumptive use* of water, is a utilization from which there is not immediate return to a surface or groundwater source. This is almost wholly the evaporation and evapotranspiration indicated as 70 percent of our annual precipitation in Fig. 3-1. Some water resource people consider this alone to be consumptive use. However, there is a small fraction of the total water used in production and processing which becomes part of the product, as in the cases of soft drinks, beer, and alcoholic liquors along with evaporation in manufacturing and public use. Note that a consumptive use is often beneficial, as indicated by the 39 percent of precipitation which waters the land for our farm crops, pasture, browse vegetation, and forests. The consumed loss of water withdrawn from streams for irrigation, industrial, and municipal uses is 101 million acre · feet, about 2 percent of our total precipitation. As shown in Fig. 3-1, that water evaporates and returns to the atmosphere. It is simply not available for immediate reuse.

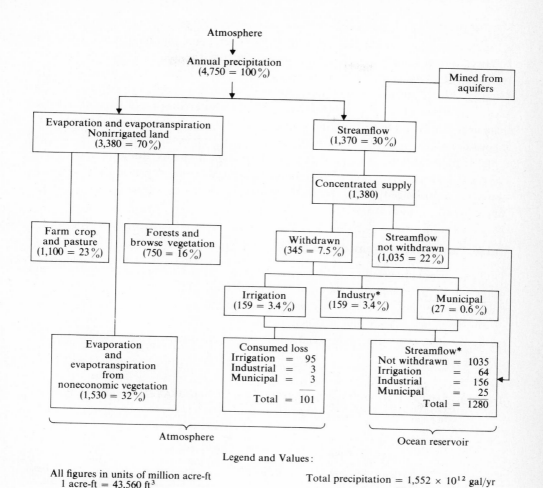

Atmosphere

Annual precipitation
(4,750 = 100%)

Mined from
aquifers

Evaporation and evapotranspiration
Nonirrigated land
(3,380 = 70%)

Streamflow
(1,370 = 30%)

Concentrated supply
(1,380)

Farm crop
and pasture
(1,100 = 23%)

Forests and
browse vegetation
(750 = 16%)

Withdrawn
(345 = 7.5%)

Streamflow
not withdrawn
(1,035 = 22%)

Irrigation
(159 = 3.4%)

Industry*
(159 = 3.4%)

Municipal
(27 = 0.6%)

Evaporation
and
evapotranspiration
from
noneconomic vegetation
(1,530 = 32%)

Consumed loss
Irrigation   =   95
Industrial   =   3
Municipal   =   3
            ‾‾‾
Total = 101

Streamflow*
Not withdrawn = 1035
Irrigation   =   64
Industrial   = 156
Municipal   =   25
                  ‾‾‾‾‾
Total = 1280

Atmosphere

Ocean reservoir

Legend and Values:

All figures in units of million acre-ft
1 acre-ft = 43,560 ft^3
1 acre-ft = 326,700 gal

Total precipitation = 1,552 × 10^{12} gal/yr
or
Total precipitation = 4,200 × 10^9 gpd

* The same water may be reused at points spaced along a single stream.

FIGURE 3-1
The fate of the annual average, 30 in, rainfall on the continental United States. [*Source*: *Abel Wolman, Water Resources, Publ. 1000B, Committee on Natural Resources, National Academy of Sciences—National Research Council, Washington, D.C.*, 1962.]

If the 7.5 percent withdrawal from streamflow and groundwater seems small as a supplement for managed use, the 0.6 percent of total precipitation for municipal use is indeed a tiny fraction, particularly as it does include the usage by many production facilities connected to public systems and the ever hopeful home lawn irrigator.   The fraction is tiny, but the quality and continued abundant supply are paramount, for this is the water of the people who make all other water uses needful.   Other beneficial uses do have more demanding quality requirements in some particular than drinking water has, for example, hardness in textile-processing water.   However, across the range of physical, biological, chemical, and radiological quality, domestic water holds the highest place.   Nor will a community allow itself to be deprived of its quantity needs for a prolonged time.   Table 3-1 shows the trends of estimated water use for major beneficial uses, from 1900 to 1975.

Public Supply Requirements in the United States

The customers connected to public water supplies in the United States are profligate water users.   It is not that they are terribly thirsty.   It is that the convenience of flush toilets and hot water for body washing is available in such a very large percentage of our dwellings.   That makes domestic use high.   About 20 percent of manufacturing-process water and commercial-service water is purchased from public supplies,

Table 3-1   THE TREND OF MAJOR BENEFICIAL USE OF WATER IN THE UNITED STATES, 1900 TO 1975,
In billions of gallons per day

Year	Irrigation	Public water supplies	Domestic	Self-supplied, industrial and misc.	Steam-electric power	Total
1900	20.2	3.0	2.0	10.0	5.0	40.2
1910	39.0	4.7	2.2	14.0	6.5	66.4
1920	55.9	6.0	2.4	18.0	10.0	92.3
1930	60.2	8.0	2.9	21.0	18.4	110.5
1940	71.0	10.1	3.1	29.0	22.2	135.4
1944	80.6	12.0	3.2	56.0	35.9	187.7
1945	83.1	12.0	3.2	48.0	28.8	175.1
1946	86.4	12.0	3.5	39.0	26.9	167.8
1950	100.0	14.1	4.6	46.0	38.4	203.1
1955	119.8	17.0	5.4	60.0	59.8	262.0
1960	135.0	22.0	6.0	71.9	77.6	312.5
1965	148.1	25.0	6.5	87.7	92.2	359.5
1970	159.0	27.8	6.9	103.0	107.8	404.5
1975	169.7	29.8	7.2	115.4	131.0	453.1

SOURCE: Water Uses in the United States, *U.S. Dept. Commerce*, *BSB*-136, January 1956.

with the other 80 percent supplied by the users, particularly the large users. The overall quantities used and their trends have been noted in Table 3-1. Table 3-2 presents public system usage in gallons per capita per day with ranges and averages. Table 3-3 presents more nearly direct personal use at home and work. The 21 gal for toilet flushing will cover four or five uses per day. The 18 gal is a comfortable tubful or a 5 to 6 min shower bath. The surprising figure is that for drinking purposes. It is about 1.5 percent of the total average per capita requirement for all uses supplied by a public system. Yet it dictates our quality standards. The drinking-water allowance includes the wastage at the tap to get a cool flow, the unemptied glass, and the drinking-fountain bypass. Public services include street flushing, park area watering, public wading and swimming pool use, and in some instances public buildings including schools and medical care facilities. The unaccounted-for water use is largely leakage. Unauthorized connections are quite rare. Pipe-joint and valve leakage in distribution systems are inevitable. Cast-iron pipe laid with joints formed on-site will leak at rates of from 100 to 500 gallons per day (gpd) per mile per inch of pipe diameter, with

Table 3-2 PUBLIC WATER-SUPPLY USE IN THE
UNITED STATES

Use	Gallons per capita per day	
	Range	Average
In home	50 to 70	50
Commercial and industrial	10 to 100	65
Public services	5 to 20	10
Unaccounted (leakage)	10 to 40	25
Total	75 to 230	150

Table 3-3 THE DISTRIBUTION OF DOMESTIC WATER
USE IN THE UNITED STATES, BY PURPOSE
AND IN RANKING ORDER

Purpose	Percentage of total	Gallons per capita per day
For toilet flushing	41	21
For hand and body washing	37	18–19
For kitchen use	6	3
For drinking water	5	2.5
For clothes washing	4	2
For housecleaning	3	1.5
For garden watering	3	1.5
For car washing	1	0.5

the high rates during cold-weather contraction.   A leaky ball cock or flush valve on a commode can pass 50 to 60 gpd.   A defective faucet can leak 10 to 15 gpd.   For systems which have all known connections metered an accounting of 85 percent is usual.   It represents total metered use for known system input.   Two factors contributing to the unaccounted-for water are meter inaccuracies and defects, and fire-fighting use.   Estimates of these factors can narrow the unaccounted-for water to 10 percent of the total production.

Water for fire fighting is a dominant requirement in estimating and providing for peak demands.   By United States practice the American Insurance Association sets the requirements for availability of water for fire fighting.   For residential areas, depending on building density, from 500 to 6,000 gallons per minute (gpm) must be provided.   The association defines a standard fire stream as 250 gpm.   Thus the residential requirement provides from 2 to 24 fire streams.   Note that a standard fire stream uses five times as much water in 1 min as a family of five would use for domestic purposes in 24 hours.   Distribution systems with pipe diameters, storage, and pumping capacities meeting American Insurance Association requirements readily meet the daily and hourly maxima for nonemergency water use.

On the average in the United States, the maximum day is 1.5 times the average day, and the maximum hour is 2.5 times the average hour.   The July evening needs of high-value suburban residential use for lawn watering is another factor.   That peak need has exceeded the designed capacities of pumping stations and transmission lines to neighborhood distribution systems in some areas of Long Island and the East Bay region of San Francisco.   Such high uses must be known to the sanitary engineers designing a water supply, as the expected maximum daily demand fixes the capacity both of lines from the raw-water-storage impoundment and of the treatment plant. The effect of lawn watering on residential water use has been studied by F. P. Lina-weaver, J. C. Geyer, and J. B. Wolff.[1]   In a residential area with three dwellings per acre, 0.2 acre of watered lawn, and a value of $25,000 per unit (1967 dollars), lawn sprinkling increases water use from 250 gpd per dwelling to 1,200, nearly a fivefold increase.

The gallons per capita per day (gpcd) required has been increasing steadily in the United States and in other parts of the world where supplies are adequate.   In the 1930s, if reliable local data should not be at hand, a design value of 100 gpcd was in wide use in the United States.   Presently, 150 gpcd is in use.   W. Hardenbergh states an increase of 1.5 gpcd each year from 1945 to 1960 with an expected leveling at 165 gpcd (Ref. 3-1, p. 49).   G. M. Fair gives a lower quantity pegged to the annual rate of population increase.   The numerical increase in gallons per capita per day equals 0.1 of the percentage of increase in population per year (Ref. 3-2, vol. 1, pp.

[1] *JAWWA*, **59**:227 (1967).

5–15).   At a relatively high urban population increase of 4 percent, there would be an increase of 0.4 gpcd each year.   Rising socioeconomic status, the great increase of central air-cooling systems using recirculated water-cooled condensers, and the increased number of public and private swimming pools produce the per capita increases.   Note that recirculating systems on refrigerant condensers and swimming pools greatly reduce water requirements, but these systems have losses by evaporation and splash-out that must be made up daily.   Recirculating water-cooled refrigerant condensers have added from 0.5 to 4.5 gpcd increases annually and from 5 to 35 gpcd increases to the maximum summer rates.   Single-dwelling-unit air coolers do not add to these increases as these use air-cooled condensers.

With 20 percent of industrial water use being met with public supplies, changes in commercial and industrial operations affect the overall demand for public water. Higher quality standards for all products, including hygienic standards for food, have pushed up water usage.   A single large chicken-processing plant in Durham, North Carolina, without recovery or recirculation uses 10 percent of the municipal supply each day.   Data in Table 3-4 for Kansas City, Missouri, on a "maximum summer day" shows where the water goes.

Public Supply Requirements in Developing Countries

While the United States considers the capacities of its urban and suburban water systems to supply air cooling systems and lawn watering, the urban areas of the developing countries of the world have more than 40 percent of their populations without access to piped water.   No piped water on the premises on which people live.   No piped water to a public outlet.   The sources available to that 40 percent are vendors,

Table 3-4   WATER USAGE ON A MAXIMUM SUMMER DAY IN KANSAS CITY, MISSOURI, IN 1954

Use	Gallons per day, millions	Percent
Total	122.8	100
Commercial and industrial	40.5	33
Air-cooling systems	31.4	25
Lawn sprinkling	22.0	18
Household	14.4	12
System losses	14.5	12

SOURCE: American Water Works Association, "Water Quality and Treatment," 3d ed., Fig. 3-4, p. 42, McGraw-Hill Book Company, New York, 1971.

rivers, local impoundments, and dug wells. "Urban Water Supply Conditions and Needs in 75 Developing Countries," by Dietrich and Henderson, states the situation as it was in 1963 (Ref. 3-3). The 41 percent of the urban population without access to piped water in the 75 countries is over 129 million people. Another 26 percent, that is, 83 million people, have the benefit of house connections. Table 3-5 details these data by three regions in percentage and in millions of people. Latin America's relatively favorable position rewards 25 years of Inter-American cooperation, which has produced strong national water-supply activities manned by a corps of capable sanitary engineers. That Latin American effort must keep pace with an annual urban population increase of 3.8 percent a year, which is adding over 75 million people to the cities in the 15 years between 1962 and 1977, and it must reduce the backlog as well. As a region, the Asian countries covered have the lowest percentage with house connections, 18 percent, and the highest, 57 percent, without access to piped water.

The *WHO* study was able to secure data on the supplies of 60 of the 75 countries to assess the quality of the water and of the water service to 245 million people, 77 percent of the total population of the 75 countries. Despite the lack of uniform standards, of strictly drawn criteria, and of detailed observations, the data in Table 3-6 form a statement of quality and adequacy in number and in degree, expressed as "good," "fair," "unsatisfactory," and "grossly unsatisfactory."

In addition to limited observations on sanitary quality measured by the WHO International Drinking Water Standards, information on continuity of service was sought. Those who have lived in renowned cities of the tropical and subtropical

Table 3-5   URBAN WATER SUPPLY, 1962
In 75 developing countries of Latin America, Africa, and Asia, showing extent and type of service

Region	Urban population supplied, 1000s						Urban population not served, 1000s	
	From house connections		From public outlets		Total served			
	No.	%	No.	%	No.	%	No.	%
Africa, subtotal	13,430	34	11,760	30	25,190	64	14,340	36
Latin America, subtotal	61,400	60	27,480	27	88,880	87	13,860	13
Asia, subtotal	32,515	18	44,180	25	76,695	43	101,055	57
The 75 countries: Total	107,345	33	83,420	26	190,765	59	129,255	41

SOURCE: Bernd H. Dietrich and John M. Henderson, *WHO, Public Health Paper* 23, Extract from Table 1, p. 38, 1963.

global belt of the world are painfully familiar with intermittent water services, frequently limited to 4 to 6 h/day. This curtails the quantity available for use depending on individual resourcefulness to fill pots, barrels, and bathtubs during the "on hours" or to have private storage legally or illegally. From the hygienic standpoint, the consequence is the complete negation of all efforts made, up to that point, to provide water free of pathogenic organisms. Once the distribution is stopped, the supply lines are not under pressure. All leakage is then into the system at joints and valves, not out from these openings. Nor is it unusual for individual connectors to pump from the system as long as their pumps draw in more water than air. Thus, the system is under negative pressure, that is, below atmospheric pressure. Contaminants are sucked into the pipes. Even without pumping, negative pressures are created in pipe networks when the supply is cut off and any connected draw is continued or attempted. Dietrich and Henderson state that 74 percent of piped public water supply in India is intermittent and that 100 percent of the services in Burmese cities is so.

For Latin America their observation is, "In this area it is known that the majority of urban consumers must put up with intermittent delivery of one type or another from their distribution systems" (Ref. 3-3, p. 15). Per capita water use in these areas is modest compared to that in the United States. It is rising, and as access becomes easier, the rate of increase accelerates. The use at public taps in Venezuela has been measured as 15 liters per capita per day (lpcd), approximately 4 gpcd. Of course, that water is hand carried to the house. Design values for public taps in use are 40 lpcd, about 10 gpcd, including waste and half that without a waste allowance. Homes with a single tap use about 40 to 60 lpcd, 10 to 15 gpcd. This water is for culinary and hand washing use. Laundry and body bathing are at the river or in

Table 3-6 URBAN WATER SUPPLY CONDITIONS IN 60 DEVELOPING COUNTRIES IN 1962 AS RATED BY WHO REGIONAL OFFICES

Rating	Countries		Urban population in countries covered	
	No.	% of total	No.	% of total
Good	3	5	12,080,000	5
Fair	4	7	15,020,000	6
Unsatisfactory	33	55	121,040,000	49
Grossly unsatisfactory	20	33	97,100,000	40
Total	60	100	245,240,000	100

SOURCE: Bernd H. Dietrich and John M. Henderson, WHO, Public Health Paper 23, Table 3, p. 44, 1963.

community laundering and bathing facilities. A self-closing limited-delivery faucet, 1 liter per valve push, reduces the single tap home use to 30 to 40 lpcd, 8 to 10 gpcd. This self-closing spring-loaded faucet is the Fordilla, designed by Richard Ford and made by the Ford Meter Box Co., Haddonfield, New Jersey. Houses with plumbing facilities of flush toilet, lavatory, sink, and laundry tub rise to 120 lpcd, 32 gpcd, with careful use, and with wasteful use and poor maintenance of valves and fittings, equal to United States domestic use of 180 to 240 lpcd, about 50 to 65 gpcd. Metering and a pay-as-you-go rate for water used curbs waste and is a moderate brake on the rate of increase. In Kingston, Jamaica, metering cut water use by one-half. In Venezuela, estimated use is doubled if the design and management does not include metering. Meters must be accompanied by an acceptable rate structure, a workable method of reading, billing, and collection, and of meter repair and recalibration.

The total cost of improving water services in the 75 developing countries is estimated by Dietrich and Henderson at $6.6 billion, United States 1960 purchasing power, a sizable sum unless compared with money spent on war. Surprisingly, the costs distributed over 15 years would not exceed 0.25 percent of the gross national product (GNP) of the 75 developing countries, Ceylon excepted. Such a financial commitment is within the investment capacity of these countries. The tough task is to develop the political and technical leadership to make water supply improvement. It requires collecting taxes, keeping profits in the country for reinvestment, and choosing unglamourous, nonmonumental public works. Pipes buried in the ground for water and sewers are poor competitors of airport terminals and hospitals as monuments of achievement of a political office.

The demand for public capital to build the infrastructure of communities that are in the crisis of excessively rapid urbanization is severely competitive. In the face of 500 million cases of disabling diseases in the world from unsafe water each year, Dietrich and Henderson offer these examples of a return from capital invested in water supplies (Ref. 3-3, p. 20).

> Information received from a number of WHO Member States provides evidence of the efficacy of safe piped water supplies in combating water-borne disease. For example, Japan, Cuba, Peru, Colombia, Pakistan, Ceylon, Madagascar, Kuwait and India have recently reported that the incidence of such diseases has markedly declined since the improvement of water supply conditions. In Japan, a survey in 30 rural areas revealed that after installation of safe water supplies the number of cases of communicable intestinal diseases was reduced by 71.5 per cent and that of trachoma by 64 per cent, while the death rate for infants and young children fell by 51.7 per cent. Another striking example was reported from Uttar Pradesh, India. There, after waterworks sanitation, the cholera death rate decreased by 74.1 per cent, the typhoid fever death rate by 63.6 per cent, the dysentery death rate by 23.1 per cent and the diarrhoeal diseases death rate by 42.7 per cent.

THE QUALITIES FOR DRINKING AND DOMESTIC USE

A user's assessment of water he is about to drink is sensory. He can observe color, turbidity, odor, taste, and temperature. There are physical characteristics. Taste may give some clue on dissolved substances such as chlorides or zinc, but he is dependent on laboratory analysis and treatment control for the chemical characteristics. Although the objectionable tastes and odors he detects may be due to biological actions, except for some rarely occurring visible biological forms, he is again dependent on others for judging the biological quality of his drinking water with the risk of disease foremost. Without instrumentation, any judgment on radioactivity is dependent on knowledge of the source and its history. The division of water qualities into biological, chemical, physical, and radioactive characteristics fits the types of analytical procedures required and provides a framework for presentation.

Biological Quality

Bacteria, protozoa, helminths, and viruses which can retain their pathogenicity in a pass through water and can be infectious through water use must be controlled. Biological forms which produce tastes and odors are primarily troublesome during raw water storage. In a distribution network occurrences of bacteria which utilize iron or sulfur require attention. Waterworks practice for producing safe water is based most firmly on the epidemiology and biology of waterborne diseases caused by bacteria which leave infected persons or carriers in feces. Table 3-7 summarizes the waterborne diseases transmitted by ingestion, grouped by type of etiological agent and ranked by likelihood of transmission.

The role of water as the route for the agents of acute diarrheas is obscured by the variety of routes for the fecal-oral transfer. Among schoolchildren and adults food is the common transfer medium. Among infants and preschoolers, direct contact, reinfection, their lack of immunity, and their nutritional state are strong influences. A variety of agents, some of low pathogenicity, are at work. These include salmonellae, enteropathogenic coliforms, Coxsackie, ECHO viruses, and ill-defined viruses. All leave the body in excreta, and all have been recovered from contaminated water. Still less certainty of a water-route transmission is attached to the recovery of the viruses of poliomyelitis and pleurodynia in contaminated waters. The epidemiological patterns of these diseases do not fit a waterborne hypothesis.

Table 3-8 lists nonpathogenic organisms of concern in water quality. The concerns are for the resultant changes in taste, odor, and appearance when such organisms are present in excessive numbers. Operational difficulties such as clogging of well screens by slimy growths of iron bacteria, and clogging of sand filters when large "blooms" of algae reach the treatment plant require vigilance for the rise in such

Table 3-7   WATERBORNE DISEASES TRANSMITTED BY INGESTION
Grouped by types of etiological agent and ranked by likelihood of transmission

Disease	Agent	Comment
Bacterial agents		
1 Cholera	*Vibrio cholerae*	Initial wave of epidemic cholera is waterborne. Secondary cases and endemic cases are by contact, food, and flies.
2 Typhoid fever	*Salmonella typhi*	Principal vehicles are water and food. Case distribution of waterborne outbreaks has a defined pattern in time and place.
3 Bacillary dysentery (Shigellosis)	*Shigella dysenteriae* *Shigella flexneri* *Shigella boydii* *Shigella sonnei*	Fecal-oral transmission with water one transmitter. Direct contact, milk, food, and flies are other transmitters. Ample water for cleanliness facilitates prevention.
4 Paratyphoid fever	*Salmonella paratyphi* *Salmonella schottmulleri* *Salmonella hirschfeldi*	Few outbreaks are waterborne. Other fecal-oral short circuits dominate. Ample water facilitates cleanliness.
5 Tularemia	*Pasteurella tularensis*	Overwhelmingly by handling infected animals and arthropod bites. Drinking contaminated raw water infects man.
Protozoan agent		
1 Amebic dysentery (amebiasis)	*Entamoeba histolytica*	Epidemics, which are rare, are mainly waterborne. Endemic cases are by personal contact, food, and possibly flies.
Viral agent		
1 Infectious hepatitis	A filterable virus, not isolated.	Epidemics are due to transmission by water, milk, and food, including oysters and clams
Helminthic agent		
1 Guinea worm disease (dracontiasis)	The roundworm, *Dracunculus medinensis*; gravid female, 1 m long, migrates to skin.	Unknown in North America. Cycle is worm larva through human skin to water to the crustacea, such as cyclops, to man's ingestion of water with cyclops in infective form.

populations and early control of them.   The appearance of any organisms visible to the eye in a glass of water, such as the crustacea, rotifera, and nematodes, is a shaking experience for all parties in United States water service, customers and suppliers alike.

Coliform bacteria are used as the index of the hygienic quality of water for several beneficial uses and for many foods.   The permissible concentrations vary for these uses, which disturbs those who feel comfortable with a firm number.   The presumption

Table 3-8   NONPATHOGENIC BIOLOGICAL FORMS OF CONCERN IN WATER FOR DOMESTIC AND FOOD-PROCESSING USES

Organism	Biological group	Occurrence	Reason for concern	Comment
Actinomycetes	Moldlike bacteria	In raw water impoundments; in distribution system.	Cause undesirable tastes and odors.	Localized problem; spores pass filters.
Algae	Phytoplankton	In raw water impoundments.	Cause undesirable tastes and odors; reduce filter runs.	Seasonal variations and "blooms."
Coliform	Bacteria	In surface waters and those receiving feces.	A measure of fecal contamination.	The index for the hygienic quality of water.
Cladocera, copepoda, isopoda	Crustacea	Predominantly in zone of recovery of polluted streams.	Reduce filter runs; occasionally get to users' taps.	Copepod cyclops transmits guinea worm larva, see Table 3-7.
Fecal streptococci	Bacteria	In waters receiving human and animal feces.	An indication of fecal contamination.	Studied as an alternate to coliform index.
Iron bacteria	Bacteria	In ground and surface water containing iron.	Produce slimy, often red, growths; clog well screens.	Levels of 0.1–0.2 mg per liter of iron are sufficient for growth.
Rotifera	Zooplankton	In zone of recovery in polluted streams; in uncovered, finished water reservoirs.	No detrimental effects reported.	May penetrate filters; some forms macroscopic.
Free living worms	Nematodes	About 7 species observed in treated, finished waters, including Diplogaster, Nais, Momhystera, and Seinura.	User rejection on sight; protect pathogenic bacteria and viruses within; odor producers.	Observed to pass slow sand filter, but not rapid type; resistant to usual chlorine doses and residuals.

is constant.   Coliform organisms are present in feces in large numbers, as many as a billion per gram.   Pathogens leave the human body in excreta.   Therefore, coliforms are presumptive evidence of the presence of pathogens in water or food. The variation in the permissible number for a particular use is dependent in part on the likelihood of pathogens surviving in company with the coliforms, as in the case of milk pasteurization, and on the expediency of control measures which only in rare instances can provide absolute protection.   The bacteriological pedigree of coliforms is straightforward.   "The coliform group comprises all aerobic and facultative anaerobic, gram-negative, non-spore-forming, rod-shaped bacteria that ferment lactose with gas formation within 48 hours at 35°C."[1]   This definition is equivalent to that used in British practice to specify the *B. coli* and in earlier United States practice for the coli-aerogenes group.   The two principal species are the *E. coli*, which are ubiquitous in all animal intestinal flora and occasionally elsewhere, and *Aerobacter aerogenes*, which are common in soil and on vegetation and usually not of fecal origin. The resultant nonspecificity of fecal origin requires knowledge of the circumstances of occurrence, of the sampling procedure used, and of the intended use of the water or food.   Professional judgment is required.   In exchange, the nonspecificity provides a margin of safety and ease of testing which a direct test for pathogens by present methods could not give.   The water would be in the distribution system, at the tap, and in use for 24 to 48 hours before the pathogen test result could be known.

The U.S. Public Health Service Drinking Water Standard of 1962 (Ref. 3-4) sets down a series of specifications to arrive at a permissible coliform density in water distribution to the public.   A minimum number of distribution system samples per month is required.   This is about 1 per 1,000 people served up to a 100,000 population, with a sharp drop in the number of samples for large cities.   For example, 325 samples per month meet the requirement for a population of 1,000,000.   There are permissible percentages of sample portions which may show gas, with provisos for the frequency with which these appear in the monthly sample series.   There are equivalent permissible occurrences of coliform recoveries when the membrane-filter technique is used.   The purpose is to establish protection sufficiently effective to limit the coliform density to about 1/100 ml.   Following probability tables of the distribution of positive and negative gas fermentation tubes, a value for the most probable number (MPN) of coliforms per 100 milliliters of water is established.   A pattern of positive and negative gas-producing sample portions in the sample series specified by the standards conforms to an MPN of about 1/100 ml.   In its origin this coliform density was derived from estimates of the occurrence of waterborne disease in the United States and of the ratios of enteric pathogens to coliforms in water.   With only

---

[1] Standard Methods for the Examination of Water and Wastewater, 13th ed., p. 662, American Public Health Association, New York, 1971.

one coliform per 100 ml in the circumstances assumed, the probability of a pathogen accompanying it is remote.   In view of this origin, H. Thomas has suggested that a higher coliform density could be accepted without a loss of safety as the incidence of typhoid fever and the number of carriers are now fewer in the United States.[1]   On the other hand, the allowable 1/100 ml may be too many in countries and regions where the incidence of enteric diseases is very high and where human excreta readily reaches the water supply.   Whatever the merits of the case, the trend of United States practice is to set a quality goal of no coliform organisms in distribution system water.   "No coliform" may be the impossible dream of the proponents of the highest quality.

Chemical Quality

The solvent property of water results in many forms of the elements being present in the dissolved state in water.   Abel Wolman has said that water is $H_2O + X$ and that the X has occupied and preoccupied waterworks people for years.   It will continue to occupy them plus toxicologists, physiologists, occasionally nutritionists, and from time to time health fadists and "crackpots."   Toxicity, reactions in normal use that are objectionable such as curdy precipitates and persistent foam, unexpected physiological responses of taste or laxative effect, appearance changes, and uncertainties of the effects of even minute traces of synthetic compounds are the reasons for concern. In the light of the number of substances which can be in water, those for which there is specific information are few.   Only nine substances are on the list of the U.S. Public Health Service Drinking Water Standards with a concentration value which is the basis for rejecting the supply.   Eight of these make up Table 3-9, along with abbreviated statements of the reasons for their inclusion and comments on the evidence of toxic effects.   In the Drinking Water Standards, the section on chemical characteristics has another grouping of desirable maximum concentrations for 11 additional items. Table 3-10 presents this group, also with an abbreviated statement of reasons for each inclusion.   These substances "should not be present in a water supply in excess of the listed concentrations where, in the judgment of the Reporting Agency and Certifying Authority, other more suitable supplies are or can be made available" (Ref. 3-4, p. 7).   It is desirable to have a supply with these characteristics below the limits, but not mandatory.

Arsenic and cyanide appear in both the basis for rejection group, with values of 0.05 and 0.2 mg/l, respectively, and on the desirable maxima list, with lower values of 0.01 mg/l for each.   The differences reflect uncertainties of toxicological judgments on margins of safety and the lack of evidence of injury to those using supplies with concentrations above the desirable maxima for arsenic and cyanide.   Issues of consensus

[1] *JAWWA*, **41**:874 (1949).

Table 3-9 TOXIC SUBSTANCES WHICH ARE THE BASIS FOR REJECTION OF SUPPLY UNDER U.S. PUBLIC HEALTH SERVICE DRINKING WATER STANDARDS, 1962

Element	Concentration above which supply should be rejected, mg/l	Reason for inclusion	Comment
Arsenic	0.05	Recognized poison; chronic effects, carcinogenic in some contacts, food intake contributory.	Skin cancer high in areas of England with 12 mg/l in drinking water; As^{+++} and As^{+++++} not essential or beneficial.
Barium	1.0	Recognized toxic effects on heart, blood vessels, and nerves from accidental, experimental, and therapeutic ingestions.	Water standard derived from occupational-exposure inhalation limit. Not essential or beneficial.
Cadmium	0.01	Acute poisoning in man via foods, increased concn. in kidney and liver of rats on water with 0.1–10 mg/l.	Individuals on water with average of 0.047 mg/l had no symptoms. Not essential or beneficial.
Chromium as hexavalent ion	0.05	Carcinogenic on inhalation; cumulative in rat tissue at level of 5 mg/l in drinking water; no toxic responses in rats for 1 yr at concn. of 0.45–25 mg/l.	No observed effect on single exam. on family of 4 in 3 yr on water up to 1 mg/l. Not essential or beneficial.
Cyanide	0.2	50–60 mg fatal in single dose; 3–5 mg/day non-injurious; 10-mg single dose not injurious.	Lethal to trout at 0.2 mg/l in 2 days; toxic limit for bluegills and sunfish close to 0.2 mg/l; chlorination converts cyanide to cyanogen chloride, which has $\frac{1}{20}$ acute oral toxicity of cyanide.
Lead	0.05	Recognized poison with daily intakes with food, water, air, and inhaled tobacco smoke. Balance maintained at total intakes of about 0.3–0.4 mg/day.	Intakes of 8–10 mg/l in water for several weeks are in the harmful range; poisoning reported from water varying from 0.04 to 1 or more mg/l; concn. as low as 0.1 mg/l is injurious to fish.
Selenium	0.01	Recognized occupational poison and cause of livestock poisoning where Se exceeds 3–4 mg/kg of food intake; high in soils and crops in some localities in north central U.S.	Definite symptoms of poisoning via water have not been identified; trace amounts believed essential for nutrition; mild poisoning in man in high-Se areas observed.

Table 3-9—*Continued*

Element	Concentration above which supply should be rejected, mg/l	Reason for inclusion	Comment
Silver	0.05	To limit additions of silver for disinfection; silver retention causes argyria, the blue-grey discoloration of skin, eyes, and mucous membranes.	Man retention data are based on therapeutic use of silver compounds; drinking water limit calculated from 1 g total body burden which produces argyria.

Note: Fluoride limits are discussed in the text.

and expedience weigh heavily in agreements on hygienic and esthetic standards. Nitrate content affects a particular population in a special water use.   There is clear epidemiological evidence that infants under 1 year who are on diets in which high-nitrate water is used to reconstitute their milk have developed methemoglobinemia. With the exception of a case in Colorado, in 1963, the reported cases have been on private-well sources.   In the Colorado exception, a baby of a family which had just moved to the town was hospitalized with methemoglobinemia.   In the previous 2 years, samples from the municipal wells showed concentrations of 35 to 40 milligrams of nitrates per liter, which gradually rose to the 60s.   A sample of the baby's formula water contained 63 mg/l before boiling and 73 mg/l after boiling.   It is prudent to set a desirable maximum for public supplies, but not so low as to put the supply in doubt without more evidence that the risk is general and higher than present evidence indicates.

Alkyl benzene sulfonate (ABS) and carbon chloroform extract (CCE) are drinking water quality characteristics which appeared in the Standards for the first time in 1962.   Both result from increasing use of synthetic compounds, the persistence of waste residues in receiving waters, and the shortening span in time and distance between water use and reuse.   Alkyl benzene sulfonate is quite specific in its origin and its undesirable characteristic.   Until 1965 it was the wetting agent component of synthetic detergents in virtually universal household and commercial use in the United States and many parts of the world.   As it is only slightly changed or removed by natural and man-made wastewater and drinking water purification processes, enough ABS was persisting in our recycled water to produce foaming at the tap in repeated instances.   There has been no evidence of toxicity or of adverse physiological effects. The risk of continued buildup and consequent limitations on water reuse is real.   Its interference with wastewater treatment processes in addition to causing massive

Table 3-10   CHEMICALS FOR WHICH U.S. PUBLIC HEALTH SERVICE DRINKING
WATER STANDARDS GIVE DESIRABLE MAXIMUM CONCENTRATIONS
These are not a basis for rejection if more suitable supplies are not available

Substance	Concentration, mg/l	Reason for inclusion
Alkyl benzene sulfonate	0.5	A nonbiodegradable component of synthetic detergents which persists through ground percolation and sewage- and water-treatment processes; foaming usual at 1 mg/l.
Arsenic	0.01	A desirable limit; see Table 3-9 for rejection limit, fivefold this amount.
Chloride	250	Proximate to salty-taste threshold; sudden increases result from sewage.
Copper	1	Essential and beneficial for metabolism; taste threshold varies from 1 to 5 mg/l; limit prevents unpleasant taste.
Carbon chloroform extract	0.2	CCE concentrations include part of the total organics in water, taste producers, toxicants, carcinogens, and wastes; water at 0.2 limit is already of poor quality.
Cyanide	0.01	A desirable limit; see Table 3-9 for rejection limit, 20 times this amount.
Iron	0.3	Essential and beneficial for metabolism, but water cannot meet the 7–35 mg daily requirement; proximate taste threshold, 2 mg/l; stains fixtures and white goods at 1 mg/l; off flavors and colors in beverages, colloidal color in some water.
Manganese	0.05	Staining of white goods by MnO_2 deposits, off flavors in beverages; limit close to the attainable removal from most waters; probably an essential nutrient with 10 mg daily intake in food; toxic on inhalation.
Nitrate	45	Private well waters with nitrates of 67–1,100 mg/l have produced methemoglobinemia in infants on milk formulated with such waters; no cases on public water service in U.S. Warn for infant formulas when nitrates exceed 45 mg/l.
Phenols	0.001	Reaction products of phenolic compounds with chlorine cause objectionable tastes and odors.
Sulfate	250	Laxative effect at 600–1,000 mg/l when magnesium and sodium are the cations.
Total dissolved solids	500	Taste and laxative effect the restraint; excess dissolved minerals in water result in poor brews of coffee.
Zinc	5	Essential and beneficial in metabolism with daily intake of 10–15 mg; emetic action at 675–2,280 mg/l; with zinc salts, milky at 30 mg/l and metallic taste at 40 mg/l. Limit is below taste threshold.

Note: Fluoride limits are discussed in the text.

volumes of foam in aeration units, has been suspected.   The soap and detergent industry resolved the ABS problem and provided considerable relief by developing and substituting linear alkylate sulfonates (LAS) in detergent formulations in 1965.   The LAS formula degrades quite satisfactorily in stabilization and purification processes, but not completely.

Carbon chloroform extract is quite the opposite.   It is the residue recovered from a large sample volume filtered through activated carbon and extracted by a chloroform distillation.   The extracted substances are not specific and their origins are multiple and widespread, but CCE gives an indication of the traces of the hydrocarbons, organic pesticides, and up to 70 percent of the phenols in the water.   Sugars, polysaccharides, proteins, and tannins are not extracted by chloroform.   The method does provide a crude index of organic residues which include compounds with toxic properties and with unpleasant tastes and odors.[1]   Although without specific identity, CCE concentrations reflect pollution loads.   The raw water of the Ohio River has ranged from 0.1 to 0.36 mg/l.   At Nitro, West Virginia, in an industrial chemical manufacturing area, the Kanawha River water has varied from 0.17 to 3.05 mg/l. The Columbia River has had only 0.024 milligram of CCE per liter.

The CCE concentration has been compared with the coliform density as a measure of the likelihood of the presence of injurious agents.   The index agents can be determined relatively rapidly and economically and provide a measurement for the surveillance of undesirable qualities for short-term and long-term changes.   Techniques to monitor trace organics are improving.   An alcohol extract of adsorbed residues on carbon filters recovers organics not dissolved in chloroform.   The American Water Works Association recommends a carbon alcohol extract (CAE) to supplement the CCE and notes that the CAE concentration will commonly be 2.5 times the CCE concentration.[2]

The values given in Table 3-10 for desirable maxima for chlorides, sulfates, and total dissolved solids are the thresholds for unfavorable taste response and laxative effects, particularly for consumers unaccustomed to the water.   Drinking Water Standards, 1962, summarizes a study by E. W. Moore with these words: "Laxative effects were experienced by the most sensitive persons, not accustomed to the water, when magnesium was about 200 mg/l and by the average person when magnesium was 500 to 1,000 mg/l.   When sulfates plus magnesium exceed 1,000 mg/l or dissolved solids exceed 2,000 mg/l, a majority [of persons questioned] indicated a laxative effect." The laxative dose of Epsom salt is 2 g.   Two liters of water with 390 milligrams of sulfates from Epsom salt per liter provides this dose.

More than 100 public water supplies in the United States distribute water with

[1] *JAWWA*, **52**:689 (1960).
[2] *JAWWA*, **60**:1317 (1968).

over 2,000 milligrams of total dissolved solids per liter.   Frequently these waters are high in calcium and magnesium, which produces hardness.   Ordinary soaps produce curdy precipitates and scums with the calcium and magnesium ions.   Incrustants of calcium sulfate and carbonate, and of magnesium hydroxide, depending on anionic concentrations, appear in hot-water lines, heaters, and cooking ware.   Those on high-dissolved-solids water take three courses of action.   They accept it with dissatisfaction. They install ion exchangers in their homes to reduce the solids.   They purchase bottled water for beverage and some cooking use.   In five California communities with dissolved solids ranging from 500 to 1,750 mg/l, 40 percent of the families were reported to be purchasing bottled water and 50 percent were dissatisfied with the public supply. Drinking Water Standards makes no specific statement on calcium or hardness and limits its statement on the related matters of alkalinity and corrosiveness to, "It should not be excessively corrosive to the water supply system."   The policy statement of the American Water Works Association on Quality Goals for Potable Water[1] covers corrosion and scaling factors along with recommended lower concentrations for many characteristics to assure a high-quality water.

Fluoride is the unique substance for which there are upper and lower concentrations in drinking water with identified injurious effects and beneficial effects for man. Over 40 years of epidemiological observations in communities on naturally high fluoride water and with total populations of 4 million people established that mottled tooth enamel, tooth discoloration, and more advanced signs of dental fluorosis occurred among users of water with fluoride ranging from 3 to 8 mg/l and above, but that these teeth showed decay less than expected.   Furthermore, in areas where the fluoride was about 1 mg/l, the decay rate was low and all signs of dental fluorosis were absent. The hypothesis that in drinking water there was an optimum concentration of fluoride which reduces dental caries by 60 to 65 percent of that in communities with little or no fluoride in the water was validated by a long series of controlled studies.   The results provided the basis for the fluoridation of public water supplies.   Figure 3-2 shows the extent of utilization of this practical and economical measure of preventive dentistry in the United States and Canada.

It is known that years of use of water containing fluoride of 8 to 20 mg/l will cause bone changes in man, although no such cases have been found in the United States.   Total daily intakes of 20 mg or more for 20 years or more will produce crippling fluorosis.   A single dose of 2,250 to 4,500 mg of fluoride is lethal to man.   This requires the intake of 5 to 10 g of sodium fluoride.   At the dental prophylactic concentration of 1 mg/l, over 1,300 gal would have to be ingested to reach a 5-g intake.

The Drinking Water Standards, 1962, states a range of recommended control limits for fluoride concentrations, grouped as "lower," "optimum," and "upper"

[1] *JAWWA*, **60**:1317 (1968).

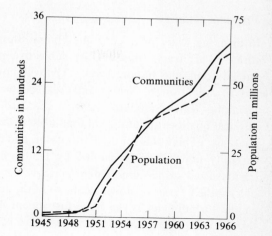

FIGURE 3-2
Communities and populations served
with fluoridated water, 1945 to 1966.
[*Source*: *JAWWA*, **60**:1199 (1968).]

with a variation in each fitted to the annual-average maximum daily air temperature
based on a minimum 5-year record.   The presence of fluoride in average concentrations greater than two times the optimum values is grounds for rejecting the supply.
Table 3-11 presents the recommended values.   To supplies below these levels, fluoride
should be added.   To supplies above these levels, fluoride should be removed.

Table 3-11   ALLOWABLE AND RECOMMENDED
CONCENTRATIONS OF FLUORIDE IN
DRINKING WATER

Annual average of maximum daily air temperatures*		Recommended control limits in fluoride concentrations, mg/l		
°C	°F	Lower	Optimum	Upper
10.0–11.9	50.0–53.7	0.9	1.2	1.7
12.0–14.5	53.8–58.3	0.8	1.1	1.5
14.6–17.5	58.4–63.8	0.8	1.0	1.3
17.6–22.0	63.9–70.6	0.7	0.9	1.2
22.1–26.2	70.7–79.2	0.7	0.8	1.0
26.3–32.5	79.3–90.5	0.6	0.7	0.8

* Based on temperature data obtained for a minimum of 5 years.
SOURCE: Public Health Service Drinking Water Standards, *U.S.
Public Health Serv., Publ.* 956, 1962, p. 8.

Physical Quality

In drinking water practice in the United States the physical characteristics are measured in arbitrary units and by subjective responses. These have been accepted, agreed upon, and standardized. The techniques are stated in Standard Methods for the Examination of Water and Wastewater.[1] All quality characteristics given in Drinking Water Standards refer to standard methods for their measurement. The physical qualities are unique in that arbitrary units are used in quality standards and in analysis. This holds for turbidity, color, and odor. Turbidity is expressed in Jackson turbidity units (Jtu), developed by D. D. Jackson in 1900 at M.I.T. He used a standardized suspension of diatomaceous earth and observed the point of extinction of a candle by peering down a column of the suspension in a dark room. The Jackson candle turbidimeter is the basic instrument for measuring standard suspensions, although it is superseded in routine analysis by a variety of electrical photometric turbidimeters. Color is standardized by a chloroplatinate solution with the disadvantage of a color-tint limitation. Odor is measured by serial dilutions with the observer sniffing from the most dilute to the first detectable level. The dilution series is indexed by threshold odor numbers. Normal butyl alcohol is used as the material to establish the series. Drinking Water Standards states no specific limit for taste. Taste is covered by the sentence, "Drinking water should contain no impurity which would cause offense to the sense of sight, taste, or smell." Taste and odor responses are mixed, subjective, and difficult to describe qualitatively and quantitatively.

Other beneficial uses of water are limited by the physical characteristics enumerated. With the exceptions of bottled beverage preparation and bathing, there are few instances of higher requirements than those for drinking water. Temperature, which has not entered in drinking standards, is an additional physical characteristic which is important for other beneficial uses. As a fundamental ecological determinant and as the governing factor in the maximum of dissolved oxygen, the primary beneficial uses influenced by temperature changes are those concerned with aquatic plant and animal culture and growth. Where limited quantities of water or manufacturing processes are involved, the user can be left with the burden of tempering the water to his requirements.

Radioactivity

There are five issues concerning radioactivity in man's intake of air, food, and water, which must be recognized in order to understand the difficulties of establishing standards. These are not wholly unique to radioactivity, but have demanded recognition to arrive at a workable management of man-made ionizing radiation emitters.

[1] 13th ed., American Public Health Association, New York, 1971.

1 All exposures to, and intakes of, radioactive sources are injurious. Therefore, every use must be necessary and beneficial, and accomplished with a minimum of exposure and release to, the free environment.

2 The chemical behavior of a radioactive element is the same as that of a nonradioactive isotope of the same element. That is, ^{32}P, a radioisotope of phosphorus, follows the same chemical pathways as normal phosphorus. Similarly, a radioisotope such as ^{90}Sr, radioactive strontium, behaves substantially like other members of the same chemical group, notably calcium. This makes the chemical behavior of radioisotopes predictable and provides valuable leads in studying their transfer in the environment.

3 Radioisotopes are measurable in extremely low quantities as their emissions of alpha, beta, or gamma produce ionizing events which can be detected by very sensitive devices and the initial signals electronically amplified, identified, and characterized. The sensitivity of measurement makes it possible to deal with concentrations of radium, for example, in picocuries per liter; 1 g of radium has a radioactivity of 1 Ci. The prefix "pico" denotes 10^{-12} of a unit. Therefore, 1 pCi/l is the equivalent of the radioactivity of 1×10^{-12} g of radium in a liter, say, of water.

4 The totality of an individual's or a population's exposure to, and intake of, radioactivity must be taken into account to determine a maximum risk that can be accepted from a particular source. Therefore, limits set for water are in the light of the necessity of accepting, in the main, larger intakes with food and a lesser degree in air. In turn, the sum of intakes must be viewed in the light of exposure to x-rays in medical and dental procedures and to gamma rays from natural background and environmental contamination, however small the latter may be.

5 All uses of radioactive materials result in some small traces being released to the free environment. This occurs in experimental and clinical use of radioisotopes, in nuclear reactor operations and the associated technology of fuel-rod manufacture and reprocessing of spent rods, in weapons testing, in tests of nuclear explosives for earth moving, in the handling of radioactive wastes of many varieties ranging from the disposal of a tissue wipe used to clear the tip of a pipette containing a radioactive solution to the discard of radioactive luminous dials from the instruments of an obsolete army tank.

In 1962 the Public Health Service Drinking Water Standards included a statement on radioactivity for the first time. Three salient items are selected, which are useful in themselves and which would signal the need for other and more specific identification in case of increases above the designated limits. These are for ^{226}Ra, a limit of 3 pCi/l; for ^{90}Sr, 10 pCi/l; and for gross beta activity, in the virtual absence

of ^{90}Sr and alpha-emitting radionuclides, a maximum of 1,000 pCi/l.   Both ^{226}Ra and
^{90}Sr are bone seekers, which in normal physiological processes deposit in the bone of
man and animals.   Radioisotope ^{226}Ra has a half-life of 1,622 years; ^{90}Sr has one of
28 years.   The half-life is the length of time required for any amount of radioactivity
to decay to one-half of the initial quantity, the unit of quantity being the curie.   The
radioisotope ^{226}Ra occurs naturally in some ground waters and in any surface water
receiving radium wastes.   The principal source of ^{90}Sr is fallout from nuclear weapons
testing, and a lesser contribution is from the low-level wastes from major nuclear energy
installations.   Table 3-12 indicates the conservative levels of the Drinking Water
Standards, as these are applicable to all people.   The recommendations of the National
Committee on Radiation Protection (NCRP), a voluntary professional group, are for
168-hour continuous exposure for occupational activities and for the persons living in
the neighborhood of the controlled areas of atomic energy plants.   The NCRP limits
are designated MPC$_w$ for Maximum Permissible Concentration in water.   The data
on tap-water concentrations of ^{226}Ra are averages from 39 cities in the United States
(Ref. 3-5, p. 152).   One city has been omitted from the radium data as the radium
content is exceptionally high.   It is Joliet, Illinois, which has recorded 6.5 pCi/l in its
deep wells and 5.8 in its tap water.   The sources of data on ^{90}Sr in 1969 and on gross
beta activity in 1968 are noted in Table 3-12.   A study of wells for radium in Maine
showed 66 pCi/l in 33 drilled wells and 73 pCi/l in 19 dug wells.   The waters of radioactive springs of the "health" resorts of the world with alleged curative powers have
shown from 100,000 to 700,000 pCi/l.   Drinking Water Standards recommends a
frequency of analysis for radioactivity as it does for other quality characteristics.   The

Table 3-12   LIMITS OF RADIOACTIVITY IN DRINKING WATER FOR THREE
POPULATION GROUPS AND CONCENTRATIONS REPORTED IN TAP
WATERS OF UNITED STATES CITIES

Radioactive characteristic	Drinking Water Standard limit, pCi/l	MPC$_w$ of NCRP for 168 h occupational exposure, pCi/l	Value for populations adjacent to an atomic energy plant, pCi/l	Tap-water concentration among U.S. cities, pCi/l
^{90}Sr	10	1,000	100	0.58–0.90†
^{226}Ra	3	400	40	0.0–0.17‡
Gross beta activity	1,000	(6,000)*	(600)*	0 to 93§

* The provisional MPC for unidentified radionuclides if ^{90}Sr, ^{210}Pb, ^{226}Ra, and ^{228}Ra are not present.
† Minimum and maximum of monthly 100-liter samples of N.Y.C. tap water in 1969, *Radiol. Health Rep.*,
11:346 (1970).
‡ Ref. 3-5 (p. 152).
§ Minimum and maximum of monthly samples of California State Health Department on 42 water supplies
and sources in 1968, *Radiol. Health Rep.*, **11**:400 (1970).

analysis for ^{226}Ra is a 7-step procedure requiring 16 days for completion.   That for ^{90}Sr is a 10-step procedure requiring 7 days for completion.   These analyses and the instrumentation required are beyond the capability of all but a few large public water supply laboratories.   These must be provided by state health department laboratories and agencies with a similar scope of service coverage.

Drinking Water Standards allows for departures from the stated limits of radioactivity where there is sufficient added detailed analytical information.   A gross beta activity in excess of 1,000 pCi/l shall be grounds for rejection of a water supply except when more complete analyses for other radionuclides show that the average daily intakes of a population conform to the radiation protection guides of the Federal Radiation Council of the United States.   Similarly, waters with more ^{226}Ra than 3 pCi/l and more ^{90}Sr than 10 pCi/l may be approved if the surveillance of total intakes from all sources, food, air, and other beverages, indicates that the intakes are within the limits recommended by the Federal Radiation Council for control action. The radiation protection guides of the Federal Radiation Council are interpreted in the chapter on ionizing radiation.

THE SOURCES AND THEIR USE

The Factors Determining Selection among Sources

There are only five prime sources of water for man's use.

1 Captured and stored rainfall in cisterns and water jars
2 Groundwater flowing from springs and artesian wells, or tapped by man-made wells
3 Surface waters of lakes and streams with or without dams to impound storage
4 Desalinized seawater or brackish groundwater
5 Reclaimed wastewater

The assets and advantages, the deficits and limitations of each are revealed in their actual use and are the determinants where costs and needs demand a rational analysis for the choice.

Captured Rain

Rainfall capture and storage produces water of high quality and variable quantity in short or long temporal cycles.   The impurities in the rain are confined to those from atmospheric washout either as suspended particulates, including radioactive ones, or as soluble gases and vapors.   The impurities in the captured rain include those washed from the capture surface, usually roofs and only occasionally a natural or artificial pad. The biological and toxic chemical contaminants are few and in very low concentrations. Dissolved minerals are so low as to cause new users to taste cistern water as "flat." Quality deficiencies can be offset by wasting the first rainfall as flushing water, by providing particulate filters between the collecting surface and storage, and by disinfection. A simple pass over a limestone bed will mineralize rain water and therefore modify the flat taste. Hard necessities have mandated rainfall dependence upon a few organized communities such as the British colony at Gibralter, localities along the Florida Keys and on Carribean islands. Rainfall collection and containment by individual households is rather frequent in Southeast Asia, in resort areas where fresh groundwater is difficult to develop, and in situations where surface waters are objectionably turbid or colored and where the upper groundwater strata are brackish. In all these circumstances, rain water is rarely used lavishly, as the storage capacity to carry from one rain to the next, particularly in a dry season, becomes very sizable. The rainfall data required to predict storage are infrequently available. In Southeast Asia the rain collection is part of a dual system of water use. It provides immediate culinary and drinking water. Bathing and laundering are done at the nearest stream or pond. Carrying water from that point for culinary and drinking needs is postponed as long as the stored rain lasts through the dry spells.

Groundwater

Groundwater is a source of splendid choice which goes to the level of magnificent when it is a spring with gravity flow to the point of need or when it is an artesian flowing well with sufficient pressure to pipe the water to the user without pumping. The Spanish colonizers of Central and South American highlands located many of their towns in response to springs which allowed gravity flow to central fountains. Many of the springs continue in use to this day and provide a starting point for piped community water service throughout the town. Springs are usually formed by surface infiltration to shallow pervious soil strata. The water in that strata then emerges at a rocky or hardpan ledge. The yields are sufficient only for small communities of a few hundred people where per capita use is small. Rarer yet are artesian flowing wells of substantial yields. Their development and use is likely to exceed the original flow so that pumping is soon required.

The virtues of groundwater are the high biological and physical qualities. The slow percolation and horizontal travel at only a few feet a day through the ground is a superb filtration removing all pathogenic forms, including viruses, and removing the causes of color, turbidity, and with a few exceptions, taste and odor. The exceptions are sulfide and methane gas content dissolved in contact with anaerobically decomposing organic matter which may be deep and ancient. The quality limitations result

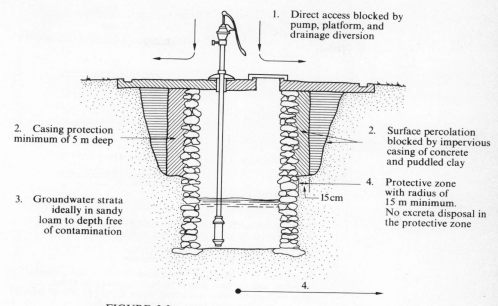

1. Direct access blocked by pump, platform, and drainage diversion

2. Casing protection minimum of 5 m deep

3. Groundwater strata ideally in sandy loam to depth free of contamination

2. Surface percolation blocked by impervious casing of concrete and puddled clay

15cm

4. Protective zone with radius of 15 m minimum. No excreta disposal in the protective zone

4.

FIGURE 3-3
The elements of protection of groundwater sources on a reconstructed dug well.
[*Source*: *WHO drawing* 8274 *modified to show contaminant blocking, Ref.* 3-8 (*p.* 109).]

from the dissolved carbon dioxide that is carried by the water through the ground as carbonic acid and acts on the soil and rock. This process of mineralizing the water brings cations of Ca, Mg, Mn, and Fe and anions such as SO_4, CO_3, HCO_3, and Cl in solution. All groundwater carries these ions. Measure for measure, the deeper the strata from which the water is drawn, the higher the concentrations. Removal to desired or recommended levels can be achieved by chemical precipitation, or by ion exchange. Sequestering by complex ion formation does not remove these objectionable cations, but does keep them from reacting to form encrustants, curds, and color.

Another attribute of a groundwater source is the ease and economy of protecting the withdrawal so that the high bacteriological and physical quality are safeguarded. Figure 3-3 shows the elemental character of well protection which can be applied to all sizes and types of wells. With a few modifications protection can be similarly applied to springs. A pump, whether hand-operated or powered, is an essential need. Bucket and rope withdrawal begins or ends with the well top open and is subject to contamination. A variant of wells to tap groundwater is the infiltration gallery. It is shown schematically in Fig. 3-4 as it merits wider use in developing countries to secure

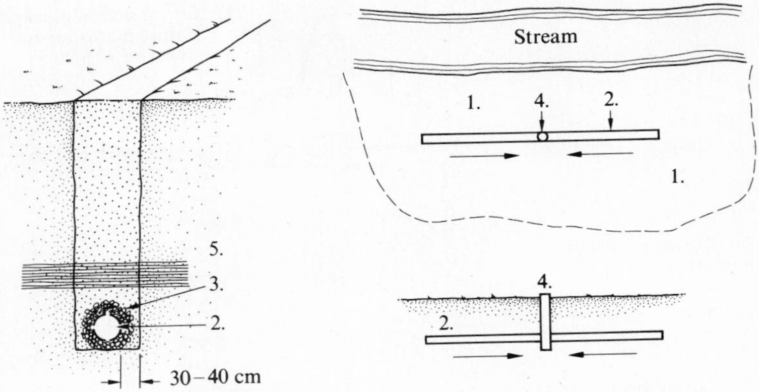

1. Sand banks beside streams offer excellent opportunities for infiltration galleries or shallow dug wells.

2. Perforated pipe should be laid on a prepared filter bed and more filter bed should be constructed over it.

3. Round 12- to 25-mm ($\frac{1}{2}$ to 1-in) stones should be laid around the pipe, and the filter should be built out away from the pipe with graded sand and gravel. Filter should be 30–40 cm (12–16 in) in thickness from pipe to extreme edge.

4. Well in middle of gallery for mounting pump and collecting water.

5. Groundwater strata.

FIGURE 3-4
Infiltration gallery beside a stream. [*Source*: *Ref*. 3-8 (*p*. 105).]

high-quality water from river and pond underbeds and to intercept groundwater drainage at the toe of slopes.

These advantages of groundwater are well recognized. The source is not only widely used but increasingly overused. The withdrawals exceed the rate of natural replenishment. The groundwater level drops permanently. The wells must be deepened or pumped harder or both. A great deal more must be learned about subsurface soil structure and the behavior of water in it. Predictions of successful well sites, of yields, of drawdown curves, and of the cones of influence on other wells in the same field are based on limited facts and incomplete theories. The concepts formulated are superior to dowsing. The latter is pure fake and fiction. The former is at least some fact and the hopeful projection of experience. No determined water searcher overlooks groundwater. Wells range from the village facility celebrated in sociological and anthropological analysis of Latin American women, to the wells in Bible story pictures, to a network of wells serving a city like Joliet, Illinois, with a radioactive water of surprising, but not hazardous, radium content. Aside from a few really large cities, the Midwest heartland of the United States depends on ground-water for farm wells; suburban home wells; private water company wells; publicly owned well systems for villages, towns, and cities; and manufacturing and food processing plants with their own wells to meet their water needs.   Most of that Midwest groundwater is hard water with the sum of Ca and Mg over 300 mg/l.   For special requirements, the well water is wholly or partially softened.   It is cheap.   It is safe. To enjoy these advantages in the near future, it will also have to be managed so that withdrawals fit replenishment.   The logging of the character of soil horizons on all drilled wells in the Midwestern states and the recording and analysis of these data by state agencies have provided useful information on the geology of groundwater.   Increasingly, records of withdrawals, yields, and depth of the water table are accumulating.   These data will provide a basis for management.   In the water-scarce economy of Israel, every well in the country is assigned a maximum withdrawal and is metered to verify the take.   Thus, withdrawals can be kept on a par with replenishment.   That means the user cannot have all the water he wishes, but only that which the source can safely and steadily provide.

Surface Water

Surface sources are the most obvious.   Those close at hand are sometimes rejected, as it is evident that the quality is bad or that the quantity is not dependable.   At this point a look at the fate of rainfall puts the first three sources in perspective, that is, rainfall capture, groundwater, and surface water.   All three arrive as rainfall.   Figure 3-5 shows the distribution of 30 in of rain per year, the United States average, among:

1 Evaporation and evapotranspiration, 70 percent
2 Groundwater storage, 10 percent
3 Surface runoff, 20 percent

In water use management, rainfall capture and storage receives skillful engineering and statistical hydrological analysis for large storage works.   The creation of an impoundment for water supply, flood control, streamflow regulation, hydroelectric power, irrigation water, or, as is now frequent, a multiple of these purposes is not a haphazard venture of rolling earth and pouring concrete to form a dam.   Rainfall, runoff, snowmelt, streamflow, and water-surface evaporation are the water parameters studied.   Soil infiltration and evapotranspiration on the watershed are examined to the extent of available information.   The records are always too short and too scant. Rarely have such data been secured for as many as 100 years in the United States. Yet a conventional storage-design factor for water supply is to guard against all but the 5 driest years in 100 years.   Clearly the factor rests on statistical projection from the data at hand.

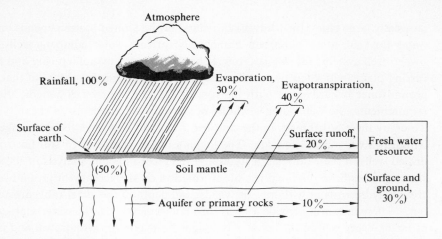

FIGURE 3-5
The division of 30 in of rainfall on the United States among surface runoff, groundwater storage, evaporation, and evapotranspiration. [*Source*: *Ref*. 3-6 (*p*. 22).]

In water use management, evaporation and evapotranspiration are being studied with the intent to control these immediate losses.   Evaporative losses from large area impoundments in hot dry climates as in the Southwest United States are from 6 to 10 ft of equivalent water depth per year.   An overall United States average is 3 ft.   As much as 35 percent of water stored for irrigation is lost by evaporation before use. Experiments to impede evaporation by applying chemicals such as hexadecanol which is spread in monomolecular layers have shown good results.   Wind and wave action disturb the layer, break it up, push it about unevenly.   This presents a yet unsolved problem.   Selective management of plant coverage is being tested to reduce evapotranspiration so that more water goes to groundwater storage.   Herbicide use on phreatophytes with high evapotranspiration rates is being tested in eastern Oregon. These plants are open-range weed growth without economic value.   Their destruction will leave more water for groundwater replenishment.   Other than these experimental efforts, 70 percent of our rainfall is subject to no management at all.   It should be noted that evapotranspiration is a beneficial use for the growth of plants and trees necessary to all living things.   Evaporation is not without benefit as a primary cooling process influencing local and general climate and weather.   Shortsighted intervention in these natural processes can produce new troubles.

Figure 3-5 sets right any first thought that most of our rainfall goes to streams, rivers, and lakes.   Twenty percent of rainfall forms streams by runoff and a portion of the groundwater sustains streamflow by surfacing and infiltration.   This 20 percent of rainfall which forms our fresh surface water enroute to the oceans is used most vigorously and usually recklessly.   Its advantages and assets for water supply are:

1   It is readily at hand for shore and bank-located communities.
2   The quantity available can be observed and, depending on the extent of hydrographic data, predicted.
3   Impoundment can be used to even out flow variations, if navigation is not a primary use.
4   Upland sources unpolluted by prior use are of high quality except for variations in turbidity and being susceptible, when stored, to algal tastes and odors and to iron and manganese accumulation in the deep reservoir zones.
5   Treatment can be fitted to raw-water characteristics and to the quality of finished water required.
6   Surface water withdrawals can be allocated, regulated, and managed under law.
7   Surface sources can be developed to provide prodigious quantities of water, albeit at the cost of treating such volumes as Chicago draws from Lake Michigan, or at the cost of conducting it long distances as New York does from its Catskill and upper Delaware watersheds.   Los Angeles surpasses the New York distances as Fig. 3-6 shows.   Its major sources are across the desert from the Colorado River, up the Sierra Nevada from the Owens Valley Project, and over 400 miles up the central valley from the Sacramento River to provide a half billion gallons of water per day from distant surface sources.

The deficits and limitations of surface sources are:

1   It is increasingly rare that surface water can be used without treatment, a minimum being disinfection by chlorination.
2   Users below the first ones along a stream and river system must cope with all sorts of waste residuals from prior use.
3   On short stream stretches and from low-volume impoundments there are flash changes in physical quality, particularly turbidity, requiring treatment adjustments.
4   Impoundments have summer and winter stratification during which the bottom waters accumulate the slowly dissolving minerals from the bottom and taste and odor compounds from the anaerobic action of benthal decomposition.
5   Impoundments are subject to algal blooms and are now threatened in a few instances with eutrophication as excessive concentrations of phosphates and inorganic nitrogen provide an over-supply of nutrients.
6   High-quality sources are to be found only at greater distances from population sources, are more competitively sought, and are more highly regarded as a valuable resource by those having a claim on such sources.   Examples of the

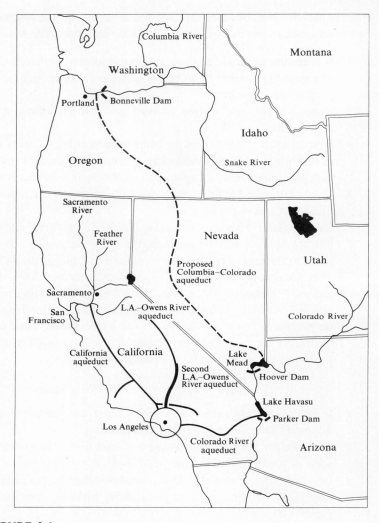

FIGURE 3-6
Water sources for Los Angeles area and proposed diversion from the Columbia
River to the Colorado River at Lake Mead. [*Source*: *From "The Metabolism
of Cities", A. Wolman. © 1965 by Scientific American Inc. All rights reserved.*]

latter state of mind are shown by the lack of enthusiasm of Northwesterners for diverting Columbia River water 800 miles to the south to the Colorado River, of northern Californians for diverting more water to southern California (Fig. 3-6), and of Canadians toward the AEC-inspired project to divert the flow of Artic-bound rivers of Canada southward to the United States.

7 As quality requirements for finished water rise and the quality of raw water deteriorates through repeated use, the necessary treatment processes must be managed more skillfully, will require larger capital investment, and will incur higher operating costs.

Desalted Water

Desalting ocean water holds the fascination of an unexpendable source for freshwater users. Desalination is the term most widely used for processes removing cations and anions from the salty waters of the seas, oceans, and ground storage. Deionization more accurately describes the process as ions are removed nonselectively according to the efficiency and characteristics of the process. More than salt, NaCl is removed. All the processes proposed require sizable energy inputs. Recent impetus has been added to process development because there has been acute concern for more water where there are more people concentrating and because nuclear reactors offer the promise of potent energy sources not dependent on cheap transportation for their fuel. Four basic processes are in use:

1 Distillation in varying degrees of complexity to achieve heat conservation and efficient separation
2 Electrodialysis, which in simplest terms is using electricity to force the separation of the ions from the water through selective plastic membranes
3 Reverse osmosis or hyperfiltration, which uses mechanical pressure across selective plastic membranes to achieve from 97 to 98 percent reductions of ion concentration in water impressed across them
4 Freezing in which the water molecules are frozen in crystal aggregates and separated, the ions being left behind in an increasingly concentrated brine solution.

Of the four, only distillation is in high volume use. Seawater has been distilled aboard ships since the days of steam power; hence the U.S. Navy has worked on such units for shipboard use and for remote bases lacking adequate sources. The unit installed by the Navy at its Guantanamo Bay base when the Cuban government cut off the land water source is a distillation system. In the United States, the other processes are in pilot plant scale, and some do produce enough water to supplement local sources. Examples of processes in use in water-scarce areas or for research are listed in Table 3-13. Further information with description of processes is in the chapter on " Saline Water Conversion " by W. E. Katz and R. Eliassen, Ref. 3-7.

The assets and advantages of desalination are:

1   There is an abundance of raw water on all coasts and over brackish ground-water zones.
2   Desalination has the promise of water for coastal arid areas for irrigation.
3   The processes are thermoelectromechanical and therefore subject to technological improvements and the economies of volume increase.

The deficits and limitations are:

1   The complexity and high energy inputs of present processes result in high unit costs.   The lowest cost yet achieved for seawater is at the Key West plant that produces water at 85 cents (U.S.) per 1,000 gal.   Brackish waters can be converted by electrodialysis for 20 to 40 cents per 1,000 gal.
2   The disposal of saline concentrates must be managed.   The average seawater contains 35,000 milligrams of dissolved solids per liter.   The waste stream from seawater conversion contains as much as 70,000 milligrams of dissolved solids per liter, with a volume from 1 to 20 times the amount of water produced.   The waste stream from brackish waters with an initial dissolved solids content of 1,000 to 3,000 mg/l contains concentrates of from 5,000 to 10,000 mg/l, which equals from 10 to 30 percent of the volume fed for conversion.   Plants located on large sea and ocean sites can use disposal by outfalls that carry the concentrates away from the intakes.   Inland sites using brackish groundwater are limited to surface disposal, evaporation beds, or ground injection.

Desalination must stand in the marketplace with other water sources.   Brackish groundwater recovery in the Southwest, particularly for irrigation, is a favorable marketplace, if all the required subsidies and collateral benefits for its use and for alternatives are examined.   Two major projects for water-scarce areas with high technological resources have been delayed.   In 1969 planning for the Balsa Island

Table 3-13   EXAMPLES OF EACH PRINCIPAL DESALINATION PROCESS IN USE, WITH LOCATION AND PRODUCTION

Process	Location	Production, gpd	Comment
Distillation, flash	Shuwaikh and Shuiaba, Kuwait	18,000,000	Oil center
Distillation, flash	Eilat, Israel	1,000,000	Arid region
Electrodialysis	Buckeye, Ariz.	650,000	Arid region
Electrodialysis	Webster, S.Dak.	250,000	Govt. research
Reverse osmosis	Plains, Tex.	100,000	Arid region
Direct freeze	Wrightsville Beach, N.C.	200,000	Govt. research

nuclear reactor facility to produce electricity and desalted ocean water for Los Angeles was stopped because of rising cost estimates.   In 1969 the Ashod project for desalting Mediterranean Sea water for irrigation in Israel was abandoned for more favorable alternative sources.   Among the sources with which desalting of the seas must compete is wastewater reclamation.

Reclaimed Wastewater

Wastewater reclamation has been the overlooked stepchild in the water resources family as "she isn't pretty at first look."   Despite that initial reaction, some impressive marriages of reclaimed wastewater and urgent need have been made.   The Back River Sewage Treatment Plant of Baltimore has been providing the Sparrows Point Works of Bethlehem Steel Company with reclaimed wastewater for process use since 1942.   It started as a war marriage at 20 million gallons per day (gpd) in 1942 and has continued with additions to 65 million gpd in 1947 and to 100 million gpd presently.[1]   The Golden Gate Park of San Francisco has been watered by reclaimed sewage of local origin for a long time.   For a short time, so have some fabled Las Vegas, Nevada, golf courses maintained greenness from thoroughly processed toilet flushings and bath waters.   At Whittier Narrows in California, wastewater is reclaimed for groundwater recharge in the Los Angeles basin at the rate of 65 million gpd and rising.   Further south in California, the Santee Project reclaims wastewater for recreational use by a series of processes: conventional activated sludge treatment, 30-day retention in oxidation ponds, surface spread to subsurface filtration galleries, and chlorination. The processed water then forms recreational lakes which provide fishing, boating, and swimming. See Fig. 2-4. From October 1956 through March 1957 the community of Chanute, Kansas, sustained its water source by recycling its treated sewage.[2] Intensive treatment including high chlorine doses maintained the bacteriological quality.   The total dissolved solids slowly rose, as the only replenishment at the raw-water intakes was the town's own treated sewage pumped upstream above the water plant.   All treatment of sewage and of the recycled water was scrupulously conscientious.   Some people reportedly did not drink the system's water, using bottled water or other beverages.   Nevertheless, there were no recognized waterborne diseases or other physiological effects in this forced trial of community wastewater reclamation for its own immediate use.

Such a drastic application of wastewater reclamation as Chanute's is not advocated by its most articulate proponents.   The case for reclamation is lucidly and concisely put by P. H. McGauhey in Ref. 3-6 (pp. 175–187).   He lists all sources, of

---

[1] *JWPCF,* **20**:15 (1948).
[2] D. F. Metzler et al., *JAWWA,* **50**:1021–1057 (1958).

which industrial and domestic return waters are most feasible, as these are at points of immediate reuse demand.   He enumerates the conventional methods of water and sewage treatment which can be applied in selected combinations and intensities, and adds a plea for engineered soil systems for which the Santee and Whittier Narrows projects are precursors.   He recognizes 11 deterrents to purposeful water reclamation, which are in part legal, in part economic, in part tradition, in part a product of pre-judgment and ignorance, but in no part the lack of technology.

Domestic sewage is the most manageable source for reclamation as only about 300 milligrams of total dissolved solids per liter are added in domestic water use, as increasingly it is already scheduled for initial treatment, and as it is in a conduit system which can be intercepted at some existing point or which can be profitably altered to reach such a point.   Direct reuse for drinking water will be the rarity.   The choices are direct reuse above ground for industry and for recreation and to a lesser degree for agriculture, as the volumes available are small compared with the need.   Mc-Gauhey states that if all the 1,000 million gallons per day of California's domestic wastes which now flow to the sea were reclaimed, that volume would meet only 6 percent of California's agricultural need for new water.   This will not hold for areas in which the high-fertility land is not farmed as intensively and is not so dependent on irrigation.   The use of sewage for irrigating crop lands is discussed in the chapter on wastes.

The second use of reclaimed domestic wastewaters is for groundwater recharge. The techniques of surface spreading, direct injection, and subsurface percolation systems are in use.   Data on their application provide improvement in use and increased certainty in predicting performance.   Such water will be added to ground-water drinking sources.   Managed and engineered, the quality and quantity of the input will be better known than that from rainwater percolation and uncontrolled return of wastes to groundwater storage.   If unrestricted groundwater withdrawals are to continue, managed replenishment is necessary.   Treated domestic wastewaters are a controllable source for recharge.   The terror of pathogen travel in homogenous soil structures has been dispelled by data given in the chapters on wastes.   The California observations at Lodi, Whittier Narrows, and Santee have been significantly reassuring including that on the removal of viruses during soil percolation.

The assets and advantages of wastewater reclamation are:

1   It can be used selectively by routing domestic sewage to a manufacturing plant for reclamation and use.
2   Treatment can be applied to produce the quality needed for a manufacturing process.
3   It can reduce the transport of water—waste, raw, and finished.
4   It can be fitted into a planned and managed system of resource use.

5 It is well fitted for groundwater recharge use and for manufacturing needs, including cooling water, with appropriate slime and corrosion control.

The deficits and limitations are:

1 It will continue to be suspect for its sanitary quality, particularly in the face of "what if" questions such as, "What if simultaneously we have an epidemic of cholera, typhoid fever, infectious hepatitis, and amebic dysentery? Will your treatment scheme produce pathogen-free water?"

2 It must confront tradition, existing restrictive regulations, and public and professional misconceptions.

3 Existing procedures to verify absolute control of all biological and chemical contaminants are not speedy; the biological techniques require days.

4 The maximum utilization of wastewater will require dual sewers to carry domestic wastes to a reclamation point and avoid adding difficult-to-remove manufacturing wastes enroute.

5 Reclaimed process water will require dual supply systems within a manufacturing plant with the risk of interconnections and with the need for additional surveillance by public health workers.

It is a characteristic of the society in the United States that the final pressure is economic. The issue is over what time span the cost versus the benefit can be perceived by experts and public alike. In that context, the presently unattractive source of reclaimed wastewater as a supplement to more attractive sources will find a place. The technology of desalination will provide techniques for which our wastewaters may prove a more suitable raw material than seawater and deep-well brines.

ATTAINING AND MAINTAINING QUALITY FOR DOMESTIC USE

A required quality for any water use can be attained by selection of a source that has that quality, by protection of the source and the delivery system, and by treatment to alter the initial quality of the raw water. For domestic use from a public supply, chlorination is the minimum treatment to protect the quality in the distribution system even when the raw water is of excellent quality at the source. Table 3-14 states the expected quality levels of raw water from the five primary sources under usual conditions, using the ranges of "excellent, ready for use"; "good, not likely to require purposeful treatment"; "fair, likely to require purposeful treatment to attain drinking water quality"; "poor, with a few exceptions requires treatment to attain a high standard of quality."

Protection of the Source

Sources are protected by blocking the drainage or infiltration of water of uncertain quality, primarily sewage; by restricting the use of land in the watershed as in the case of upland reservoirs; by close sanitary supervision of sewage and wastewater disposal on the reservoir watershed and of upstream users on rivers; and by limiting use of water supply impoundments by prohibiting the use of water supply reservoirs for swimming, boating, and water skiing.   These measures are not all equally rational or equally effective.   The objective is to maintain the quality of the raw water as it was at the time of first development and to prevent its deterioration by irresponsible prior user's discharges, including wastewater discharges that enter the ground strata.   The safeguards in use are directed toward managing bacterial contamination and overt color and suspended pollutants.   The time is at hand to develop procedures to limit chemical and radioactive contaminants.   The latter is already under supervision in the United States by licensing radionuclide use, nuclear reactor operation, and radioactive waste disposal.   Analogous control has not developed for toxic chemicals and suspected carcinogens that enter water supply sources in factory wastewaters or in runoff from forest and cultivated land receiving repeated applications of stable pesticides and herbicides.   A rise in indices of chemical pollution in heavily used United States

Table 3-14   QUALITY RATINGS OF RAW WATER SOURCES UNDER USUAL CONDITIONS PRIOR TO TREATMENT

Source	Quality factor				
	Bacteriological	Physical	Toxic chemicals	Other chemicals	Hardness
Captured rain	Good	Good	Excellent	Excellent	Excellent
Groundwater	Excellent	Excellent	Excellent*	Fair	Poor
Surface water:					
Upland reservoirs	Excellent	Variable	Excellent	Fair	Good
Lakes	Good	Good	Excellent	Fair	Good
Rivers	Fair to poor	Variable	Fair	Poor	Fair
Water for desalting:					
Oceans and seas	Good	Good	Fair	Poor	Fair
Brackish ground	Excellent	Good	Good	Poor	Poor
Wastewater for reclamation:					
Domestic	Poor	Poor	Good	Good	Good
Industrial	Good	Poor	Poor	Poor	Variable

* In rare instances, arsenic, radium, or nitrates are in groundwater.

surface waters is shown in surveillance studies by such tests as the carbon-chloroform extract and the carbon-alcohol extract of organic residues in large-volume water samples.

Groundwater requires a high degree of source protection as it is often used without chlorination. Figure 3-3, which shows the elements of protection, is supplemented by Fig. 3-7 to illustrate the application of the principles to a deep well. The earth and cement-grout seals around well casings and spring boxes must be secure against penetration by leakage along side walls. This protection is made more secure by sloping and ditching to make local drainage flow away from the source. The issue of distances from excreta disposal facilities is examined in the chapter on wastes. Cistern and spring protection are detailed in Ref. 3-8 (pp. 104 and 119).

The protection of surface sources is difficult, and its intensity is variable. The oldest upland watersheds in New England are wholly owned by the water authorities and wholly subject to their control of entry and use, not only of the impounded water, but of the drainage area making up the watershed. At the other end of the spectrum is Cincinnati, Ohio, with its intakes in the Ohio River, which receives the wastes, domestic, manufacturing, and agricultural, of everything upstream, including that of Pittsburgh, Pennsylvania; the Miami River draining the heavily populated and used land of southeast Ohio; and the Kanawha River, the industrial drain of Charleston and Nitro, West Virginia; and all the manufacturing complexes downstream. Cincinnati's protection of its source rests in the power of the tributary basin states and their interstate creation, the Ohio River Valley Stream Sanitation Commission (ORSANCO), to hold pollution loads and volumes to a level which can be removed by good treatment facilities and by conscientious operation and control at the waterworks. Between the ends of the system are natural lakes from which the source protection can be provided by the control of sewage discharge. The control may be the absolute prohibition of discharge or the requirement of a degree of sewage treatment to keep the lake in high-quality water that is easily treated to meet drinking water standards. This applies not only to small lakes and to small communities. Chicago's sequence in the use of Lake Michigan water has been:

1   Use Lake Michigan as it was, as any stalwart pioneer did.
2   Build the Chicago drainage canal to keep its wastewaters out of the lake and to divert them to the Gulf of Mexico through the Mississippi River system.
3   Chlorinate the lake water before drinking it.
4   Build the largest and most automated rapid sand filtration plant in the world to keep the lake water safely drinkable.

This sequence of increasing the intensity of protection and of treatment will have to be repeated in other high-density populated areas even with adequate management of liquid and solid wastes on the surface and groundwater drainage areas.

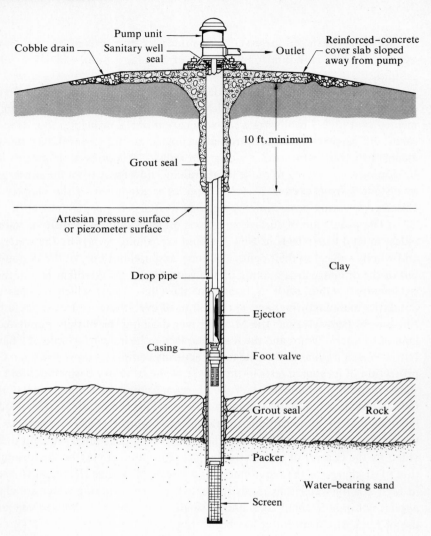

FIGURE 3-7
Protection of a deep well source. [*Source*: "*Manual of Individual Water Supply Systems*," *U.S. Public Health Service, Pub. 24, p.* 38, *1962.*]

Desalted water has been used on too limited a scale to define requirements of source protection and postdesalting procedures to guarantee a water of high hygienic quality and of ready consumer acceptability.   Present use situations leave no source alternatives.   Desalted water is not yet competing with alternative sources.   On the face of it, processes in use produce a water of drinking quality in biological, physical, and chemical characteristics.   The product is close to distilled water.   Two complaints have appeared.   It tastes flat.   It is corrosive to metallic pipes and fittings. Both are readily corrected.   Remineralize the water, and raise its pH by the addition of lime.   In a public system, chlorine will be needed for biological growth control in the mains, fluorides for caries prevention, and likely, lime or soda ash, or both, for corrosion control.   Results and observations will differ from those of more familiar surface and ground waters.   Major uses of desalted water for irrigation and manufacturing will not require drinking standard quality.   Such uses, particularly for genetically selected plant life, will permit moderately salty water well above drinking tolerances.

Source protection of wastewaters scheduled for reclamation does seem paradoxical, as the practice of marking certain wastewaters for particular reuse after selected treatment has just begun.   Domestic wastes scheduled for cooling-water use require treatment which will not increase slime growths and foaming in cooling towers and tube condensers.   Commercial laundry wastes high in detergents are unsuited for such use and require segregation.   Wastewater high in stable toxic compounds are not fit for groundwater recharge.   Therefore, such manufacturing and, at times, agricultural wastewaters containing such toxic compounds must be rejected.   The source protection of wastewaters considered for reclamation has two components:

1   The selection of wastewaters most easily treated to the required quality
2   Surveillance to keep the drain lines restricted to carrying selected water to the point of treatment and reuse and to prevent clandestine discharges of wastes that cannot be conditioned by the processes in use.

Treatment Processes for Quality Goals

Where did it all begin?   In 1883, an Englishman in Bengal found that the Hindu system of medicine according to Sus'ruta, covering hygienic lore from 2,000 B.C., recommended, " Impure water should be purified by being boiled over a fire, or being heated in the sun, or by dipping a heated iron into it, or it may be purified by filtration through sand and coarse gravel and then allowed to cool."   That Englishman may have been aware that since 1802 the water supply of Paisley, Scotland, had been filtered and that London water purveyors in 1828 began filtering the Thames River water to make it less lethal for drinking.   Probably he would have taken a dim view of the report that Richmond, Virginia, built a water purification plant in 1832, and been not at all surprised that the plant failed.   He would well be surprised at the state of affairs in 1969.   His homeland has a high level of safe water throughout urban and rural areas with 99 percent of the total population on public piped water.   The United States has its share of deficiencies, but 80 percent of its people in communities of over 25 are on public water.   In Calcutta, where he published his findings, the desirability and feasibility of a metropolitan water development is still under discussion, while cholera makes its spasmodic and seemingly erratic appearance in that densely peopled urban conglomerate.   In the United States, the techniques of water treatment were refined from 1895 to 1915 by such men as William Sedgwick, Allen Hazen, Earle Phelps, and George Fuller.   The refinements were more certain in hydraulic and bacteriological results than in chemical effects.   Large and effective plants were built that applied the unit processes of aeration, plain settling, chemical coagulation and flocculation, sedimentation, slow and rapid sand filtration, chlorine disinfection, softening, and corrosion control.   A post-World War I group brought more precise science and engineering to the processes to lower costs and to increase efficiency.   The group included such men as John Baylis, Abel Wolman, Lynn Enslow, Thomas Camp, Gordon Fair, W. F. Langelier, Charles Gilman Hyde, and A. P. Black.   Some of these continue in very active professional practice.   Their monuments are already secure.

Table 3-15 relates the quality of raw water, expressed in concentration ranges of principal contaminants and pollutants, to three levels of treatment.   The first three quality constituents measure organic wastes from man, and from agricultural and manufacturing industries.   Fresh domestic sewage in the United States will have a biochemical oxidation demand (BOD) of 200 to 300 mg/l.   Complete conventional sewage treatment will provide an 80 to 95 percent reduction.   The plant effluent will have a BOD ranging from 10 to 60 mg/l.   Time and dilution provide the reduction to the levels of Table 3-15.   The dissolved-oxygen levels required for game fish and their accompanying aerobic biota are those shown in Table 3-15, even those of the " poor source " column.   The next four constituents are chemical with pH an overall index of the chemical mix, chlorides for salinity taste, fluorides for dental benefits, and phenolics for chlorinous taste products and as a rough tracer of organic chemicals in the water.   The last two, color and turbidity, are physical qualities.   Water in the ranges of the " good source " is well managed for its hygienic quality.   Such sources are free of heavy pollutional loads and are readily treated for drinking.   The " more than " for 8 of the 12 constituents under " poor source " permits a decidedly contaminated and polluted raw material.   The dissolved-oxygen requirement of 4 mg/l ensures that the source is not deoxygenated, not anaerobic and, to be hoped, in recovery. To produce, consistently, water of drinking quality, a treatment plant for poor source water must be carefully designed for hydraulic and chemical performance, must treat water at rates within its design capacity, must have its rates of chemical dose promptly adjusted to raw-water changes, and must have its product continuously monitored for its biological, chemical, physical, and radiological characteristics. The margins for overload, for failure to respond to changes, and for failure to monitor the effluent quality are quite small.

A water treatment plant is an engineered series of unit processes fitted to the characteristics of the raw source and the defined quality of the finished water. It is sized hydraulically in each of its unit processes to a determined rated output, usually in millions of gallons per day. Engineering choices in sizing the flash-mix and floc-culating units and the flocculated water flume permit future addition of settling basin and filter units to expand capacity. Flexibility is provided by routing the water through the plant with bypasses and, less frequently, recirculating lines. In United States practice, water treatment plants are remarkably similar to one another in such details as layout, treatment methods, chemicals used, hydraulic controls, dosage equipment, and laboratory facilities.

Figure 3-8 shows the flow sequence of water treatment processes. Those in common use are solid lined. Those in less frequent use are dash lined. The usual

Table 3-15   RANGES OF PROMULGATED STANDARDS FOR RAW-WATER SOURCES OF DOMESTIC WATER SUPPLY

Constituent	Excellent source, requiring disinfection treatment only	Good source, requiring usual treatment such as filtration and disinfection	Poor source, requiring special or auxiliary treatment and disinfection
BOD (5-day), mg/l:			
Monthly average	0.75–1.5	1.5–2.5	*>2.5
Max. day, or sample	1.0–3.0	3.0–4.0	>4.0
Coliform MPN/100 ml:			
Monthly average	50–100	50–5,000	>5,000
Max. day, or sample	Less than 5% over 100	Less than 20% over 5,000	Less than 5% over 20,000
Dissolved oxygen:			
Average, mg/l	4.0–7.5	4.0–6.5	4.0
Saturation, %	75 or better	60 or better	
pH average	6.0–8.5	5.0–9.0	3.8–10.5
Chlorides (max.), mg/l	50 or less	50–250	>250
Fluorides, mg/l	†<1.5	1.5–3.0	>3.0
Phenolic compounds (max.), mg/l	None	0.005	>0.005
Color, units	0–20	20–150	>150
Turbidity, units	0–10	10–250	>250

* >, *more than.*
† <, *less than.*

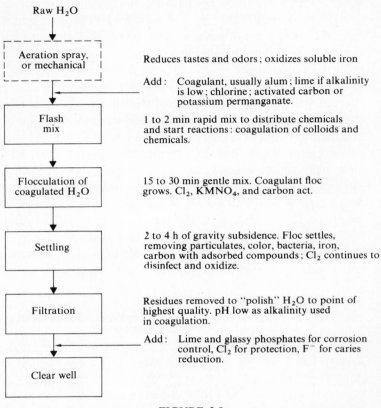

Raw H_2O

| Aeration spray, or mechanical | Reduces tastes and odors; oxidizes soluble iron |

Add :   Coagulant, usually alum; lime if alkalinity is low; chlorine; activated carbon or potassium permanganate.

| Flash mix | 1 to 2 min rapid mix to distribute chemicals and start reactions: coagulation of colloids and chemicals. |

| Flocculation of coagulated H_2O | 15 to 30 min gentle mix. Coagulant floc grows. Cl_2, $KMNO_4$, and carbon act. |

| Settling | 2 to 4 h of gravity subsidence. Floc settles, removing particulates, color, bacteria, iron, carbon with adsorbed compounds; Cl_2 continues to disinfect and oxidize. |

| Filtration | Residues removed to "polish" H_2O to point of highest quality. pH low as alkalinity used in coagulation. |

Add :   Lime and glassy phosphates for corrosion control, Cl_2 for protection, F^- for caries reduction.

| Clear well |

FIGURE 3-8
Flow diagram of water treatment processes.

points of chemical dosage are shown, and the results of the process stated qualitatively. Occasionally, plain settling precedes aeration to gain subsidence of particulates from high-turbidity water and to equalize raw-water changes.   The structure cost and labor cost of cleaning a large basin have made this choice rare in new works.   Labor costs rather than technological advantages have been decisive in making changes in water treatment processes and process control in the United States since World War II.

Calcium carbonate is the analytical convention for expressing hardness, the sum of Ca and Mg ions in solution.   There is some change of these during coagulation, settling, and filtration, but the change is not sufficient to "soften" waters whose hardness is 250 to 300 mg/l or more.   In large works, the economical method is to add lime and sodium carbonate to precipitate the Ca as $CaCO_3$ and the Mg as $Mg(OH)_2$.

This "lime-soda" process is effectively integrated with the unit processes of flocculation and settling.   In smaller works, particularly where the source is high-quality well water, the Ca and Mg are removed by a pass through ion exchange beds under pressure.   Synthetic resins have supplemented and replaced natural zeolites such as "green sand."   Sodium is the replacement ion.   Therefore, the sodium content rises in the softened water.   The beds must be regenerated with concentrated salt solutions.

The unit processes of water treatment have been applied with admirable results without a full understanding of their chemistry and physics.   The biological aspects other than bacterial kill are less significant but no better known in their mechanisms.   This ignorance of the refinements of the reactions and the processes has two explanations:

1 Water, as used, is $H_2O + X$, with the X being a bit different in each instance and within itself, as runoff and percolation conditions change.
2 Engineers, particularly civil engineers choosing the sanitary speciality, have taken up the task of developing water and waste treatment methods.   Their chemistry and biology are new, second, borrowed skills.   Their physics must be applied on a different scale than for dam and truss design.

It is remarkably fortunate that since the beginning of this century sanitary engineering has benefited from the inquiring, challenging minds of such men as Allen Hazen, George Fuller, Abel Wolman, Thomas Camp, H. W. Streeter, and Gordon M. Fair.   Since World War II, a new genera has appeared to develop the scientific team attack, particularly on university campuses and in national laboratories.   With recognized neglect of others, a few are cited: Donald J. O'Connor at Manhattan College, Harold A. Thomas at Harvard, P. H. McGauhey at Berkeley, D. A. Okun at the University of North Carolina, H. B. Gotaas at Northwestern, Ernest Gloyna at the University of Texas, John C. Geyer at Johns Hopkins, Rolf Eliassen at Stanford, and Don Bloodgood at Purdue.   These teaching and research groups are providing knowledge of mechanisms—chemical, biological, and physical—which make the best use of present processes and give a basis for rational design of new ones.   Valuable contributions continue from consulting offices, as illustrated by the published studies by Paul Haney of Black and Veatch, by H. E. Hudson of Hazen and Sawyer, and by Thomas Riddick of Thomas Riddick and Associates.   All of it is needed to meet the squeeze of population and urban-technological growth on relatively fixed water resources.

The solid-lined processes of Fig. 3-8 are examined briefly for their phenomena.

Flash or rapid mixing   The coagulant, most usually alum, $Al(SO_4)_3 \cdot 18H_2O$, is driven into the colloidal materials identified as color and fine particulates.   The speedy mechanical mix gives the chemical forces of attraction free and immediate play.

Synthetic organic polymers are in limited use as additives to enhance the action.   The other chemicals being added get uniform distribution.   In the terms of the physical chemist, this is the point of coagulation.   Electrically driven agitators in small rectangular chambers are the choice for flash mixing provided that maintenance is certain, replacement parts cheap and readily available, and power reliable and low in cost. Without these advantages, over-and-under or end-around baffled channels will do an acceptable job and will serve as flocculators as well.   These are well suited for most of the plants needed in the developing countries.   The first few seconds of encounter between the coagulant and the colloids in suspension are critical.   Polymers must be formed immediately and the polymer adsorption started rapidly.   Instantaneous mixing and accurate dose are needed.   The complexity of the process and its importance are described by C. R. O'Melia.[1]

Flocculation   Baffled channels accomplish the job without short circuiting, at the price of 2 or 3 ft of elevation head.   These plus operational flexibility and the space requirement have made mechanically paddled basins the choice in the United States. During this slow and gentle mixing, the barely visible floc grows to feathery white agglomerates up to a half inch in their longest dimension.   With floc growth, there is chemical engagement of Fe, Mn, Ca, and Mg; colloidal attraction; mechanical enmeshing of large particles, including bacteria; and surface adsorption of ionic, colloidal, and suspended particulates.   Concurrently the first chlorine dose is acting on chemical materials by oxidation and substitution and addition reactions, and is killing biological forms.   The chlorine action prepares some material for floc inclusion. Activated carbon adsorbs the soluble components of off tastes and bad odors on the extensive surface of its fine particles.   When potassium permanganate is used in place of carbon, the permanganate ion acts by straightforward oxidation of the taste and odor producers.   The choice between the two rests in the results to be produced on the particular water in that plant.   If it is the segregation of the desirable from the undesirable, purification is accomplished by coagulation and flocculation.   There is the need to separate the impurities on the floc; hence settling and filtering follow.

Sedimentation   Gravity and time for it to act on the floc are all that are needed for the slow settling from the quiescent, slowly moving water as it flows through the sedimentation basin.   The intent is that the vector of the downward settling particle and the forward flowing water will intersect the basin bottom before the far end is reached. The behavior is not solely determined by the forces of gravity, bouyancy, and friction as there is the continued agglomeration of floc during the slow descent.   Large particles overtake small ones and coalesce to continue flocculation.   Without knowing the intricacies of the physical and chemical actions at work, early designers recognized

---

[1] *Public Works*, **100**:97 (1969).

the superior removal in deep basins and called for depths of 12 to 18 ft.   During the 2 to 4 hour detention, forward velocity is 0.5 to 3 feet per minute (fpm).   Wind and sun heat produce basin currents, and hydraulic oddities at inlets and outlets disturb the orderly movements hoped for at the drawing board.   The settled sludge slides into steeply sloped hoppers, which form the basin bottom, and is held there for flushing at 2 to 4 month intervals.   It is also removed by bottom scrapers moving continuously at 1 fpm to a drawoff channel at the inlet end.   It is disposed of in a sewer or nearby stream.

Radial-flow circular basins with mechanical continuous settled-solid plows are in use.   These are similar in design to units used for sewage settling and are in like manner often called clarifiers.   These configurations have been adapted to provide "solids contact processes" in which mixing, coagulation, flocculation, the separation of solids from water, and the continuous sludge removal are contained in a single structure.   A suspended sludge blanket is held about the center well.   All water and the newly formed floc pass through it, providing a floc conditioning.   Some of these patented units provide for returning a portion of the settled sludge to hold a uniform blanket in suspension.   This is in accord with experiments of recirculating settled solids in conventional basins to gain better floc.   The process demands careful hydraulic design, chemical dosage fitted to the raw water, and a high level of operational skill.   Two beautiful water treatment plants using this process have been incorporated in the 400-year-old Canal Isabel II water system supplying metropolitan Madrid. Figure 3-9 shows a solids contact process schematically.   In the United States such units have been used for the lime-soda softening method to reduce hardness.   With rare exceptions conventional settling and solids contact processes are followed by filtration.

Filtration   Whatever may have been the thought of the first ones who cleaned water by letting it seep through a bed of sand or other granular material, a filter depends only weakly and lastly in importance on mechanical straining for retaining the filth.   What then are the forces at work?   Figure 3-10 is a cutaway view of the concrete box and its contents which is a typical rapid sand filter unit.   A single plant may have from four to dozens of such units operating in parallel.   The filter bed of 24 to 30 in depth of sand is carefully sieved to sizes specified by two parameters:

1   Effective size (E.S.) is the grain size in millimeters, such that 10 percent by weight are smaller and correspondingly 90 percent are larger.   In United States practice an E.S. of 0.40 to 0.65 mm is used.
2   Uniformity coefficient (U.C.), which fixes the spread of grain size, is the ratio of the 60 percent size to the 10 percent size.   Thus, half the sand will be between the 10 and 60 percent sizes.   A U.C. of 1.3 to 1.7 is used for rapid sand filter beds.   The parameters are useful for specifying any granular filter material.

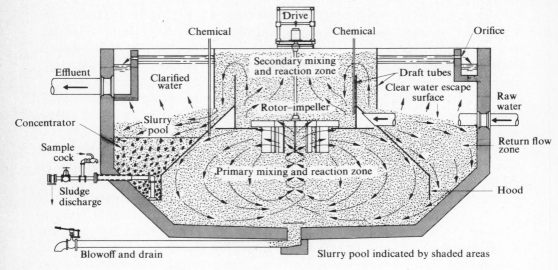

FIGURE 3-9
A schematic drawing of a solids contact process unit for mixing, coagulating, flocculating, and settling water. [*Source*: *Infilco Drawing* 7*RD*-1825-*A*1, *Westinghouse Electric Corp., Infilco Div.*]

The sand layer rests on a 12 to 18 in bed of gravel sized from $\frac{1}{16}$ to 2 in.   The interstices in such a sand bed are not small enough to do the size removals accomplished by mechanical straining.   The efficiency of removal by fine granular beds is due to mechanisms of adsorption, further flocculation, sedimentation in the tiny pore spaces, and finally, straining, particularly as the *schmutz* accumulates in the upper inches of fines.   Filtration is a contact process with the action between the residual floc and filter grain surfaces and, importantly, the floc particles already deposited. The sand grains acquire a sheath of floc.   The upper 6 in of bed of a conventional filter does the removal of the particulates.   A well-coagulated, flocculated, and settled water comes onto a filter with about 2 Jtu and leaves with 0.2 Jtu or less.

A number that had been well enshrined in United States waterworks practice for half a century was the filtration rate of 2 gallons per square foot of bed area per minute. It stemmed from George Fuller's studies in 1895 which showed that rates from 1 to 5 were effective, with 2 satisfactory and dependable.   Two got into handbooks and regulatory agency design standards.   In the last 15 years exceptions have been granted to filter at 3, 4, and 5 gal/(ft^2)(min) to:

1 Take advantage of improved coagulation, flocculation, and settling.
2 Test new filtering materials, such as anthracite coal particles under plant conditions.

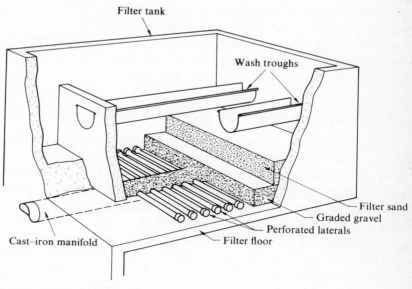

FIGURE 3-10
Cutaway view of a typical rapid sand filter. [*Source*: *ASCE, AWWA, CSSE, Water Treatment Plant Design, AWWA*, 1969, *p.* 128.]

3 Get maximum use of automatic continuous recording turbidimeters on filtrates which sound alarms and can close the influent valve when a filter breakthrough signals a loss of efficiency.

4 Save added capital investment in additional filters, as going from 2 to 4 gal/ $(ft^2)(min)$ doubles the flow-through of existing filters and halves the area required for new ones.

Slow sand filters, which are a good choice for communities in the developing countries, require extensive bed areas as these have a through-put rate of $\frac{1}{30}$ that of rapid filters.   An acre, about 40,000 ft^2, of slow sand filter beds produces 4 million gpd. An acre of rapid sand filter beds produces 125 million gpd at 2 gal/$(ft^2)(min)$.   What then commends slow sand filters for the medium and small cities of developing countries?   Plain settling often suffices for pretreatment.   The assemblage of mechanical devices for coagulation and flocculation is eliminated.   Purchase of chemicals and laboratory control of dosage are eliminated.   Backwashing is eliminated.   The intervals between cleanings are 30 times as long, say 3 months.   Cleaning is by surface skimming by hand with the help of sand-recovery washers of simple design, readily made locally.   The same unit can be used to select and separate local bank-run sand for the building of the original bed (Ref. 3-2, vol. 2, p. 27-14).   The parameters of the bed are an effective size of 0.3 mm and uniformity coefficient of 2.5 with a half-unit range either way.   All the cost factors, which favor rapid sand filters in highly developed communities, produce the choice of slow sand filters for the many developing communities of the world.   Two precautions are:

1   Do not apply water with a turbidity over 40 Jtu.
2   Control algal blooms at the source or in the plain settling basin.

Slow sand filters are scheduled for the sanitation museum in the United States, while a breed of variants of the classical rapid sand filter are in test.   As a departure from conservative practice, the treatment plants at the Hanford Atomic Energy Works near Richland, Washington, use a mixed-media bed, graded sand below at specific gravity 2.65, and coarse anthracite coal particulates at specific gravity 1.5 above the sand.   This provides a downflow first through a coarse layer.   As it has a lower specific gravity, on subsidence after backwash the coal is restored to its top position. The Hanford units have been operated by coagulating directly on the filters.[1]   Precise coagulant dose, flash mix, and polyelectrolyte addition are needed to prepare the water for mixed-media filtration.   Further refinements of grading from coarse at the top to fines at the bottom are in use.   Three or four materials make up the bed, with layers of the fine, high-specific-gravity particulates at the bottom and layers of large, low-specific-gravity particles at the top, which produces a uniform grading of coarse to fine from top to bottom ready for downflow.   In the United States over 100 plants using mixed-media beds for public and industrial water treatment have been put in operation since 1962.   All use polyelectrolyte dosage to control floc formation and to get the maximum filtration in the pass from large to small voids.   Diatomaceous earth filters, developed by the U.S. Army for field water purification, are in wide use in this country to filter recirculated water in swimming pools.   Cost of the filter feed and the ease of crackage, slippage, and breakthrough of the filter cake are undesirable attributes for use in public water purification.

Chemical Reactions of Alum Coagulation and Chlorination

Alum coagulation and chlorination are the principal chemical water treatment processes.   The chemical reactions of these and present understanding of these reveal the empirical character of water treatment.   Each had been in use with considerable effectiveness before the theory of chemistry was brought to bear on it.

Alum coagulation   Filter alum is $Al_2(SO_4)_3 \cdot 18H_2O$.   It reacts with alkaline ions, primarily HCO_3^-, CO_3^{--}, and OH^-, to produce a floc.   This means that the colloids

---

[1] W. R. Conley, *JAWWA*, **53**:1473 (1961).

have been destabilized and are prepared for settling and filtration. As the alkaline ions are removed in the reaction, the pH goes down. In many waters at low turbidities and at the alum dosages used, a simple $Al(OH)_3$ floc is formed. With good flocculation and settling facilities and control, this floc produces very satisfactory removals by gentle mechanical enmeshing. The process has been described as "sweep floc action." In water of higher turbidity, destabilization of colloids at proper alum doses takes place through the action of the aquo complex ion. One example of a hydrolytic reaction which results in forms which destabilize colloids is

$$Al(H_2O)_6^{+++} + H_2O \longrightarrow Al(H_2O)_5(OH)^{++} + H_3O^+$$

This illustrates the complexity of the ions that are formed and active. For an extended examination of this action, see O'Melia.[1]

Other investigators have evidence that one or more of the following multivalent polymeric cations are formed:

$$Al_6(OH)_{15}^{+++} \qquad Al_7(OH)_{17}^{+++} \qquad Al_8(OH)_{20}^{+++} \qquad Al_{13}(OH)_{34}^{+++++}$$

These complex ions alter the behavior of colloids by a process called *bridging* and by affecting the charge states. These mechanisms explain the destabilization in high-turbidity waters.[2] The chemistry of very dilute aqueous solutions is complicated. Behavior changes with slight qualitative and quantitative differences in ionic makeup. Few chemists have been called to study these matters as the economics are not pressing. The use of more costly polyelectrolytes will require more knowledge of coagulation reactions.

Chlorination John L. Leal reported on the routine use of chloride of lime to kill bacteria in the Jersey City public water supply in 1908. Within 10 years many plants throughout the United States were adding chlorine. The results were frequently uncertain as the nature of chlorine reactions in water were known incompletely and dosage was haphazard. The paper by Abel Wolman and Lynn Enslow in 1919, Chlorine Absorption and the Chlorination of Water, is reprinted in Ref. 3-9 (p. 42). It illustrates the efforts of a state health department staff to reconcile records and results of chlorine use among a couple of dozen public supplies. It states, "The importance of the absorption of so-called 'active chlorine' by different waters is somewhat ill defined in its relation to disinfection or the elimination of objectionable bacterial life." In the 50 years which followed, numerous investigators have contributed to the chemistry of chlorination of water.

[1] *Public Works*, **100**:97 (1969).
[2] J. W. Moffett, The Chemistry of High-Rate Water Treatment, *JAWWA*, **60**:1255 (1968).

When elemental chlorine reacts with water free of ammonia, organic nitrogen, other organics, and reduced inorganics, the following reversible reactions occur:

$$Cl_2 + H_2O \rightleftharpoons HOCl + H^+ + Cl^-$$

at a pH above 3, the reaction is wholly to the right

$$HOCl \rightleftharpoons H^+ + OCl^-$$

The HOCl, hypochlorous acid, and OCl^-, hypochlorite ion, are the free available chlorine which provides quite rapid bacterial kills. The lower the pH, the more of the free chlorine is HOCl and correspondingly the more effective the killing power of a given concentration, as indicated by the curve in Fig. 3-11. In usual waterworks practice, the first chlorine dose is at coagulation, which carries the pH to 6.5 or less. At pH 6.5 and at 20°C (68°F), 90 percent of the free chlorine is HOCl. The acid HOCl has a higher killing efficiency than OCl^- by the ratio of about 80:1. Without making a temperature correction, Fig. 3-11 shows that less free chlorine than 0.006 mg/l would kill 99 percent of *E. coli* at pH 6.5 in 30 min. In a flocculating and settling basin sequence, the pH would be favorable and time ample. However, there would be a few other chlorine reactions underway, the same ones which raised doubts in the minds of Wolman and Enslow in 1918 on the relation of chlorine absorption and disinfection.

Among the reactants demanding chlorine in raw water to form chloramines are ammonia and organic nitrogen.

$$NH_3 + HOCl \longrightarrow NH_2Cl + H_2O$$

This monochloramine production predominates at a pH above 6 and at a molar ratio of chlorine to ammonia of 1:1 or less.

$$NH_2Cl + HOCl \longrightarrow NHCl_2 + H_2O$$

Dichloramine is produced in much smaller amounts than monochloramine at equimolar concentrations of chlorine and ammonia and at the same pH and temperature.

$$NHCl_2 + HOCl \longrightarrow NCl_3 + H_2O$$

This formation of nitrogen trichloride is slight in normal pH ranges until nearly all the ammonia has been acted upon, which means the *breakpoint* is at hand.

Other chlorine reactions produce organic chloramines, traces of substitution and addition products with organic compounds, the oxidation of Fe^{++}, Mn^{++}, NO_2^-, and H_2S, and of unidentified taste and odor components. These reactions are the reason for the versatility of chlorine for water treatment. The chlorine requirement to carry all these reactions to completion is the chlorine demand. Good practice is to

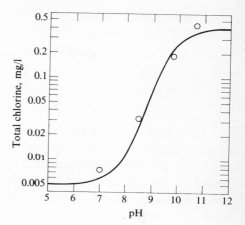

FIGURE 3-11
The concentration of free available chlorine required for 99 percent kill of *E. coli* in 30 min at 2 to 5°C. [*Source: Ref.* 3-2, (*vol.* 2, *p.* 31-38).]

provide enough chlorine and contact time to meet the demand so that a free, available chlorine residual remains to sustain disinfection.   The oxidation of ammonia so that there is no concurrent mono- or dichloramine requires about 2 moles of chlorine per mole of ammonia.   This is about a ratio of 10:1 by weight.   Chlorinating to the required concentration is breakpoint chlorination.   It guarantees a free, available chlorine residual.   For speedy disinfection in distribution systems, and in swimming pools, breakpoint chlorination is necessary.

WATER FOR RECREATION

Recreational uses with particular protection and control are swimming in natural sites, water skiing, surfing, and boating, artificial pools for swimming and wading, and fishing.   For most of these uses Ref. 3-10 provides extensive background information and presents utilitarian judgments.

Natural Waters for Swimming, Skiing, and Surfing

The treasured bit of the American past, "the old swimming hole," presents an epidemiological and bacteriological paradox.   So do the expanses of beaches along Chicago's Lake Michigan front, and the variety of river, sound, and ocean beaches in and about New York City.   Coliform MPN values shoot up into several thousand per 100 ml; yet there are no devastating waterborne disease outbreaks among the swimmers.   Even among closely observed summer camp groups on lake and river sites, there has been only one reported outbreak, that of bacillary dysentery in a camp on an Indiana lake.   The lack of a correlation between high coliform counts and the presence of disease among swimmers raises three questions:

1   What is the origin of the coliforms observed?
2   How much ingestion of water is there during swimming?
3   Are swimmers healthy specimens with a good chance of having a high resistance to waterborne infections?

This lack of a correlation prompted the U.S. Public Health Service to do epidemiological-environmental field studies at Chicago beaches in 1948, on Ohio River beaches at Dayton and Bellevue, Kentucky, in 1949, and on the Long Island Sound beaches at New Rochelle and Mamaroneck, New York, in 1950 in saline tidal waters. The epidemiological index was any illness, respiratory, ear, eye, skin, or gastrointestinal.   The water quality index was the total coliform MPN.

The findings summarized by A. H. Stevenson[1] showed:

1   Swimmers had a higher overall incidence of all illnesses than nonswimmers.
2   Those swimmers under 10 years of age had a 100 percent higher incidence of illness than those over 10.
3   Of the illnesses reported, 20 percent were gastrointestinal; 50 percent were eye, ear, nose, and throat ailments; and the balance were skin and others.
4   On the Chicago beaches after three successive days with coliform MPNs over 2,300/100 ml, there was for a time a significant increase in reported illness.
5   On the Ohio River, the gastrointestinal illness rate was substantially higher than in the other groups studied.   When the median coliform density of the Ohio rose to 2,700/100 ml, a significant increase in disease was reported.

The National Technical Advisory Committee on Water Quality Criteria used these findings to set a bacteriological limit for primary-contact recreation waters, that is, for water uses during which ingestion occurs: swimming, skiing, surfing, and wading. The limit set is in terms of fecal coliforms.   In a minimum of 5 samples in 30 days, the fecal coliforms shall not exceed a logarithmic mean of 200/100 ml, nor shall more than 10 percent of total samples in 30 days exceed 400/100 ml.   How did these numbers evolve from the Public Health Service studies?   "An epidemiologically detectable health effect" level was cited as 2,300 to 2,400 coliforms per 100 ml.   Later, Ohio River water studies showed that 18 percent of total coliform were fecal coliform. That moves the detectable health effect level for fecal coliforms to 400/100 ml.   A factor of safety moves it to 200/100 ml.   Furthermore, the Committee cites the findings of the Santee, California, project on sewage renovation.   That data showed one plaque-forming unit per milliliter can be expected in treated sewage, with one

[1] *AJPHA*, **43**:529 (1953).

virus particle per 10,000 fecal coliforms. Thus, "A bathing water with 400 fecal coliforms per 100 ml could be expected to have 0.02 virus particles per 100 ml (one virus particle per 5,000 ml)." (Ref. 3-10, p. 12.) The implication is that viruses will be at very low concentrations in natural waters with 200 fecal coliforms per 100 ml.

The variables in natural waters are too great to permit so fixed a guide value. The "sanitary survey"—a diligent search for the sources of recent human excreta discharged into water that is being assessed for its relative hygienic safety—has an absolute requirement that a professional judgment be rendered. Even in that process, the expediencies of living in a real world must be accepted. This is borne out in the comparison of the TVA's ranking of swimming sites along its chain of man-made lakes in the still relatively undespoiled Tennessee River basin and the classification adopted by the Board of Health for waters in New York City. The City Board sought to protect its poor, who can get to the beaches by subway, from the risks of waterborne disease, but did not want to deny these millions an escape from their hot, crowded tenement streets to shore breezes and a cooling dip in waters much below pristine wilderness quality. Table 3-16 summarizes the stance of the two agencies. The coliform bacteria content of the water is the initial criterion, but the "sanitary survey" is used in both instances for further classification. The New York Board takes its final stand on positive epidemiological evidence of illness before the last step of prohibition.

A second guide line of the National Technical Advisory Committee on Water Quality Criteria is on the range of pH of primary-contact recreation waters. One of its members, Professor Eric Mood of Yale University, has carefully documented the effects of the pH of swimming waters on eyes. The lacrimal fluid of the human eye maintains a pH close to 7.4 with complex organic buffering agents. Excessive exposure to liquids of other pH exhaust the buffer and a variety of irritations and visual disturbances of blurring, rainbows, and tearing result. A range of 6.5 to 8.3 pH is recommended with provisos for exceptional natural causes and with limits on discharging buffering wastes to waters outside the range.

Swimming Pool Waters

"Swim in Drinking Water" is the advertising message of Wallace and Tiernan, a large United States manufacturer of chemical dosing machines for water and food processing. Modern recirculation purification systems for pool water can achieve that with filtration through pressure sand or diatomaceous earth filters and disinfection, usually with chlorine from gas cylinders or calcium hypochlorite formulations. With proper design, construction, and operation, such systems can produce water with coliform counts and turbidity readings equal to drinking water. The question is, "Is that good enough?" Certainly it is for protection against transmission of gastrointestinal disease during pool use.   But drinking water quality is not directed to the factors in pool use which influence eye, ear, nose, throat, and skin disorders and infections.   In fact, any set of water quality standards for pool water may be no more than secondary contributors to a defense line against these.

The biological fact is that man is poorly equipped for prolonged aquatic exposure.   He has too many body openings exposed.   His membrane coatings are not developed for such exposure.   His skin is barely satisfactory for land exposure without considerable cover.   His thermal adaptive responses are poor for water immersion. With these deficiencies in mind, the reasons that have been given for the high incidence of eye, ear, respiratory, and skin disorders among swimmers are:

Table 3-16   A COMPARISON OF THE CRITERIA AND CLASSIFICATIONS OF SWIMMING WATERS BY THE TENNESSEE VALLEY AUTHORITY AND THE BOARD OF HEALTH OF NEW YORK CITY

N.Y.C. Board of Health	Total coliforms, MPN per 100 ml	Tenn. Valley Authority
	Under 50	Preferred sanitary quality.
	50–500	Normal contamination from surface wash; satisfactory if free of detrimental sewage; sanitary survey and epidemiological data do not indicate human fecal contamination.
Class A, Group 1, approved; sanitary survey and epidemiological data satisfactory.	Under 1,000	
	500–1,000	Somewhat suspicious and dangerous if in proximity to fresh sewage.
	Over 1,000	Not recommended unless san. survey shows the reason for high density and that its cause is found to be harmless.
Class A, Group 2, approved; epidemiol. data satisfactory; san. survey shows pollution increasing.	Over 1,000, but under 2,400	
Class B, not recommended, but *not* prohibited; san. survey shows sewage on beach and in water; epidemiol. data satisfactory.	Over 2,400 and 50% of samples over 2,400	
Class C, prohibited; epidemiol. data disclose evidence of infection incident to using the beach.		

1 Washing away of normal protective coatings, including the eye's lacrimal fluids.
2 Autoinfection by existing microflora after the protective coatings are reduced or by pressure penetration as for ear infections.
3 Chilling the body, which reduces resistance to infections.
4 Some transfer of mucous from man to man before the pool disinfectant can penetrate the encapsulating material to kill infectious organisms;
5 A combination of these factors with ample variation among individuals and conditions.

To these are added the extra-pool-water contacts of wet decks, floors, shower stalls, dirty footbaths, and on occasions, common towel and swimsuit reuse without adequate laundering.

The American Public Health Association's committee on swimming pools and other bathing places have recommendations which are revised from time to time. The last official recommendations are of 1957, with a suggested ordinance and regulations in 1964. The recommendations for bacteriological quality of pool water are:

1 Not more than 15 percent of samples shall have a total of undifferentiated bacterial colonies that is more than 200/ml.
2 Not more than 15 percent of the samples shall have any positive coliform portions.

The recommendation on disinfection is that the pool water have a free available chlorine residual of 0.4 to 1.0 mg/l. Efforts to update recommendations on disinfectants have not resulted in approved agreement to 1970. The bacteriological requirement is not satisfactory as the time of sampling, frequency of sampling, and place and number of sampling points are not specified. Without a number and frequency specification, the requirement cannot be interpreted as an MPN.

The literature on the bacteriology of swimming pool water is replete with proposals and studies on more sensitive bacterial indices than the coliform. *Streptococci* and *Neisseria* species have been found in pool water. The number of streptococci has been correlated with swimmer loads, disinfectant concentrations, and coliform recoveries. The failure of new proposals to be adopted is:

1 There is no compelling epidemiological emergency or even evidence to favor one index organism over another.
2 Pool use is still largely seasonal; no health jurisdiction has a large number of public pools to control, and therefore it is most convenient to handle pool samples by the same methods as other water samples.

In a like vein, chlorine is the disinfectant choice for pool waters, as assistance in its use is readily available from water departments and equipment or material suppliers. It is familiar to health department sanitarians and engineers. A variety of reliable feeders from liquefied gas and hypochlorite solutions sources are marketed in a broad price range. Its disadvantages are the dissipation by ultraviolet action in a pool under heavy swimmer loads on hot sunny days, and the odor of chlorinous complexes when dosage is not skillfully adjusted to changing demands. The competing agents, iodine, bromine, and chlorinated cyanurates, have not been widely adopted despite the advantages which outweigh their individual disadvantages. The most extensive work in laboratory and field testing and development of these agents has been on iodine by A. P. Black and his associates of the University of Florida.[1]

For Fish, Shellfish, and Waterfowl

Water quality to support these forms of life has commercial, recreational, and esthetic values to man egocentrically. More vitally, it is a determinant in species survival which man influences knowingly or unknowingly in his use of water as a resource or as a waste sink. The complex of physical and biochemical factors which support all aquatic life and the waterfowl dependent on it, and which assures their reproduction, is just beginning to be known. The aquatic life now evolved has some tolerance for the natural cyclic variations of temperatures, tides, and flows. The range of tolerance is not great for any species and dismayingly narrow for some, with dissolved oxygen and fish an example. Man-made changes may be only moderately disturbing or drastically disrupting, immediately obvious or slow in changing an existing balance. The variety of conditions which can upset the balance for one species is multiplied by the responses set off in other species dependent on the first by predation or symbiosis or on environmental modifications maintained by the first species. A review of requirements covers the essential chemical and physical factors, including the conditions needed for light penetration to power photosynthesis, and the obviously detrimental pollutants and contaminants that destroy life.

Temperature is a determinant of the biological regime which gets established. The maximum temperatures recommended for several fish species is given in Table 3-17 (Ref. 3-10, p. 33). The temperature rises and rates of rise determine whether a species stays in a habitat. Lake fish move away if possible when the temperature rise is more than $3°F$ (or $1.5°C$) above an existing ambient level. River fish can withstand a rise of $5°F$ ($3°C$). Saline water fish can tolerate a $4°F$ ($2°C$) change in the cool months, September to May, in the north temperate zone, but only a 1 to $2°F$ (0.5 to $1°C$) in the summer months, June through August, in the north temperate zone. Rises of $1°F/h$ (or $0.5°C/h$) or more can be disastrous and even make an escape impossible. Fish have been observed to become torpid in waters of rapidly rising temperature, and to abandon efforts to swim to cooler waters.

[1] For reprints, address the Chilean Iodine Educational Bureau, Inc., 120 Broadway, New York, N.Y. 10005.

These consequences along with the replacement of existing regimes with an altered biology fitted to higher temperatures have aroused concern for thermal overloads, particularly from electricity generating stations. Furthermore, nuclear-fueled stations of present designs must dissipate from 25 to 30 percent more heat than fossil-fueled plants of equal generating capacity. With the expectation that in the United States before 2000, one-half of our total electricity will come from nuclear-fueled stations, thermal loads from condenser cooling waters will have to be handled differently than at present. As inland lake populations are most sensitive to temperature rises and such waters have limited circulation, generating plants on lakes have been most suspect.[1] Power demands will impose solutions. Alternatives are:

1 Air-cooled condensers with the handicaps at present result in cooling towers with massive structures, high evaporative losses, localized fogs, and some radioactive releases
2 Man-made cooling ponds of immense size, presumably with special variances on what water quality and aquatic environment must be maintained
3 Continued work to develop nuclear-reactor heat-utilization systems with smaller amounts of heat to be dissipated

Table 3-17 PROVISIONAL MAXIMUM TEMPERATURES RECOMMENDED AS COMPATIBLE WITH THE WELL-BEING OF VARIOUS SPECIES OF FISH AND THEIR ASSOCIATED BIOTA

34°C	93°F	Growth of catfish, gar, white or yellow bass, spotted bass, buffalo, carpsucker, threadfin shad, and gizzard shad
32°C	90°F	Growth of largemouth bass, drum, bluegill, and crappie
29°C	84°F	Growth of pike, perch, walleye, smallmouth bass, and sauger
27°C	80°F	Spawning and egg development of catfish, buffalo, threadfin shad, and gizzard shad
24°C	75°F	Spawning and egg development of largemouth bass, white and yellow bass, and spotted bass
18°C	65°F	Growth or migration of salmonids and egg development of perch and smallmouth bass
13°C	55°F	Spawning and egg development of salmon and trout (other than lake trout)
7°C	45°F	Spawning and egg development of lake trout, walleye, northern pike, sauger, and Atlantic salmon

Note: Recommended temperatures for other species not listed above may be established when necessary information becomes available.
SOURCE: Water Quality Criteria, Natl. Tech. Advis. Comm. Secr. Inter. Rep., table 3-1, 1968, p. 33.

[1] Dorothy Melkin, "Nuclear Power and Its Critics: The Cayuga Lake Controversy," Program Sci., Technol. Soc., Cornell Univ., Ithaca, N.Y., 1970.

4 Heat recovery systems as by soil heating, for large hothouses for year-round horticulture
5 Controlled discharges to benefit an existing or acceptable ecosystem by thermal enrichment

The minimum dissolved-oxygen concentrations for maintaining a good variety of aquatic life is from 5 to 7 mg/l for fresh waters, a minimum of 5 mg/l for coastal ocean reaches, and of 4 mg/l for estuaries. Waterfowl require that boundary-waters' bottom deposit remain aerobic, as anaerobic conditions produce botulinus bacteria infections in water birds that are bottom feeders. Freshwater species do best in waters with total dissolved solids under 1,500 mg/l. Saline-water regimes remain stable when the isohalines do not shift more than 10 percent in a body of water. Isohalines, defining zones of equal salinity, are analogous to equal-elevation contour lines. The pH range of freshwaters with a varied biological distribution is 6 to 9. For saline waters the range is narrower, 6.5 to 8.5. The mixed biota which feeds waterfowl grows well during the summer in a pH range of 7.0 to 9.2. The carbonate cycle is reflected in pH and alkalinity. Its orderly participation in the energy cycle requires that in freshwaters the total alkalinity not drop below 20 mg/l, and that for waterfowl habitats a bicarbonate alkalinity range of 30 to 130 mg/l be stable with fluctuations of less than 50 mg/l from natural conditions. Man-made structures and alterations of channels change currents and tides. Unless basin geometry and freshwater inflows are substantially maintained, changes in biological regimes will occur. In all these matters, what changes are acceptable is a continuous and bitter controversy between conservationists and the economic developers to whom man's use, and theirs particularly, is paramount and overriding.

Light penetration maintains photosynthesis by phytoplankton which provide food and nutrient balance and release oxygen. Turbidity, color, and surface filth reduce transparency. For good photosynthesis 10 percent of the surface incident light should penetrate to a 6-ft depth. Wild waterfowl are most sensitive to this need as their food depends on it. Their tolerance is a 5 percent penetration to the 6-ft level. Light penetration is readily estimated by lowering a Secchi disc until it cannot be seen. The disc is 20 cm in diameter with two white and two black quadrants.

Injurious conditions are those which despoil the habitat so that the usual forms of life leave or disappear, those which change the nutrient balance, and those which bring specific toxicants into the area and kill off one or more species. Settleable and floatable solids and oil in persistent visible amounts start off the sequence of driving out aquatic life or they alter it drastically. One early result is tainted flavors in the eatable fish in commercial and game catches. The nutrient balance is the product of at least five phenomena:

1   The carbonate cycle
2   The nitrogen cycle
3   The phosphate cycle
4   The level of photosynthesis
5   The maintenance of aerobic processes

There are optimal ratios of NO_3^-/N and PO_4^{--}/P for varied regimes.   As the balance becomes tipped some species become predominant and the environment becomes unfavorable for many others.   The rise in phosphates in lakes of low replacement, as Wisconsin glacial lakes, of vast shallows as Lake Erie, or of very ancient origin as Lake Constance in Europe have produced a nutrient cycle highly favorable for great increases in algae growth.   This is *eutrophication*, from the Greek word *eutrophos* meaning "well nourished."   In very long time cycles of geological dimensions, all lakes move that way.   The recycling and building up of phosphates is a factor. Recent Canadian studies suggest that to incriminate phosphates alone is a simplification.   Man's increment of phosphates from heavily fertilized field runoff, from detergents, and from treated domestic sewage speeds the process.   The algae bloom is an overabundant phosphate feeding, with other life unable to keep the balance.   This can be readily observed in artificial farm ponds in which the owner fertilizes the pond directly in hope of speeding fish growth.   The overfed algae blot out everything else and cover the pond with an unattractive green slime.

The specific toxicants of aquatic life include several of the notorious culprits that appear in our food and air, as well as water.   There are the heavy metals, Cu, Hg, Pb, and Zn, the cyanides, ammonia, and the residues of pesticides, weedicides, and surfactants.   Certainly the heavy metals have been in water since the cycle of life began and are a part of the evolutionary process.   It would be most useful to know the amount of mercury and other heavy metals there is in fish tissue from waters not subject even to small wastage from man.   The issue which must now be faced is the increased quantities of toxicant wastes and the concentration of dumpers in certain regions of the world.   An example is the mercury discharge into the Baltic Sea, which has a very low water throughput.   The combination of discharges and low throughput has overwhelmed the assimilative capacity of the aquatic environment of the Baltic Sea for certain toxic forms of mercury.   Reports of the meticulous efforts of scientists over the world to delineate these phenomena are in *Chemical Fallout* (Ref. 3-11), the proceedings of an international conference on toxicity at the University of Rochester, New York, in 1968.   Water Quality Criteria (Ref. 3-10, pp. 39–96) provides detailed data in a systematic way on the quality requirements briefly cited here for fresh and saline aquatic life and waterfowl.   From the present tribulations on environmental quality there must come the prudent use of the assimilative capacity of the environment for all forms of man's wastes.

Man's Adverse Effects on Recreational Waters

The conservationists dramatically and pictorially have appealed, and now frequently capture our support by calling to our attention the results of man's pollutants on wild-life dependent on clean water for survival. The oil-soaked waterfowl, the dead up-turned fish, the green slime on lakes, and the trash-laden beaches are well displayed in newspaper and magazine photographs and on the TV screen. These are realities. Some are one-shot, acute episodes of offshore oil- and gas-well blowouts and leaks, of oil-transport-tanker collisions, groundings, breakups, or fires, of spills from flooded waste-lagoons, of storm or earthquake dismemberment of man-made structures built to hold our wastes in storage. Others are the uncovering of long-standing practices of offshore disposal of unwanted materials. In the United States the Department of Defense has had to meet the people's consternation that its subordinate agencies have been literally dumping toxic gases and waste oil into the world's oceans as a matter of course. Large industries and municipalities use the ocean for their waste residuals, particularly sludges from treatment processes. Frequency and quantity are the items which kill the game.

Far more subtle and capable of more lasting damage are the waste-disposal habits of those who use recreational waters most intensively. These are the boating devotees, ranging from offshore sailing to houseboat anchoring, and the onshore resort cottage and cabin dwellers on ocean beaches, on the margins of man-made and natural lakes of all sizes, and in the mountain retreats on upland streams. In these settings man keeps on generating his wastes, his own excreta and the liquid and solid wastes from his eating, drinking, and washing. Again it is the frequency or intensity and the quantity which make unconcerned disposal impossible. Henry Thoreau did not need to concern himself with his wastes' polluting Walden Pond. The thousands who now share that beautiful site each year must do so even if at the necessity of suf-fering the compulsory restrictions imposed by the Town of Concord, an institutional creature of some of the thousands.

The point is well made by considering the disposal of human excreta from boats on inland waters in the United States. The number of people, of boats, and of the hours onboard and the length of travel has increased enormously in the last 10 years. The U.S. Coast Guard had 4.9 million boats registered in 1970. About 10 percent of these had toilets of some sort. Obviously a very large percentage are open runabouts with no practical means of toilet facilities and presumably on short-run use. Marinas have become a United States weekend and vacation institution. These are community anchorages for watercraft of all sorts from cabin cruisers to houseboats. Originally conceived as a place to go from, these facilities are increasingly a place to go to—for the weekend. Observations of the North Carolina Wildlife Protection Service, con-firmed by marina managers, are that many patrons on North Carolina inland lakes never castoff, start a motor, or raise a sail for their weekend stay. The marina is a compact floating village, much like those in parts of Southeast Asia.

Such marina use and clusters of resort homes present difficult waste disposal needs as there usually is no planning at the start. Often there is little thought of growth or intensity of use. The thing just grows and staggers from inadequate roads to the lack of parking space to poor drainage to the need for fire protection, water supply, and waste control and disposal. Only electrical power comes rather easily. These situations are not solely in the United States. These are repeated and are intensifying in beautiful natural areas outside of the capital cities of South and Central America, such as Lakes Amatitlan and Atitlan in Guatemala, along the Mediterranean coves of Italy, France, and Spain, and in the mountain retreats of Norway. Advanced planning and controlled land and water use are the necessary price to prevent ruin of the very resources which make these places attractive and precious. Ingenious application of the principles of environmental hygiene and community organization are needed. Illustrations are the construction of community waterlines and sewers about Lake Lure, North Carolina, before land sale was started in the 1930s; the modification of jet-airliner recirculating flush toilets for small cabin-cruiser and camper-trailer installation by the Monomatic Company of California; the decision of the government of Norway to establish a unit of the health services to develop and implement methods for the environmental sanitation and protection of a variety of vacation and resort facilities. In the United States, the Public Health Service and the National Park Service have worked together for many years to meet such needs in our national park areas, using both sophisticated and simple procedures.

WATER FOR AGRICULTURE

Farmstead water needs including drinking-culinary use and livestock watering are readily met in all but the most arid regions. The quality criteria for farmstead use are those for drinking water. Dairy-farm water requires concentrations of iron and copper of not more than 0.1 mg/l, which is less than Public Health Service Drinking Water Standards. The bacteriological quality for dairy-farm use must meet the needs of on-farm bulk storage tanks and in-place milk piping. To prevent the buildup of undesirable bacterial growths which cause "ropy" milk and off-flavors, the cleaning water should contain no more than 20 bacteria per milliliter and not more than 5 lypolytic and proteolytic bacteria per milliliter. One of the boons of the milk sanitation efforts that began in the United States in the 1920s was safe, abundant water under pressure for the farm family as it shared the improved supply required for the milk house and dairy barn.

Livestock water should be comparable to human-use water in permissible toxic element content. Fluoride content for cattle should not exceed 2.4 mg/l. Farm animals can tolerate total dissolved solids to 10,000 mg/l, which is 1 percent. Poultry prefer water with total dissolved solids not in excess of 3,000 mg/l. Algae blooms on watering ponds are objectionable. Livestock water should be free from infectious quantities of pathogenic microorganisms and parasites. Among those which cause trouble are:

1 Bacteria: salmonella, *Bacillus anthracis*, leptospira, and clostridia
2 Viruses which cause pox, hog cholera, blue tongue in sheep and cattle, and three not present in the United States—foot-and-mouth disease, Teschen's disease of swine, and African horse sickness
3 Parasites: flukes and strongyloids are likely to be waterborne, roundworms occasionally, and tapeworms rarely.

The sign of trouble is infection in the livestock. Control requires isolation and elimination or treatment of the sick, and finding alternative water sources. Prevention depends on cleanliness, good nutrition, and on not crowding barns, yards, pens, fields, or watering places.

Irrigation is the tremendous agricultural water use. Figure 3-1 shows that in the United States it equals industrial water use at 159 million acre · feet per year, 3.4 percent of the country's total annual rainfall. Irrigation use is increasing in the United States, spreading eastward as a routine practice on high market crops such as vegetables and tobacco. The increase is worldwide as higher yields are sought from semiarid lands and new areas are cultivated to feed rising populations. The bitter paradox is that each step in irrigation worsens the very quality of the water most vital to its function. A low-salinity water is necessary for irrigation, as the concentration of salts in arid soils must be leached so that the plant root systems have selectively lower concentrates in the water to move up into the plants by capillarity for nutrition and eventually transpiration. In semiarid and arid regions, the first step of collection during rainy seasons and of storage in reservoirs exposes large surfaces to evaporation. In the western United States annual evaporative losses are about 35 percent of the total reservoir capacity. At 15 million acre · feet per year, these losses at the reservoir are nearly 10 percent of the country's annual irrigation use. Worse yet, the salts are concentrated with a loss of leaching capacity. Evaporation continues along the usual distribution system of main canals, subcanals, and laterals. Transpiration by plants in and along these channels further concentrates the salts in the water as it heads for its leaching task. There's a repeat, of course, during the field spread.

In regions where these waters are used again and again along the drainage basin, with due allowance for seepage into the earth and for replenishment by lower tributaries, the concentration of salt mounts. To compensate, larger quantities of water are applied to gain the minimally needed leaching to produce a crop. These phenomena have been long studied by agricultural scientists. The concentration of salts and its effect are expressed by:

1 SS, the solute suction or osmotic pressure of the soil water
2 EC_e, electrical conductivity of the saturation effect
3 SAR, sodium absorption ratio

Crops are well identified in terms of salt tolerance. Celery, green beans, most clovers, and most of our fruit trees are examples of crops with a low salt tolerance. Beets, spinach, barley, cotton, date palm, and most grasses have a high salt tolerance. Detailed listings with EC_e ranges are in Ref. 3-10 (p. 150).

The importance of the SAR is that it provides an indicator of the effect of sodium on the soil. The effect is very drastic as it is a reduction of the soil's permeability to air and water. When the sodium concentration is high in ratio to the calcium and magnesium, the soil becomes plastic and sticky. This phenomenon along with salts left by evaporation destroyed the yields of the fertile soils of ancient Mesopotamia after centuries of irrigation. The problems of waterlogging of the irrigated land of the Indus River in West Pakistan in our times are the same. With the concentrations in milliequivalents per liter, the SAR is an integer by

$$SAR = \frac{Na}{\sqrt{(Ca + Mg)/2}}$$

An SAR of 8 is satisfactory, 12 to 15 is marginal, and over 20 is very disadvantageous. The SAR in combination with total salt content determines the suitability of a water for irrigation. With higher salt content, higher sodium concentrations can be accepted (Ref. 3-10, pp. 164–166).

There are 20 elements from Al to Zn for which desirable maxima have been recognized. These include phytotoxins such as As, Be, Cd, Cr, Co, Pb, Li, Mn, Ni, V, and Zn. Others have effects on certain species for which limits are set, such as Al, B, Cu, Mo. Of these, boron has been most troublesome in irrigation waters. Boron up to 0.5 mg/l is an essential nutrient. There are gradations of crop tolerance to 4 mg/l, beyond which the water is unsatisfactory. High-boron waters come off the California coastal range and from the Hot Creek area in Owens Valley on the eastern slope of the Sierra Nevada in California. For a classification of crops as tolerant, semitolerant, and sensitive to boron, see Ref. 3-10 (p. 153). Data on the effects of herbicide residues on crops are in a table, Levels of Herbicides in Irrigation Waters, in Ref. 3-10 (pp. 158–159); these cover 15 compounds. The quotation that follows summarizes the issue on insecticide and herbicide residues (Ref. 3-10, p. 157).

There is little evidence to indicate that under normal use insecticide contamination of irrigation water would be detrimental to plant growth or accumulate in or on plants in toxic concentrations.   Herbicides, on the other hand, could be harmful to crop growth if misused.   Since many herbicides break down in water, permissible limits should be established for the point of application to crops.

The very purpose of irrigation is to leach salts from the soil; therefore, total dissolved solids increase.   With this, the other components which rise are hardness, chlorides, sodium in ratio to calcium and magnesium (the SAR), phosphorous content, and usually turbidity, color, taste, and odor.   In short, irrigation use causes a degradation of quality.   About one-third of the flow diverted for irrigation returns to the usable resource pool of surface water or groundwater.   It varies from one-fifth to three-fifths, with one-third an average.   The rest returns to the hydrological cycle as vapor by evaporation and transpiration.   As the vapor carries virtually no dissolved solids, a threefold salt concentration would be the minimum expected in the returned water.   In fact, the concentration factor is from 5 to 10 as the water is used more than once along a major basin, as much of the return flow is less than one-third and as the percolating water gains ionic content by solution and ion exchange.   Part of the increment is the nitrates and phosphates from fertilized fields.   That load is also carried by rainfall runoff and adds to the nitrate and phosphate nutrition of surface waters.   When in excess as for low-circulation lakes, the addition is a contributor to eutrophication.

In arid and semiarid areas, streamflow is meager most of the year, and shallow groundwater is limited.   The returned irrigation water with its five- to tenfold increase in dissolved solids and other degraded qualities gets very little dilution.   It is a pollution that is less evident than organic pollutants which deoxygenate the receiving waters and produce visible and smellable changes.   These inorganic loads from irrigation use are a long-term degradation.   This impairs the quality for downstream irrigation reuse and for other beneficial industry use requiring a low content of dissolved solids and for public supply without the added costs of demineralizing.   McGauhey (Ref. 3-6, pp. 65–66), cites the dilemma of the San Luis Drain in California.   This is a vast diversion of water to the head of the San Joaquin Valley in California for irrigation, for groundwater supplementation, and for the public and private needs of an increasing population.   The great volume of wastewater will be so increased in salt content that adding it to the San Joaquin River will deteriorate the quality of the groundwater strata replenished by riverbed percolation and will alter the salinity of the San Francisco Bay at the mouth of the San Joaquin.   On the matter of returned irrigation waters, McGauhey writes:

> The unfortunate prospect at this point in time is that agricultural use of water will contribute in a major way to the long-term decline in the mineral quality of the water resources in some areas unless better systems for managing the quality of its return

waters are forthcoming. . . . [He sees] but little preparation in either policy or technology for upgrading the quality of return waters from agricultural use.

Coming from a sanitary engineering teacher and investigator with a distinguished record for his creative and imaginative work, that is sheer pessimism.

WATER FOR INDUSTRY

A prediction for 1980 is that United States industry will use 360 billion gallons of water per day, agriculture 150 Bgd and municipal use (public supplies) 36 Bgd.   While all uses are rising, industry use is rising faster.   In 1960 industry accounted for 50 percent of the total daily 325 Bgd.   In 1980 the predicted 360-Bgd use by industry is based on 65 percent of a total 550 Bgd.   These are prodigious amounts of water.   It is further customary and impressive to state industry's water use in gallons per unit of product. Examples are from 12,000 to 16,000 gallons per automobile built; from 1,400 to 65,000 gallons per ton of steel, from 2 to 50 gallons per gallon of crude oil refined, from 120 to 650 gallons per glass bottle formed, from 15 to 300 gallons per pound of synthetic rubber made, and 20,000 gallons per ton of bleached pulp and paper.   A look at the wide ranges shows that use depends on ease of availability.   The low figure for steel is that of the Kaiser Fontana Plant in Southern California.   There, every drop of water is worked through recycling and recovery, as sources are scant.   The high figure is typical of steel works in the Pittsburgh area where the abundant flow of the Allegheny and Monogahela Rivers join to form the mighty Ohio.

Ninety-one percent of the water used by industry is taken for use "as is," although additives may be used to control slimes and corrosion.   Only 9 percent is treated on site or taken from the public supply to meet special quality requirements. The reason for this is that 90 percent of industry's use is for condensing and cooling. Only 8 percent is process water in direct contact with the raw and finished materials. There is 2 percent which is boiler feed water.   All but a few percent of industry's needs are met by water far from drinking quality.   Thirty per cent of its water is brackish with dissolved solids from 1,000 to 35,000 mg/l.   Nor is recycling new to industrial water use.   Fully 45 percent of its use is recycled water, particularly in refrigeration condensing systems and cooling ponds.   In these, the losses are confined to evaporation.

To industry, water is a raw material which must be of a quality fitted to its use. Whenever it can be used as it is, that is the choice.   The availability of water suited to needs is a consideration in plant siting.   Water used in textile dyeing is near distilled water in quality.   Water used in rayon manufacture must meet a maximum turbidity of 0.3 unit.   Bleached chemically pulped paper requires a water equal to Drinking Water Standards for manganese, 0.05 mg/l, and not more than one-third the standard for iron.   Water for brewing beer must be adjusted to a pH of 6.5 to 7.   Soft drink bottlers use water at Drinking Water Standards passed through activated carbon filters to remove all traces of tastes and odors.   Canned-food process water requires drinking water quality, with particular attention to F^- and NO_3^- content for baby foods. Boiler-feed-water requirements are increasingly demanding as the system pressure rises.   The quality of water fed to the boilers of fossil-fueled generating stations is virtually at the levels of detectability of our water analysis methods, that is, zero by test; dissolved solids 0.5 mg/l; dissolved oxygen 0.007 mg/l; silica, aluminum, copper, and iron each at 0.01 mg/l.   However conscious of the quality of water entering the plant, management in the past has discharged the used water in whatever condition the traffic would bear.   The needs of downstream plants crowded into a tightening water economy, public expectations and demands, and slowly a stiffer backbone in the regulatory agencies, together, are bringing changes.

POSSIBLE CHANGES AND DEVELOPMENTS

Water demand and use will continue to rise.   Quality goals will be held high by the initiative of the professional societies.   Epidemiological evidence of waterborne viral diseases, of carcinogenesis, and of low-level toxicant damage will be sought, with poor prospects for success by present methods.   The lack of evidence will confound the problem of legal standards based on requirements of firm rational evidence of damage. Two alternative approaches are that of defining the assimilative capacity of the environment for man-made wastes and that of returning to Phelp's " rule of expediency." The latter is the rule of applying all the sanitary and hygienic know-how which is technologically feasible, economically possible, and socially necessary.

Organizational changes should be the consolidation of geographically contiguous supplies now under individual local jurisdictions, and often by private efforts for residential subdivisions.   Two pressures are required to produce joint planning, joint development, and joint operation: (1) the " dry-up " of high-quality, easily accessible sources with dry-up either literal, or an overuse with marked deterioration of yield and of quality; (2) the rise in cost of local operations and of new capital, causing a re-examination of the advantages of scale and of skilled management.   The administrative patch-work of water and sewer services around the urban centers in this country derive from the concept of local independence.   Density of people and intensity of water use and volume of water discharge make that expression of independence costly, and make the concept of interdependence one of social benefit and, in time, of economic necessity.   All this fits the objectives of water resource management.   Examples of regional development and management of water resources are in England and Israel. Examples of urban-area water supply systems which are not confined by city limits are the *Aqua Potable de Lima* in Peru and the Canal Isabel II that provides for all the metropolitan area of Madrid.   The southernmost state of Brazil, Rio Grande do Sul, has had a statewide organization to develop and operate a network of town water services for over 35 years.

The adoption of dual or triple distribution systems, set in a hierarchy of quality-use classes, would be a revolutionary change wholly altering criteria for source selection and use.   A community would have one distribution system for drinking, culinary, and personal use, a second for toilet flushing, car washing and lawn watering, a third for fire-fighting water.   Commercial and manufacturing supply would be fitted to quality needs.   An analysis of the economics can show the limit of elaboration of multiple distribution.   P. D. Haney and C. L. Hamann have stated the case in Dual Water Systems.[1]   D. A. Okun has examined it favorably in Alternatives in Water Supply, for the 1968 meeting of the American Water Works Association.[2]   For sanitary control authorities the concept raises nightmares of interconnections and of mistaken uses.   The addition of a repulsive color or taste to nondrinkable water is one answer.   The idea raises pleasant dreams of source use.   The high-quality sources go to personal domestic use.   Reclaimed wastewater goes for toilet flushing and lawn sprinkling.   Partially desalted or natural seawater and brackish groundwater goes to fight fires and wash streets.   The idea is not novel.   At the start of this century, Boston had a fire-fighting water system of saltwater pumped from the bay.   The use of reclaimed Baltimore sewage by the Sparrows Point Steel Works has been noted. McGauhey's thoughts on wastewater reclamation require dual distribution systems at least in the locale of manufacturing users.   Many factories have well supplies for process water, and public connections for personal use and standby process supply. Los Angeles has had a successful experience in controlling dual supplies, which was set up after grievous episodes of waterborne disease outbreaks among factory workers. Standby sources for fire-fighting are frequent.

Multimedia filters with the use of polyelectrolytes to eliminate flocculation and settling basins are examples of the product of unit-processes research by the chemical engineers.   The chemical engineer's approach differs from that of the hydraulic performance analysis of the treatment processes by the civil engineers.   Papers by Werner Stumm and Charles R. O'Melia on filtration, and by Thomas R. Camp on sedimentation show these two approaches.   Gordon M. Fair's incisive writing comes from a mind capable of synthesizing the biology, chemistry, and hydraulics of water and wastewater treatment.   The application of electronic analytical equipment, of automated controls, and of high-rate unit processes accepting high-cost chemicals, must be utilized to offset the rising cost of labor and of new capital to expand existing works.

[1] *JAWWA*, **57**:1073 (1960).
[2] *JAWWA*, **61**:215 (1969).

With suspicions aroused by increases in the quantities and the varieties of organic traces present in raw water, more sensitive and more discriminating detection methods will be widely applied and will be extended.   Sophisticated methods requiring expensive analytical instruments can be applied to such pollutants now.   For efficiency and economy, such analytical services are already available in some state health and water-control laboratories and in regional laboratories of Federal agencies.

A bacteriological technique for differentiating coliforms from warm-blooded animals from other sources, by 44.5°C incubation on a membrane-filter-contact agar in a submerged water bath is in limited use.   The enriched agar contains an indicator of aniline blue and the sodium salt of rosolic acid.   Fecal coliforms of warm-blooded animals appear as blue colonies.   Other coliform colonies appear gray to cream.[1]   In over 3,000 checks of blue colonies from natural waters by Standard Methods procedures, over 90 percent showed the characteristics of fecal coliform.   Coliforms which produce the gray-to-cream colonies by Geldreich's method come from soil, plants, insects, old sewage, and long-standing pollution.   Widespread testing of the bacteriological method on a diversity of waters is needed to determine its reliability and consistency.   The media is commercially available.

AN APPRAISAL OF MAN'S MANAGEMENT OF WATER

The First Level: Prevention of Disease Transmission

The rationale of managing drinking water has been in development and use in urban Europe and in most of North America for a century and a half; in Central and South America for about 50 years in the capital cities, and extending to other cities and towns in the last 25 years; in Japan since the 1900s; and in an assortment of population centers which at various times have been the foci of colonial efforts for trade, political, or natural resource value.   In every instance, waterborne disease transmission has dropped to barely reportable levels.   The occasional outbreaks are found on investigation, to be caused by operational lapses, not by flaws in the rationale of control. The information on the fate of viruses is incomplete.   It does show substantial removal by present treatment methods.   Certainly there are not massive doses of virus being issued at water taps.   The evident exception of New Delhi, India, in November 1955 requires comment, as reports in United States literature have been from particular and limited viewpoints.

[1] E. E. Geldreich et al., Fecal-Coliform-Organism Medium for the Membrane-Filter Technique, *JAWWA*, **57**:208 (1965).

R. Viswathan wrote the 29-page section on the epidemiology of the outbreak of infectious hepatitis in Delhi.   Bear in mind that the rise in cases was first noted the first week of December by medical authorities.   Viswathan says (Ref. 3-12, p. 29):

> The epidemic was evidently caused by massive infection occurring from 13th to 17th November 1955 and partly on 11th and 13th November.   The pathogenicity of the icterogenic agent was, in all probability, modified by the extra protective measures taken during the period from 12th to 17th November 1955.   The incubation period for the disease during this epidemic was consequently longer than usual. . . .

From early December 1955 into January 1956 there were 7,000 reported cases. Epidemiological investigation covered 3,786.   A sample survey estimated 29,300 frank cases of icterus.   A drainage canal which sewers 200,000 people enters the Jumna River a short distance downstream from the Wazirabad Pumping Station, which pumps and treats at the intake to supply 90 percent of the Delhi–New Delhi urban population.

The chloride content of the Jumna raw water was a constant 5.6 to 5.7 mg/l from November 1 to 10.   The drainage-canal water was 160 mg/l.   On November 11 the chloride content at the intake rose to 12.7 mg/l, on the twelfth to 25 mg/l, on the thirteenth to 60 mg/l, on the fourteenth to 80 mg/l, on the fifteenth to 90 mg/l.   On the sixteenth when an intake change was completed, the chloride content dropped to 60 mg/l.   From the eleventh to the sixteenth there was visible evidence of canal water back-circuiting upstream during low-flow river conditions and of its being drawn into the intakes.   On the eleventh, the alum dose was promptly raised from 0.57 gr/gal (9.8 mg/l) to 3.26 gr/gal (55 mg/l).   The chlorine residual was 0.2 mg/l on the twelfth and was brought up to 0.8 mg/l on the thirteenth.   The digging to bring the water of the Jumna from the opposite bank to avert the back-circuiting was completed on the sixteenth.   These protective efforts were taken 3 weeks before the case reports suggested an approaching epidemic.   Coliform results were confusing during the first days of November, as both samples and controls showed positives.   Coliform tests after November 12, when chlorine residuals had been brought up, were satisfactory.

The water and health authorities can be faulted for a lack of vigor in pressing for funds to move the intake from its hazardous location close to the canal discharge.   The original design and construction in the early 1900s required channel clearing to prevent back-circuiting during low flows in the Jumna.   Back-circuiting was not new.   Few water and health authorities anywhere stand faultless in acting upon recognized hazards with dispatch.   The Delhi authorities acted directly on the routine laboratory results and began digging long before a case of infectious hepatitis was laid at the intake.   The action taken, limited in the light of consequences 3 to 8 weeks later, must have reduced the mass of the viral dose immediately and attenuated it toward zero thereafter.   A trip to India is not necessary to meet a lapse in water hygiene control. Keene, New Hampshire, 1959; Ravena, New York, 1960; Riverside, California, 1965 ;

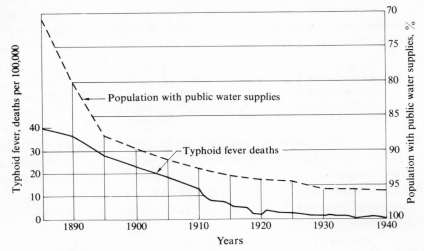

FIGURE 3-12
The relation of the typhoid fever death rate to the percentage of the population with public water supplies in the state of Massachusetts. [*Source*: *Ref.* 3-3 (*p.* 21); *WHO Drawing* 2848.]

or Madera, California, 1965, will do.   Continued vigilance demands a sanitary conscience.   This is what taxes for a state health department must buy and what the payers must demand.   Professional service is not a cut-rate buy.   It can be only delivered by well-educated, well-paid men and women.   The record of such public servants in running water services is that of the near disappearance of waterborne communicable diseases in their communities.   Figure 3-12 is the record of Massachusetts from 1885, correlating the drop in typhoid fever as the population without public water supply was reduced from over 80 percent in 1885 to 3 percent in 1940. There is limited supporting data to show that the need for ample water easily accessible is as important as the quality in the distribution system to reduce diarrheal diseases, particularly among children.   Studies in migrant farm-workers' camps in the central valley of California showed diarrheas to be lowest in the camps that had a tap and shower or toilet in each cabin, to be higher in those with only a tap in the cabin, and to be higher by a factor of 4 where there was no plumbing in a family cabin.[1]   Hollister's observations substantiated those of James Watt's in California in 1950, and of W. H. Stewart's in Georgia in 1955.   A protective level of personal hygiene depends on adequate and accessible water.

[1] A. C. Hollister et al., Influence of Water Availability on Shigella Prevalence in Children of Farm Labor Camps, *AJPH*, **45**:354 (1955).

Toxic chemicals in water are an issue of renewed concern.   Every feasible effort must be made to eliminate irresponsible actions which increase these.   At the same time the toxicant intake from water must be kept in perspective and examined in relation to intakes with food and air.   It is paramount to know why a particular action is taken and what the consequences, positive and negative, will be.   It may be proper for the Michigan Legislature to ban DDT to protect the lucrative Coho salmon in Lake Michigan.   But to support a propaganda roll to ban DDT from the world while hundreds of millions of people depend on it to eradicate malaria is inhumane.   There has been no mass poisoning of a population because of toxic chemicals in their water supply.   There is no epidemiological evidence to support the premise that chronic diseases of cancer and the circulatory system are due to the chemical content of public water.   It is prudent to limit all such substances in all intakes of water, food, and air, each weighed and each control examined for its costs and benefits, immediate and local, long-term and global.   Useful guide values and a considered discussion on toxic chemicals, other compounds, coliforms, and physical characteristics are in Ref. 3-10 and in a waterworks journal article.[1]   A rational approach to permissible toxic chemical concentrations in water extrapolated from toxicological data on inhalation is offered by H. E. Stokinger and R. L. Woodward.[2]

The Second and Third Levels: Comfort, Convenience, and Esthetics and Safeguarding the Ecological Balances

The development and provision of hygienic water supplies are fully compatible with the objectives of man's comfort, convenience, and esthetics and in general of safeguarding ecological balances.   The last does present confrontations between those wishing to keep natural wildlife sites wholly undisturbed and those wishing to use such sites for watersheds and impoundments.   Development solely for public water supply use is seldom an issue as areas are small.   Multipurpose developments flooding many square miles and inundating sites of natural beauty and wildlife habitat are not subject to reasoned compromise.   These must be fought to a choice in the political arena.   An articulate democracy must choose between Glen Canyon as a visual esthetic pleasure or as a vast water container.   In the case of Glen Canyon, the latter prevailed.

Excepting the toxic chemicals, the quality requirements for physical and chemical characteristics of domestic water are directed to comfort, convenience, and esthetics. The quality goals of the American Water Works Association[3] move these to new levels seeking consumer approval.   Some services will have great difficulty in achieving these goals because of source quality or of limitations of treatment facilities.   It is precisely

[1] *JAWWA*, **61**:133 (1969).
[2] *JAWWA*, **50**:515 (1958).
[3] *JAWWA*, **60**:1317 (1968).

to support efforts to overcome these difficulties that the association endorsed the quality goals. Where public supplies fail to meet public expectations, bottled water is introduced and sales increase. Those who can afford the luxury of buying bottled water are the very same ones who would exert local political influence and pay the tax or water rate increases with the least sacrifice to bring the public water to their desires of quality. To fail to reckon with that influence and effect is to pile another second-class label on the lower socioeconomic group and to widen the gap between the haves and have-nots.

REFERENCES

3-1 HARDENBERGH, WILLIAM, and EDWARD B. RODIE: "Water Supply and Waste Disposal," International Textbook Company, Scranton, Pa., 1961.

3-2 FAIR, G. M., J. GEYER, and D. A. OKUN: "Water and Wastewater Engineering," vol. 1: "Water Supply and Wastewater Removal," 1966; vol. 2: "Water Purification and Wastewater Treatment and Disposal," 1968; John Wiley & Sons, Inc., New York.

3-3 DIETRICH, BERND H., and JOHN M. HENDERSON: Urban Water Supply Conditions and Needs in Seventy-five Developing Countries, *WHO, Public Health Paper* 23, 1963.

3-4 Public Health Service Drinking Water Standards, 1962, *U.S. Public Health Serv. Publ.* 956, 1962.

3-5 EISENBUD, MERRIL: "Environmental Radioactivity," McGraw-Hill Book Company, New York, 1963.

3-6 MCGAUHEY, P. H.: "Engineering Management of Water Resources," McGraw-Hill Book Company, New York, 1968.

3-7 American Water Works Association: "Water Quality and Treatment," 3d ed., McGraw-Hill Book Company, New York, 1971.

3-8 WAGNER, E. G., and J. N. LANOIX: "Water Supply for Rural Areas and Small Communities," *WHO, Monogr. Ser.* 42, 1959.

3-9 WHITE, GILBERT F. (ed.): "Water, Health and Society," Selected Papers by Abel Wolman, Indiana University Press, Bloomington, 1969.

3-10 National Technical Advisory Committee to the Secretary of the Interior: Water Quality Criteria, U.S. GPO, 1968.

3-11 MILLER, M. M., and G. G. BERG (ed.): "Chemical Fallout," Thomas Publishing Company, Inc., New York, 1969.

3-12 VISWATHAN, R., et al., "Infectious Hepatitis in Delhi 1955–56: A Critical Study," *Indian J. Med. Res.*, **45**, Supplementary No., January 1957.

4

DISPOSAL OF EXCRETA AND WASTEWATERS

THE NEED

Of the 27 communicable diseases designated in Appendix A as transmitted by environmental agents and vectors, 10 are sustained in man by the pathogens that leave in the excreta of an infected person, and find their way by water, food, or soil to another human being.   Man's continued careless handling of his own excreta maintains these diseases in man.   On the face of the matter the first line of defense seems to be easy and perfect.   Manage human excreta so that none of it reaches our drinking water or our food.   Keep it off the ground surface, and keep it inaccessible to any animals, including insects and birds, which can keep the pathogens in circulation.   Figure 4-1 demonstrates how a pit type of privy accomplishes these hygienic objectives.   At least 2 billion rural people have yet to take this personal step of health protection by isolating their own excreta so it cannot reinfect them with the roundworms, hookworms, flatworms, protozoa, bacteria, and viruses.   Figure 4-2 shows that the septic tank system achieves these hygienic objectives admirably with the comfort and convenience of a water-carried disposal which is easier to keep clean and free of odors.   The ill-repute of septic tank systems is not their hygienic failure, but their failure as a disposal process, squeezed into small lots in soils of limited permeability.   Additionally, the septic tank

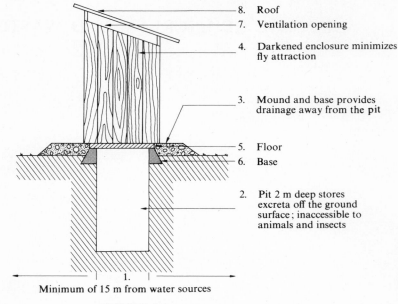

8. Roof

7. Ventilation opening

4. Darkened enclosure minimizes fly attraction

3. Mound and base provides drainage away from the pit

5. Floor

6. Base

2. Pit 2 m deep stores excreta off the ground surface; inaccessible to animals and insects

1.
Minimum of 15 m from water sources

FIGURE 4-1
How a pit privy provides for the hygienic disposal of excreta.

system is a curious combination of unit processes which was initially intended for rural farm families and has shown itself to be ill-fitted to suburban land use and suburban water usage.

Indeed it is paradoxical that the sanitary pit privy provides more certain hygienic containment of the pathogens of cholera, salmonellosis, shigellosis, typhoid and paratyphoid fevers, amebiasis, schistosomiasis, hookworm, ascariasis, trichuriasis, and infectious hepatitis than the sewerage systems of cities, large and small, with and without sewage treatment facilities. Water-carried sewage transport and disposal systems do not in a direct way meet the hygienic criteria for excreta disposal of keeping it out of your water supply, off the ground surface, and inaccessible to animals. However, the pathogens in sewage are in an alien and hostile environment. The dilution factors favor lowering the mass of the dose. In recognized and required circumstances, the sewage can be disinfected by chlorine before discharge to the receiving waters. For built-up communities where water supply makes water-carried sewage disposal practical, the protection against communicable disease of fecal origin depends, not primarily upon the management of excreta disposal, but upon safeguarding the water and food supply and upon a higher level of personal hygiene than can be practiced in a rural setting with hand-carried water. Water-carried sewage and disposal by

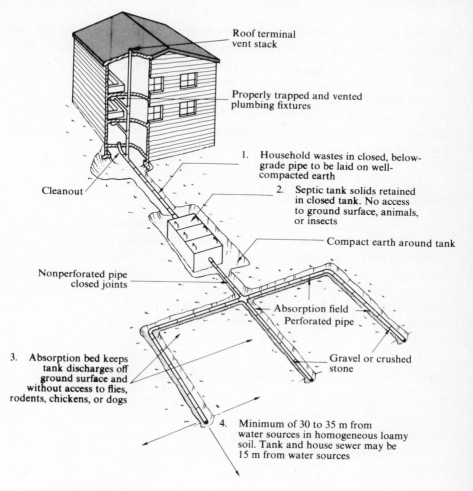

Roof terminal
vent stack

Properly trapped and vented
plumbing fixtures

Cleanout

1. Household wastes in closed, below-
    grade pipe to be laid on well-
    compacted earth

2. Septic tank solids retained
    in closed tank. No access
    to ground surface, animals,
    or insects

Compact earth around tank

Nonperforated pipe
closed joints

Absorption field
Perforated pipe

3. Absorption bed keeps
    tank discharges off
    ground surface and
    without access to flies,
    rodents, chickens, or dogs

Gravel or crushed
stone

4. Minimum of 30 to 35 m from
    water sources in homogeneous loamy
    soil. Tank and house sewer may be
    15 m from water sources

FIGURE 4-2
How a septic tank system provides for the hygienic disposal of excreta. (*Modified
from Ref. 4-7, pt. 1, p. 25.*)

dilution are adequate safeguards against recycling hookworm, ascaris, and trichuris
among the contributors.   Irrigation use of sewage and fertilizer use of raw sludge
does expose a secondary population to infection with such intestinal parasites.[1]
Figure 4-1 requires 100 percent privy use by all at all times.   It does not happen.
In tropical and subtropical areas, the toddlers, age 2 to 5, are difficult to manage, as

[1] H. Shuval, Sanitary Aspects of Water Reclamation and Reuse Practice in Water
Deficient Areas, *WHO, W. Pol.*, WP/67.2, 1967.

they are mobile but not easily habituated to privy use.   The gains in the case of the helminthic infestations of ascaris, hookworm, and strongyloids are more likely to be in the reduction of worm loads rather than the number of persons showing positive stools.   For example, in Egypt the prevalence of ascariasis was 73 percent in certain villages without latrines and 72 percent in similar villages with latrines.   However, a more encouraging change occurred in hookworm with a prevalence drop from 87 percent to 47 percent.   Even incomplete privy use provides a benefit of reduced worm loads per person.[1]

DILUTION AND POLLUTION

About one-quarter of the 100 to 150 grams of feces produced per person per day is bacterial cells.   These are many billions of organisms from each person.   Coliform organisms are at an output of 300 billion per capita per day.   A typhoid carrier will discharge an equal number of *Salmonella typhosa* bacilli.   An amebic carrier will discharge millions of cysts of *Entamoeba histolytica* daily.   Similarly, there are large numbers of virus bodies from cases and carriers of viral diseases.   A hookworm case with a grave infestation of 300 worms will discharge 8,000 eggs per gram of feces. In 100 grams of feces, the output is 800,000 eggs daily.

The Composition of Sewage and the Dissolved-oxygen Dilemma

Of course, human excreta is only one component of domestic sewage, with the wastes of personal washing, household cleaning, and home food preparation adding to the dissolved and suspended, organic and inorganic materials in the carrier water.   Despite the recognized and established infective character of domestic sewage, it is not

Table 4-1   APPROXIMATE COMPOSITION OF MEDIUM-STRENGTH DOMESTIC SEWAGE BASED UPON A WATER CARRIAGE OF 80 GPCD

Solids	In mg/l			5-day 20°C BOD, mg/l	Estimated counts of coliform per 100 ml
	Total	Organic	Inorganic		
Total	800	450	350	200	100×10^9
Suspended	275	175	100	150	
Settleable	175	50	125	70	50×10^9
Nonsettleable	100	70	30	80	50×10^9
Dissolved	525	275	250	50	

[1] *WHO, Tech. Rep. Ser.* 379, 1967, p. 31.

the microorganisms, pathogenic and nonpathogenic, which are used to determine whether there is adequate dilution in the receiving stream. It is the nature and behavior of the surprisingly small 0.08 to 0.1 percent of total solids by weight in domestic sewage. Table 4-1 is the average composition of a domestic sewage in the United States with concentrations in milligrams per liter or parts per million by weight for the types of solids present. Note that with only 0.08 to 0.1 percent of impurities and 99.92 to 99.9 percent of water, sewage has a standard of purity which matches some advertised commercial products. Of the total solids, it is the organic half, some 500 mg/l, which give sewage its unique attributes. These organic solids, dissolved, suspended, and settleable, enter into the biological activity of the receiving waters. These become the foodstuff for a wondrously complex and interdependent system of plant and animal life. The processes are aerobic so long as there is sufficient dissolved oxygen (DO) in the water. The end products will then be stable oxidized forms of carbon, nitrogen, sulfur, and phosphorous. There will be no odors or unsightly scum and sludge which accompany uncontrolled anaerobic decomposition.

Table 4-2 SOLUBILITY OF OXYGEN IN WATER AT SELECTED TEMPERATURES

Temperature $°C$	$°F$	Dissolved oxygen, mg/l
0	32	14.6
4	39	13.1
8	46	11.9
12	54	10.8
16	61	10.0
20	68	9.2
24	75	8.5
30	86	7.6

Table 4-3 AEROBIC AND ANAEROBIC END PRODUCTS OF THE ORGANIC CARBON, NITROGEN, SULFUR, AND HYDROGEN IN DOMESTIC SEWAGE

Through aerobic stabilization in presence of DO				Through anaerobic decomposition in absence of DO
	CO_3^{--} ←	CO_2 ←	C →	CH_4 and CO_2
NO_3^- ←	NO_2^- ←	NH_3 ←	N →	NH_3
	SO_4^{--} ←	S ←	S →	H_2S
	H_2O ←	H ←	H →	organic by-product or NH_3
	PO_4^{---} ←	P ←		

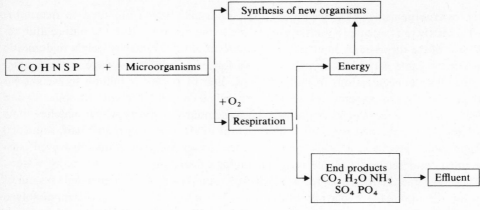

FIGURE 4-3
Synthesis and energy production in the biological oxidation of organic matter.

Table 4-2 presents the maximum solubility of oxygen in water for the temperature given. The limit of meeting pollution by dilution is the DO resources of the receiving water. The BOD of the sewage is exerted rather speedily. Replacement of the DO utilized is from the relatively slow process of natural reaeration at the surface and by the oxygen produced by photosynthesis of aquatic plants.

Table 4-3 is a schematic simplification of the end products of the aerobic stabilization and of the anaerobic decomposition of the elements C, N, S, H, and P which, along with O, make up the organic compounds in sewage. These are present initially as carbohydrates, proteins, and fats. These compounds become the food for the living processes of energy production and protoplasm synthesis of bacteria, and in turn of higher forms of aquatic life, with fish at the apex of the pyramid of life.

Biological Actions on Sewage

Figure 4-3 schematically shows the action of the microorganisms feeding on the wastes in the presence of oxygen. The process of respiration produces the stable oxidized end products and energy. This energy is used in the synthesis of new protoplasm for new cells from the waste materials. It is a simultaneous operation of a cafeteria and maternity ward. It is feeding and reproducing with the beneficial end of stabilizing the putrescible organic matter.

Examples of the chemical reactions of these processes are:

1 Plant photosynthesis

$$6CO_2 + 6H_2O \xrightarrow{\text{light}} C_6H_{12}O_6 + 6O_2$$
$$\text{glucose}$$

2 Energy from a carbohydrate

$$C_6H_{12}O_6 + 6O_2 \xrightarrow{\text{aerobic}} 6CO_2 + 6H_2O + 674 \text{ kcal}$$

3 Hydrolysis and deamination of a protein

$$
\begin{array}{cc}
H_2C & H_3C \\
\| & \| \\
H_2N-C-COOH + H_2O \longrightarrow & C-COOH + NH_3 \\
\text{amino acid of serine} & \| \\
& O
\end{array}
$$

$$\text{pyruvic acid} + \text{ammonia}$$

Note the ammonia release.   The pyruvic acid can now pass through a cell wall.

4 Action of nitrifying cells

$$NH_3 + O_2 \xrightarrow[\text{via } NO_2^-]{\text{bacteria}} NO_3^- + H_2O$$

5 Anaerobic action on glucose

$$C_6H_{12}O_6 \longrightarrow 2CO_2 + 2C_2H_5OH + 22 \text{ kcal}$$
$$\text{ethyl}$$
$$\text{alcohol}$$

6 Methane-producing bacteria

$$2C_2H_5OH + CO_2 \xrightarrow{\text{anaerobic}} 2CH_3COOH + CH_4$$
$$\text{acetic acid} \quad \text{methane}$$

7 Further action on acetic acid

$$CH_3COOH \xrightarrow{\text{anaerobic}} CH_4 + CO_2$$

In addition to the primary requirements of the food and microorganisms, there are protein enzymes produced by the bacteria.   The activity of these enzymes is influenced by temperature, pH, and the concentration of the organic compound rather specific to a particular enzyme.   Some of the bacteria have actions which are unique to their species.

8 Pigmented photosynthetic bacteria capable of inorganic oxidation on sulfide

$$3H_2S + 6H_2O + 6CO_2 \xrightarrow{\text{light}} C_6H_{12}O_6 + 3H_2SO_4$$
$$\text{glucose}$$

9 Chemosynthesis by nitrosomonas

$$2NH_3 + 3O_2 \longrightarrow 2HNO_2 + 2H_2O + \text{energy}$$

10 Chemosynthesis by nitrobacter

$$2NO_2^- + O_2 \longrightarrow 2NO_3^- + \text{energy}$$

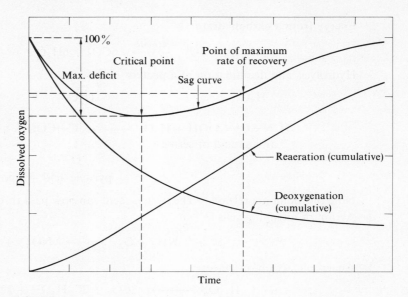

FIGURE 4-4
The DO conditions in a stream under a waste load producing deoxygenation and the response of reaeration. [*Source*: *Ref.* 4-3, *p.* 174.]

These actions provide the raw materials and the energy for the life in the stream, beginning with microorganisms and moving through the algae. These in turn are food for the plant-eating mayfly nymphs, which are food for minnows. Pike feed upon the minnows. This type of cycle depends on a DO resupply which meets the BOD of the stabilization processes. Dissolved oxygen is required for fish life. Carp, which are bottom feeders, can survive in waters with DO of 1 to 2 mg/l. Game fish such as bass and trout require DO minima of 4 to 5 mg/l.

Deoxygenation of a stream or lake is accomplished not solely by the production of the foul odors of H_2S, NH_3, and the mercaptans, but by the extinction of the aerobic life cycle with its variety of bacteria, plankton, insects, and fish. Bottom deposits accumulate. Anaerobic microorganisms take over.

Deoxygenation, Reaeration, and the BOD in a Stream

Figure 4-4 records two events in a stream which has received domestic sewage at a point at which it was saturated with oxygen. As the biochemical oxidation process gets under way, there is a progressive cumulative deoxygenation measured from the saturation point. This deoxygenation curve is the curve of the BOD reaction. As a saturation deficit appears, reaeration begins. The net DO resulting from the two events traces an oxygen sag curve. As long as the point of minimum DO remains above 4 or 5 mg/l, the stream will have a flourishing aerobic biota. Should it drop to 2 mg/l, most aerobic forms will deteriorate. At 0 ppm anaerobic processes will prevail. It is not unusual to have anaerobic or near anaerobic conditions at the stream bottom where the organic waste sediments have overwhelmed the available DO reserves. At the same time, at shallower depths, aerobic conditions are sustained.

The BOD test defines the oxygen which is used by the bacteria while they utilize the sewage as their food and energy source. As it is a measure of a living process, time and temperature must be specified. The standard test in the United States since 1936 specifies 5 days at 20°C (BOD$_5$). The procedure is simple, but good technique is essential to secure consistent results. In the case of domestic sewage, 2 to 10 percent of sample is diluted into well-aerated, buffered dilution water in two BOD bottles. The DO in one is determined immediately. The second is incubated at 20°C for 5 days along with one bottle containing only dilution water, termed a *blank*. There must be some DO remaining in the sample at the end of the incubation, for the difference between it and the initial test is the oxygen utilized. The blank provides correction information. For domestic sewage, the naturally occurring bacteria provide the starter inoculum, or seed. Industrial wastes and chlorinated effluents usually require a " seed " with the blank dilution water treated the same way. Other tests of sewage strength are for the chemical oxygen demand (COD) and total oxidizable carbon (TOC).

The BOD test provides a measure of the amount of biologically oxidizable material in the sewage. It is a measure of the pollutional load being placed on the stream. In the case of a BOD test of the receiving water itself, the existing pollutional load is estimated. It provides a means for predicting the course of the aerobic stabilization in a stream and with reaeration data the likelihood of maintaining aerobic conditions. Over half a century of work has gone into the BOD test and the study and analysis of its meaning and behavior. As early as 1909, Phelps recognized that the biochemical oxidation of sewage followed the pattern of a monomolecular chemical reaction. This means that in each time interval, say 1 day, a fixed percentage of the oxidizable matter remaining undergoes biochemical oxidation. The percentage is about 20.6 per day for domestic sewage.

Using data from BOD tests of the Ohio River studies by E. J. Theriault and H. Hommon, besides their own, H. W. Streeter and E. B. Phelps stated in 1925, "The rate of the biochemical oxidation of organic matters is proportional to the remaining concentration of unoxidized substance, measured in terms of oxidizability." With L as oxidizable substance, in mathematical symbols,

$$-\frac{dL}{dt} = KL$$

the reduction in L in time change t is a constant proportion of the oxidizable substance. This integrates to $\ln L_t/L = -Kt$ and converts from natural logarithms, base e, to base 10 as

$$\log \frac{L_t}{L} = -0.434Kt = -kt$$

substituting k for $0.434K$. In exponential form, $L_t/L = 10^{-kt}$ states that the fraction remaining equals 10 to the $-kt$ power. The k is the reaction constant, which is 0.1 at 20°C, and t is in days. For 1 day, $L_t/L = 10^{-0.1(1)} = 0.794$, the fraction remaining unoxidized; $1 - L_t/L = $ the fraction oxidized, $1 - 0.794 = 0.206$. This fits Phelps' observation of 1909, based on a different test of oxidation rates, the relative stability test, that 20.6 percent of the remaining oxidizable substance was used in biochemical oxidation each day. The BOD test measures the biochemical oxidation of organic wastes by bacteria in the presence of oxygen. Phelps' formula and the modifications and refinements by others have been useful in predicting the behavior of streams under pollutional loads and reaeration conditions. The circumstances portrayed in Fig. 4-4 can be expressed in an analogous way mathematically. A reaeration constant must be provided, often based on limited information. The integrated form of the oxygen-sag curve developed by Streeter and Phelps is a precursor to the use of mathematical models in water pollution. They used it in 1925 to predict conditions in the Ohio River below Pittsburgh at low water flows under summer temperatures.

Such formulas are used to estimate the effects of BOD loads on streams and are used by water pollution control agencies to allot stream use for waste discharges and to determine the degree of treatment required to maintain a desired stream condition. The factors which must be known are the stream's deoxygenation and self-purification characteristics and the DO deficits at the low, critical point of the sag curve and at the point of waste discharge. To determine the DO deficit, the low-flow hydrology of a stream must be known.

The Fate of Intestinal Bacteria in a Stream

The practical limits of pollutional loads on streams are determined by the oxygen balances required to prevent extinction of the aerobic biota, including fish, and to prevent the esthetic and economic offense of creating an open sewer. In the United States few stretches of stream adjacent to large sewered communities remain with sufficient rates of flow to dilute the intestinal bacterial loads of raw sewage to a concentration at which a downstream community could use the water for drinking without treatment. The criteria for the coliform content of raw water range from between 50 and 100 organisms per 100 ml, when disinfection is the only treatment applied, to between 50 and 5,000 when complete treatment is applied.[1]   As a first approximation, dilution water of 5 ft^3/s is needed per 1,000 sewered population to maintain aerobic conditions.   The per capita per day coliform contribution is about 300 billion.   These factors will result in a coliform content of 25,000/100 ml, which is 500 times the low range value of 50 coliforms per 100 ml for a satisfactory raw-water source.   Fortunately, the coliform population of a stream does not remain static.   Organisms of human origin die away rather rapidly in a stream.   This aspect of "self-purification" of a stream is a welcome safeguard.

In 1904, E. O. Jordan and associates[2] found that *S. typhosa*, the pathogen of typhoid fever, survived from 5 to 8 days in Lake Michigan water, and from 3 to 4 days in the heavily polluted water of the Chicago River.   Houston made test-tube observations of the survival of typhoid organisms in Thames River water at various temperatures.   With an initial concentration of 103,000 organisms per milliliter, he observed the following survivals at the end of 1 week: 0°C, 47,766; 5°C, 14,894; 10°C, 69; 18°C, 39; 27°C, 19; 37°C, 5.   The 2-week survival numbers in the same temperature order were 980, 26, 14, 3, 0.1, and 0.   Two deductions from these data have been supported by other evidence.   Organisms from the human intestine survive longer in low-temperature, clean waters than at higher temperatures or in polluted waters.

In 1924, W. H. Frost and H. W. Streeter (Ref. 4-1) reported extended studies of the survival of Cincinnati's coliform contribution to the Ohio River water en route downstream 123 miles to Louisville's water intakes.   The death-rate patterns found were not quite in accord with a first-order monomolecular reaction or with Harriet Chick's observations of disinfection rates.   There appeared to be two populations of coliform.   One made up 99.51 percent of the total with a death-rate constant of 0.467 in the summer months, with a resultant 50 percent reduction in concentration each 0.64 day.   The second grouping, which made up 0.49 percent of the total population, was more resistant.   It displayed a death-rate constant of 0.0581, with a resultant 50 percent reduction each 5 days.

Figure 4-5 shows the coliform death-rate curves for cool and warm weather conditions in Ohio River water.   Note that the cool-weather curve is a straight line for the first 2 to 5 days, and the warm-weather curve is so for the first 5 days.   The rapid die-away populations predominate in the data.   The departure from a straight-line plot on semilogarithmic scales, which characterizes first-order reactions, reflects the slower rate of death of the second population grouping.

The benefits of this die-away of coliform in natural waters can be estimated by recalling and applying the fact that in seven time intervals of 50 percent reductions, there is a 99 percent decrease from the initial concentration.   For the 0.64-day 50

---

[1] J. E. McKee and H. W. Wolf, "Water Quality Criteria," California Water Board, 1963, p. 93.
[2] *J. Infect. Dis.*, **1**:641 (1904).

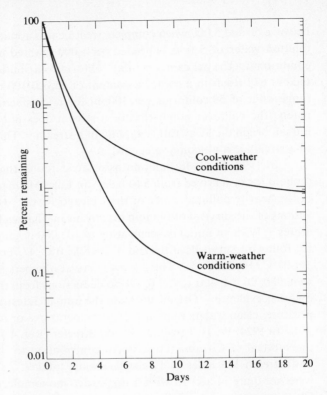

FIGURE 4-5
Death-rate curves of coliform organisms in the Ohio River. (*Source*: *Ref.* 4-3, *p.* 217.)

percent reduction, the 99 percent decrease is reached in 4.5 days. For the smaller fraction with a 50 percent die-away period of 5 days, 35 days are required to reach a 99 percent reduction of their initial population.

SEWAGE TREATMENT AND PROCESS CHOICES

All the natural processes of a stream's self-purification can be compressed in time and in space in a series of one or more sewage treatment unit processes. The processes are those of settling, of anaerobic decomposition of the settled and separated solids, and of bio-oxidation of the nonsettleable and dissolved organic material. In a sewage treatment plant, these natural processes are accelerated, controlled, and supplemented by such procedures as digested-solids drying and chlorination of the plant effluent. Chemical coagulation and precipitation are rarely used, with such special applications reserved for industrial wastes. Mechanical devices such as microstrainers for solids removal and sludge centrifuges for dewatering are in increasing use to provide high capacities in a small space.

Main-stream Processes and Their Effects

Table 4-4 summarizes the three treatment actions that are commonly applied to sewage in the main stream through a treatment plant. Sedimentation is simple subsidence, and when applied to raw sewage is termed *primary settling*. The essential mechanics of the process were stated by Allen Hazen in 1904[1]. Modern sewage settling basins are frequently circular with horizontal flow radiating from a center inlet to a peripheral notched collection weir. The settled material, sludge, and any floating solids or scum

Table 4-4   MAIN-STREAM PROCESSES OF SEWAGE TREATMENT
AND THEIR EFFECTS

Treatment action	Process	Sewage constituent effected	Cumulative percentage removed	Sequential step required
Sedimentation	Primary settling	Settleable solids BOD Bacterial count	35–65 25–40 50–60	Sludge digestion, dewatering, and final disposal
Bio-oxidation in each process here listed has been preceded by primary settling	High-rate "trickling filters"	Settleable solids BOD Bacterial count	70–90 65–95 70–95	Secondary settling and digestion, dewatering, and final disposal of the additional sludge
	Activated sludge	Settleable solids BOD Bacterial counts	80–95 85–95 90–95	Secondary settling, thickening, digestion, dewatering, and final disposal
	Intermittent sand filters	Settleable solids BOD Bacterial counts	90–95 85–95 95 and over	None
Disinfection	Chlorination of settled sewage	Settleable solids BOD Bacterial count	35–65 in primary settling 25–40 in primary settling Plus 90–95	None

[1] *Trans. Am. Soc. Civil Engrs.*, **53**:63 (1904).

are continuously removed to a collection sump for periodic pumping to a sludge digester. There are a variety of sludge- and scum-removal mechanisms applied to circular as well as square and rectangular basins. Vertical flow tanks are in use and frequently are equipped to provide gentle agitation in the inlet zone to conglomerate or flocculate the solids. In United States practice many tank arrangements with their mechanical devices are protected by patents and labeled with proprietary names. This is also the case for other sewage treatment units.

Bio-oxidation is precisely the same phenomenon as aerobic stabilization in a stream, contained and arranged to accelerate the process and to a hopeful degree to control it. Table 4-4 lists the two most widely used bio-oxidation processes, high-rate "trickling filters" and activated sludge. Intermittent sand filters are listed because of their simplicity and notably high efficiency. Note that they require no sequential step. As large land areas are required and bed surface cleaning requires much labor time, intermittent sand filters have become limited in the United States to small populations, including institutions such as schools and hospitals too distant for economical public sewer connection. Public works engineers and health officials of developing countries should make their acquaintance with intermittent sand filters more intimate, along with their acquaintance with oxidation ponds. Additional process applications of bio-oxidation not listed in Table 4-4 are low-rate trickling filters, contact beds, and contact aerators.

Disinfection by chlorination is a final main-stream process which is used in some locations seasonally to maintain the bacteriological quality of swimming waters, and at the same time to protect the property values and recreational usefulness of waterfront areas. It also has its place in reducing the bacterial loading on waters that must shortly be reused as drinking water sources, particularly on streams during low, dry-weather flows. In sufficient doses, chlorine reduces the BOD by direct oxidation of some organic compounds. It also combines with nitrogen compounds and other organics by substitution and addition reactions. It has been stated that 1 milligram of chlorine per liter will satisfy as much as 2 milligrams of BOD per liter. This is optimistic.[1]

Other processes applied to the main stream through a plant which are not listed in Table 4-4 precede primary settling. Grit chambers are used for removal of sand and grit in a quick-acting settling channel which allows the subsidence of coarse particulates of specific gravities near that of sand, 2.65, down to sizes of 0.2 mm. The purpose is to protect pumps and prevent the accumulation of inert grit in sludge lines and digesters. Where sewers collect both sanitary sewage and storm water, grit chambers are needed. Bar racks intercept rags and floating debris in sewage as it enters the plant by a pass through openings of $\frac{1}{2}$ to $1\frac{1}{2}$ in between steel bars. The purpose is

---

[1] W. B. Snow, *Sewage Ind. Wastes*, **24**:689 (1952).

to protect pumps, to prevent unsightly and troublesome flotation in settling tanks, to keep such materials out of sludge lines and tanks.   To minimize handling, automatic scrapers are fitted to the intercepting racks, which carry the screenings to a grinder. The grindings drop back into the sewage stream.   Mechanisms which integrate the interception and grinding in the sewage flow channel are in wide use, designated by such trade names as Comminutor and Barminutor.   Grease-removal skimmers with air-induced flotation are provided in localities where considerable amounts of oil and grease are in the sewage.   Figures 4-6 and 4-7 show schematic flow diagrams of sewage treatment plants.   The solid lines are the principal processes, and the dashed lines indicate the supplementary ones.

A Comparison of Bio-oxidation Treatment Methods

Table 4-5 states the means by which four bio-oxidation processes are provided oxygen, and the form or location of the biologically active mass.   Figure 4-8 diagrams the means by which the three components—organic matter, oxygen, and biological life—are brought together in the four processes.   The gelatinous mass of biological life is clearly visible as a film on the rock of trickling filter beds, and as a suspension in a sample from an activated-sludge tank.   The *zoogloea* is made up of bacteria embedded with other forms of life to make up a transparent gelatinous mass, literally "living glue."   Bacteria active in the process are *Bacillus cereus*, *Escherichia intermedia*, *Paracolobacterium aerogenoides*, *Norcardia acintomorpha*, and species of *Flavobacterium* and *Pseudomonas*.   Ciliated protozoans colonized on the films and flocs, and free swimming forms consume the bacteria and stimulate a continuous renewal of the bacterial population.   Among the protozoa are *Euglena*, *Colpidium*, *Vorticella*, *Amoeba*, and *Paramecium*.   In the film-covered rocks of trickling filters are the bloodworm, *Chironomus*; the sludge worm, *Tubifex*; the larvae and pupae of the filter fly, *Psychoda*; and the water springtail, *Podura*.   Similar biological hierarchies are at work in inter-

Table 4-5   THE ESSENTIAL PROVISIONS OF FOUR BIO-OXIDATION PROCESSES

Process	Source of oxygen	Biologically active mass
Trickling filter	Natural ventilation	Film on rock surfaces
Activated sludge	Bottom diffusion aeration or mechanical air entrainment	Activated-sludge suspension
Intermittent sand filter	Air displacement and entrainment in the bed	Active films on sand granules
Stabilization ponds	O_2 by photosynthesis plus surface aeration	Suspended bacteria, protozoa, algae, and larger plants

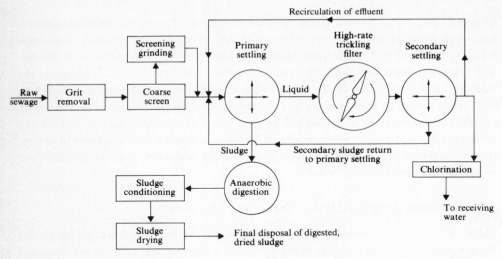

FIGURE 4-6
Schematic flow diagram of high-rate trickling-filter sewage treatment plant.

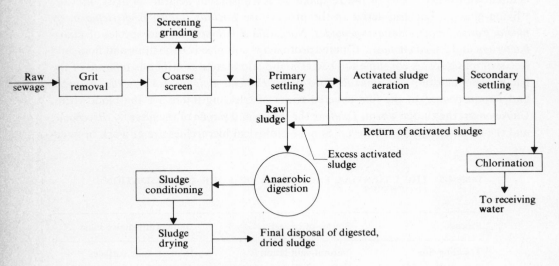

FIGURE 4-7
Schematic flow diagram of an activated-sludge type of sewage treatment plant.

mittent sand filters and in stabilization ponds.   Fungi play a role in the processes which has not been well defined.   The bacterial action is at the cell surface with the enzymatic absorption of nutrients from the sewage and the release of waste and by-products as the food is utilized for energy and the synthesis of new cells.   This synthesis of organic material forms new solids.   Some of the new solids are the constant new growth and renewal of the active biological mass.   Some is the end debris of the process.   As noted in Table 4-4 and as shown in Figs. 4-6 and 4-7, there must be a secondary settling basin for the new solids formed in the trickling filter and the activated-sludge system.

Trickling filter is not an apt term for the high-rate bio-oxidation process that carries that label.   The process is not one of filtration in the mechanical sense of the word.   Nor are applications of 10 million gal/(acre)(day) trickles.   Such a rate is approximately 200 gal/(ft^2)(day), equal to about 13 in for the day in rainfall.   Some United Kingdom authors favor the term " bacteria bed."   That description is limiting, as bacteria make up only part of the activity.   " Bio-oxidation stone bed " describes the process and arrangement.   In like manner, bio-oxidation sand bed describes the intermittent sand filter.

High-rate trickling filters were developed from standard or low-rate units.   In 1927 H. N. Jenks began experiments on recirculating the settled effluent through the bio-oxidation unit.[1]   The benefit is that of a more uniform feed to the biological mass. The active colony is subject to less fluctuation of nutrients and of feeding periods, and to lessened shocks of chemical changes from sludge discharges of unusual wastes. High-rate units have wholly replaced standard units in new installations in the United States, and have found wide use for many industrial wastes for which a suitable biological mass develops.   Activated sludge units are quite susceptible to shock loads. Failure to maintain an adequate suspended-solids concentration in the aeration tank, say from 1,500 to 2,500 mg/l, and an adequate oxygen supply for the raw load applied results in solids that do not settle easily.   The efficiency of settling is reduced.   Solids carry over with the plant effluent.   There is a poor seeding of the influent.   Biologically, there is a different population established.   The condition is termed *bulking*. It results in a loss of treatment efficiency.

Bio-oxidation of the carbonaceous material is a two-step process.   First, there is the sorption of the nutrients into the biological mass.   Second, there is the utilization of the nutrients in the presence of sufficient oxygen.   The intermittent sand filter provides for these by the cycles of dosing once per day and "resting," during which the second step proceeds.   In high-rate trickling filters, the processes appear to be concurrent, with the biological mass securely anchored to the rock bed.   In activated sludge, the system is a more delicate arrangement.   The returned activated sludge

[1] *Sewage Work J.*, **8**:401 (1936).

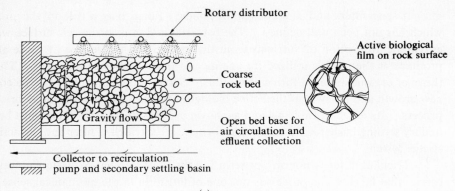

Rotary distributor

Active biological
film on rock surface

Coarse
rock bed

Gravity flow

Open bed base for
air circulation and
effluent collection

Collector to recirculation
pump and secondary settling basin

(a)

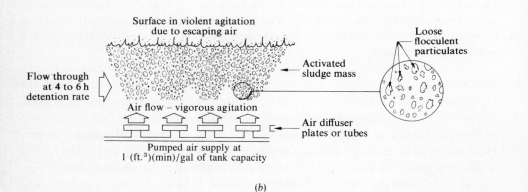

Surface in violent agitation
due to escaping air

Loose
flocculent
particulates

Activated
sludge mass

Flow through
at 4 to 6 h
detention rate

Air flow – vigorous agitation

Air diffuser
plates or tubes

Pumped air supply at
1 (ft.^{3})(min)/gal of tank capacity

(b)

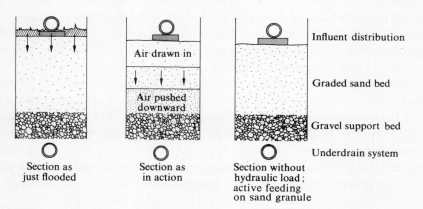

Air drawn in

Air pushed
downward

Influent distribution

Graded sand bed

Gravel support bed

Underdrain system

Section as
just flooded

Section as
in action

Section without
hydraulic load;
active feeding
on sand granule

(c)

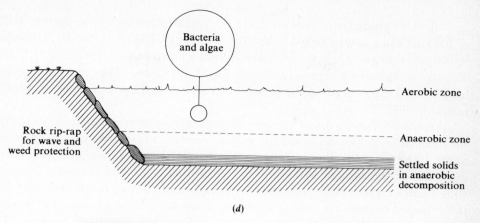

(d)

FIGURE 4-8
Schematic cross-sectional diagrams for four bio-oxidation processes for stabilizing sewage: (a) trickling filter, (b) activated sludge, (c) intermittent sand filter, (d) oxidation pond. (*After WHO Drawing 70805 in E. F. Gloyna, "Low-Cost Wastewater Treatment," draft, fig. 5-1, WD/67.2, pp. 5–11.*)

must provide the seed to the entering sewage. There must be the nutrient sorption and subsequent utilization. The product of the utilization is new activated sludge, which is a floc that separates readily in the secondary settling basin. The two steps go on sequentially in the violent agitation of the aeration tank, except for the short quiescent period in the settling tank. In the face of incoming sewage which does have variable characteristics, the balance which must be maintained requires operational skill and experience. The same biological actions go on in streams, lakes, and the aerobic zones of stabilization ponds in a highly dispersed state without the appearance of floc and film. This is the first stage of bio-oxidation. The second stage, nitrification, is discussed under "Extended Aeration." The biological dynamics of these processes are well described by R. E. McKinney (Ref. 4-2, chaps. 19–22).

Up to this point, BOD has been expressed in mg/l or ppm by weight of oxygen. The concentration of 8.34 pounds per million gallons of water is 8.34 per 8,340,000 pounds of water (1 gal = 8.34 lb); hence it is equal to 1 ppm or 1 mg/l. For a known volume of sewage and BOD, the required oxygen can be stated in pounds in a given unit of time. Conversely, the capacity of treatment processes to provide oxygen for the BOD can be expressed in pounds per day per some unit of treatment volume. From such loading factors, the sanitary engineer designs the process in accord with the known or estimated volumes and BOD strength of sewage to be treated.

Biochemical oxygen demand can be expressed in another way which is particularly useful for equating industrial wastes with domestic wastes. It is the population equivalent (PE) stated in pounds per day.   For domestic sewage with an average BOD_5 of 200 mg/l and a flow of 80 gpcd, the PE is 0.13 lb/day, 80 gpd = 300 l/d; 300(200) = 60,000 mg or 60 g or $\frac{60}{454}$ = 0.13 lb/(capita)(day).   For combined sewage, a multiplier of 1.4 covers the added organic load carried by storm water.   Thus combined, sewage has a PE of 0.18 pound per capita per day.   From 0.17 to 0.2 pound per capita per day is used for PE.

Table 4-6 shows a use of PE to express the relative costs of land and of facilities for three treatment methods and for varying sizes of sewage communities expressed as PE.   The use of PE permits the inclusion of industrial and agricultural wastewaters expressed on the basis of BOD in estimates of total load to be treated.   Despite a considerably higher cost for land, the facilities for stabilization ponds are about one-third the cost of complete biological treatment and about one-half the cost of primary treatment, consisting of raw-sewage settling and separate digestion of solids.   The economy of putting together as many contributors as possible to constitute the sewage community is evident with drops of 50 percent in the dollars per PE for treatment facilities as the sewage rises from 1,000 to 10,000 PE.

Irrigation

The application of sewage to the land surface directly or with presettling, once widely practiced in Europe, still continues in Edinburgh, Paris, and Berlin.   It is used by over 130 communities in the Southwest of the United States.   There are over 150 sewage

Table 4-6   COSTS OF LAND AND OF TREATMENT FACILITIES BY POPULATION SIZE OF 1,000, 10,000, AND 100,000 FOR THREE MEANS OF TREATMENT

	Cost in U.S. dollars per population equivalent*		
	Primary settling and digestion	Complete biological treatment	Raw-sewage stabilization ponds
Land cost	$ 1.25	$ 1.20	$ 3.10
Treatment facilities			
For 1,000 PE†	40	65	18.5
For 10,000 PE	20	33	12
For 100,000 PE	10	17	7

* Cost ratios remain about the same.   Increase dollar values by 60 to 75% for 1972–1973 equivalences.
† PE is population equivalent, at 0.17 pound of BOD per day.
SOURCE: H. C. Clare and D. J. Weiner, Economics of Waste Stabilization Lagoons in Region VI [of Public Health Service], Waste Stabilization Lagoons, *Public Health Serv. Publ.* 872, 1961, pp. 57–67.

utilization projects by land application in Israel, where the water economy requires that 20 percent of all sewage flow be reused. Melbourne, Australia, has used land disposal since 1893 and now has 27,000 acres of land for the disposal of the whole of the sewage of its population of 2 million. In comparison with the United States, the per capita flow in Melbourne is low, about 40 gpcd, but the sewage is strong with a BOD_5 of 500 mg/l and suspended solids of 450 mg/l. In effect, approximately the same waste load is carried in one-half the quantity of water.

Land application may be in the form of ultimate disposal by evaporation, transpiration, and infiltration without any channeled runoff to a stream. Alternatively, it can be a treatment process with an open-channel or underdrain collection of the treated filtrate discharged to receiving waters. It is not a haphazard discharge without consideration of soil characteristics, slopes, distribution channels, control gates, recognition of bio-oxidation requirements or limitations on crops which may be grown. When used as a treatment process with the collection of the effluent, land application most nearly resembles intermittent sand filtration.

Irrigation is a practical method for handling sewage when the following conditions prevail:

1 A large area of quite level land is available at low cost.
2 A method requiring the minimum of equipment is desirable for economic or foreign exchange reasons.
3 There is low rainfall making the reuse of wastewater beneficial.
4 Stream capacity for dilution disposal is low either seasonally or throughout the year.
5 There is incentive to recover at least part of the cost of disposal by returns from the crops grown.

Excessive loadings, insufficient resting periods for the bio-oxidation to be completed, and poor soil permeability and drainage must be avoided, as these produce water logging of the soil and consequent failure of the process. The water table must be maintained well below the root systems of the cover crops to ensure normal growth.

Land application has attributes which merit careful consideration for use by growing urban communities of the developing countries. The five criteria cited above for practical utilization are not so rigid as to prohibit modification to meet pressing requirements of water conservation, increased crop production, and the need to limit equipment purchases and maintenance. The restrictions that are imposed by the evidence of the survival of pathogens have been discussed. These can be fitted to the types of crops grown and the processing, even simple storage, which follows the harvest. It is true that the eggs of *Taenia saginata*, the beef tapeworm, are in raw sewage and even in well-digested sludge. The application of these to grazing land exposes cattle to the infection and can route the parasite back to man in his rare roast beef.

An outbreak of diarrhea via the public water supply of Madera, California, was traced to sewage infiltration into a wellhead sump that had been left unprotected following repairs. The sewage passed via gopher holes from an irrigated pasture under a road into the sump and down the uncapped casing.[1]   Despite the risks and occasional blunders, there is no overwhelming epidemiological evidence that pathogens make their way in heavy infective doses and produce large numbers of cases of human disease by the use of sewage and its partly treated products for land application.   The calculated risk can be absolutely minimal through the exercise of professional judgment in the planning and operation of sewage irrigation, in the selection of crops grown, in spacing the harvest, and in postharvest handling and processing.

Extended Aeration and the Second Stage of BOD

Package Sewage Treatment Plants earn their name by being designed and constructed as a single integral unit, frequently as a single steel structure of compartmented tanks. The process is a modification of activated sludge process by extended periods of aeration.   Termed *extended aeration*, this treatment method is in increasing use for motels, interstate-highway restaurant and service stops, schools removed from public sewer services, resort and recreation areas, mobile-home parks and suburban housing subdivisions.   Their utility for such places is marked by these characteristics:

1   A BOD removal of 85 percent and upward and suspended-solids removal of 60 to 65 percent can be achieved.

2   Operational manpower time averages about 2 h/day.

3   Initial costs solely for the treatment facility range from $60 to $250 per person served.   In an average-density housing development, this cost will be from $200 to $600 per house, a readily absorbed cost for middle- to high-value houses.

4   Electric-powered air compressors or mechanical aerators have a high power cost of over $100 per million gallons of sewage treated.   Offset by low labor costs, this charge is passed on to the people served.

5   There is no separate digestion of sludge.   In some instances, the excess sludge is discharged with the effluent.   To protect stream resources, usually the excess wasted sludge is held for periodic pumping to tank trucks for haulaway, preferably to a municipal sewage treatment plant or supervised land disposal.

6   The basic processes can be supplemented by additional treatment as indicated in Fig. 4-9.

7   Such facilities are well suited for interim use pending land development resulting in annexation to a city, the formation of a sanitary district, or the extension of a trunk sewer serving multiple subdivisions.

[1] *JAWWA,* **58**:1465 (1966).

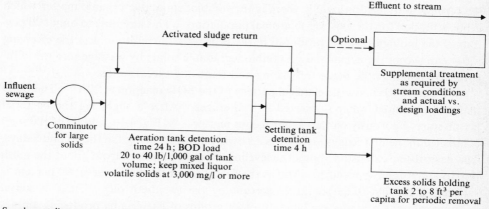

Supplemental treatment which can be provided:
1. Chlorination and discharge
2. Stabilization pond and discharge
3. Intermittent sand filter and discharge

FIGURE 4-9
Basic flow diagram of extended-aeration sewage treatment plant, the package plant.

8   A definite plan and policy for the management of the plant must be set, covering costs of operation and maintenance, amortization and replacement funds, operator training and supervision, and in the case of housing subdivisions, legal means for governmental authorities to guarantee to home buyers and renters the responsibility of the parties originally building the facility and operating it as a utility.

Extended aeration provides a useful means for a further examination of bio-oxidation and the mechanisms of BOD.   Figure 4-9 is a basic flow diagram of the extended aeration method.   Table 4-7 compares conventional activated sludge with extended aeration.   The appeal of extended aeration for use in isolated installations is the elimination of primary settling and sludge digestion.   As nearly as possible, the activated and oxidized solids are continuously recirculated.   Hypothetically, the solids are carried to the point of an "ash," wholly stabilized, which can be wasted to the stream in the effluent.   This is the objective of the high air volumes, long detention time, and continuous, nearly 100 percent recirculation of the suspended solids.   The hypothetical end of all solids as an ash is not attained for hydraulic and biological reasons.   Some of the biodegradable organic matter is not perfectly coagulated, flocculated, or settled during the processes, and goes out to the stream with the liquid effluent.   Some escapes hydraulically by not settling or because of short-circuiting in the settling unit. Additionally, there is the nonbiodegradable organic matter which is not a fit food for the existing microbial population. This amounts to about 20 percent of the biological solids produced in the process. Therefore, unless the receiving water can accept the accumulating nonbiodegradable solids by wastage into the effluent, provision must be made for storing and removing excess solids.

Figure 4-10 shows the classical pattern of the BOD reaction at 20°C. The BOD of freshly polluted water is exerted in two stages. After a slight lag the bacterial action starts vigorously on the carbonaceous matter. In Fig. 4-10, a BOD of 100 mg/l is satisfied in the first 5 days. There is a slowing down to 32 mg/l in the second 5 days. The dashed-line extension shows the leveling-off as it continues from about the tenth day to about the twenty-fifth. This is the first stage of the BOD curve; 90 percent is satisfied in the first 10 days, and 99 percent by the twentieth day. These bacterial actions make the proteins available for other groups of bacteria by producing amines and ammonia. Nitrosobacteria convert these to nitrites. In turn, the *Nitrobacter* group converts the nitrites to nitrates. The actions become vigorous at about the tenth day at 20°C, with a second acceleration of the rate of oxygen use. During days 10 to 15, the use is 24 mg/l with part going to the first-stage carbonaceous action. During days 15 to 20, the use is 49 mg/l before a leveling-off to an even rate of use at 20 days. At higher temperatures the time spread is shortened, and at lower temperatures it is lengthened.

Table 4-7 A COMPARISON OF CONVENTIONAL ACTIVATED-SLUDGE TREATMENT AND EXTENDED AERATION AS USED IN PACKAGE PLANTS

	Activated-sludge treatment	Extended aeration
Coarse solids screened and ground	Yes	Yes
Primary settling	Yes	No
Separate sludge digestion	Yes	No*
Detention times, hours:		
In aeration tank	6	24
In secondary settling	2	4
Loading BOD_5, lb/1,000-gal tank capacity	3–8	20–40
BOD_5 removal, %	80–95	85
Suspended-solid removal, %	85–95	60–65
Nitrate concentration in effluent, mg/l	0.1–6	up to 30
Air provided, ft³/lb BOD_5 removed	750–1,000	1,500–3,000
Sludge % recirculated to aeration tank	20	As nearly 100% as operating conditions permit

* Unsatisfactory operating results have caused many state control agencies to require sludge separation treatment and disposal. Aerobic digestion is being used to meet the requirements.

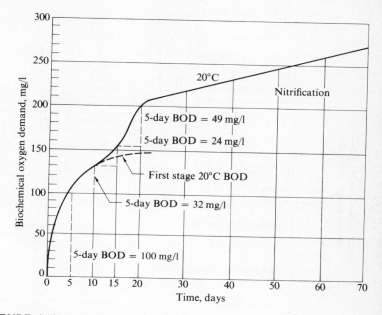

FIGURE 4-10
Curve of BOD carbonaceous and nitrification stages at 20°C. [*Source*: *G. M. Fair, J. C. Geyer, and D. A. Okun, "Elements of Water Supply and Wastewater Disposal," p. 644, John Wiley and Sons, Inc., 1971.*]

In conventional activated sludge, the nitrification stage of bio-oxidation is barely entered.   In low-rate trickling filters and intermittent sand filters, the nitrification stage is reached with resulting high nitrate concentrations in the effluents.   Similarly, in extended aeration, nitrification is well established as there is an excess of air, relatively low organic loadings, and long contact time.   The formation of nitrates creates an operational problem of decreasing pH in the aeration tank and of rising sludge in the settling compartment.   The fact that the nitrification stage has been reached confuses the interpretation of BOD_5 tests of the effluent.   High BOD values in the effluent are observed, as the nitrifying organisms enter the action immediately instead of being virtually absent during the first 5 days, the usual test period.   In such test conditions at least part of the high rate displayed in Fig. 4-10 from the tenth to the twentieth days is concurrent with the carbonaceous stage, days 1 to 5.   The nitrates in the effluent of extended-aeration plants are, however, an asset in the receiving stream's oxygen economy.   The nitrates can be a source of oxygen and can delay or offset anaerobic stream conditions.   It is for this reason that sodium nitrate is sometimes spread to provide an oxygen source in stabilization ponds and anaerobic streams.

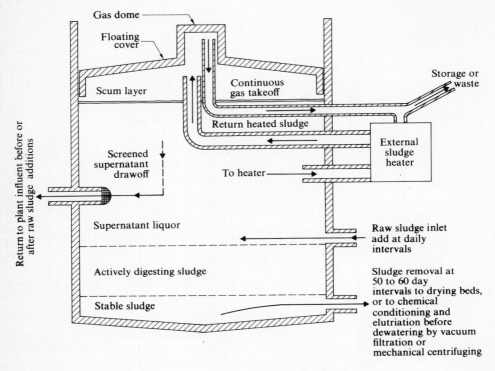

FIGURE 4-11
Schematic view of a sludge digester.

Anaerobic Processes

In contrast with extended aeration, which achieves the stabilization of sewage solids by aerobic action, are the anaerobic processes for the conversion of the solids to liquids, gases, and residual stabilized solids. These actions go on in treatment plant digesters; in the settled solids in septic and Imhoff tanks; in anaerobic stabilization ponds; in the settled solids in streams, "sludge banks," or, more elegantly, benthal deposits; and in streams where the DO is zero. The process is anaerobic in that DO is not present. Chemically, however, the process is a concurrent reduction and oxidation in which the microbiological respiratory processes are intermolecular and intramolecular. In digesters and tanks, the process is largely bacterial with only a few ciliates, colorless flagellates, and amoebae present. In anaerobic waters, fungi, protozoa, worms, and insect larvae participate. The bacteria are not all true anaerobes. They are facultative types which adapt to aerobic or anaerobic conditions. Among these are such familiar bacteria as *Bacillus subtilis, Clostridium perfringens, Escherichia coli,* and *Staphylococcus aureus.*

In all its manifestations, anaerobic stabilization is a slow process. Present developments of high-rate digestion in cycles of 6 and of 20 days are to be compared with 50 to 60 day retentions in conventional heated digesters, Fig. 4-11, and the behavior of benthal deposits in which fresh material requires 1.5 years to reach a 90 percent stabilization and an additional 5.5 years for the next 90 percent stabilization of the remaining decomposables. The processes are of the same nature as those which have converted vegetation to peat, coal, oil, and natural gas, for which the time is expressed in geologic eras.

The reactions of anaerobic stabilization are a series of intricate steps in which bacteria elaborate both extracellular and intracellular enzymes. Enzymes, which are complex proteins, have specific actions in preparing material for passage through the cell wall, achieving the passage and use, and acting as energy transfer agents. The illustrative reactions, in words and chemical symbols, are parts of an extended series and are simplifications. These are presented to provide some clues to an understanding of the biochemistry of anaerobic stabilization.

1 Further action on a carbohydrate product at an acid pH

Pyruvic acid → acetyl methyl carbinol + carbon dioxide

$$2CH_3COCOOH \longrightarrow CH_3COCHOHCH_3 + 2CO_2$$

2 Action on a saturated fatty acid

Fatty acid + water → carbon dioxide + methane

$$C_nH_{2n}O_2 + \frac{n-2}{2}H_2O \longrightarrow \frac{n+2}{4}CO_2 + \frac{3n-2}{4}CH_4$$

3 General protein decomposition in words only

Protein → proteoses → peptones → peptides → amino acids

4 A specific protein intermediate, an amino acid

Glycine + hydrogen + water → acetic acid + ammonia + water

$$H_2CNH_2COOH + 2H + H_2O \longrightarrow CH_3COOH + NH_3 + H_2O$$

5 Methane fermentation

A compound, H_2A, activated by methane bacteria + carbon dioxide
→ the compound A less its hydrogen atoms + methane + water

$$4H_2A + CO_2 \longrightarrow 4A + CH_4 + 2H_2O$$

Temperature increases speed up sludge digestion to a limit which coincides with the thermal death point of many of the active bacteria. Primary sludge digests 1.5

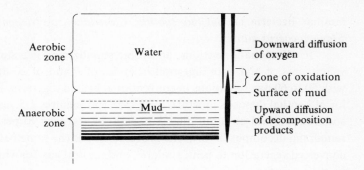

FIGURE 4-12
Anaerobic and aerobic actions of sludge deposits in streams. (*Source*: *Ref.* 4-3, *fig.* 7, *p.* 122.)

times as rapidly at 40°C as at 25°C.   Activated sludge digests 2.2 times as rapidly at 40°C as at 25°C.   At 40°C there is a shift with a slowdown of organisms which perform well from 15 to about 37°C.   This is the mesophilic range for organisms fitted to moderate temperatures.   Above 40°C there is another spurt to about 55°C, which describes the range of thermophilic, heat-loving, organisms.   In practice, the use of efficient digester gas for heating makes it possible to maintain a digestion temperature of 32°C (or 90°F).   This is a satisfactory point in the mesophilic range.   It provides a temperature at which about 90 percent of gas production can be attained in 30 days of digestion.   Empirical observations have emphasized the importance of keeping digesting temperature within 2 or 3°F of that chosen for operation, optimally a point between 85 and 95°F.   It is the uniformity of temperature within this range that is important.   In practice, sludge thickening before transfer to the digester and sludge mixing while in the digester are beneficial to achieve and maintain good digestion.

Anaerobic stabilization ponds are in use ahead of aerobic and facultative ponds in warm climates and experimentally in Costa Rica for abattoir wastes.   No algae grow in these.   High BOD loads of 3,000 lb/(acre)(day) and short retention times of 1 day or less have produced good results in the tropics, where the sludge temperature will be between 20 and 25°C.   Removals of 70 percent of the BOD have been reported. The values are improved performance of the aerobic stabilization ponds which follow; increased loadings on, or reduced sizes of, these ponds; and the elimination of floating sludge on them.   The establishment of alkaline fermentation in an anaerobic pond and the return of from 10 to 40 percent of the effluent from the facultative pond eliminates the release of sulfides.   The hydrogen sulfide is held as a hydrosulfide ion. Sulfur bacteria grow and fix the sulfide as elemental sulfur.   In time there is digested sludge accumulation which requires removal or the abandonment of the pond.

Figure 4-12 shows the unique character of benthal deposits. Anaerobic processes are active in the settled sludge, which is compacted with depth. The gaseous products leave by solution in the case of CO_2 and by bubbling to the surface in the case of the slightly soluble CH_4. The liquefaction products diffuse to the sludge-water interface. Very much like digester supernatant liquor, these exert a high BOD and therefore deoxygenate the water at the boundary. With the DO replenished by downward diffusion, oxidation of the liquefaction products is achieved. As this means of stabilization is very slow, deposition conserves the oxygen resources of a stream, provided the water above is not totally deoxygenated for long periods of time by the soluble and nonsettleable solids load. Efforts to formulate equations to predict the effects of benthal deposits on a stream's oxygen economy have had to take into account the rate of oxidation in the sludges and the rate of deposition. G. M. Fair developed an approximate empirical equation for the daily oxygen demand of benthal deposits. Phelps makes practical use of it in an analysis of benthal loads in a 10-acre millpond receiving 100,000 gallons of wastes per day from a New England textile mill (Ref. 4-3, p. 126). In effect, Phelps had an anaerobic stabilization pond for some months of the year, distributing the overall load on the stream below.

INDUSTRIAL WASTEWATERS

Of all the water that industry uses, including cooling water for thermal power generators, only 0.2 percent is estimated to leave the premises as part of the product. Assuming evaporative losses to be about 2 percent, there remains a gigantic daily discharge of water that is changed in some way. As the cooling water quantity is at least 90 percent of the total discharge and it is changed only in temperature, only about 10 percent of the total water used is changed in biological, chemical, or physical characteristics of color, turbidity, foaming, taste, or odor. If there were absolutely no separation or treatment of such wastes, industry would be discharging about 6,000 billion gallons of water per year polluted to some degree. What is objectionable about these wastes? What are the sources? For whom and for what purpose is protection sought? What means of control and treatment can be used? Who will pay the bill?

Objectionable Components of Industrial Wastewaters

Table 4-8 lists eight components of contaminants and pollutants all of which industrial wastewaters carry in common with domestic wastewaters. These vary, of course, with their source and the extent of water and waste care within the manufacturing plant before discharge. The biodegradable organics, expressed in BOD_5 in milligrams per liter, reach levels 100 times that of the 250 to 300 milligrams per liter of domestic sewage.   Some highs are wastes from grain and molasses distilling, 20,000 to 30,000; from sulfite cookers in pulping for paper, 15,000 to 25,000; and from brewery slop, 11,500. Levels of 2,000 are reached in wastes from beet sugar refining, canning, milk and meat processing.   These high BOD_5 values are from soluble carbohydrates.   The specific

Table 4-8   OBJECTIONABLE COMPONENTS OF INDUSTRIAL WASTEWATERS, THEIR EFFECTS, AND TYPICAL SOURCES

Component group	Effects	Typical sources
1 Bio-oxidizables expressed as BOD_5	Deoxygenation, anaerobic conditions, fish kills, stinks	Large amounts of soluble carbohydrates: sugar refining, canning, distilleries, breweries, milk processing, pulping, and paper making
2 Primary toxicants: As, CN, Cr, Cd, Cu, F, Hg, Pb, Zn	Fish kills, cattle poisoning, plankton kills, accumulations in flesh of fish and mollusks	Metal cleaning, plating, pickling; phosphate and bauxite refining; chlorine generation; battery making; tanning
3 Acids and alkalines	Disruption of pH buffer systems disordering previous ecological system	Coal-mine drainage, steel pickling, textiles, chemical manufacture, wool scouring, laundries
4 Disinfectants: Cl_2, H_2O_2, formalin, phenol	Selective kills of micro-organisms, taste, and odors	Bleaching of paper and textiles; rocketry; resin synthesis; penicillin preparation; gas, coke, and coal-tar making; dye and chemical manufacture
5 Ionic forms: Fe, Ca, Mg, Mn, Cl, SO_4	Changed water characteristics: staining, hardness, salinity, encrustations	Metallurgy, cement making, ceramics, oil-well pumpage
6 Oxidizing and reducing agents: NH_3, NO_2^-, NO_3^-, S^{--}, SO_3^{--}	Altered chemical balances ranging from rapid oxygen depletion to over nutrition, odors, selective microbial growths	Gas and coke making, fertilizer plants, explosive manufacture, dyeing and synthetic fiber making, wood pulping, bleaching
7 Evident to sight and smell	Foaming, floating, and settleable solids; stinks; anaerobic bottom deposits; oils, fats, and grease; waterfowl and fish injuries	Detergent wastes, tanning, food and meat processing, beet sugar mills, woolen mills, poultry dressing, petroleum refining
8 Pathogenic organisms: B. anthracis, Leptospira, toxic fungi, viruses	Infections in man, reinfection of livestock, plant diseases from fungi-contaminated irrigation water; risks to man slight	Abattoir wastes, wool processing, fungi growths in waste treatment works; poultry processing wastewaters

chemicals that make up groups 2 to 6 in Table 4-8 are primary toxicants such as As, CN, Cr, Cd, Cu, F, Hg, Pb, and Zn; acids and alkalines which disrupt pH buffer systems in natural waters; concentrations of disinfectants, such as chlorine, formalin, hydrogen peroxide, and phenols, sufficient to kill aquatic microorganisms; ionic forms which change water quality, such as Fe, Ca, Mg, Cl, and SO_4; and oxidizing and reducing agents which can produce undesirable changes in the receiving water, such as ammonia, nitrites, nitrates, sulfides, and sulfites.

Components of industrial wastes which are physically evident raise violent objections. Floating solids, foam, coloring agents, materials and reactions which cause turbidity are high on the complaint list. Odoriferous materials, whether they are in the waste, are subsequent reaction products after discharge, or are from the anaerobic decomposition of settled solids, are offensive in themselves and frequently a sign of other heavy pollutional effects. Fats, oils, and grease add to visual objections and have direct effects on fish and waterfowl, including some instances of tainted flavors in the flesh. Group 8, pathogenic organisms, has not been an evident problem in industrial wastewaters. Anthrax and leptospirosis transmissions are possible. Virus transmission from poultry-processing wastewaters may be possible. Direct animal contact is much more the route of animal to man transmission of such diseases.

Manufacturing operations that generate objectionable chemical wastes are metal cleaning, pickling, and plating; bleaching and dyeing; and pulping. Food processing operations that are prominent contributors are canning of fruits and vegetables; cane and beet sugar refining; milk and milk product handling; breweries, distilleries, and confectionery goods. Textile manufacture, including synthetic fibers; the pharmaceutical industry, including antibiotics; and laundries are contributors of high alkaline and high BOD_5 loads. Oil refineries and gas and coke works are heavy industries that have large quantities of phenols, oils, ammonia, and cyanides in their disposal inventories. Acid mine wastes from worked-out and active coal mines and the leachings from tailings piles of mines and ore refineries are chronic sources of stream pollutants. No manufacturing waste is really clean.

Protection for Whom and for What Purpose?

The control and management of industrial wastewaters must have a beneficial justification. The center column of Table 4-8 does not indicate that industrial wastes are a threat to man's health. On a "what if" basis, the threat of carcinogens, cumulative chronic toxicants, and animal viruses can be invoked. There is neither experimental nor field epidemiological evidence to support the what-if hypothesis. Should it come to that, there would be less expensive alternatives to provide man with safe drinking and culinary water than cleaning up all industrial wastewaters. Fish provide the major evidence of being a victim of polluted waters. Deoxygenation, specific toxins, and sudden temperature rises cause fish kills. The number of reported fish kills from all causes in the United States is 400 to 500 per year. Reduced catches and lower reproduction rates over a period of years have been recorded in Midwest United States rivers, in West Germany, and in the U.S.S.R. The gradual change of a river or lake environment with deterioration for some fish species has been observed and documented. Bottom deposits, anaerobic conditions, and the release of toxicants in organic complexes have been noted. An early observation of mercury in fish tissue came from studies in Swedish lakes in which mercury entered fish in a methylated form found in bottom deposits. The mercury came from industrial wastes. Lesser forms of zooplankton and phytoplankton change with pollutant changes. A few prosper under the new conditions. Some mollusks have been found to have a longer growing season in waters heated by industrial discharges.

There is even a place for anaerobic forms. The deterioration of aerobic regimes is not due solely to industrial wastewaters. Domestic and mixed municipal sewage put their measurable oxygen demand on streams and lakes and add carbonates, nitrates, and phosphates, all useful nutrients if not in excess. In stream stretches that are anaerobic, the variety of species decreases from that in cleaner waters, often to 10 percent or less of the clean-zone number. The relatively few that are fitted to the zero DO have an abundant food supply which results in large densities of a few species. Examples of such organisms are the rat-tailed maggot, an ugly larva of the dronefly; the sludge worm, a red tubiflex; bloodworms of the *Chironomus* species; and the sow bug or water log louse. All are bottom feeders, adapted to anaerobic conditions. The field biologist has betrayed his preference for the variety and color of the aerobic conditions by labeling the anaerobic forms with distinctly unattractive names.

Streams carrying acid mine drainage are at pH below 4 with clear red- or copper-colored water. Fish and all but a few plants such as the cattail die in such water. But there is plenty of life in these acid streams. Bloodworms, caddis flies, certain mosquitoes, and beetles do very well. There is an abundant population of protozoa and algae, although the variety is limited. Life persists under a wide spectrum of chemical and physical conditions. It may not be in the way man perceives to be normal. Man's wastes and particularly certain of his industrial wastes radically change biochemical environments. To the cursory look, life has been wiped out. It may not be so. Customary life regimes have been killed. New ones are formed from survivors fitted to the special conditions.

There then remains resource conservation as the reason for controlling industrial wastes. There is the value of the water itself for downstream users. Under the English common law doctrine, the riparian property owner may use a stream water so long as he returns it unimpaired. Industry within its own community has a selfish interest in protecting the quality of one of its raw materials—water. It shows that interest when the noose tightens, when good quality water becomes hard to get and when the cost of special water treatment rises.

The depreciation of property for residential use, resort sites, and recreational development is a tangible resource loss due to gross pollution of streams and lakes. In the past, too often stretches of a river and reaches of lakes have been written off as large open municipal and industrial sewers.   Such has been the history of the Delaware River from Trenton, New Jersey, to the Atlantic Ocean, and of the south shore of Lake Erie from Cleveland to Buffalo.   Now comes the second look as there are fewer places for more people to satisfy larger water-use needs and as the pollution effects become repulsively intolerable to a heightened sensitivity.   This esthetic requirement that our water be attractive has no dollar value unless translated into recreational use, but it is gaining a powerful political value identified as the conservationist clout in lobbying and voting.

Control and Treatment of Industrial Wastewaters

There are four options, not mutually exclusive, for the management of industrial wastewaters.   These are:

1 Control at the point of generation within the plant
2 Pretreatment for discharge to public sanitary sewers
3 Discharge to public sewers for combined treatment at the municipal treatment works
4 On-site treatment with discharge to receiving waters or for reuse either on-site or by others and either as is or with further treatment to meet special requirements.

Management often prefers option *3* even at the cost of special charges, as it avoids getting into waste treatment as a plant responsibility.   Resort to option *4* is not as wide as may be thought.   It is estimated that there are about 3,000 industrial wastewater treatment plants in the United States.   There are many more partial-treatment procedures, falling under option *2*, to modify wastewaters before discharge to public sewers.

Control at the Point of Generation

Control at the point of generation within the plant requires a water-use and wastewater consciousness in all levels of management.   This is not usual as those are not high among management's concerns.   A good consultant who periodically inventories water and wastewater handling is a productive participant in this practice. Working with process and plant engineers, the consultant zeros in on the obnoxious components at their origin, isolates these, and seeks means to prevent their joining main waste streams. Separate treatment of such wastes as plating-room drainage, interception of oils and grease in separators, neutralizing strong acids and alkalies immediately, settling or screening solids while still in low flow volumes are examples of the technique. In most instances these procedures result in a recovered concentrate that must be handled. Occasionally useful material can be recovered. Usually burning or burial is the resort.

Wastewaters from which coarse solids have been screened or settled can be re-used, either cycled back into the process or routed to lower-quality uses. Holdup tanks and ponds are less sophisticated means to equalize discharges to avoid slugging a treatment plant and to gain some advantage of settling, neutralization, or self-oxidation in the mixed mass. Blind lagoons are widely used where land values are low. Liquid loss is by seepage and evaporation. If odors and groundwater contamination are not risks, lagooning can be used. Fencing to keep out domestic animals, pets, and people is needed. Protection against flooding and dike failure are part of design, construction, and maintenance. High dissolved inorganic solid wastes such as brines and alkalies can be handled by lagoons. High-toxicity wastes should not be lagooned. Flooding, structural failure, and uncertainties of seepage make such disposal too risky.

Pretreatment

Pretreatment to prepare for discharge to public sewers is often a concomitant to isolating the waste at the point of generation. Pretreatment of large volumes of waste, even a plant's total flow, is done by interception of screenables or settleables, or both, to reduce gross solids loads on streams, sewers, and treatment plants. Examples are found at poultry dressing and meat packing plants, tanneries, canneries, beet sugar mills, and ore refineries and mills. More elaborate means are needed to reduce BOD loads. One technique is recirculating roughing filters. These are trickling filters in which an oxidizing zoogloea develops which can feed on a waste material at high concentrations and with characteristics which overwhelm a usual municipal bio-oxidation unit. The roughing filter reduces and modifies the BOD to a point at which it can be handled in combination with other mixed municipal wastes. Milk processing, cannery, paper mill, and pharmaceutical wastes are among those treated by roughing filters. Chemical precipitation, despite the cost of the coagulant and the necessary disposal of sludge has been used on textile and low-level radioactive wastes. Ferric chloride is an effective coagulant of alkaline high-color textile wastes. Neutralization of acid and alkaline wastes is a frequent pretreatment. Often it is done to protect sewers from rapid deterioration and to avoid discharge of corrosive wastes into municipal sewers. Pretreatment methods and facilities must keep pace with in-plant changes of materials and processes which change wastewater volumes and characteristics.

Combined Treatment at the Municipal Treatment Works

Combined treatment of industrial and municipal wastewater becomes a special technique when the wastewater of a single plant or group of plants is a major fraction of the total municipal sewage or when it has unique characteristics of high BOD, acidity-alkalinity, color, suspended solids, or toxicants.   Except for residential areas, all public sewers receive some wastes from commercial, service, and the smaller manufacturing establishments.   Even these should be subject to charges based on volume, BOD, a specified pH range, or acidity-alkalinity content, and to regulations for the exclusion of materials which interfere with treatment.   The issue becomes different when the volume and characteristics of the industrial wastewaters become a recognized determinant in the design, construction, and operation of the municipal treatment works. Table 4-9 gives the salient items of five agreements in which particular industrial wastewaters were dominant considerations in combined treatment facilities.   All but the Bayport, Texas, installation are combinations of industrial wastewaters and domestic sewage.   The Bayport contributions will be largely other industrial wastes.   Two have been unsatisfactory experiences in which the governmental partners have been left "holding the bag."   In reviewing such agreements, E. B. Besselievre (Ref. 4-4, p. 143) states three conditions which must be specifically spelled out to protect all participants.   These cover:

1   Waste volumes and characteristics
2   A schedule of financing and of charges
3   Provisions for increments in volumes and for changes in composition and characteristics that require new capital for additions and modifications in sewers and in treatment facilities.

The two failures listed in Table 4-9, Worcester and the Passaic Valley Sewerage Authority, are described by Besselievre.   The successful cases are Bound Brook, New Jersey, and Longview, Texas.   The latter provides a surprising contrast in the managerial policy of the same corporation's actions in Winston-Salem, North Carolina.   Only after serious overloads on the Winston-Salem sewage treatment plant which produced fish kills in the Yadkin River and legal action by the downstream city of Salisbury in 1970, did Jos. Schlitz Brewing Company take steps to reduce its discharges to the city sewers by installing centrifuges to remove solids.

On-site Treatment of Industrial Wastewaters

A wide variety of industrial wastes are treated by conventional sewage treatment methods.   In complete treatment, fine screens, grit chambers, or chemical precipitation are often used before primary settling.   A frequently used bio-oxidation method is high-rate recirculating trickling filters. High BOD is a frequent industrial waste characteristic. Several have already been noted. Besselievre lists 31 sources of industrial wastes satisfactorily treated by trickling filters. There is a selective development of a biological colony on the filter beds which utilizes wastes as unlikely as formaldehyde, phenols, and pickle factory residues as its food. Such filters have been favored, as these withstand shock loads and usually recover well from such events. Pulp and

Table 4-9 EXPERIENCES WITH COMBINED MUNICIPAL AND INDUSTRIAL WASTEWATER TREATMENT PLANTS

Location	Participants	Nature of the wastewater	Year started	Terms of agreement	Operator and results
Bound Brook, N.J.	Amer. Cyanamid Co. and Somerset-Raritan Valley Sewerage Authority	Heavy chemical; domestic from townships	1958	Capital 4.5×10^6 from Amer. Cyanamid; 1×10^6 from SRVSA.	Amer. Cyanamid; SRVSA pays oper. fee of about $10,000/yr. Flow: industrial, 21 million gpd; domestic, 4 million gpd.
Longview, Texas	Jos. Schlitz Brewery and the city	High BOD and solids from brewery	1966	Brewery 4.9 million gpd; city 1.1 million gpd.	City owns and operates plant.
Bayport, Texas	Humble Oil Co. and industrial park tenants	Petrochemical wastes	1969	Biologically treatable wastes accepted to 40 million gpd capacity.	Humble Oil Co.; users pay fees.
Worcester, Mass.	Steel plant and city	Metallurgical wastes and municipal sewage	About 1910	Inadequately defined as to steel waste volumes and character of these; city "stuck."	City had to bear all costs of increased volumes and treatment changes.
Passaic Valley Sewerage Authority, N.J.	Textile mills and towns	Textile wastes and domestic sewage	1958	Textile mills to discharge 10% untreated to interceptor sewer, 90% to be treated; character not stipulated; the Authority has been "stuck."	Passaic Valley Authority; the untreated 10% from the mills was by volume and was the strongest, least-treatable wastes.

paper mills, petrochemical plants, and pharmaceutical factories, all of which put out strong wastes in large volumes, use trickling filters for on-site treatment.   For new treatment works, designers favor the "complete mixing" type of activated-sludge treatment.

Trickling filters require large land areas.   Rock beds are costly to place properly. Industry has found answers in light-weight plastic filter media of diverse patterns which provide large honeycomb voids and ample surface area.   Such plastic forms are stacked vertically as high as 50 ft in light-weight open structural frames.   Trade names for these media and materials are Surfpac, Dowpac 10, Saran, Flocor, and Koro-seal.   Most are polyvinyl chloride plastics with forms that provide large void spaces of 94 to 95 percent; they are light, 3 to 5 lb/ft^3, and have good surface areas, 25 to 40 ft^2/ft^3.   This surface area compares well with Raschig rings, slag, and rock, which range from 20 to 30 ft^2/ft^3.

Activated sludge as the bio-oxidation process in industrial waste treatment plants has not been widely used in its classical form.   Variants of it have been useful.   One has been *contact stabilization*, which provides a short time for the mixed-liquor aeration of the incoming wastes and returned sludge.   This is followed by a separation of the activated sludge and a long aeration of it in a separate chamber for up to 24 hours.   It is this continued aeration of the separated sludge, an activated sludge, which is the contact stabilization.   That well-aerated, stabilized sludge is then returned to the incoming waste stream.   There is virtually no sludge drawoff.   This process has been very effective for high-BOD pulp and paper wastes.   It is suitable for similar wastes in which there are no substances which are toxic to the biological life that makes up the activated sludge.

A second variant of activated sludge has been termed *complete mixing*.   There are long aeration periods, no sludge drawoff, and feed of the influent throughout the aeration-mixing tank.   This complete mixing of the raw influent with the activated sludge mass provides a uniform dilution and distribution of any changes of influent. The entire microbial population can feed uniformly on the fresh material.   Bessel-ievre reports that the process has handled penicillin culture wastes with BODs to 6,000 mg/l, 20 times the BOD of domestic sewage; has reduced phenol concentrations from a range of 2,000 to 3,000 mg/l to less than 0.1 mg/l; and has treated cotton kiering and bleaching wastes from textile mills with BOD reductions of an influent of 450 mg/l to an effluent of 3 mg/l.   These remarkable BOD removals are well above the 90 to 95 percent that well-operated conventional activated-sludge plants produce.   It is at the cost of pumping large amounts of air through the wastes for longer periods.

Land disposal by direct spraying of grasslands and woodlands and by ridge and furrow irrigation is used for many high-organic-content wastes.   Coarse solids are usually intercepted.   As easy access to large areas is necessary, food processing plants in rural areas and often with seasonal operation have resorted to land disposal.

These have included dairy products, citrus fruit processing, canneries, cattle-feed-lot and stockyard drainage, meat and poultry dressing, and pulp and paper mills. Besselievre lists 21 types of wastes for which land disposal has been used. Application cannot be haphazard, as there are bad results from overloading poor soils such as waterlogging, ponding, stenches, insect hordes, and in the case of some food wastes, rats.

Oxidation ponds are used for raw wastes, settled wastes, and bio-oxidized and settled wastes. The last has been called *polishing*. Ponds are used singly or in series. The series can extend to three, an initial anaerobic pond followed by an aerobic pond and finally a polishing pond. Large areas are required even for single ponds. Aeration is usually left to the natural actions of air-water solution and photosynthesis. Where more oxygen is needed because of increased loads or unforeseen oxygen demands, mechanical aeration by surface or underwater rotors or porous Saran tubes at the pond bottom have been used. The Saran tube method is called Air Aqua and is provided by the Hinde Engineering Company of Highland Park, Illinois. Besselievre lists 100 types of wastes treated in oxidation ponds. He gives notable successes of petrochemical plants, roofing-felt wastes, a winery, tomato processing, a Costa Rican slaughterhouse, canneries, two Georgia textile mills, and an Indiana metalworking plant which has four ponds in series to get a BOD reduction from 200 to 4 mg/l.

Whatever may be used of these conventional methods, solids must be confronted. These accumulate from fine screens, grit and presettling tanks, secondary settling tanks, and at the bottom of oxidation ponds. The solids can be left in the ponds as long as odor conditions and floated deposits and scum remain tolerable. Even then the pond can be abandoned and filled if feasible. In the other instances there must be a regular removal of solids, usually some processing, and finally disposal. The first-round choices are aerobic or anaerobic digestion, dewatering, and burial, or dewatering and direct burning in gas-fired furnaces. Some well-dewatered sludges can be burned in conventional incinerators with other mixed combustible wastes. Sludges can be dewatered by vacuum filters, centrifuges, filter presses, or flash drying. The final inerts from flash driers have usefulness for soil sealers if ponds are on-site or nearby. Otherwise, the material goes to fill or burial. Any sludge that does not produce nuisances of odors, fly or rat attraction and breeding, or mosquito breeding can be lagooned. Land area must be close by and cheap. Transport can be by tanker or pipeline. Soil conditions and geology must be known to be certain that seepage and leaching do not impair groundwater quality and future use.

As industry has wastewaters of unusual characteristics and has the special skills of its own engineering and scientific staff who are very knowledgeable of the production processes and materials, it is not surprising that unconventional treatment methods have been developed and are in use. Innovations have resulted from joint work of plant staff, consulting engineers, and waste treatment equipment manufacturers. Economic, regulatory, and occasionally community pressures motivate the search for new methods to save land area, reduce capital costs, and circumvent the need for another staff task of operating conventional wastewater treatment plants. Higher operating costs of unconventional methods are accepted to gain such advantages. An advantage that is not overlooked in the new day of environmental consciousness is that of enhancing the corporate image by advertising waste control efforts to the point of glamourizing them.

A series of examples of unconventional approaches with their brief identification follow. Details can be found in Besselievre (Ref. 4-4), in the references he cites, and in current readings in the *Journal of the Water Pollution Control Federation*, particularly in its annual review of the literature in the June issue of each year.

1 Adsorption of wastes is not a municipal practice. Industry has found it feasible to use activated carbon to adsorb organic compounds and to regenerate the carbon. In German practice, beds of common reeds with high porosity, 23,000 pores per square centimeter, have been used to adsorb phenols.

2 Flotation and foam separation can be done by aeration or gasification with or without the feeding of foaming agents. Oils, greases, and emulsified organics respond to this method. By taking a leaf from the ore milling techniques, flotation is used for separating fines of colloidal size of metallics and inorganics. Besselievre gives 11 examples.

3 Electrodialysis has been an industrial unit process since its application in Europe in 1915. It is used to improve orange juice, remove minerals from molasses and cane syrup, and desalt cheese whey. So it was another step to use the separation of ionic content across charged membranes to modify wastewaters with the benefit of recovery of reuseable material. Electrodialysis works to recover nitric and hydrofluoric acid from stainless steel pickling liquor, and pulping liquor from organic mixes.

4 *Reverse osmosis* is a somewhat unfortunate term for a process that meets the requirements of a very high removal of contaminants or pollutants. The term reverse osmosis makes more sense when we recall that osmosis is the pass of low-dissolved-content water through a semipermeable membrane to dilute a concentrated solution. Reverse osmosis is the passage of molecules selectively from the concentrated side through the membrane to the dilute side. It occurs naturally for some molecular forms through semipermeable membranes. Reverse osmosis can be made to occur for many molecular forms and some viruses by using selective membranes and by applying pressure from the concentrate side. Pressures used in wastewater purification by reverse osmosis are a modest 50 psi or less with rates of 10 to 40 gallons per square foot of membrane. Reverse osmosis has been satisfactory for separating toxic ions from plating wastes, recoveries on chemical and pharmaceutical wastes, organic removals from vegetable and animal wastes, and acid recovery from pickling liquors. Costs are high. The initial costs of units are estimated at $10 to $20 per square foot of membrane surface provided. There is a requirement of 0.25 to 0.5 hp per 1,000 gallons treated per day. Membrane life is from 6 to 12 months.

5 Injection wells have gained an unsavory reputation because their use at the Rocky Mountain Arsenal, Colorado, to dispose of toxic fluids has raised two serious questions. That installation injects 800 gpm to strata over 12,000 ft deep under a pressure of 2,000 psi. The questions are

(a) Is the travel of the toxicants in these strata known?
(b) Is the injection causing seismic stresses with resulting strains capable of initiating earthquakes?

There are about 100 injection wells for industrial waste disposal in use in the United States to get rid of toxic materials; brine waste; organics from pharmaceutical, chemical, and petrochemical plants; phenolic, coal-tar, sulfide, and high-odor wastes; and concentrated acid and caustic wastes. An answer must be found to the questions:

(a) Who has the right to use this particular form of the assimilative capacity of our environment for wastes?
(b) Who has the responsibility to control such subterranean disposal sites?

The Pennsylvania State Sanitary Board accepted the solution of the Hammermill Paper Company for its waste disposal by injection wells. These penetrate a brine-bearing limestone at a depth of 1,600 ft. Four wells are receiving 2 million gpd. It is estimated that in 50 years only, an area of 1.25-mi radius will be affected. The federal water quality control officials stated their opposition to injection wells for wastewater disposal in 1970.

6 Predigestion is an anaerobic processing of high-BOD wastes in which the whole waste stream goes to a digester at 95°F for 1 to 10 days as the first treatment step. It has been used on brewery, winery, and meat packing wastes. Reductions of 75 to 97 percent of BOD have been obtained on wastes with BODs of 1,000 to 30,000 mg/l with high organic solids.

THE DISPOSAL OF HUMAN EXCRETA WITHOUT SEWERS

Sewers provide a network of pipes for the water-carried transport and collection of human wastes, storm water in combined systems, and varying amounts of trade wastes. Where such a system does not exist, human wastes disposal can be made by:

1 A pit privy or one of its variants
2 Retention containers with frequent collection or with chemical control permitting delayed removal
3 Short water transport for solids separation and digestion in a septic tank or cesspool, and liquid effluent disposal by subsurface irrigation or infiltration, or by a stabilization pond
4 Indiscriminate ground- and water-surface disposal.

A minimum of two-thirds of the world's people use one of these four methods. A vast majority of them continue on method four. In yet another paradox of human behavior, so do the passengers of the world's most luxurious trains packaged in streamline-shaped stainless steel with tinted glass, conditioned air, and fluorescent lighting.

The Pit Privy and Its Variants

Figure 4-1 shows the isolation of human excreta in a pit privy. Figure 4-13 presents variations which are intended to improve odor and fly control. In the bored-hole variant, the groundwater table is penetrated. The reduced volumetric pit capacity is presumed to be offset by liquefaction products discharging to the groundwater. It may happen in very coarse sands and gravel, but not in fine sands and loam, where clogging sets up in 2 to 3 months.[1] Tropical temperatures do speed digestion. The need for special equipment to bore the hole and the inability of a rural family to replicate the hole without a drilling rig make the bored-hole latrine a poor choice for rural excreta control. The water-seal latrine provides fly and odor control superior to the pit privy. It does require a smooth finish to the concrete bowl and about 1.5 to 2 liters of water to clear the trap after each use. It is not fitted to freezing temperatures or to places where seasonal or continued water scarcity requires hand carrying the family's water ration long distances. The aqua privy is a rather elaborate variation as it requires an impervious receiving vault, usually a gas vent, and an overflow to a second pit for seepage to a subsurface irrigation line, or collectively to a sewer and stabilization pond.

Figure 4-14 is a schematic summary of the extensive and intensive studies by Caldwell and Parr,[2] and by Dyer, Baskaran, and Sekar of the movement of bacterial contaminants and chemical pollutants from pits in which human excreta have been deposited. In the studies of three pits which penetrated the groundwater table, the movement of coliforms is remarkably limited. Even in direct contact with the groundwater the maximum advances of *E. coli* observed were 10, 35, and 12 ft. In

[1] B. R. Dyer, T. R. Baskaran, and C. C. Sekar, *Indian J. Med. Res.*, **33**:23 (1945).
[2] E. L. Caldwell and L. W. Parr, *J. Infect. Dis.*, **61**:148 (1937); and **62**:225, 272 (1938).

Type of pit, pit lining, base, and floor recommended by the
U. S. Public Health Service, superstructure not included to show
floor and riser with cover.

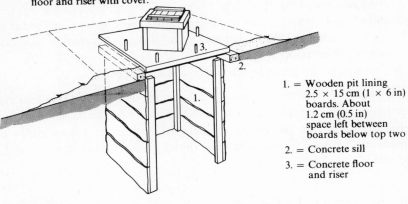

1. = Wooden pit lining
2.5 × 15 cm (1 × 6 in)
boards. About
1.2 cm (0.5 in)
space left between
boards below top two

2. = Concrete sill

3. = Concrete floor
and riser

Typical bored-hole latrine
with squatter slab

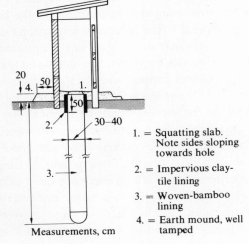

Measurements, cm

1. = Squatting slab.
Note sides sloping
towards hole

2. = Impervious clay-
tile lining

3. = Woven-bamboo
lining

4. = Earth mound, well
tamped

Water seal slab used in Ceylon

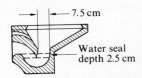

Water seal
depth 2.5 cm

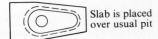

Slab is placed
over usual pit

FIGURE 4-13
The pit privy and its variants. (*Source*: *WHO drawings* 7131, 7456, *and* 7459,
Ref. 4-5, *pp.* 46, 90, *and* 96.)

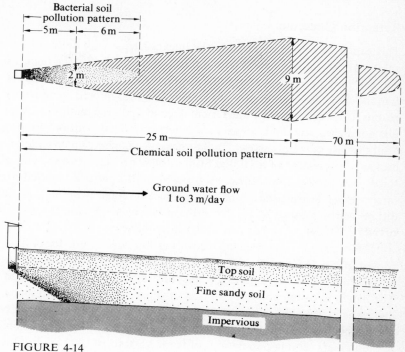

FIGURE 4-14
The movement of bacterial contaminants and chemical pollutants from pit disposal of human excreta. (*Source: Ref.* 4-5, *p.* 30.)

each case there is a subsequent regression as soil clogging and biochemical action get under way.   The soil conditions were sandy loams with some clay, generally finer than sand beds used for water filtration.   In pits that did not penetrate the groundwater, typical of 95 percent or more of the pit type of privies, *E. coli* never reached a point 5 ft from the pit in the groundwater stream.   In a pit with the groundwater table from 12 to 15 ft below its bottom, no *E. coli* moved as much as 1 ft vertically downward or laterally from the pit.

Wagner and Lanoix (Ref. 4-5) provide a comprehensive guide to the selection of pit methods of excreta disposal and the procedures of organizing, executing, and following up pit-privy campaigns.   The important mission is to get the human feces off the ground surface by putting it into a pit.   This will substantially reduce individual worm loads among a couple of billion people who for all or part of a year are scarcely able to feed themselves, let alone share their meager food with an intestine full of worms.   Much the same applies to reducing schistosomiasis by keeping feces and urine out of surface waters so that the schistosome cannot begin another cycle through the snails in the water.

Retention Containers

This caption covers a range from the bucket latrine with daily collection to the recirculating flush toilet units on jet aircraft. Hypothetically, the bucket latrine or "box and can" method can accomplish a sanitary disposal of human excreta. Wagner and Lanoix (Ref. 4-5) summarize the difficulties encountered in practice. Large populations, rural and urban, in the Orient depend upon the method. Analysis shows that it is not a cheap method, for there is collection, transportation, and ultimate disposal, as in the case of solid wastes. In Southeast Asia, where an unskilled laborer earns the exchange equivalent of a United States dollar per day in town, and one-half to two-thirds that rurally, the cost ranges from $4 to $15 per pail handled per year, with the family served bearing the added costs of bucket replacement and repair. Such expenditures warrant a search for alternative means by a community service in communities of over 2,000 people and by some privy alternative in smaller communities.

The custom and need of recovering human excreta for soil fertilizer are well rooted in the Orient. Procedures for composting the excreta with other refuse and animal manure, or for digesting it anaerobically, have been developed and are in use. The handling to the point of compost or digestion is difficult to manage in a sanitary and esthetic way, but at least the composted or digested product can be pathogen free and innocuous in odor and appearance for farm use. In Japan, some 20 central digestion plants serving populations of from 3,500 to 100,000 are producing a stabilized humus by the same procedures as anaerobic sludge digestion at sewage treatment plants. H. B. Gotaas (Ref. 4-6) details compost methods which produce an agriculturally useful product for single families and for communities.

The caustic-soda chemical toilet never came into wide use in the United States. It made a brief appearance in many Midwestern rural schools before the electric power line came down the road and placed running water and septic tank systems within reach. Today's version of the chemical toilet is in commercial aircraft and private pleasure boats. A combination of emulsifiers and deodorants permit the recirculation of small quantities of water through a self-contained fine screening and flushing system. One such unit used aboard boats has only 4 gallons of water in the circuit which can provide for 80 flushings with the correct chemical charge. A pump-out and recharge every 5 days is recommended. For commercial passenger aircraft, pump-out and recharge is usual after a day's flying. These units have no connections with the potable water service aboard the craft.

Septic Tank Systems

About 1860 Louis Mouras developed the Mouras Automatic Scavenger in France. It was a closed vault with a water seal which "rapidly transformed all excremtitious matter" to a liquid state. A fellow countryman, Abbé Moigno, studied the process under glass in the laboratory in 1881. He conjectured, "May not the unseen agents be those vibrions or anaerobes which, according to Pasteur, are destroyed by oxygen, and only manifest their activity in vessels from which the air is excluded?" Thus the *fosse septique* was developed, and the nature of its action recognized in France. Septic tanks first appeared in the United States in the 1890s. Professor A. N. Talbot built one in 1894 at Urbana, Illinois, and used his observations to design a 22,000-gal unit which began to serve neighboring Champaign in 1897. In 1899 the Lawrence Experiment Station, Massachusetts, on the basis of studies of a two-compartment 250-gal tank, reported that continuous operation was better than a batch loading, with a 47 to 60 percent removal of organic matter measured by the oxygen-consumed test. A septic tank system has two components, an impermeable compartment and a provision for liquid effluent discharge to the subsoil. Figure 4-2 shows a typical installation in which the effluent goes to subsurface irrigation lines. Essential design criteria are indicated.

By the 1920s, in the United States, the Agricultural Extension Services of many of the Land-Grant Colleges had demonstration models and bulletins to assist farmers who had made the step to indoor flush toilets by building septic tank systems. In 1928, E. Lehmann, R. C. Kelleher, and A. M. Buswell published their studies on the family septic tank in Illinois.[1] Their findings are valid to this day, and little with practical effect has been added since on tank sizes, compartmentation and baffling of inlet, connecting and outlet pipes. The tank serves simultaneously as a settling unit and as a storage and digestion unit for scum and sludge. The second function determines its volume, dimensions, and structure. The greater the depth, the less is the disturbance of the sludge. Baffling improves scum retention. Compartmentation provides a secondary unit to resettle and to digest further any solids which are carried from the first compartment.

The detailed studies of the U.S. Public Health Service from 1947 to 1953 (Ref. 4-7) confirmed good recommended factors for tank design and put these on a much more rational data base, provided much useful information on performance, dispelled some folklore, and revealed that the behavior of the liquid effluent in subsurface soils is dependent on the soil characteristics, which are usually very diverse and frequently not compatible with the task of effecting the absorption of large quantities of water still burdened with organic matter. The results of these studies which could be put to practical application, along with all available recorded and voiced experience, are embodied in the 1967 revised Manual of Septic Tank Practice, of the Public Health Service (Ref. 4-8). Adherence to the procedures in the manual will result in a satisfactory sewage disposal device. The notoriety of septic tank systems for poor performance in suburban residential areas in the United States results from urban

[1] *Illinois State Water Surv. Bull.*, **27** (1928).

volumes of sewage being imposed on a refractory subsoil on small lot sizes.   As David Lee, formerly Chief Sanitary Engineer of Florida has observed, " It has been the case of a country girl coming to the city and getting into trouble in a hurry."

The Public Health Service field observations on sludge accumulation and the effects of compartmentation on solids behavior in experimental tanks conform to uncontrolled anaerobic digestion.   Sludge accumulates during the first year at the rate of about $3\frac{1}{2}$ ft^3 per capita, 26.5 gal.   Digestion gets under way and compaction occurs so that in the next 5 to 6 years the rate drops to about $1\frac{1}{3}$ ft^3 per capita annually and levels off thereafter.   A check on sludge and scum accumulations at the end of 3 years and each year thereafter, with pump-out when the sludge clear space is less than 1 or $1\frac{1}{2}$ ft in tanks with a surface area of 25 ft^2, will extend the service life of the absorption lines.   Pump-out should leave some settled solids to seed renewed digestion without a lag phase.   Do not scrub, flush, or disinfect.

Figure 4-2 shows the relation and function of the soil absorption lines.   Seepage pits can replace a tile type of lines where the groundwater table is at least 4 ft below the pit bottom and there is homogeneous porous sand of an effective size of about 0.2 mm and uniformity coefficient of about 1.5.   These lines dispose of the liquid by infiltration through the trench bottom and wetted sides, by transpiration through plant and grass cover, and by evaporation through the soil cover.   The unstable dissolved and suspended solids must be managed by biological action.   The action is probably a combination of anaerobic, facultative, and aerobic systems.   Until serious overloads and soil clogging sets in, thin films of organic matter very likely behave as benthal deposits.

The determination of the required absorption area by a soil percolation test was first used by Henry Ryon of the New York State Health Department.[1]   He based his ratio of percolation test absorption to absorbable load in an operating system, upon the performance of absorption systems which failed or were about to fail after 20 years of use.   This resulted in applied loads of about one-fiftieth of the percolation test's hole absorption capacity expressed in gallons per square foot per day.   The validity of Ryon's work has been borne out by the Public Health Service studies (Ref. 4-7, pt. 2, pp. 54–55).

Careful technique in making soil percolation tests is an absolute necessity.   Soil characteristics are so variable even in a single lot, that unless the immediate area is well known, a minimum of six replicate tests should be made.   Complete wetting of the hole is necessary to reach the condition of saturation and swelling of the soil before readings are made.   The readings at the end of repeated wettings are those of an equilibrium state and are the reliable ones.   Soil percolation tests are very time-

---

[1] Henry Ryon, Notes on the Design of Sewage Disposal, with Special Reference to Small Installations, Albany, N.Y., 1928.

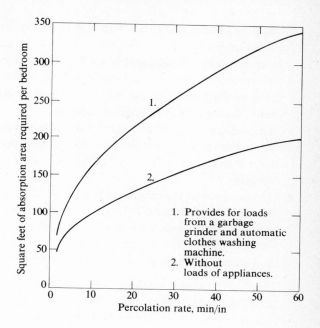

FIGURE 4-15
Absorption area required for private residence for observed percolation rates into saturated, swollen soils at equilibrium. (*Source*: *Ref.* 4-8, *p.* 9.)

consuming, but provide the only practical means of establishing soil absorption capacity. The objective procedures (Ref. 4-8, pp. 4–6) must be followed to produce dependable information. Figure 4-15 plots percolation rates in minutes per inch of water-level drop in the test hole versus square feet of area of absorption-trench bottom required per bedroom for private residences. This curve is for use where United States water consumption and sewage strength prevails, particularly for suspended solids. Curve 1, Fig. 4-15, provides for garbage grinders and automatic clothes washing machines. Curve 2 is for United States homes without these appliances. Percolation-test absorption-area data for other rates of water use are in Part 3, p. 3, of Ref. 4-7.

Six Observations on the Behavior of Septic Tank Systems

1 Seeding eliminates a lag in starting solids digestion in new tanks. It is most desirable in tanks receiving ground garbage from the outset. It is not a necessity for tanks receiving mixed household wastes without garbage. Cultures and enzymatic mixes are not needed.

2   Resting absorption fields is helpful in restoring absorptive capacity.

3   Vegetation over absorption areas helps to reduce infiltration loads by evapo-transpiration.   Root penetration is rarely a problem.

4   Synthetic detergents in normal quantities of household use are not harmful to tank performance.   These may have a long-term detrimental effect on soil structure causing an acceleration of clogging.

5   The sodium, calcium, and magnesium salts in household water-softener regeneration discharges are not detrimental to sludge digestion in the tank.   These may have a long-term detrimental effect on soil structure causing an acceleration of clogging.

6   The addition of the caustic-soda type of "cleaners" to tanks is very detrimental to system performance.   The caustic soda liquefies the sludge, causes flotation, causes excessive solids discharge to the absorption field, and raises the pH which inhibits established digestion.   The caustic soda in the tank effluent damages soil structure which causes an acceleration of clogging.

In the central and southern parts of Africa, stabilization ponds have been used to receive the effluent from septic tanks.   This disposal method has been used in conjunction with communal facilities for excreta disposal, bathing, and laundry in African village housing projects, in conjunction with family unit septic tanks and aqua privies combining discharges from tanks to sewers on very low grades to stabilization ponds. Pond size requirements are modest.   Using three ponds in series with a 4-ft depth, the area required for central African conditions have been 14 ft^2 per person for the primary pond and 7 ft^2 per person for each of the secondary and tertiary ponds.   On the primary ponds, BOD_5 loadings of 450 lb/(acre)(day) have been handled without scum flotation.   The economy, the sanitation achieved, and the ease of maintenance make the system very favorable for use in tropical areas.[1]   Pond edges must be faced with concrete or cleared frequently of vegetation.   Pathogens do not survive. Mosquitos do not breed in the ponds which have peripheral vegetation cleared. Snail vectors of schistosomiasis do not propagate in stabilization ponds.

POSSIBLE CHANGES AND DEVELOPMENTS IN MANAGING HUMAN EXCRETA

The first modern valve water closet was devised in 1596 by Sir John Harrington.   It found no market and had to be reinvented and patented by two additional Englishmen, Alexander Cumming in 1775 and Joseph Bramah in 1778.   This time, the convenience

---

[1] G. V. R. Marais, New Factors in the Design, Operation and Performance of Waste-Stabilization Ponds, *WHO Bull.* 34, 1966, p. 737.

of water-carried waste took hold and gained slow ascendency. Henry Wadsworth Longfellow is credited with installing the first valved flush toilet in the United States in 1840. By 1850 Windsor Castle and the White House had such facilities. Most of these early installations discharged to cesspools. In fact, in many American and English cities, connection to the storm drains was prohibited, as in Boston until 1833 and Philadelphia until the 1850s. A large fire in 1842 in Hamburg set the stage for a rehabilitation which included an extensive system of sanitary sewers. In the United States sewers for sanitary wastes were planned and built in Brooklyn in 1857 to 1858, Omaha in 1872, and in Boston following the Hering Report of 1881 (Refs. 4-9 and 4-10). In this evolution, sewers for rain runoff became combined sewers, while in some areas of the same city separate systems developed, one for sanitary wastes to the sanitary sewers and one for the storm water to the storm sewers. Even in well-planned separate systems storm water enters the sanitary sewers by infiltration and by illicit connections. All manner of liquid wastes enters sewer systems from homes, public buildings including hospitals, commercial and manufacturing places, animal feed yards, and meat and poultry dressing plants. The existing patterns, a little over a century in development, place severe economic and social constraints on technological changes and developments in managing waste at the source, in transportation, in reclamation, and in treatment. Excepting some industrial situations, the carrier water is of drinking quality until a valve opening converts it from supply to waste.

This brief historic look at water-carried sewage makes the statement of Professor P. H. McGauhey of the University of California more comprehensible and the dilemmas in making changes more dolorous.

> If sewage were discharged without any treatment whatsoever, we should be sending a 2000-ton train of water, on which we lately spent a great deal of money in purifying, to transport a single ton of organic solids. Worse yet, in the more common case of well treated sewage, one good burro could carry all that is required of this half million gallons of water. Furthermore, we throw away the train at the end of a single trip. It is in line with our heritage of waste, but it is without parallel in the history of transportation (Ref. 4-11, p. 429).

If the water we presently use on a seeming one-way trip is too valuable, what alternatives can be considered?

In Transportation

In an appendix, Combined Sewers, in the Tukey Report (Ref. 1-5), J. C. Geyer and L. Katz briefly comment on 12 means by which the problem of combined sewer overflow during high-intensity storms can be attacked. Three concern the sewers: separation, larger interceptors to reduce shore-front overflows, and sanitary express sewers running directly to treatment plants and bypassing existing combined mains. One proposal under study is macerating sanitary sewage on-site and transporting the suspension under pressure through small-diameter pipes hung within existing sewers.   Two of the Geyer-Katz suggestions are on rainfall runoff control, and two are for better maintenance and monitoring of existing overflow control devices on combined sewers. The latter is a sizable task as New York has 218, Chicago 362, and Cleveland 420. The English method of passing storm water through standby settling tanks and subsequently treating the holdup is cited as a means to reduce treatment plant peak loads and diversions without treatment.   Other suggestions noted are for reducing the volume and the solids of sanitary sewage at the source, with slim hope of doing either, and for structures along the sewers to store storm water peaks and to treat sewage en route to the plant.   Storage structures are feasible, with their required cleanout of settled grit and muck an issue.   Treatment en route is now practiced to the extent of chlorination to prevent deoxygenation.   Settling could be done readily.   One sewer maintenance problem is the settlement of grit and coarse solids during dry-weather flows in lines designed for storm flows.   But settling means a second handling to remove the solids.   Aeration en route to initiate bio-oxidation is a possibility. Improved mechanical aerators and even tonnage oxygen in combination with sewage pumping stations, where these exist, might be used.   Chemical additives to increase sewer-flow capacities, to improve treatability, and to reduce BOD are in experimental use.[1]

One aspect of wastewater reclamation, which has been pointed out by McGauhey, is transportation, that is, delivery of the raw wastewater to the point of reclamation and use before it has a myriad of untreatable pollutants added to it.   For industrial uses, these pollutants are more likely to be of industrial waste origin such as cyanides, phenols, acids, alkalies, heavy-metal ions, and dye stuffs.   In such cases, the domestic sewage should go by an express sewer to the user, who would provide all the treatment steps required to produce the quality of water his use requires.   The transport system has a vital role in reclamation.   In McGauhey's terms, the train would be reused at the end of that particular trip.   By selective loading en route, passengers who would be difficult to remove at the end of the line would be denied transportation.

In Treatment

Technology exists for the restoration of wastewater to very high purity.   The bill is a high one when ionic manipulation becomes a step, for that requires chemical precipitation, ion exchange units, and the less developed methods of osmosis, reverse osmosis, or electrodialysis.   More will happen along this pathway when the quality of readily available water deteriorates to the point that social and economic pressure produce political responses for more conservation and reuse of existing sources.   A question that must be met is that of the undefined health hazards of water reuse.   The issues of

[1] D. A. Okun, *J. Water Pollution Control Federation*, **43**:2177 (1971).

virus survival and trace chemicals are easily raised, but difficult to answer definitively. The epidemiological evidence on the risks of waterborne viruses is reassuring, even in the case of infectious hepatitis.   On the chemical side, the intakes of the suspects are very much larger in many foods and in air than in water.   Lead, arsenic, selenium, and nitrates are examples of that.   Suspected carcinogens raise the specter of damage which may come only after decades of cumulative exposure.   One mission of the Public Health Service's Environmental Health Sciences Research Center in North Carolina is to study long-term effects of long-residence trace environmental contaminants.

Residues of nondegradable pesticides, herbicides, and other chemical contaminants are of a like nature.   Until the biological evidence is clearer, prudent management of the environment requires the same course as is being followed for radioactive wastes.   Costly and often heroic efforts must be made to hold the discharge to the free environment to an absolute minimum, frequently to the minimum levels of sampling and analytical techniques.   The fate after use of nondegradable agricultural chemicals in surface runoff and soil infiltration is scarcely known quantitatively.

At high levels of inorganic nitrogen and phosphates in ratios which are not certain and in the presence of a variety of trace metallic ions, a lake becomes nutrient rich, eutrophic.   The results are algal "blooms," and their subsequent death and decay with deoxygenation of the lower water strata.   Such conditions impair appearance, produce difficult taste and odor problems, and are rather self-perpetuating as the decayed matter reenters the cycle.   Water from fields that are chemically fertilized and sewage treatment plant effluents are added sources of inorganic nitrogen and phosphates.   Some 4 billion lb of detergents with 20 to 30 percent phosphate content are produced annually in the United States.   Most of this is discharged as waste.   One solution being explored by the Soap and Detergent Association, which sponsored the development and adoption of the LAS soft detergent to replace ABS hard detergent, is the substitution of nonphosphate compounds as detergent builders.

Table 4-10 shows the patterns of inorganic nitrogen and phosphates in source waters and sewage effluents and the percentage of removals by conventional bio-oxidation plants and by a series of tertiary treatment processes.   Lake Tahoe, California, is a high-value resort area.   To prevent its progressive deterioration by eutrophication, all lakeside sewage is intercepted and carried through the processes of *1, 2,* and *4* in Table 4-10.   High aeration rates have been found to increase phosphate uptake into activated sludge, so that process alteration may be useful in some instances.   The diversion of sewage effluents past a lake has been in use at Lake Monona, Wisconsin, since 1935, and was started at two other Wisconsin lakes in 1959 and at Lake Washington, Seattle, in 1965.[1]   On a pilot plant scale, studies of advanced or tertiary

---

[1] E. G. Fruh, *J. Water Pollution Control Federation,* **38:**1449 (1967).

processes for wastewater renovation were begun by the Public Health Service and are continuing under the Federal Environmental Protection Agency to determine design factors, costs, and operating problems.   Anion exchange, carbon adsorption, electrodialysis, distillation, and chemical precipitation are among the processes being tried.

Other Developments

As the cycle between water waste and water use becomes shorter in time and distance, more use is being made of wastewater reclamation for industry, for irrigation, for groundwater recharge, and for surface-water conservation in man-made ponds. Wider reuse is feasible, including some in high-density suburban apartment projects requiring dual supply lines for nonpotable purposes.[1]   Anaerobic processes can be engineered and managed more closely as the biology and chemistry of these become better known.   High-rate digestion, and the use of septic tanks and anaerobic ponds ahead of aerobic and facultative stabilization ponds are steps in that direction.

Methods which are low in facilities costs and minimal in mechanical equipment are urgently needed throughout the developing countries and in many sections of the United States.   The needs of unsewered rural communities which are just beginning to grasp for piped water, if not in their homes, at least near them, must be met.   In

Table 4-10   INORGANIC NITROGEN AND PHOSPHATES IN SOURCE WATERS AND SEWAGE TREATMENT PLANT EFFLUENTS, AND PERCENTAGE REMOVALS BY TREATMENT PROCESSES

	Inorganic nitrogen	Phosphate-phosphorous
In source waters	0.5–1 mg/l	0.1–3 mg/l
In sewage effluents	20 mg/l Range 20–50 mg/l	16 mg/l Range 1–20 mg/l
Percentage removable:		
1 By conventional treatment	50%	10%
2 By lime-alum coagulation and rapid sand filtration	0%	85%
3 By electrodialysis	20%	2%
4 By adsorption	5%	0%
Cumulative removal	75%	97%

SOURCES: Tukey Rep. (Ref. 1-5, p. 184), 1965; and Spilhaus Rep. (Ref. 1-6, p. 193), 1966.

[1] D. A. Okun, *J. Water Pollution Control Federation*, **43:**2174 (1971).

the warm and tropical climates the water seal privy with a pit lined only when soil conditions require it and a very modest superstructure of local materials and building methods is an economical and sanitary method for rural areas.   There is another vast and growing mass of unsewered people in the urban centers of the developing countries. These are the overflow from the rural areas, who are landless, whose hands are not needed on the land, and who sense some better life in the cities.   They crowd into the worst of existing housing and spill over into squatter shack communities, called *hutments* in India, *favelas* in Brazil, *barreadas* in Spanish-speaking countries.   Their precarious water supply is luxurious in comparison to their waste disposal facilities. Some intermediate means between pit type privies and conventional flush toilets and wastewater sewerage is needed.   Communal facilities combining bathing, laundering, and excreta disposal have been used in El Salvador communities.   Among alternatives which need field trials are short-run, covered surface channels to stabilization ponds with and without prior solids separation, solids separation and discharge to streams during the rainy seasons, and to shallow evaporation ponds or to land irrigation in the dry seasons.   Whatever scheme is undertaken, education must precede and maintenance must follow.

AN APPRAISAL OF MAN'S MANAGEMENT OF HIS OWN EXCRETA AND WASTEWATERS

The First Level—Prevention of Disease Transmission

The epidemiology of the diseases transmitted by failures to manage human excreta is well defined.   There are large gaps in numerical information on these diseases among the people in the underdeveloped countries.   Examples are the incidence of diarrheas in children under 5 and of schistosomiasis in those up to adolescence.   Sample studies in Guatemala on the diarrheas, and in East Africa on schistosomiasis show these to be high in number and to cause a continuous sapping of energy required for physical and mental growth.   These are among the obscure drainoffs of the human resources and social vitality of these populations.

The simple hygiene of the pit disposal of human excreta is not practiced among some 2 billion people of the world, most of whom live by subsistence-level farming. Well-organized local public health services can mount and sustain activities to promote privy construction and use.   This has been demonstrated in the southeastern United States from 1912 to 1940, in the Amazon region of Brazil from 1943 to the present, and in Thailand from 1955 to the present.   In Thailand a half million privy units, mostly of the water seal type, were built from 1961 to 1967.

The suburban expansion in the United States found sanitarians and sanitary engineers technically somewhat uncertain about septic tank systems, particularly in judging soil adsorption characteristics.   The Public Health Service studies have been of great value in systematizing our technical rationale.   Administratively, local government has been quite unprepared and often unwilling or unable to manage land development for housing.   The deficiencies and waste in organizing sanitary services are only one part of a conglomerate arising from attempts to meet the needs for traffic control, transportation, schools, recreation, health facilities, and police and fire protection.   The underlying conflict is within ourselves, for it involves the choice between independence and interdependence at a series of social levels—the individual, the neighborhood, and the layers of community government.   In the organization of sanitary services the economics of long-range planning and development of services for large population groups on contiguous land areas must be emphasized.   Great urban centers throughout the world confront suburban organization and development. Great Britain and the U.S.S.R. offer useful patterns for study.

Sewered urban areas are on a treadmill in which each forward step is rolled back. Sewer construction barely keeps up with increases of population and of intensity of land use.   Sewage treatment plant construction barely keeps up with the added loads on the capacity of receiving water to dilute and to assimilate the treated effluents. Despite the construction of new plants and improvements in the old ones in the metropolitan area around New York City, the quality of the waters of New York Harbor continue to deteriorate in increases in coliform densities.   These are saline waters without use as a drinking water source, but they are still useful for swimming and fishing at points close to large concentrations of people with the least economic resources to travel long distances for relief from the intensities of their slum and blighted neighborhoods.   The pattern of deterioration of water quality is not unique to New York Harbor.   It extends to our vast inland lakes, our trunk rivers of the Midwest and South, and their tributaries.   These are vital sources for domestic and industrial water, and they are becoming increasingly the source and ultimate disposal point of irrigation water.   The management of the waters of the Tennessee and the Ohio valleys by the Tennessee Valley Authority and the Ohio River Stream Sanitation Commission provides learnable lessons.   The effort of assessing the optimum utilization of the waters of the Delaware River basin succinctly reported in Ref. 1-6 by a cost-benefit analysis demonstrates an approach which may raise the level of selfish use to considerations broader in geographical area and longer in time span than has been the American tradition.

The ticking of the epidemiological and sociological time bomb of the unwatered and unsewered thousands crowding on squatter land in and about the cities of South and Central America, of Southeast Asia, and only to a lesser degree, in Central Africa has been noted.   The inadequate suggestions made for possible solutions must be examined and extended to better ones.

The Second Level—Comfort, Convenience, and Esthetics

Rural and village people in the underdeveloped countries have been slow, by our measure, to recognize the convenience and esthetic benefits of the pit disposal of their excreta, quite aside from any acceptance of the "germ theory" of diseases. The failure to use and to maintain privies has been high. In parts of Thailand, cited above as having a successful construction program, as many as one-third of the units go unused. Apparently, the units are built to please the local health worker and earn neighborly merit without use being part of the bargain. Water scarcity during the dry season causes water seal privies to go unused. What makes particular social behavior culturally acceptable will engage sociologists, and in the case of health habits, the health educators, on many fronts for many years. Privy use is only one of them. In the Amazon region a monthly visit to each family by the "guarda sanitario" has produced good usage and maintenance. There, in turn, it was necessary to keep up the interest and the morale of the "guarda sanitario." Each one in the responsibility ladder needed the assurance that the one above him cared about his actions and appreciated them.

Esthetics have provided considerable leverage in gaining support for pollution control in streams, in estuaries, and even on ocean fronts. In the last case, visible floating human waste will send the bathers out of the water as fast as sighting a shark fin. The boaters and water skiers are ready allies for clean water when their accessible areas are threatened. The convenience and economic value of the use of attractive waters for recreation are closely related. In part, these can be assigned dollar values in balancing the costs and benefits of pollution control.

The Third Level—Safeguarding the Ecological Balances and Conserving Our Resources

For all but the prosperous rural farm areas, the recovery of human excreta and decomposable organic solid wastes by sanitary composting is a beneficial recovery of humus and low-grade fertilizer for soil improvement. Long practiced in China and Japan, an improved method is applicable to rural cluster villages common in India and Southeast Asia. In similar vein, but on a different scale, there is the use of sewage for cropland irrigation. Large cities in the dry-wet season climatic cycle can utilize their wastewaters for land irrigation to augment food production either directly by selected crops, or indirectly through forage crops and animal grazing. Melbourne, Australia, and Israeli communities have been cited along with cities in Texas and the southwestern United States and areas in California. The hygienic risks are manageable.

A major impetus for clean streams in the United States has been wildlife conservation. Until recent years, the need has been to regulate the pollution loads so that the DO did not fall below fish needs, and to regulate and monitor specific inorganic toxins such as cyanides and copper. New sources of potent poisons for aquatic life are industrial wastes and agricultural land runoff containing residues of pesticides and herbicides. The recognized fish kills have been the result of industrial discharges, accidental or unmanaged, from points of manufacture of these materials. But each user adds a trace. The nutritional imbalance caused by excesses of inorganic nitrogen and phosphates in wastewaters discharged to lakes accelerates eutrophication. The algal "blooms" establish disorder in a desirable ecological balance. The main sources are the wastes of users of phosphate-based detergents, and an undetermined contribution from runoff and seepage from land treated with nitrate-phosphate-potassium fertilizers. Beyond these specifics, there is the place of wastewater reclamation in conserving water resources. The use of wastewaters for groundwater recharge is in use on Long Island in the East, at Midwest points, and in the Los Angeles basin. Wastewater recovery has been shown to be practical and economical in particular circumstances varying from the use of Back River Sewage Treatment Plant effluent in Baltimore by the Bethlehem Steel Plant at Sparrows Point, a few miles away, to the Santee Project of San Diego where a major benefit is the recreational facilities including swimming. Some early signs of eutrophication at the Santee Project underscore the necessity of continued study of all phases of wastewater behavior. Much information is needed to undertake and manage wastewater reuse economically, with the minimum risk to health and without serious esthetic offense. A variety of studies underway in this country and abroad, engaging a wide spectrum of professional skills, will produce the technology. An equal effort is needed in the equally or more difficult task of bringing about changes in social values and in governmental structures and services in managing our environment. That requires the action of all who perceive good and are prepared to make sacrifices to achieve it.

REFERENCES

4-1 A Study of the Pollution and Natural Purification of the Ohio River, vol. 3, sec. 6, *U.S. Public Health Serv. Bull.* 143, 1924.

4-2 MCKINNEY, ROSS E.: "Microbiology for Sanitary Engineers," McGraw-Hill Book Company, New York, 1962.

4-3 PHELPS, EARLE B.: "Stream Sanitation," John Wiley & Sons, Inc., New York, 1944.

4-4 BESSELIEVRE, E. B.: "The Treatment of Industrial Wastes," 2d ed., McGraw-Hill Book Company, New York, 1969.

4-5 WAGNER, E. G., and J. N. LANOIX: Excreta Disposal for Rural Areas and Small Communities, *WHO, Monogr. Ser.* 39, 1958.

4-6 GOTAAS, H. B.: Composting, *WHO, Monogr. Ser.* 31, 1956.

4-7 Studies on Household Sewage Disposal Systems, *U.S. Public Health Serv.*, *Publ.* 397, pt. 1, 1949; pt. 2, 1950; pt. 3, 1955.

4-8 Manual of Septic Tank Practice, *U.S. Public Health Serv.*, *Publ.* 526, rev., 1967.

4-9 REYNOLDS, R.: "Cleanliness and Godliness," George Allen & Unwin, Ltd., London, 1943.

4-10 COHN, M. M.: "Sewers for Growing America," Certainteed Products, Inc., Ambler, Pa., 1966.

4-11 ISAAC, P. C. G. (ed.): "Waste Treatment," Pergamon Press Ltd., London, 1960.

5

OUR AIR ENVIRONMENT

ENCOUNTERS WITH CONTAMINATED
AND POLLUTED AIR

The mixture called air, depending on locale and time, contains the molecules and particulates of thousands of different materials initially separable into chemical materials and biological forms. The dusts and fumes are included in chemical materials, although a given dust particle may be a complex conglomerate of minerals and adsorbed gases and vapors. The dispersed states of the chemicals are gases, vapors, dusts, or fumes. If these produce identifiable pathology in man, animals, or plants, the chemicals are classed as toxic. There is then a lengthy array of chemicals in our air supply which are considered nontoxic, or which to now have not been identified as toxic. The chemical contaminants and pollutants in air are not solely man-made. Even without the biological materials, there are dusts, particulate nucleii such as from sea-salt spray, and gases from natural organic decay and of volcanic, groundwater, and geothermal origins. These natural sources are of importance in understanding the global background of air impurities and the natural mechanisms of assimilation of these materials. Man's accelerating demand and production of energy in some areas of the world have created multiple and varied sources of materials that are discharged into the local air envelope as wastes.   Certainly, at least in those areas, man-made sources outstrip natural sources in amounts and in variety.   The question is: "Are the assimilative processes that result in an acceptable ecological equilibrium at risk of being overwhelmed?"   To begin to answer that question, the effects that must be observed, measured, and interpreted are:

1   Those on man's health and well-being and on his property
2   Those on the changing characteristics of the environment about him, including its support of animal and plant life on land, in the water, and in the air
3   Those on the very makeup of air itself
4   Those on the atmosphere's consequent response to the terrestrial, oceanic, and cosmic energies with which the earth's air cover is in continuous interaction.

Our concern and our knowledge of biological forms in air have been rather confined to those particularly associated with specific pathology.   Examples are the distribution of the virus of psittacosis from birds to man, of known pathogenic bacteria in surgical operating, in recovery and aftercare rooms, and in intensive-care units in hospitals.   Or the concern has been to mitigate the misery of those allergic to airborne pollens and dusts.   Pathogenic airborne fungi producing such diseases as coccidiomycosis and blastomycosis have been identified.   There is some evidence that minute, even microscopic aerophytes in continuous suspension function in atmospheric reactions.   One hypothesis for explaining the disappearance of carbon monoxide in air postulates aerophytic action.

Man encounters contaminants and pollutants in his air supply in six distinct situations.   These are:

1   In routine work, toxic gases, vapors, dusts, and fumes are generated in a number of specific manufacturing operations and in an increasing number of farm and service trades requiring the use of chemicals.   Usually the toxicants are discrete and known.   The pathology is usually specific and identified as an occupational disease.   A major concern of industrial hygiene and occupational medicine is the prevention and management of occupational diseases.
2   The community air supply has always had some contaminants and pollutants of natural origin.   Man and other mammals evolved a respiratory system which has protective mechanisms to defend them against inhaled impurities.   That system must have been in the making before man began to manage fire as a controlled energy source.   With that, man added smoke of his making in his hut, tent, or cave and to the air of his village.   He now puts his respiratory protective actions to severe tests by concentrating himself, his activities, and his airborne wastes in conurbations.   There are records of widespread failures of pulmonary protection identified as air pollution disasters or episodes.   There are indications of

individual failures after long exposure resulting in chronic bronchitis, emphysema, and lung cancer, sufficiently numerous to constitute epidemiological evidence of injury from polluted air.

3   There are acute encounters arising from collisions, derailments, and fires.   The last are most frequent, with the risks of carbon monoxide, oxygen deprivation, and smoke inhalation.   Smoke may now include the combustion products of synthetic fibers and plastics.   These synthetics often contain organic chlorides which can produce hydrogen chloride, phosgene, or phosgenelike compounds of high toxicity.   Large quantities of toxic gases and liquids are in transport by tank trailers and tank railroad cars.   In 1970 derailments of such freight cars put two small towns, one in Illinois and one in Mississippi, in peril.   Evacuation was required as gas releases, fire, and explosions followed the rail wrecks. Large manufacturing-plant fires and explosions hold similar threats of community disaster.   The New Jersey petrochemical complex near New York City has had two major threats, one a land explosion and fire at a processing plant in 1971.   One was a collision of tanker ships in Kill Van Kull between Staten Island and New Jersey in 1966.   Heroic, skillful, well-equipped men managed to contain these fires and explosions with a minimum loss of life and property. Less readiness is usual in many cities and towns along our transportation routes.

4   In the United States there are an estimated 5 million people particularly sensitive to certain air contaminants and pollutants.   The best known are the ragweed reactors, who suffer the misery of their allergic reaction when the ragweed pollen becomes airborne or who flee to pollen-free areas.   Major metropolitan newspapers, such as *The New York Times*, print pollen counts daily during the risk months.   It is estimated that allergens cause 10.5 million days of work absenteeism per year in the United States.   Airborne algae and protozoa have been added to the list of allergens.   Many cities have scheduled weed eradication and cover-crop planting of unused land to bring relief to its allergic citizens.   A very different group of people particularly susceptible to air pollutants are those with a history of cardiorespiratory limitations.   These cardiorespiratory cripples suffer the most severe distress during high concentrations of air pollutants, and some die.   Among the 17 deaths in Donora, Pennsylvania, during an air-pollution episode in late October 1948, the common factors were preexisting cardiorespiratory disease and being old.   The ages of the dead ranged from 52 to 84 with a mean of 65 (Ref. 5-1, p. 5).   If vital statistics trends continue, many of us are likely to meet these specifications.   The quality of the community air supply will be a matter of life or death when we become aged and have had a round or two of cardiorespiratory disorders.

5   That airborne pathogenic organisms are a cause of human disease has been obfuscated by the ease of transmission of the same organisms by person-to-

person contact, by various sorts of carrier states, and by autoinfection. The last implies that we already have the pathogen in our bodies and that changed conditions in our bodies permit infection. While the role of airborne pathogens in the general free environment remains uncertain, there is evidence of true airborne transmission in the peculiar environments of hospitals, nursing homes, and pathogenic research laboratories.

6   A final possible encounter with potent air contaminants is in warfare. As a uniform is no longer required to be an active participant in combat action, chemical and biological agents to kill or to immobilize people are designed with

Table 5-1   A COMPARISON OF EXPOSURE AND EFFECT FACTORS FOR TOXIC GASES, VAPORS, DUSTS, AND FUMES IN THE OCCUPATIONAL SETTING AND IN THE COMMUNITY AIR SUPPLY

	In the occupational setting	In the community air
Those exposed	Adults, predominately males, sufficiently healthy to get to the job.	All who are breathing, from the newborn to those near the end of life in all stages of health and sickness.
Exposure time	Usually limited to 40 h/week, 5 days/week, 50 weeks/year; frequently intermittent exposures during work periods; hence the body has elimination and recovery time.	Continuous; elimination and recovery time depend on periods of very low to zero concentrations and on leaving polluted area.
Exposure levels	May be measurable fractions of threshold limit values (mg/m^3 magnitudes).	Generally very low at limits of instrumental and analytical sensitivity ($\mu g/m^3$ magnitudes).
Exposure materials	Usually single toxicants of known origin, known to management and workers; hazards usually identified and some protection provided; usually freshly formed and released.	A mixture of primary pollutants from multiple and varied sources, and of secondary pollutants formed in the air by physical and chemical actions from the primaries; origins and hazards not readily identifiable; often unknown to those exposed.
Effects of concern	Specific pathology in the worker Increased risks of accidents Reduced productivity Increased costs of compensation insurance.	Nonspecific respiratory impairment Increased irritation of nose, throat, and eyes Reduced well-being Reduced visibility and increased accident risk Physical damage to property and increased depreciation Injury to plants and animals Esthetically displeasing Long-term ecological effects, including climatic changes.

all of us included as targets. There is some consolation in the nations of the world's seeming to have agreed to cease and desist from the use of chemical-biological (CB) agents. In 1970 to 1971 the orderly and safe disposal of stockpiles of CB materials was underway in the United States in accord with a 1969 order of President Nixon's. It is ironic that the preparation of a United States stockpile of the virus of Venezuelan equine encephalitis (VEE) for CB war provided the only ready countermeasure against an epizootic of VEE among horses in Texas counties along the Mexican border in the summer of 1971. As countermeasures are prepared along with offensive measures, the U.S. Army had a supply of VEE vaccine which was released for use on exposed horses.[1]

Occupational exposure and an impure community-air supply share a growing body of scientific knowledge, professional practice, and expertise. Instrumentation and analytical methods range from identical to similar. The toxicology and epidemiology of the two have a large common ground. Some of the differences are evident in Table 5-1.

TOXIC GASES, VAPORS, DUSTS, AND FUMES PRODUCING OCCUPATIONAL DISEASES

Occupational diseases produced by inhalation are a specific pathology, each caused by a specific airborne toxicant. Most frequently the disease is identified by the intoxicating agent, as carbon monoxide poisoning, benzol poisoning, and silicosis from silica dust. In terms of the number of cases of occupational diseases reported per year, the problem seems small compared with deaths and injuries from accidents at work. However, when the number of cases is related to the number at risk from a specific poison, the problem of the worker exposed is seen on a correct base. All men in a metalworking shop are not exposed to chromic acid mist. It is only those in the electroplating department.

Occupational diseases fall into two time-concentration patterns. There are those which have transient effects with quick recovery from relatively high concentrations in short periods of time. Many gases and organic vapors produce that pattern. The body's capacity to tolerate or to eliminate the inhaled contaminant is temporarily overwhelmed. The second type is made up of those whose effects are cumulative, with a slow onset of symptoms from relatively low concentrations over weeks, months, or years of exposure. Tables 5-2 and 5-3 present each a grouping of selected substances providing, respectively, acute exposures with transient effects and prolonged

[1] *Natl. Obs.*, July 19, 1971.

Table 5-2 SELECTED SUBSTANCES PRODUCING TRANSIENT EFFECTS FROM EXCESSIVE CONCENTRATIONS, IN PERIODS OF LESS THAN 1 DAY

Substance	Inhaled form	Source of exposure	Substance	Inhaled form	Source of exposure
Ammonia	Gas	Chemical manufacturing	Hydrogen cyanide	Gas	Fumigation, chemical manufacturing
Carbon monoxide	Gas	Combustion processes	Hydrogen sulfide	Gas	Oil refining, coal mining
Chlorine	Gas	Chemical manufacturing	Sulfur dioxide	Gas	Acid manufacture, ore smelting
Hydrocarbon mixtures	Vapor	Solvents and thinners	Perchloroethylene	Vapor	Degreasing, dry cleaning
Petroleum benzine	Vapor		Trichloroethylene	Vapor	Degreasing and extraction
Petroleum ether	Vapor	Grease extraction	Zinc oxide	Fume	Brass and bronze founding, welding and burning on galvanized metal
Gasoline (benzol-free)	Vapor	Fuel handling			

Table 5-3 SELECTED SUBSTANCES PRODUCING CHRONIC EFFECTS FROM CUMULATIVE EXPOSURES IN PERIODS RANGING FROM MONTHS TO YEARS

Substance	Inhaled form	Source of exposure	Substance	Inhaled form	Source of exposure
Benzene	Vapor	Solvent and chemical use	Mercury and its salts	Vapor	Electric apparatus, agricultural chemicals, chemistry labs.
Carbon tetrachloride	Vapor	Solvent and chemical use	Nitro benzene	Vapor	Chemical manufacture
Carbon disulfide	Vapor	Rayon manufacture	Chromic acid	Mist	Chrome electroplating
Asbestos	Dust	Asbestos cloth manufacture	Silica	Dust	Drilling, grinding, cutting, and milling on material containing crystalline silica
Arsenic	Dust	Insecticide manufacture and use			
Beryllium	Dust	Metallurgy	Uranium	Dust	Mining and metallurgy
Lead	Dust and fume	All lead use suspect			

exposures with cumulative chronic effects.   In particular circumstances, such as exposure to a very high concentration or an individual hypersusceptibility, the substances grouped as chronic-cumulative, silica and asbestos dust excepted, can produce injury in a single exposure.

Toxic Gases and Vapors

Physical behavior   Gases, in molecular dispersion, and vapors, aggregates of near molecular size, follow the *ideal gas law* $PV = nRT$.   This simple formula relates pressure, volume, number n of moles, temperature T on an absolute scale, and the gas constant R.   The numerical value of R depends on the combination of units used for the four terms P, V, n, and T.   The formula provides for calculation among weight, temperature, volume, and pressure of gas.   In industrial hygiene it can be used to estimate gas and vapor concentrations from solvent losses and gas releases and dilution air volumes required.   It is needed to prepare known concentrations in air for instrument calibrations.   Its use has been facilitated by convenient conversion tables.

An erroneous assumption that is presented occasionally is that gases and vapors of high-molecular-weight compounds settle.   If it is based on the heavy molecules' behaving in air like chunks of lead in water, the assumption is contrary to the kinetic theory of gases.   In accord with theory, molecular movement is a function of temperature.   If it is based on the notion that the vapor or gas produces a parcel of air-vapor mixture which has a high density ratio in reference to air, the assumption does not take into account the arithmetic of the situation.   For example, a change of 1 percent [or 10,000 parts per million (ppm)] by volume of CCl_4 causes a change in the vapor density of the mixture in air from 1.000, the reference density for air, to 1.043.   The difference of 0.043 has a negligible effect on the behavior of the mixture.

Air movement or its absence is significant in the dispersion and dilution of gases and vapors.   Very moderate velocities of 50 fpm, a barely perceptible draft, will speed evaporation of volatile solvents and disperse the contaminant.   Enclosed spaces, sumps, pits, tanks, and manholes, without natural or mechanical ventilation are serious hazards for the accumulation of high concentrations of noxious gases and vapors.   Deaths upon entering sewage sludge sumps, abandoned wells, dead ends of mines, fermentation vats, and silos occur primarily from the oxygen deficiency in the atmosphere.

Physiological action of gases and vapors   Henderson and Haggard's classification (Ref. 5-2) of gases and vapors into three physiological responses, asphyxiation, irritation, and anaesthesia or narcosis, brings order to an initially bewildering array of actions and effects.   Subdivisions of the three groups are needed to cover differing modes of asphyxiation, differing sites of irritation, and the effects in addition to narcosis produced by the organic vapors.   Table 5-4 is a modification of Henderson and Haggard's classification and presents examples of each action.   The zone of the respiratory tract affected is directly related to the solubility of the gas, with those that are highly soluble producing immediate irritation in the upper passages.   The slowly soluble ones penetrate to the lungs and produce delayed reactions.

   Urban populations are almost constantly exposed to carbon monoxide, CO, from gasoline engines, fossil-fuel burning, and their individual tobacco smoking. Therefore, special note is made on CO.   The mechanism of intoxication is the reversible combination of CO with the blood hemoglobin to form carboxyhemoglobin.   As a result, the hemoglobin is not available for oxygen transport.   The onset of this

Table 5-4   PHYSIOLOGICAL ACTION OF TOXIC GASES AND VAPORS

Groups	Subgroups	Mode of action	Examples
A Asphyxiants	1 Simple	Oxygen deficiency in air and lungs.	CO_2, N_2, CH_4
	2 Chemical	Oxygen deficiency in blood.	CO
		Oxygen use blocked in the cell.	HCN, $(CN)_2$
B Irritants	1 Highly soluble	Irritate nasal passages and trachea.	NH_3, H_2SO_4, HF, HCl, formaldehyde
	2 Moderately soluble	Irritate lower trachea and bronchia.	Cl_2, SO_2, Br_2
	3 Slowly soluble	Irritate bronchioles and alveolar sacs.	Oxides of N, O_3, $COCl_2$
C Anesthetics	1 Simple anesthetic	Deepening depressant action on central nervous system without complications.	Gasoline (benzene-free)
	2 Anesthetic action plus organ damage	Severe single exposure or repeated exposures cause additive damage to liver, kidneys, heart, or intestines.	Ethanol, ketones, ethers, CCl_4, tetrachloroethane, $CHCl_3$, and solvents containing CCl_4 admixture or impurity
	3 Anesthetic action plus blood changes	Severe single exposure or repeated exposures cause additive damage to blood-forming system.	Benzene, and solvents containing benzene admixture or impurity
	4 Anesthetic action plus nervous system effects	Repeated exposures cause additive damage to the nervous system.	Methyl alcohol, carbon disulfide

chemical asphyxiation is subtle and without provocative signs such as irritation, coughing, or shortness of breath.   As the reaction is reversible, there is an equilibrium which is reached in 5 or 6 hours for concentrations of 200 to 600 ppm of CO by volume, and in 15 to 30 min for concentrations of 3,000 to 5,000 ppm.   At equilibrium, the ratio of carboxyhemoglobin to oxyhemoglobin is between 210 and 300 to 1.   This expresses the greater combining affinity of CO for hemoglobin.   This was observed by C. G. Douglas, and J. S. and J. B. S. Haldane, in 1912.   Extensive observations, including human volunteer exposures, have provided data for expressing the effects of time and concentrations to predict symptoms and percentage of CO hemoglobin in the blood.   Similarly, blood findings can be used to estimate the environmental conditions.   For concentrations up to 100 ppm, each part per million produces 0.16 percent of COHb in the blood.   Therefore, COHb% = CO in parts per million (0.16).   Accordingly, a 30 ppm exposure for several hours will produce an equilibrium value of 30(0.16), or about 5 percent.   This is a value found in the blood of habitual cigarette smokers, although they are not under a continuous 30 ppm exposure. Rather, they are taking from 200 to 800 ppm with each smoke inhalation.

Toxic Dusts and Fumes

Physical behavior   Dusts are particulates produced by shattering, abrasion, and cutting.   These actions result in sizes which remain airborne from a matter of a few seconds to many hours, and result in an enormous aggregate surface area for their mass.   The suspension in air time and particle size determines the likelihood of the dust particle's being inhaled and its penetration and retention in the human respiratory system.   The surface area increase results in increased solubility, increased volatility, increased chemical activity, increased adsorptive capacity, and a decreased ease of wetting.

The unit of measure for dusts is the micron (μm), one-thousandth of a millimeter, 1×10^{-6} m, or one twenty-five-thousandth of an inch.   Those who have peered at bacteria under a microscope will recall bacilli of 5 to 7 μm.   Size and density determine settling behavior, a critical matter in the inhalation risk.   The patterns for a density of 1 are:

1   Particles over 5,000 μm settle in accord with gravity acceleration.   These have no physiological significance as they drop from the respirable zone immediately.
2   Particles from 0.1 to 5,000 μm settle at a constant velocity for a given particle size.   Those below 10 μm settle at such a relatively slow velocity that they are inhaled.   Their behavior after entrance to the respiratory system is important.
3   Particles under 0.1 μm show Brownian movement and are in permanent suspension as are molecular and near molecular sizes.   True dusts do not have such small sizes.   Fumes and smoke do, and sizes go as low as 0.01 μm.

In still air, particles from 9 to 200 μm settle in accord with Stoke's equation. Corrections are required for smaller sizes and for shape, as spheres are assumed.   The equation states that for a uniform density, the free-falling speed varies as the square of particle size.   Stoke's equation is of practical use for predicting the penetration and retention of particulates of other densities in the respiratory tract.   This is done by determining the equivalent aerodynamic diameter.   Table 5-5 uses water, silicon dioxide, and uranium oxide in particulate sizes to illustrate equivalent aerodynamic diameters.   Read vertically for the equivalents among the three substances.   The fourth-column entries state that a particle of uranium oxide dust 0.35 μm in diameter and a particle of free silica 0.62 μm in diameter have the same aerodynamic behavior as a droplet of water 1.0 μm in diameter.   This parameter is useful, as the physical behavior of a particulate in the respiratory tract is a function of its settling characteristic, which can be predicted from its equivalent aerodynamic diameter.

Some benchmarks on particle sizes are useful.   The unaided eye can see sizes down to 100 μm.   The microscopic range is from 0.2 to 10 μm.   A 325-mesh screen, 325 openings per inch, passes particles up to 30 μm.   Fog is water in 1 to 45 μm size, while rain drops are from 450 to 5,000 μm.   Metallurgical dusts and fumes are from 0.001 to 100 μm.   Zinc oxide fume is from 0.1 to 0.4 μm.   Flour-mill dust size ranges narrowly around 10 μm.

The dynamic behavior of fine particulates is illustrated by crystalline, free silica and coal dust.   Settling velocities of less than 1 fpm show the very slow removal by gravity of the sizes below 10 μm.   These are the sizes which enter the respiratory tract. *Stirred settling time* is the period required for one-half of the particles of the stated size and specific gravity to drop from a 7-ft level after dust generation stops.   The respirable sizes under 1 μm remain suspended for 8 to 16 hours.   *Stopping distance* is a measure of the "throw" that the kinetic energy of generation, as, say, from a grinding wheel, imparts to the particulates.   For particles under 10 μm it is less than 1 in.   For particles of 1 μm and less, the throw is 0.01 in for silica and 0.005 in for coal dust.   The small-sized particles are not being hurtled away from the worker at a dust-generating

Table 5-5   THE EQUIVALENT AERODYNAMIC DIAMETERS OF WATER, SILICON DIOXIDE, AND URANIUM OXIDE

Material	Density	The equivalent aerodynamic diameter, μm*						
H_2O	1	0.5	1.0	2.0	3.0	5.0	7.0	10.0
SiO_2	2.6	0.31	0.62	1.24	1.86	3.10	4.34	6.20
U_3O_8	8.4	0.17	0.35	0.69	1.03	1.73	2.42	3.45

* Read vertically for equivalent diameters.
SOURCE: Ref. 5-4 (p. A-2-5).

operation to the extent that his breathing zone is clear of respirable sizes.   The respirable sizes are staying right with the worker, lingering in his breathing zone.

Fate of particles in the respiratory system   The phenomena of penetration and retention of particulates is a function of equivalent aerodynamic size.   The physiological effects are dependent on the chemical actions between the inhaled material and the body.   The physical behavior by particle size is summarized.

1   Particles over 10 μm are captured in the nasal chambers by impaction.   Mouth breathers lose part of this protection.   Rapid, heavy breathing enhances it.   The beneficial removal continues down to 5 μm, but decreases.   Mucus discharges remove them from the respiratory tract.

2   Particles from 5 to 2 μm settle in the middle respiratory passages, the trachea and bronchia, as the increasing cross-section area produces diminished velocities.   Unimpaired ciliary action removes them.

3   Particles making the passage to the lungs are totally removed in the lung air spaces down to 2-μm sizes.   This is not beneficial as the particles are trapped in the lungs.   Defensive mechanisms of the lung tissue cannot cope with some dusts.

4   In the lung air spaces, the removal and retention decreases for particle sizes from 2 to 0.5 μm.   These intermediate sizes remain suspended and are carried out on the tidal movement of breathing.

5   For particles below 0.5 μm, the pattern reverses.   As the size of Brownian movement is reached, retention increases.   The forces of diffusion precipitation drive the particle to the lung surfaces, where the body's defenses must meet the invasion.

6   For sizes from 1 to 2 μm the percentage of particles which penetrate to the lung air spaces and which are retained there is at a maximum.[1]

Thus in terms of particle size the task of the industrial hygienist is defined.   It is not in the very large and sometimes visible sizes above 5 μm, as they do not penetrate to the lung.   Nor is it in the near ultramicroscopic sizes about 0.5 μm which are not retained.   Industrial dusts have only very small fractions in sizes below 0.5 μm.   Control measures, particularly filter devices and sampling instruments, must be at their peak efficiencies for particle sizes above 0.5 μm and below 5 μm.

Fumes, as the term is used in industrial hygiene, are a distinct form of airborne particulates.   Fumes are formed by the reaction of vapors or gases on release to the air.   Metallic fume forms when the vapor from molten metal cools, oxidizes, and coalesces.   The appearance of zinc oxide above a hot zinc pot or during the founding

---

[1] J. H. Brown, K. M. Cook, et al., Influence of Particulate Matter in the Human Lung, *Am. J. Public Health*, **40**:450–459 (1960).

of brass and bronze is a vivid example. Chlorinated waxes, used for impregnating wire insulation, vaporize, cool, and condense to form fine particles producing a fume. Fume formation by chemical reaction of gases in air occurs occasionally. Ammonia and hydrogen chloride gas combine to form ammonium chloride fume. Freshly formed fumes agglomerate strongly, increasing particle size. Thereafter behavior is like that of dusts.

Physiological behavior The body reacts to a respiratory invasion of dust by a series of defenses. As the penetration advances down the respiratory tract, these are:

1 The cough reflex
2 Turbinate impaction
3 Ciliary action to move the deposited material back out to be expectorated or swallowed
4 Macrophage phagocytosis of particles precipitated in the lung tissue
5 Filtration through the alveolar walls into the lymph nodes

The aerodynamic equivalent diameter of the particle is the major determinant of the defense provoked. For particulates which are dissolved after deposition and which follow the blood path, the interaction of the solute with the sites of accumulation and in the organs of excretion determines whether the solution from the lung is a successful defense or a transfer of the invader to a more vulnerable tissue. For example, if lead and its compounds remained as a benign deposition in the lung tissue, the body would fair better. As the lead dissolves and enters into circulation, a bewildering number of symptoms involving the blood, the muscles, the gastrointestinal and central nervous system appear.

There are three patterns of effects from the inhalations of dusts and fumes. There are effects upon the lung tissue and lung function resulting from the deposition of dust. For three of these lung conditions, the name of the disease identifies the cause: silicosis from free crystalline silica, asbestosis from asbestos, and talcosis from talc. Other changes in the lung picture are described as pneumoconiosis with such dusts as amorphous silica, coal dust, and natural graphite involved. These effects develop after 10 to 20 years of exposure, and show specific pathologies recognizable from symptoms and radiograph by experienced physicians.

The second pattern is that of systemic effects resulting from the absorption of the dust and fume from the lungs after deposition. In some instances the scene of injury is the respiratory tract as for beryllium, chromates and chromic acid mists, and nickel and its compounds. Antimony and cadmium oxide fumes produce effects in the lungs and on the liver and kidneys, respectively. Manganese oxide may produce a pneumonitis, but its main effect is on the central nervous system. Arsenic, lead, and yellow phosphorous cause no lung damage, but produce injury to other organs after absorption.   These patterns are more aptly described as poisonings, which are some-times acute and rapid from short exposures to high concentrations.

The third pattern is a benign effect with no recognized damage by deposition in the lungs or upon absorption in the body.   Examples of dusts producing this pattern are Alundum, iron oxides, limestone, synthetic graphite, and starch.   Impurities of injurious compounds in the inert dusts or nuisance particulates markedly alter the risk. Their absence must be verified if exposure to high concentrations of the inerts is accepted.

The Measurement of Exposure

Air sampling with direct-reading instruments which give immediate information on existing concentrations of toxic substances, or with collection devices which provide samples for subsequent analysis, is the principal means for determining the environ-mental exposure risk of workers using recognized occupational poisons.   Bulk samples of raw materials and products are useful to determine the identification of a toxicant, for example, the presence of benzene in gasoline, of lead in an alloy, and of the free silica content in a mother rock or in a "rafter" sample of settled dust.   Air samples are taken for analysis for a specific toxicant to determine the need for control measures before there is damage.   In the cases of suspected or alleged on-the-job impairment, the purpose of the measurement is to determine the validity of the injurious exposure.   In both instances, all available medical information should be secured and evaluated by competent, experienced medical persons.   These methods presuppose the existence of a reliable bank of data on which to base a judgment on whether the sample information indicates a hazardous exposure.   Industrial hygiene and toxicology practice has developed the data for such comparisons and judgments. For inhalation, many of these results of experience and research are in the list of threshold limit values (TLV) as disarmingly simple numbers (Ref. 5-3).

Air sampling   An air sample which produces useful, revealing, and reliable informa-tion requires that it be taken for the injurious substance at the point of exposure and for a time to make it representative of the inhaled air and its contaminant.   If inhala-tion estimates are not the goal of the sampling, this should be clear in the mind of the sampler and those who subsequently use the results produced.   In air sampling the identity of the toxicant and any possible interfering substances must be known, and the cycle of operation or process must be observed.

The point of sampling bounds the interpretation of results in terms of the quan-tity of contaminant inhaled.   A breathing-level sample taken at the worker's position, and following his movements for the time it takes to complete a typical job, closely approximates his inhalation concentration.   Instrument limitations frequently prevent such monitoring of the breathing zone.   Sampling at a fixed point near the process where the worker is required to be for a considerable part of the time gives a range of the concentration of contaminant release.   Such positioning is well suited for samples taken to determine the effectiveness of process controls such as exhaust ventilation or wet methods to prevent the dispersion of contaminants.

A sample of the ambient air in the workroom, taken without reference to a particular process, position, or time in a cycle, represents the exposure for all the workers in that shop area.   It is useful to validate group complaints and to ensure that contaminants are under control.   At the points of generation and release, there will be higher concentrations.   These points must be observed and sampled separately.

The variety of sampling devices available to the industrial hygienist for many substances permits a choice of a grab sample or of an extended-time sample.   The grab sample represents the exposure experienced for a few seconds or, at most, a minute or two.   A grab taken at the time of most active release, such as during the unloading and recharging of a ball mill, approximates the peak of exposure.   A series of grabs taken through a cycle of position, operation, and time provides information for estimating a time-weighted average exposure value.   Grab samples are useful to determine if a contaminant is present and whether a collection sampling for laboratory analysis is warranted.

The most frequent type of extended-time sampling is a collection of a contaminant for later analysis.   It inherently averages the exposure.   There are a limited number of portable instruments which continuously indicate the contaminant concentration in the sample stream, with the advantage of showing variation and duration of exposure.   Such instruments are often restricted to a single toxicant or a class of them, such as carbon monoxide or the chlorinated hydrocarbons.

The results of air sampling and the reliability of their interpretation are no better than the calibration of the instruments used and the abilities of the analyst handling a collection type of sample.   There must be periodic calibration of instruments for the rate of air flow and for response to known concentrations.   As a minimum the analyst must be given an amount of sample fitted to the sensitivity of the methods used and information on any suspected interferences.

Air sampling instruments   Instruments for sampling dusts and fumes depend on one of the following physical mechanisms for separating the particulates from the air: impingement in a liquid, impingement on a slide, electrostatic precipitation, thermal precipitation, filtration, centrifugation, and settling.   The choice of one of these mechanisms in designing a particular instrument is governed by the intended use.   For particulate counting by direct microscopic observation, impingers, thermal precipitators, and settling chambers are used.   For sizing by weight fractions, a series of centrifugal separators or miniature cyclones is used.   For determinations of weight

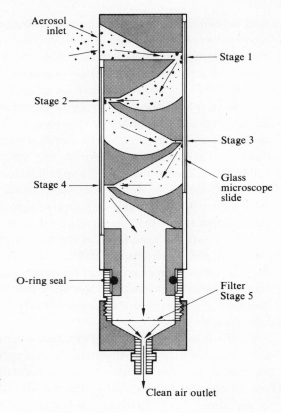

Aerosol inlet

Stage 1

Stage 2

Stage 3

Stage 4

Glass microscope slide

O-ring seal

Filter Stage 5

Clean air outlet

FIGURE 5-1
Collection and sizing of dusts by dry impingement on a series on microscope slides mounted in a cascade impactor. [*Source: Union Industrial Equipment Company, Fall River, Mass*]

per air volume, electrostatic precipitators and filters are used. Devices dependent on optical effects of airborne particulates have had very limited use in industrial hygiene practice. There is one very expensive instrument in custom production which depends on light backscatter to a photomultiplier tube. It has the attractive capability of simultaneously sizing selectively and indicating the particulate count. This provides a direct readout of size and concentration. Figures 5-1 to 5-3 show three collection instruments.

Instruments for sampling gases and vapors are either collection devices for later analysis or direct-reading devices. The collectors may use absorption into a liquid with known solubility and chemical reactivity for the substance sampled, or condensation in freeze-out traps cooled by dry ice or liquid nitrogen. Such collection trains can be assembled from stock chemical glassware. There are the disadvantages of being cumbersome and fragile for field use. These can be offset in part by the use of plastic ware.

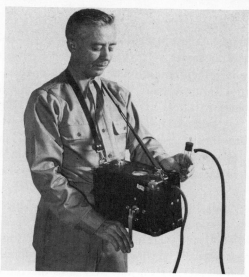

FIGURE 5-2
Collection by wet impingement in a midget impinger. Air flow provided by four-cylinder hand-powered pump usually at 0.1 ft³/min. [*Source: Mine Safety Appliance Company, Pittsburgh, Pa*]

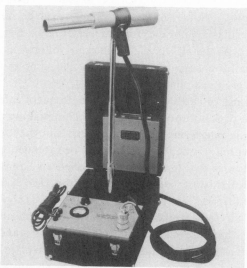

FIGURE 5-3
Collection by electrostatic precipitation. [*Source: Mine Safety Appliance Company, Pittsburgh, Pa*]

The direct-reading instruments are ingenious applications of the physical and chemical properties of gases and vapors. The variety of these devices, their sensitivity, their reliability, and usually their cost have all increased in recent years. They have also tempted those without knowledge of the instrument's limitations and with little experience in air sampling, to assess hazardous exposures. These devices are single-purpose, responding to a single contaminant such as CO, O_3, SO_2, or to an analogous group such as hydrocarbons or chlorinated hydrocarbons. Manufacturers have gained some versatility by using the same air pump and readout panel to detect and measure more than one substance by routing each through its own reaction and response path.

One group of direct-reading instruments depends on a reaction between the contaminant and a sensing system which produces heat, electrical changes, or optical changes. An example of each is given: the heat of burning a combustible gas or vapor along a wire increases the resistance of the wire, which alters a balanced Wheatstone bridge; the soluble gases such as NH_3, HCl, and SO_2 alter the conductivity of an aqueous sensing cell; mercury vapor absorbs ultraviolet light at 253.7 nm and reduces the beam intensity entering a phototube.

A second group of direct-reading devices is colorimetric. A known contaminant reacts with a sensitive chemical to produce a color proportional to concentration. The sensitive chemical can be impregnated on granules of silica gel, glass or ceramic, in a glass tube. The first such tube was devised for CO in 1920. There are now tubes for 150 toxic gases and vapors. Some sensitive chemicals can be impregnated on filter surfaces, paper or molecular membrane, for use wet or dry. Some are used in solution for bubbler contact with the air sample. Since air volumes as little as 50 ml are sufficient to produce a color change in these devices, the samples are grabs and subject to the limitations of grab sampling.

Good technique in the use of detector tubes requires frequent calibration of the suction device, use of known concentrations to acquire skill in making the color comparison, knowledge of existing interfering gases and vapors and the tube response to these, and use of the tube within its shelf life, which can be extended by refrigerated storage. With these precautions detector tubes in experienced hands will produce readings within 10 percent of existing concentrations in the grab. A detailed and practical description of air sampling instruments is in Ref. 5-4.

The interpretation of any environmental sample is the application of professional judgment. It is not the mere comparison with a set of standard numbers, however valid these may be. For air samples a sound judgement requires that the conditions and circumstances of sampling be known, particularly any variations from the usual. The type of damage which is produced by excessive exposure must be known and considered in interpreting results and framing recommendations. With these in mind, the exposure measured can be compared with the TLV of the American

Conference of Governmental Industrial Hygienists (Ref. 5-3), the hygienic guides of the American Industrial Hygiene Association, and other sources of industrial toxicological data pertinent to the compound and processes confronted.

The units used for expressing concentrations of airborne contaminants in industrial hygiene practice are:

1 For gases and vapors, parts per million by volume (ppm). It is useful to note that 0.01 percent equals 100 ppm. Alternatively, TLV values for gases and vapors are also given in milligrams per cubic meter of air (mg/m^3).

2 For dusts which produce lung damage by discrete-particle interaction, the number of millions of particles per cubic foot, as for crystalline and amorphous silica. For metric units, millions of particles per cubic meter is used.

3 For fumes and dusts which act in accord with the weight inhaled and retained, milligrams per cubic meter are used.

The Control of Toxic Gases, Vapors, Dusts, and Fumes

Industrial hygiene control measures are grouped as (*1*) substitution of materials, (*2*) methods and process changes, (*3*) good housekeeping, (*4*) personal protective devices and washup facilities, (*5*) general dilution and local exhaust ventilation. Choices and decisions on these methods require a comprehensive knowledge of the processes in use. Experience provides much of this, but the exchange of information with management and labor adds to understanding and facilitates acceptance and utilization of control recommendations.

Substitution of nontoxic or less-toxic materials used in processes is the most certain control. It is most easily understood by noting the examples given in Table 5-6. Its acceptance depends on the substitute material's serving nearly as well as, or

Table 5-6 EXAMPLES OF THE SUBSTITUTION OF NONTOXIC OR LESS–TOXIC SUBSTANCES FOR HIGH–HAZARD MATERIALS IN OCCUPATIONAL EXPOSURE

High-hazard material	Replace with less- or nontoxic ones
Benzol (benzene)	Toluene, xylene, naphtha
Carbon tetrachloride	Trichloroethylene, methyl chloride
Gasoline containing benzol	Gasoline free of benzol
Mercury in hat making	Nonmercurial carroting compounds
Lead paint pigments	Titanium dioxide
Silica grinding wheels	Carborundum wheels
Silica parting compounds in foundries	Nonsiliceous compounds
Carbon tetrachloride in dry cleaning	Tetrachloroethylene, perchloroethylene
Sandblast	Steel shot or water jet, calcined lime
Tetrachloroethane	Amyl acetate
Ground flint	Powdered alumina

better than, the toxic original.   More active engagement of production people in searching for and considering alternative materials would eliminate more toxic substances from the workplace.

Changes in processes are directed at reducing the generation and release of the toxicant, limiting its dispersion, and limiting the area requiring control.   Examples of reducing toxicant release are replacing the spraying of lead paints with brush painting, reducing the amount of lead burned on automobile bodies by close seam welding and use of plastic fillers, replacing high-speed grinding on lead with hand filing, and replacing dry drilling, grinding, and sanding with wet methods.   Three of the examples are for lead uses, in which the exposure has produced poisoning so frequently that the higher labor costs of slower methods are accepted.

Wet methods to reduce dust release are effective.   John Leyner added water injection to his pneumatic drill in 1898, one year after the introduction of his dry drill. The step was an easy one as the drill already had a hollow core and air supply to blow out the hole and partially cool the drill steel.   Wide use of wet drilling was not achieved until 1920, as satisfactory drill steel alloys were not available for such use. By that time Leyner's pneumatic drill with dry-hole air-jet cleaning had earned the title of "the widow maker" among drillers (Ref. 5-5, p. 1001).   Water is used to reduce dust by wetting down muck piles before loading and hauling, by sprays at conveyor-belt transfer points, in wet grinding and polishing, and by infusion into mine faces before barring down and removal after blasting.   Wet methods are readily acceptable, as the life of drill steel is extended and abrasive wear of machinery is reduced.   The limitations are caking and undesirable moisture content which affect subsequent processes or product quality.

The enclosure of processes limits the dispersion of the toxic materials.   The handling of large volumes of highly toxic and explosive compounds in the petroleum and chemical industries is possible by fully enclosed continuous flow systems with a minimum of open-vat, batch operations.   Pneumatic and screwdrive conveyors reduce the dust dispersion and material loss of open belts.   There are instances of enclosure being supplemented by ventilation and protective respirators, as in the cleaning rooms for castings.

The isolation of operations using or releasing toxic substances from general work areas reduces the number exposed and limits the area of control and special supervision.   Examples are shake-out stations in foundries, electroplating rooms in metalworking shops, mercury-amalgam handling rooms in transistor battery making, spray painting shops.   In these cases there is a need for additional control by ventilation at specific operations.

Good housekeeping may not be an exciting method, but it is an effective one, particularly for reducing dust concentrations.   It reduced lead dust concentrations to acceptable levels in an overcrowded, rush-scheduled drop forge shop of a large aircraft factory during World War II. The emphasis is on cleaning methods, cleaning schedules, and cleanable surfaces. This means wet methods, dust-suppressant sweeping compounds, vacuum cleaning, immediate cleanup of spills, and the use of impervious surfaces and coved corners. It requires a well-supervised janitorial squad provided with good equipment, operating on scheduled coverage, and using cleaning compounds fitted to the filth to be removed.

Respirators are often thought to be a quick and easy answer to hazardous inhalation exposures. No respirator has yet been designed which can be worn for more than 15 to 20 min, comfortably and without interfering with work. Even under the duress of emergency and rescue operations, respirator use cannot be extended for long periods. Its place and purpose in regular work is to protect against high concentrations from intermittent operations of short durations. A respirator must be fitted to the man's facial contours and adapted to the toxicant. The U.S. Bureau of Mines list of approved respirators can be used to select one which safeguards against the exposure encountered. Check the approval numbers on each mask and filter, cartridge, or cannister to verify that the proper equipment is on hand or in use. Respirators must be clean and maintained in usable condition.

Protective clothing such as gloves, shoes, boots, aprons, and goggles must similarly be fitted to the man and the exposure. Changes, cleaning, and repair must be provided to assure use and to ensure protection. Facilities for hand washing, face washing, and body bathing and their use reduce dermatitis, skin absorption, and ingestion from contaminated hands. The need for the facilities and the habit are underlined by the fact that dermatitis is the most frequently compensated occupational disease, and that one-fourth of the substances on the TLV list for inhalation are also absorbed through the eyes, mucous membranes, and the skin (Ref. 5-3).

Ventilation—General Dilution and Local Exhaust

The objectives of general dilution ventilation and of local exhaust ventilation in the occupational environment are the same, the prevention of injurious concentrations of toxicants in the breathing-level air of workers. The means of the two are wholly opposite. General dilution ventilation depends upon the introduction of enough uncontaminated air to dilute continuously the quantity of the contaminant released so that there is no hazardous buildup of concentration. Local exhaust ventilation depends on capturing the contaminant at the point of release and removing it from the work area before it mixes with the room air.

General dilution ventilation The amount of clean air required to dilute a known quantity of air contaminant for which a threshold limit, or acceptable concentration, has been established in volumetric units is defined by

$$\text{Acceptable concentration} = \frac{\text{rate of contaminant release, cfm}}{\text{rate of dilution air, cfm}}$$

If CO is released at 1 cfm from a gasoline engine, and 50 ppm is the TLV for an 8-hour exposure,

$$50 \text{ ppm} = \frac{50}{1,000,000} = \frac{1 \text{ cfm, CO}}{x \text{ cfm, dilution air}}$$

$x = 20,000$ cfm, the quantity of air which will dilute the contaminant to a safe level, provided there is uniform distribution of the air and perfect dispersal of the contaminant before the breathing-level zone of workers is reached.   The example exposes the disadvantages of general dilution ventilation.   The rate of generation of the contaminant must be quite uniform.   Nearly perfect mixing must take place.   Large air volumes are required unless the particular contaminant is of low toxicity and permits the inhalation of high concentrations without injury.   As uniform generation and perfect mixing are rarely the characteristics of a workplace, from three to ten times the ideal air volume must be provided.

The universal gas law $PV = nRT$ provides the means for estimating the volume of vapor generated from a known or estimated volume or weight of solvent loss in a process.   To facilitate calculations, industrial hygiene books and manuals provide convenient formulas for estimating the volumes of contaminant generated and the volumes of dilution air required (Ref. 5-6, p. 2-1).   However, there is no substitute for the professional judgement required to evaluate the percentage of solvent loss to the air, the rate of fume generation, and the degree of uniformity of contaminant generation and of mixing.

The volume of the room in which the operation goes on does not enter into formulas for estimating the dilution air volume.   The notion that it should is encountered and is a carry-over from expressing dilution ventilation of spaces with fixed maximum human occupancy, such as schoolrooms and theaters, in terms of room-volume air changes per hour.   In industrial processes, the room, at best, provides only an initial volume of clean air for diluting the initial release at start-up.   This volume will be found to be small in comparison with the dilution air needed during continuous operation.

For the control of occupational toxicants, general dilution ventilation is best applied for operations using solvents of low evaporation rates and with high TLV. Table 5-7 contrasts the air volumes required to dilute the vapors from 1 pint each of two highly toxic solvents, carbon disulfide and carbon tetrachloride, and two moderately toxic solvents, ethyl ether and turpentine.   As large volumes of clean air are needed, the requirements of fan power, distribution ducts and grills, conditioning for temperature and possibly humidity are high.   There are advantages of flexibility in process layout and in materials used, and the benefit of warm weather cooling and process heat removal, which are not attributes of local exhaust ventilation systems.

Local exhaust ventilation   This method has the marked advantage of containing the contaminant at the point of generation and removing it from the work area by a suction opening and ductwork.   The air stream can then be put through an air cleaner so that the contaminant does not become a contribution to community air pollution. In some situations, the air may be recirculated to reduce conditioning costs.   About 80 percent of control recommendations for inhalation hazards are local exhaust ventilation.   Therefore, an understanding of its limitations is necessary to minimize bad design, poor installation, poor maintenance, and improper use of exhaust hoods.

Good understanding begins with the geometry of blowing and sucking air and the projection of the equation of continuity $Q = AV$, into free air space.   Figure 5-4 shows the dramatic difference in airflow patterns on the discharge side and suction side of ducts.   On the discharge side there is a jet pattern which retains its shape and velocity for some distance, so that at a distance of 30 diameters of the opening there is still 10 percent of the discharge velocity remaining.   On the intake or suction side, the velocity inward is a scant 10 percent of the inlet velocity just 1 diameter from the opening.   Figure 5-5 helps to clarify this apparent paradox, although it is limited to two-dimensional representation.   A theoretical point as source of suction influences an infinite series of spheres defining a boundary of points under equal negative pressures impelling the air molecules toward the hood opening.   All air velocities are determined by $Q = AV$; the quantity, in cubic feet per minute, through a cross-sectional area A, in square feet, is a velocity V, in feet per minute (fpm).   As the area of a sphere is $4\pi r^2$, or approximately $12r^2$, increasing the radius from 1 to 2 units increases the boundary area from 12 to 48 square units.   Therefore, if 1,440 cfm of air is being drawn into a suction source, considered a point source, the velocity 1 ft away is $Q/A = V$, or $\frac{1440}{12} = 120$ fpm.   At 2 ft it is $\frac{1440}{48} = 30$ fpm.   The critical question is,

Table 5-7   CONTRAST OF AIR VOLUMES REQUIRED TO DILUTE THE VAPORS FROM 1 PINT EACH OF TWO HIGHLY TOXIC SOLVENTS AND TWO MODERATELY TOXIC SOLVENTS

Solvent	Toxicity shown by TLV, ppm	Vapor, ft^3/pint, at 70°F	Dilution air required, ft^3/pint evaporated
Carbon disulfide	20	6.7	335,000
Carbon tetrachloride	10	4.2	420,000
Ethyl ether	400	3.9	9,700
Turpentine	100	2.6	25,500

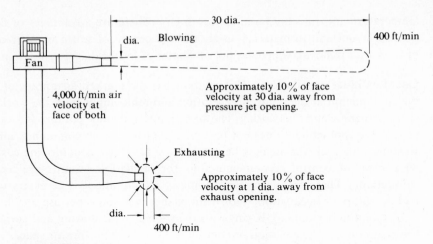

FIGURE 5-4
Jet discharge and suction intake velocity patterns. [*Source*: *Ref*. 5-6, *p*. 1-5.]

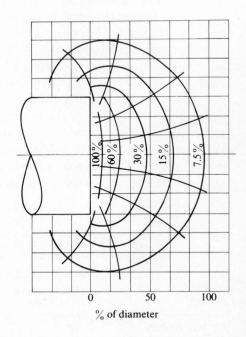

FIGURE 5-5
Equal velocity contours about a point source of suction. [*Source*: " *Exhaust Hoods*," *J. M. Dallavalle*, 1946, *by permission of Industrial Press, Inc*.]

What is the minimum velocity required to capture the contaminant? Table 5-8 states the range of capture velocities required for four intensities of contaminant release, from no release velocity into quiet air, as in quiescent evaporation, to particulate release with high kinetic energy into turbulent air, as in grinding. Note that the example would provide a zone of control for the first two classes of release for a distance of 1 ft, but that the 30 fpm at the distance of 2 ft is below the minimum velocity needed to capture contaminants in the most quiescent release conditions.

Industrial exhaust ventilation designers have ingenious shapes of exhaust hoods, flanged and fitted to the processes to maximize the zone of control with the minimum rates of flow and minimum energy requirement to move the air toward and into the exhaust opening. Reference 5-6 details the techniques and design data for hundreds of industrial operations and processes. The design of local exhaust systems is a rewarding application of fluid mechanics. Beyond the hood, provision must be made for an optimum transport velocity, a minimum of friction requirement in bends and transitions, the selection of an efficient fan, a proper air cleaner where required, and enough makeup air.

The benefits of good design and of conscientious construction and installation can be lost readily by improper use, by negligent maintenance, and by adding hood openings without regard to the original design. The most frequent improper use is working outside of and beyond the zone of effective capture velocity. Proper maintenance of ventilation systems requires the same attention as for production equipment. The ventilation systems are part of the productive facilities and must be systematically checked.

Table 5-8 THE RANGE OF CAPTURE VELOCITIES FOR TOXIC GASES, VAPORS, DUSTS, AND FUMES GENERATED BY INDUSTRIAL PROCESSES

Condition of dispersion of contaminant	Examples	Capture velocity, fpm
Released with practically no velocity into quiet air	Evaporation from tanks, degreasing	50–100
Released at low velocity into moderately still air	Spray booths; intermittent container filling, low-speed conveyor transfers, welding, plating, pickling	100–200
Active generation into zone of rapid air motion	Spray painting in shallow booths, barrel filling, conveyor loading, crushers	200–500
Released at high initial velocity into zone of very rapid air motion	Grinding, abrasive blasting, tumbling	500–2,000

SOURCE: Ref. 5-6, p. 4-5.

Hygienic Standards for the Concentrations of Toxic Gases, Vapors, Dusts, and Fumes in Workplace Air

In the mid 1930s Warren Cook, then an industrial hygiene engineer with a large insurance company, compiled a list of concentrations of toxicants in air that were believed safe to inhale in a normal workweek without injury.   By 1940 the California Industrial Accident Commission had printed such a list for advisory use.   In 1947 the American Conference of Governmental Industrial Hygienists published its first list, then termed Maximum Allowable Concentrations.   It has continued to prepare such a list of threshold limit values, or TLV, annually (Ref. 5-3).   The 1971 edition lists nearly 400 substances which are encountered in workroom air.   The publication is the result of the deliberations of a committee of 14 or 15 toxicologists, engineers, physicians, and scientists engaged in industrial hygiene practice.   Reference 5-7 documents

Table 5-9   LOCAL EXHAUST–VENTILATION DESIGN OBJECTIVES

Objective: To optimize the energy requirement and the work output of the system

A Needed	B Meet the need by
1 Required capture velocity at the point of generation	Most efficient hood shape and flow rate through it which gives the capture velocity
2 Minimum entry requirement	Using hood shape which approaches streamline flow and yet provides 1 above.
3 Transport velocity in duct to prevent settling, abrasion, and excess noise	Dimensioning duct to required flow rate Q to get required velocity V by $Q = AV$.
4 Minimum energy requirement for friction in ductwork	Holding velocity to that required to transport contaminant; approaching smooth flow in turns, transitions, and branch entries
5 Efficient fan	Careful choice of fan inlet and outlet; fan sized to flow rate and total pressure requirement at optimum point on fan curve; fan type suited to the system
6 Efficient air cleaner to remove particulates; gas and vapor removal dependent on specific needs	Selecting type needed to remove the contaminant, sized to require minimum energy to put air through the cleaner unit
7 Makeup air to prevent creating negative pressure in the workspace	Providing a sufficient number of openings to the outside for entry air, tempering and conditioning it to seasonal and process requirements

in summary statements for each toxicant the exhaustive examination of evidence which the committee makes to reach its recommended values.

The Hygienic Guides of the American Industrial Hygiene Association are a series of comprehensive data sheets prepared on particular compounds, covering physical, chemical, and toxicological facts, uses in industry, methods for sampling and analysis, and reference sources.   These are published in the journal of the association as they are developed or revised, and then printed as separates and as a loose-leaf collection. The American National Standards Institute, Health and Safety Committee, issues detailed bulletins on particular substances.   Similarly, the Manufacturing Chemists' Association and the American Chemical Society prepare health and safety information on selected compounds.   Several leading corporations prepare data sheets on their products and materials.

The TLV of the American Conference of Government Industrial Hygienists assumes that there is a dose-response curve like that in Fig. 9-10.   It is ogive with a nil or very slight response for low intakes even if continued throughout the work period. This does not mean that the TLV number is an absolute "effect, no-effect" level. Some individual workers may be distressed at lower exposures.   Others may withstand higher concentrations.   The TLV number is a guideline point.   It is a benchmark from which to make a professional judgement on a risk.   There are assumptions concerning the person at risk which include the following:

1 He is in normal health with adequate nutrition and rest.
2 He is a working adult aware of his exposure.
3 He is under observation of management.
4 He works a schedule of 8 h/day, 5 or 6 days a week.
5 He has normal physiological functions for handling low-level intakes of toxic substances.

The TLV committee makes provision for three types of exposure and response. These are time-weighted daily averages, ceiling values for exposures of about 15 min, with consideration of absorption through the skin, eyes, and mucous membranes contributing to inhalation exposure.   The committee expresses a strong caveat concerning the use of its values outside the United States.

The information base for TLV levels are in six groups.   These are:

1 Epidemiological studies over a period of months or years correlating environmental exposure and clinical medical data.   Such studies are well suited to compounds producing cumulative, chronic effects during long-time, low-level exposure.   Among such studies completed by the U.S. Public Health Service in the last 40 years are conditions and effects of exposure to:

      Free silica dust in quarrying, mining, and pottery making
      Lead dust and fumes in storage battery manufacture

Manganese dust in ore refining
Mercury vapor in hat manufacture
Chromate dust in chromate ore refining
Uranium ore dust and radon gas in mining and milling
Chromic acid mists in electroplating
Asbestos dust and fibers in asbestos fabric manufacture

2 Investigation of cases and complaints, using medical and environmental data. Examples are those dependent on assembling data from many reported experiences. This has been done for zinc oxides, benzol, and cadmium. Another approach is the study of plants where new materials have caused problems. Examples are carbon disulfide in rayon manufacture, lead tetraethyl, and beryllium.

3 Animal exposure experiments to determine toxicity, dose response, metabolic paths and products is the basis for a large part of the information on organic compounds. Phenol, methanol, ketones, vinyl chloride, methyl bromide, and chlorinated hydrocarbons are examples of compounds studied by animal exposures. Such exposure tests are a means of establishing ranges of response for acute effects; means of observing side and delayed effects other than narcosis. A frustrating dilemma of test results is the extrapolation from animal response to prediction for man.

4 Human exposure experiments have been quite limited   There have been experimental exposures to CO, as the effects are easily reversed, and to ammonia, as irritation levels in the upper respiratory tract are immediate.   There have been ingestion studies of DDT on human volunteers to observe storage in fat variations with intake changes.

5 Sensory responses to irritants, odorants, and simple narcotics by human test panels can set exposure values. On-the-job conditions show the adjusted worker withstanding higher concentrations than the laboratory test subjects.

6 Analogy with compounds of like chemical structure and composition is of some help. Similarities among chlorinated hydrocarbons and aliphatic and aromatic compounds do exist and have been observed, as have similarities among organophosphate pesticides. Analogy can provide the basis for a first-round estimate to be checked with experience in use.

In using TLV levels, three matters must be borne in mind:

1 That the TLV is a guide in making a professional judgement
2 That the consequences of exposure in excess of the TLV varies from long-term damage to transient irritation
3 That environmental and individual factors must be weighted

OUR COMMUNITY AIR

Since he adopted fire—whether to cook his catch, to warm his body, or to ward off threatening animals—man has been an air polluter. His step of "busting the sod" to plant crops opened the land surface to man-made erosion by water and wind. From there on he became a maker and user of things and materials. In the last hundred years he has become the master and user of thermal, electrical, and nuclear energy. Each step in the creation and use of these energies is attended by some unutilized form of energy or matter, designated as waste. This has been allowed to go to the free environments of water, land, and air until the consequences have become intolerable because of threats to man's health and comfort, deletrious effects on plants and animals he needs or cherishes, or esthetically offensive conditions that impair the pleasant responses to our surroundings. In the last 10 to 15 years there has been an intensely sharpened public concern for the quality of our community air supply. An increasing number of people glower at a smoking stack, no longer accepting it as a sign of productive prosperity. A snoutful of motor vehicle exhaust at a pedestrian crossing or bus stop is accepted with a grimace. Some aspects of polluted water and ill-managed land can be avoided by not looking at it, using alternatives, or staying away from it. The only escape from the local air envelope, except for indoor respites of rarely available filtered and deodorized supplies, is to get out of the area. Perhaps there is an intuitive awareness of our precarious dependence on air for survival. It is stated that man is able to survive without food for 5 weeks, without water for 5 days, but without air for only 5 mintutes. It has been stated that he requires 30 pounds of air per day, compared with 3 pounds of food and $4\frac{1}{2}$ pounds of water per day. That 30 pounds of air translates to 400 ft^3, or over 11 m^3. The minute concentrations of airborne pollutants become more consequential when volume of air breathed is calculated. The geometric mean for suspended particulates in United States air is about 100 $\mu g/m^3$. That results in about 1 mg/day for respiratory disposal by one means or another or for retention of some fraction of it. The sources, behavior, effects, measurement, and control of air pollutants are presented mainly with dependence on United States data.

Sources of the Five Primary Pollutants

Table 5-10 and Fig. 5-6 show the magnitudes of five primary emissions in the United States: carbon monoxide, particulates, hydrocarbons, nitrogen oxides, and sulfur oxides. These data are from the 1966 National Emissions Inventory (Ref. 5-8, p. 9). Four of the five man-made sources are identified and one is natural, forest fires. The total of 210 million tons/year is a staggering quantity. It is 1 ton for each of us. About 180 million tons is released in gaseous or vapor state. Carbon monoxide forms 100 million tons of these gases and vapors.   By applying $PV = nRT$, the carbon monoxide tonnage converts to 2.75×10^{12} ft^3, or about 80 billion m^3 of carbon monoxide at 1 atmosphere of pressure and 25°C (77°F).   Our high degree of mobility of people and things requires discharging over 90 million tons of wastes to our air.   The exhaust pipes of over 100 million motor vehicles are the major source of transportation pollutants.   The unburned hydrocarbons and nitrogen oxides require further attention, as these primary pollutants become photochemical reactants to produce secondary pollutants.

About 70 percent of the sulfur oxides are emitted from stationary combustion sources.   These are boilers consuming sulfur-bearing coal and oil.   Nearly three-quarters of the 31.2 million tons of sulfur dioxide are emitted from fossil-fueled electricity generating stations.   At the present doubling of electricity use each 10 years in the United States, to keep down sulfur oxide pollution the alternatives are removal from the stack gases, nuclear-fueled power plants, desulfurized oil and coal, or a reduction in the rate of increase of electricity use.   Of all particulates 60 percent are from the stationary combustion of fuels and from industrial processes.   Several air cleaners remove particulates with efficiencies of from 75 to 95 percent.   At a cost, some like percentage of particulates can be removed from a myriad of waste stacks. The collected 12 to 15 million tons will be transferred to the solid wastes column for further disposal or recovery.   It should be noted that solid waste-disposal accounts

Table 5-10   ESTIMATED EMISSIONS OF FIVE PRIMARY AIR POLLUTANTS IN THE UNITED STATES FOR 1966 FROM FIVE MAN-MADE AND ONE NATURAL SOURCE

Source	Millions of tons per year					
	Carbon monoxide	Particulates	Hydrocarbons	Nitrogen oxides	Sulfur oxides*	Total
Transportation	64.5	1.2	17.6	7.6	0.4	91.3
Fuel combustion in stationary sources	1.9	9.2	0.7	6.7	22.9	41.4
Industrial processes	10.7	7.6	3.5	0.2	7.2	29.2
Solid-waste disposal	7.6	1.0	1.5	0.5	0.1	10.7
Miscellaneous	9.7	2.9	6.0	0.5	0.6	19.7
Total	94.4	21.9	29.3	15.5	31.2	192.3
Forest fires	7.2	6.7	2.2	1.2	(†)	17.3
Total	101.6	28.6	31.5	16.7	31.2	209.6

* For the year 1967.
† Negligible.
Note: Nitrogen oxides expressed as nitrogen dioxide, and sulfur oxides expressed as sulfur dioxide.
SOURCE: Progress in the Prevention and Control of Air Pollution, Sen. Doc. 91-64, March 1970, p. 9.

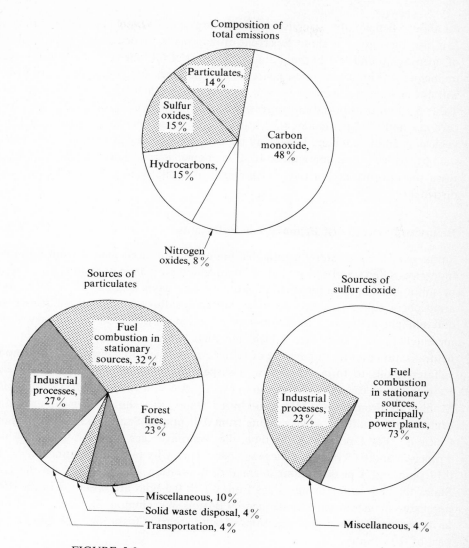

FIGURE 5-6
Five primary air pollutants as percentages of total emissions, and the sources in percentages of sulfur dioxide and particulates. [*Source: Danger in the Air—Sulfur Dioxide and Particulates, U.S. Public Health Serv. NAPCA. Publ.* 1, 1971, p. 3.]

for about 5 percent of total emissions, with the predominant portion carbon monoxide. It is also the source of about 5 percent of man-made particulates. A successful ban of open dump and leaf burning and full control of all types of incinerators—central municipal and industrial ones, apartment house types and backyard trash burners— will not make more than a 5 percent dent in man-made emissions. The raw data in Table 5-10 on transportation sources, and the fractions of carbon monoxide, hydrocarbons, and nitrogen oxides shown in Fig. 5-6 underline the gasoline-fueled motor vehicle as an air polluter. As many peoples strive to match United States personal mobility by having an internal-combustion-engined automobile, it is time to share with them the information on the concomitants of traffic deaths and disabilities and of dirtied air.

Behavior and Fate of Primary Air Pollutants

Sulfur oxides are a readily identifiable pollutant, produced mainly from burning the inorganic sulfides and sulfur-bearing organic compounds in coal and oil. The ratio of sulfur dioxide to sulfur trioxide in combustion gases is about 25 or 30:1. In the atmosphere, sulfur dioxide is slowly converted to sulfur trioxide with moisture content and sunlight influencing the oxidation. With moisture present, sulfur trioxide immediately forms sulfuric acid, which contributes to haze. Particulate absorption and neutralization occur. A complex of sulfuric oxides including metallic and ammonium sulfates results to form an aerosol, a suspension of liquid and solid agglomerates. Rain and snow carry the suspension to earth. A 6-year record of the Continuous Air Monitoring Program (CAMP) in 6 United States cities shows the mean annual concentrations of sulfuric oxides ranging from 0.01 ppm in San Francisco to 0.18 ppm in Chicago. For 1 percent of the time, the 5-min averages exceeded 0.09 ppm in San Francisco and 0.68 ppm in Chicago. New York City has had an annual average of 0.17 ppm and a peak 24-hour average concentration of 0.38 ppm. In the United States the high sulfur oxide values from 0.1 to 0.5 ppm are observed in the densely populated industrialized area defined by Boston, Washington, St. Louis, and Chicago at its corners. The largest quantities of sulfur-bearing fossil fuels are burned in that part of the country.

The fate of the over 100 million tons of carbon monoxide released in the United States remains an enigma. It is estimated that the rest of the world releases approximately another 100 million tons/year. If carbon monoxide accumulated, the emission of 200 million tons/year is calculated to raise the atmospheric concentration by 0.03 ppm/year. Careful measurements show no such rise. Direct chemical reaction of carbon monoxide with oxygen and with water at ambient temperatures happens far too slowly to account for carbon monoxide removal. At ambient temperatures these direct reactions are calculated to occur once in 10^{15} collisions. Explanations for removal that have been advanced are based in part on theoretical conjecture and in smaller part on experimental observations. The mechanisms hypothesized are:

1 Oxidation in the lower atmosphere by reactive species such as radicals, excited oxygen atoms, and singlet molecular oxygen[1]
2 Oxidation in the upper atmosphere to carbon dioxide in the high intensities of far ultraviolet radiation (Ref. 5-9, vol. 1, p. 181)
3 Contact with moist soil and utilization by anaerobic methane-producing bacteria such as *Methanosarcina barkerii* and *Methanobacterium formicum*

The annual mean concentrations of carbon monoxide in the air of the cities in the Continuous Air Monitoring Program in the United States range approximately from 5 to 15 ppm. Five-min highs range approximately from 40 to 60 ppm. On maximum days, values range approximately from 10 to 30 ppm. These sampling stations are at street level in downtown traffic. The concentrations are sufficient to increase carboxyhemoglobin in the blood during prolonged breathing. For traffic police, route drivers, and taxi drivers, the maximum-day concentrations are a significant fraction of the occupational TLV for carbon monoxide of 50 ppm.

Carbon dioxide has not been considered a pollutant, although it is the major component of fossil-fuel stack gases. A complete burning of pure carbon will produce a dry flue gas of 21 percent carbon dioxide and 79 percent nitrogen. The estimates of the earth's carbon dioxide balances are $2{,}300 \times 10^9$ tons in the air; $150{,}000 \times 10^9$ tons dissolved in the oceans; 200×10^9 tons of carbon dioxide added to the air over the years by man's carbon fuel burning, now accelerated to the rate of 9×10^9 tons of carbon dioxide additional per year; 60×10^9 tons of carbon dioxide used per year in plant photosynthesis, all of which is eventually returned to the air or soil moisture by daily respiration or the long-term decay of dead plant life. Is man's fuel use altering the balances? The present average concentration of carbon dioxide in air is about 300 ppm. There is evidence that man's combustion processes are now increasing that concentration at the rate of nearly 1 ppm each year. More precise data are:

1 From 1890 to 1965, the carbon dioxide has increased from 290 to 314 ppm. The increase of 24 ppm in 75 years is an average of 0.3 ppm/year.
2 From October 1959 to March 1962, carbon dioxide concentrations at the Mauna Loa Observatory, Hawaii, increased from 313 to 315 ppm, an increase of 0.06 ppm/month or 0.7 ppm/year.[2]
3 Observations in Paris since 1891 show that the 1891 to 1900 annual average of 320 ppm increased by only 1 ppm for the period of 1901 to 1909. The 1954 to

[1] B. Dimitriades and M. Whisman, *Environ. Sci. and Technol.*, 5:219 (March 1971).
[2] B. Bolin and C. D. Keeling, *J. Geophys. Res.*, 68:3899 (1963).

1964 value rose to 351, a 30 ppm increase in 55 years, about 0.6 ppm/year. Within the 10-year period of 1954 to 1964, the moving 5-year annual averages were 348 ppm in 1954 to 1958, and 354 ppm in 1959 to 1964.   The 5-year increase was 6 ppm, or over 1 ppm/year (Ref. 5-9, vol. 1, p. 30).

The consequences of increased carbon dioxide in our air is that carbon dioxide and water vapor absorb infrared radiations both from the sun and from the back-radiation from the earth.   The absorbed radiation is in turn reradiated.   The water-vapor–carbon dioxide canopy in the atmosphere acts like the glass cover of a green-house and produces the " greenhouse effect " of maintaining the earth's surface temperature.   The increase in carbon dioxide is expected to raise the earth's ambient temperatures.   One careful calculation predicts a 1.5°C (2.7°F) increase if the carbon dioxide concentration doubles from 300 to 600 ppm.   There is evidence that part of such infrared increases will be offset by increased haze produced by condensation nucleii and sulfur dioxide from other components of man's air pollutants.   The long-term ecological disbalances are threats that require continued precise measurement of the chemical and physical changes and study of the mechanisms of the existing equilibria (Ref. 5-9, vol. 1, pp. 392–395; vol. 3, pp. 13–14).

Particulates, in air pollution nomenclature, include the solids and liquids dispersed in air with a size range from small molecules to diameters up to 500 μm. Particles of these sizes may settle in a few seconds or remain suspended for months. Those larger than 1 μm have measurable settling velocities but are readily stirred by air movements.   Adsorption of gases and vapors on particulates, oxidation, condensation, and photochemical reactions produce changes from the original states.   Particulates include the air pollution we see as smoke, dust, haze, and mists.   The visible pollution results from two things.   There are particle sizes seen by the naked eye, about 100 μm, the size of the period for this sentence.   There are light effects of dispersion, reflection, and selective color absorption that our eyes readily detect as reduced visibility, haze, and red skies at sunset.

Particles larger than 10 μm are products of mechanical processes, grinding, spraying, abrasion by the movement of vehicles and people, and wind erosion and pickup.   Particles from 1 to 10 μm are smoke, other combustion products, process dusts, and sea salt.   Particles below 1 μm originate from combustion and condensation.   Those from $\frac{1}{10}$ to 1 μm are largely combustion products and the result of photochemical reactions.   Those below $\frac{1}{10}$ μm, a submicroscopic size found in urban air, are minute combustion products.   With the random motions of gas molecules, these very small particles collide frequently and form larger particles rapidly by sorption and nucleation of gas molecules and adhesion with other particles (Ref. 5-10, p. 12-2–12-3).

Particulates are separable by sampling into two types.   The settleables can be collected in dust-fall jars usually exposed for a week to a month. The suspended particulates can be collected on glass fiber filters by high-volume samplers operated for 24 hours. The settleable solids concentrations, called *dust fall*, are stated in tons per square mile per month, or milligrams per square centimeter per month. Table 5-11 gives the " cleanliness index " of dust-fall values used by Allegheny County, which includes Pittsburgh, Pennsylvania. Figure 5-7, on dust fall in seven United States cities from 1935 to 1965, shows that Pittsburgh moved from the classification " heavy " by 1955 to that of " moderate," 20 to 40 tons/(mi^2)(month) [0.7 to 1.4 mg/(cm^2)(month)]. Note that by 1960 only New York City remained above 50 tons/(mi^2)(month). That was a dramatic reduction from New York City's initially graphed high of 150 tons/(mi^2)(month) in 1944. The change from coal to oil or gas for residential and office building heating and for a very large number of commercial and manufacturing boilers produced the declines shown in Fig. 5-7. The principal components of dust fall are materials lost on ignition (the soot), oxides of silicon, calcium, iron, aluminum, and sulfates. Dust fall is not a useful index of overall particulate pollution or of the general quality of a community air supply. It is a measure of air-transported filth.

Suspended particulates are defined by the sampling apparatus and the filters used. It is the airborne material which is drawn into the sampler intake and retained on its filter that is identified as suspended particulates. For the high-volume sampler, shelter, and filter used in the United States, particles with an aerodynamic equivalent greater than 1 and a diameter of 100 μm cannot enter the shelter. It is calculated that 90 percent of the particles collected by the standard device are less than an aerodynamic equivalent of 1 and diameter of 16 μm. Such particulates remain suspended for appreciable periods, are readily moved by air currents, and do not settle near the emission source (Ref. 5-9, vol. 1., p. 83). Concentrations are expressed in micrograms per cubic meter. The collected material cannot be classified by size, as it is matted and agglomerated on the filter. It can be divided into water-soluble and other

Table 5-11 GUIDELINES FOR DUST FALL IN
ALLEGHENY COUNTY, PENNSYLVANIA

Classification	Dust fall	
	tons/(mi^2) (30 days)	mg/(cm^2) (30 days)
Slight	0–30	0–0.7
Moderate	20–40	0.7–1.4
Heavy	40–100	1.4–3.5
Very heavy	>100	>3.5

SOURCE: Allegheny County Health Dept., Pittsburgh, Pa.

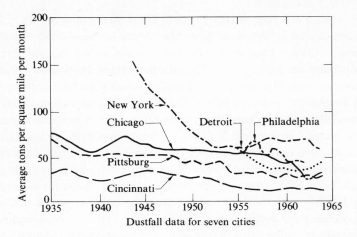

FIGURE 5-7
Dust-fall data for seven cities in the United States, 1935 to 1965. [*Source*: *Physicians' Guide to Air Pollution, American Medical Association*, 1968, *p.* 9.]

solvent fractions and into inorganic and organic fractions. It can be analyzed for many inorganic and organic chemical identities. Benzene-soluble organics, sulfates, and nitrates make up from 15 to 20 percent of the total collection. Some 15 metals from antimony to zinc have been detected in routine samples, with iron, lead, and zinc the most abundant. Abundant, in this case, means iron up to 2 $\mu g/m^3$ and lead and zinc up to 1 $\mu g/m^3$. Aliphatic hydrocarbons are found in a weight ratio thirteen times as great as aromatic hydrocarbons. To get whole integer values for discrete organic compounds, it is necessary to state concentrations in micrograms per 1,000 m^3. For example, benzo-α-pyrene, a recognized carcinogen, has been reported in composited monthly suspended particulate samples in a range of concentrations from a low of 0.25 $\mu g/1,000$ m^3 to a high of 31 $\mu g/1,000$ m^3.[1]

Table 5-12 groups the National Air Sampling Network suspended-particulate data for 1964–1965 on 300 United States cities into five groups of 60 each by concentration ranges in micrograms per cubic meter. Only those cities in the lowest fifth are acceptably free of suspended particulates. About 80 percent of the lowest group are cities of under 100,000 people. Suspended particulates appear to be directly proportional to population and population density. For the United States, the annual geometric mean for suspended particulates in urban areas ranges from 60 to 200 $\mu g/m^3$. Nonurban areas show concentrations of from 10 to 60 $\mu g/m^3$. The maximum 24-hour

[1] E. Sawicki et al., *Am. Ind. Hyg. Assoc. J.* **23**:137 (1962).

average concentration in urban areas is generally about three times the annual geometric mean, although instances of seven times the annual value have occurred (Ref. 5-10, pp. 12-4, 12-5).

Hydrocarbons, nitrogen oxides, and ozone interreact by photochemical processes. A. J. Haagen-Smit was the first to identify these constituents and reactions in 1954 in unravelling the intracacies of Los Angeles smog. The primary source of hydrocarbons and nitrogen oxides in United States cities is the gasoline-fueled motor vehicle. This can be spoken of simply as the motor vehicle, since 99 percent of those in the United States are gasoline-fueled despite about a million diesel-fueled trucks and buses. Prior to 1963 when the United States had 90 million motor vehicles, it was estimated that their annual pollution contribution was 12 million tons of hydrocarbons and 6 million tons of nitrogen oxides. Additionally, there were 66 million tons of carbon monoxide and a million tons each of sulfur oxides and particulates released per year. For each automobile, R. W. Hurn states that observations based mostly on 1956 to 1966 models in routine stop-start driving at an average speed of 25 mi/h (40 km/h) showed the average United States car put out 1,400 ppm of hydrocarbons, 850 ppm of nitrogen oxides, and 310,000 ppm (3.1 percent) of carbon monoxide. The hydrocarbon emission equals 3.3 percent of the gasoline supplied to the engine (Ref. 5-9, vol. 3, p. 59).

There are other sources of hydrocarbon emission in any community. These include evaporation in gasoline handling, paint drying, dry cleaning, and industrial use of cleaning solvents. Any manufacture and handling of such materials adds its evaporative losses. Oxides of nitrogen are formed in any high-temperature combustion, so there are multiple sources of it in any community. Station data of the Continuous Air Monitoring Program show the hydrocarbons in our downtown-traffic-level urban air to be at an annual geometric mean of 2 to 3 ppm. The maximum-five-min-duration values are from 17 to 20 ppm. The respective values for nitric oxide, NO, and nitric dioxide, NO_2, are each in hundredths of parts per million for

Table 5-12 RANGES OF SUSPENDED–PARTICULATE CONCENTRATIONS IN 300 CITIES BY FIFTHS

Highest fifth	136–245 $\mu g/m^3$
Next highest fifth	106–134 $\mu g/m^3$
Middle fifth	93–105 $\mu g/m^3$
Next lowest fifth	77–92 $\mu g/m^3$
Lowest fifth	38–76 $\mu g/m^3$

SOURCE: Mel Weisburd, Physician's Guide to Air Pollution, *AMA*, 1968, p. 10.

the annual mean; in tenths of a part per million for the maximum days; and from $\frac{1}{4}$ to $1\frac{1}{3}$ ppm for the maximum five-min-duration values.   Why the great concern for these two classes of pollutants?   It is not their direct effects as entities that warrant concern. These are the primary input reactants of an intricate series of photochemical reactions which produce irritants and oxidants.   The irritants produce pain in the respiratory passages and eyes of man and presumably animals.   The oxidants change the appearance and growth of vegetation for the worse and change the structure of rubber and synthetic fabric in appearance, structural strength, and usefulness.   A look at photochemical reactions in the air explains how minute quantities of pollutants can produce major pollution problems, and provides an experience in physics and chemistry applied to the mess we are brewing in our air, our water, and on and in our land.

Secondary Air Pollutants by Photochemistry

The information in Fig. 5-8 is the result of the painstaking study of Los Angeles smog for which A. J. Haagen-Smit of the California Institute of Technology provided the key solutions.   Although it is hardly simple at first look, Fig. 5-8 is a simplified schematic flow diagram of an intricate process.   If it only answered the question of the source and cause of the damage from Los Angeles' air pollution, it would be worthy.   It is now evident that Los Angeles reached the conditions first.   It has prolonged periods of air stagnation.   It has abundant sunlight.   It has more than abundant sources of the primary pollutant inputs of hydrocarbons and nitrogen oxides from its overabundant motor vehicle numbers and use.   In its development and growth, Los Angeles skipped lightly over mass transportation as an option for its people and since has practically abandoned it.   Several cities of the world have conditions one and two, air stagnation and abundant sunlight, at least in season.   These cities lack the motor vehicles.   The candidates include Lima, Peru; Rio de Janeiro, Brazil; Bombay, India; Bangkok, Thailand.   Tokyo already has all the inputs and the problem.   The problem may be masked in our older cities, New York, Chicago, St. Louis, London, and Paris, by smoke and sulfur dioxide.

The photochemistry of smog begins its sequence with some oxides of nitrogen, in the upper-right box of Fig 5-8.   The yellow-brown molecules of nitrogen dioxide absorb one or more of Planck's quanta in the blue and near-ultraviolet frequency and dissociate to nitric oxide and monatomic oxygen.   The ultraviolet, which in the lower atmosphere is at a frequency of 1×10^{15} Hz (290 nm) or less, is also absorbed by oxygen molecules.   The absorbed energy is not enough to break the bond of the oxygen molecule, O_2.   It is enough to produce an excited state.   Some of the monatomic oxygen joins diatomic oxygen to form the triatomic form, ozone.   These three, monatomic, excited diatomic, and triatomic oxygen, feed into the oxidant pool shown in the large, middle-right box.   Ozone is a very active participant in our air.   The reason

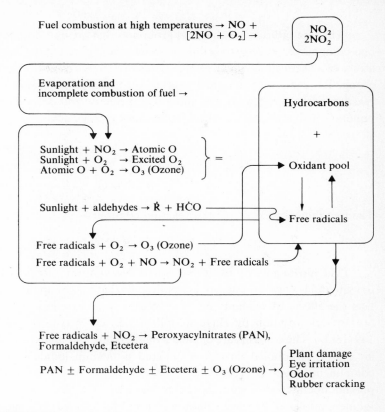

FIGURE 5-8
A schematic of the photochemistry of smog. [*Source: Seymour Tilson, Air Pollution, Int. Sci. Technol., June*, 1965.]

that the ultraviolet in the lower atmosphere is in wavelengths of more than 290 nm is that the short-wavelength ultraviolet has been absorbed in ozonosphere, a layer of air high in ozone, 10 to 20 mi above the earth.

Another important input into the large, right-middle box are free radicals. Aldehydes are a partly oxidized form of aliphatic hydrocarbons. Formaldehyde is the simplest and best-known one. There are aldehydes in combustion gases, including vehicle exhaust. More are formed in the air as the oxygen forms combine with the hydrocarbons. The important reaction is the absorption of ultraviolet and possibly visible light by the aldehydes, which results in their dissociation into two free radicals, the alkyl group and the HCO. This feeds into the free-radical pool in the large, right-middle box. The hydrocarbon pool is provided by the polluters. All this would be quite enough. But as Fig. 5-8 shows, there are further steps that make the processes cyclically regenerative.

The free radicals are chemical groupings that are not recognized as stable molecular compounds; nor are they ions, as there is *no* ionic charge.   A dot over one of the atoms of a chemical formula, as $H\dot{C}O$, indicates a free radical.   The free-radical alkyl group, R, reacts with diatomic oxygen to form a peroxy radical, ROO.   It is very reactive with nitrogen oxides and other primary and secondary, partly oxidized, pollutant hydrocarbons, alcohols, ethers, and organic acids.   Example reactions are

$$ROO + NO_2 \longrightarrow ROONO_2$$
$$ROO + SO_2 \longrightarrow ROOSO_2$$
$$ROO + O_3 \longrightarrow RO\cdot + 2O_2$$

The free radical $RO\cdot$ of the last reaction continues

$$RO\cdot + NO_2 \longrightarrow RONO_2 \qquad \text{peroxyacyl nitrite}$$

The nitrite goes on to $RONO_3$, peroxyacyl nitrate, PAN.   This last is a strong irritant and is one of the secondary pollutants that makes up the oxidants.   Figure 5-8 lists the effects of oxidants on man, plants, and materials.   Further discussion on atmospheric reaction by Haagen-Smit and L. G. Wayne is in Ref. 5-9 (vol. 1, pp. 149–186).   The oxidants are defined by a sampling and analytical method in which an air sample is bubbled through a buffered potassium iodide solution.   The oxidant components, such as organic peroxides, ozone, hydrogen peroxide, and chlorine, if present, liberate iodine from the iodide solution.   The color change due to the liberated iodine is measured by spectrophotometer and interpreted by standard concentrations.

The Effects of Air Pollutants

The wastes man releases into the air change the composition of the air he breathes. Depending on the waste constituents and their concentrations, his health and well-being are affected.   Occasionally the recognized effects are so acute and dramatic that they are identified as a high-air-pollution episode.   With varying susceptibility to particular constituents and sensitivity to particular ranges of concentrations, plants and animals are damaged.   The most evident and least-disputed meteorological effect of air pollutants is that of forming haze and reducing visibility.   With his ground and air mobility man finds reduced visibility, at minimum, an inconvenience to road and air traffic and, at most, an added risk of collisions and crashes.   Finally, there is the damage to, and depreciation of, property.   The damage is by specific actions of pollutants on material surfaces and to fabrics, including simple soiling.   The depreciation is the net effect of persistent, recurring dirty air, which restricts desirable and acceptable uses of land and buildings to producing low returns, which results in low market values.   These effects will be examined with particular attention to the five ubiquitous pollutants of our industrial, urban, automobile-transported society and economy.   These pollutants are the sulfur oxides, particulates, carbon monoxide, photochemical oxidants, and hydrocarbons.   Other pollutants with specific actions for one or more of the effects, such as airborne fluorides, sulfides, beryllium, and lead compounds, are noted.

Effects on man's health   The etiology of injury to people from breathing a community air supply impaired in quality by contaminants and pollutants is based largely on associative epidemiological evidence.   As epidemiological evidence is usually not much more than circumstantial evidence, the evidence that is associative is less firm, less certain, less able to demonstrate specific causes and specific effects.   Faced with demands for precise, replicate quantitative data on causative concentrations and resultant mortality, morbidity, and pathology, our best epidemiologists cannot satisfy those who will not act until air tight evidence is provided.   The nature of the case that can be made for convicting dirty air as damaging to man's health is set forth as (1) the occurrence of acute air pollution episodes, (2) the relations between polluted air and several respiratory diseases, (3) the evidence of damage from recognized toxicants, and (4) the interpretation of toxicological observations from various sources on the quality of the community air supply.

ACUTE EPISODES   The best-known acute air pollution episodes that the world has experienced in the last 40 years or so are summarized in Table 5-13.   Except for Poza Rica, there are common factors among conditions, probable causes, and the recognized effects.   During the inversion stagnations with marked accumulations of smoke particulates, sulfur oxides, and fog, the cardiovascular "cripples" and those with a history of respiratory limitations were the readiest victims of death and severe illness.   Most of these were aged.   Donora provides an example of a community medical care emergency.   Ten percent of the city's population sought care at hospital, clinic, or physician's offices.   Poza Rica provides an example of a failure in handling a toxic material in large-scale chemical processing and the consequences that can be inflicted on a "company town" in a short time.   Note that the hydrogen sulfide release lasted less than a half hour.   Episodes similar to those of London, 1952, London, 1962, the Meuse Valley, and Donora occurred in New York City in 1953, and during the period of November 27 to December 10, 1962, in Washington, Philadelphia, New York City, Rotterdam, Hamburg, and Osaka (Japan).   The last period is concurrent with the London, 1962, happening.   The conditions in the cities named were similar to those in London during the same period, but apparently less intense and less damaging.   Roueché gives the Donora event his usual dramatic and captivating treatment in The Fog (Ref. 5-11, p. 173).

Table 5-13   ACUTE AIR POLLUTION EPISODES THE WORLD HAS EXPERIENCED

Place	Time	Effect and number	Conditions and probable cause
Meuse Valley, Belgium; coke ovens, blast furnaces, steel, glass, zinc, and sulfuric acid plants	Dec. 1–6, 1930	60 deaths, "thousands ill," coughing, breathlessness, chest pain, eye and nose irritation experienced.	Inversion, stagnation in 15-mi river valley for 1 week; smoke and irritant gases; sulfur oxide, sulfuric acid mist, and fluorides suspected; estimated sulfur dioxide 25–100 mg/m^3 (10–40 ppm).
Donora, Pa., U.S.; zinc smelter, wire coating mill, steel mill, sulfuric acid plant	Oct. 27–31, 1948	6,000 of 14,000 population ill, 1,400 sought medical care, 17 died; coughing, sore throat, chest constriction, burning and tearing eyes, vomiting, nausea, excessive nasal discharge.	Temperature inversion and fog along horseshoe-shaped valley of Monongahela River; Sulfur oxides, smoke, and zinc compound particulates present; sulfuric acid mists likely; estimated sulfur dioxide of 1.5–5.5 mg/m^3 (0.5–2 ppm).
Poza Rica, Mexico; petrochemical plant, hydrogen sulfide recovery system	4:45 A.M.–5:10 A.M., Nov. 24, 1950	22 deaths; 320 hospitalized, acute hydrogen sulfide poisoning, unconsciousness, vertigo, severe irritation of respiratory tract, loss of sense of smell.	Low inversion layer, fog, weak winds; hydrogen sulfide released when burner on 4-day-old sulfur recovery plant failed under increased hydrogen sulfide flow rate; release lasted for only 25 min.
London, England	Dec. 5–9, 1952	3,500–4,000 deaths in week of Dec. 5–12 in excess of expected norm of like weeks; causes of death, chronic bronchitis, bronchopneumonia, and heart disease; increased hospital admissions for respiratory and heart disease.	"Pea soup" fog and temperature inversion covered most of the U.K.; smoke and sulfur dioxide accumulations in stagnated air; reported smoke highs of 4.5 mg/m^3 and, sulfur oxide highs of 3.75 mg/m^3 (1.4 ppm).
London, England	January 1956	1,000 excess deaths charged to a pollution episode.	Extended fog conditions similar to 1952 episode; resulted in Parliament's passing Clean Air Act.
London, England	Dec. 5–7, 1962	700 excess deaths and increased illness charged to a pollution episode; emergency medical care plan functioned.	Severe fog and inversion; sulfur dioxide levels higher than in 1952, but particulates were lower; alert system operated.

RESPIRATORY DISEASES   H. Heimann summarizes his monograph, Air Pollution and Respiratory Diseases, with these words:

> Air pollution, as it exists in some of our communities, contributes significantly as a cause or aggravating factor for the following medical conditions: acute respiratory infections, chronic bronchitis, chronic constrictive ventilatory disease, pulmonary emphysema, bronchial asthma, and lung cancer.   (Ref. 5-1, p. 17.)

Acute, nonspecific upper-respiratory disease includes the common cold, acute tonsillitis, sore throat, acute bronchitis, acute sinusitis, laryngitis, and asthmatic attacks.   Heimann cites studies in Maryland as early as 1950, in the U.S.S.R. in 1957, in Great Britain, and in Japan showing associations between air pollution at moderate levels commonly found in our communities and the frequency and duration of acute, nonspecific, upper-respiratory disease.   He cites animal exposure studies from which a most significant finding is the loss or reduction of an important respiratory clearance mechanism.   Irritants inhaled produce increased mucus secretion, but at times the mucus thickens.   More importantly, the movement of the hairlike cilia is slowed and even stopped.   These changes mean less effective removal of material from the surfaces of the respiratory airways.

Chronic bronchitis has been much more widely recognized in Great Britain than in the United States.   In Great Britain it accounts for 10 percent of all deaths and over 10 percent of all industrial absences for illness.   Using the British definition of chronic bronchitis as a chronic productive cough on most days for 3 months of each of 2 successive years, one case-finding study in the United States revealed that 21 percent of a group of men 40 to 59 years of age had chronic bronchitis.   Based on the experience and findings of nine British investigations and studies, Heimann states:

> (1) Chronic bronchitis mortality rates are associated with the following community air pollution indexes: population density, amount of fuel use, sulfur dioxide air levels, settled dust measures, airborne dust measures, and decreased visibility; (2) Aggravation of the condition, in the form of acute irritations, have been observed among British postmen employed in the more highly polluted areas, gaged by decrease of visibility; (3) Other things being equal, postmen who work outdoors lose more time from such illness than those who work indoors; (4) On days of higher pollution, a panel of chronic bronchitics kept under regular observation show a worsening of their illness.   The circumstantial evidence, therefore, ties air pollution in a causal relationship to chronic bronchitis.   (Ref. 5-1, p. 12.)

Chronic constrictive ventilatory disease is a condition that can be detected by pulmonary function tests in which the person under test blows.   It may have its onset without symptoms or signs of other respiratory disease.   There is increased airway resistance.   That condition has been induced in laboratory exposures of animals and man to irritant air pollutants such as the sulfur oxides at concentrations found in a polluted community air supply.   A western Pennsylvania study of two towns of under 1,000 people showed increased airway resistence in the town with greater pollution

(Ref. 5-1, p. 13).   The condition is also found among heavy smokers.   The risks of such constricted ventilation may be small for an otherwise healthy person.   These become larger with the appearance of other cardiorespiratory disorders in the same person.

Emphysema is the condition in which the thin walls of the alveoli, the air sacs at the termini of millions of bronchioles in our lungs, have lost their elasticity and so tear. The excess capacity of normal lungs, about sixfold the base requirement, to provide our body oxygen is lost irreparably.   The distended air sacs do not squeeze to exhale. Their oxygen–carbon dioxide exchange usefulness is ended.   The victim breathes 25 to 30 times per minute, compared with a normal 16, but does not get enough oxygen. From 1965 to 1969 the number of new cases of emphysema seen by physicians in the United States nearly doubled from 267,000 to 510,000.   The number of deaths in the United States from emphysema more than tripled from 7,728 to 24,420 in the 10 years from 1959 to 1968.   These data are from 1971 reports of the National Tuberculosis and Respiratory Diseases Association.   A very large number of emphysema cases have been heavy cigarette smokers.   Exposure to lung irritants, gases, dusts, and fumes occupationally and in dirty community air, and repeated illnesses of bronchitis, chest colds, and respiratory infections contribute to the development of emphysema.   The Report on Smoking and Health to the Surgeon General by the U.S. Public Health Service in 1964 was unequivocal in this statement:

> Cigarette smoking is the most important of the causes of chronic bronchitis in the United States.
> For the bulk of the population of the United States the importance of cigarette smoking as a cause of chronic bronchopulmonary disease is much greater than that of atmospheric pollution or occupational exposure.[1]

The updated report of 1967 reinforced these observations.   Nevertheless there is agreement that after chronic cough and shortness of breath set in, cigarette smoking and breathing polluted air increase the severity of chronic chest diseases.

Lung cancer poses several dilemmas in relating its alarming increase during the last 50 to 70 years in most countries, particularly among men, to the quality of the community air supply.   The cause of lung cancer is not known, although cancer can be induced in experimental animals by introducing identified carcinogens in specific ways.   Factors that are believed to contribute to the increase of lung cancer are improved diagnosis, increased life span, genetic constitution, race, viral diseases, and occupational exposure.   There is agreement on three things: The disease is increasing, and more people die of it, and cigarette smoking is a major factor in the increase.   The role of community air pollution remains conjectural despite some associative epidemiological evidence that there is more of the disease in urban areas than there is in rural

---

[1] If You Have Emphysema or Chronic Bronchitis, *U.S. Public Health Serv. Publ.* 1726, 1964, p. 5.

areas and among those who migrate from low-prevalence areas to high ones. There has been a search for an "urban factor," and data have been assembled to associate it with lung cancer among urban dwellers. The evidence is such that two recognized authorities looking at the same data arrive at rather different conclusions. These differences are clear in their statements, although both have words that allow latitude for change. Heimann states:

> These bits and pieces of circumstantial evidence lead to the reasonable conclusion that air pollution is indeed one of the factors contributing to the increasing occurrence of lung cancer. (Ref. 5-1, p. 17.)

J. Goldsmith in a vigorously disciplined discussion of Effects of Air Pollution on Human Health (Ref. 5-9, vol. 1, pp. 547–615) carefully and circumspectly reviews the epidemiological evidence on the urban factor as a cause of lung cancer. He states (Ref. 5-9, vol. 1, p. 574):

> In summary, the available evidence supports a migration and an urban factor as contributing in a minor way to the complex of causal factors affecting lung cancer rates. The available evidence has failed to support the hypothesis that exposure to community air pollution is a causal factor. Personal air pollution from cigarette smoking is certainly a major causal factor; occupational air pollution is (in a few occupations) likely to be a causal factor; and domestic air pollution simply has not been studied sufficiently.

The idea of the urban factor rests on the higher concentrations of pollutants in urban air than in rural air, on the reduced sunshine and ultraviolet light, and on the increased cloudiness and fog in the urban areas. The extent of these differences is stated in Table 5-14. Goldsmith provides information and comment on several

Table 5-14 QUALITY FACTORS OF URBAN AIR IN RATIO TO THOSE OF RURAL AIR EXPRESSED AS 1

Urban	Quality factor
10	Dust particles
5	Sulfur dioxide
10	Carbon dioxide
25	Carbon monoxide
0.8	Total sunshine
0.7	Ultraviolet, winter
0.95	Ultraviolet, summer
1.1	Cloudiness
2	Fog, winter
1.3	Fog, summer

SOURCE: Seymour Tilson, Air Pollution, *Int. Sci. Technol.*, June 1965.

studies on lung cancer and the urban factor.   He gives the reported data on some of the studies in three tables and one figure.   He then puts the case to test by citing five consequences which should follow a strong urban factor in lung cancer.   These consequences have not been observed.   Goldsmith's chapter is rewarding to read and well worth discussion.

TOXICANTS   The evidence of health effects of recognized, identified, and measured toxicants in the community air supply has been assembled and painstakingly analyzed by the National Air Pollution Control Administration, since December 1970 re-organized as the Office of Air Programs of the Environmental Protection Agency. The analyses and findings are published as a series of Air Quality Criteria and provide the bases for national air quality standards (Ref. 5-12).   To mid-1971, the series covered sulfur oxides, particulate matter, carbon monoxide, photochemical oxidants, oxides of nitrogen, and hydrocarbons.   The data provide additional support on health effects.   The data and observations on them are summarized for sulfur dioxide and particulates in Table 5-15, for carbon monoxide in Table 5-16, and for photochemical

Table 5-15   SOME OBSERVED HEALTH EFFECTS OF SULFUR DIOXIDE AND PARTICULATES

Concentrations of sulfur dioxide			Concentrations of particulates		
$\mu g/m^3$	ppm	Measured as	$\mu g/m^3$	Measured as	Effect that may occur
1,500	0.52	24-h average	......	....	Increased mortality
715	0.25	24-h mean	750	24-h mean	Increased daily death rate; a sharp rise in illness rates among bronchitics over age 54
300–500	0.11 – 0.19	24-h mean	Low	24-h mean	Increased hospital admissions of elderly respiratory disease cases; increased absenteeism among older workers
600	0.21	24-h mean	300	24-h mean	Symptoms of chronic lung disease cases accentuated
105–265	0.04–0.09	Annual mean	185	Annual mean	Increased frequency of respiratory symptoms and lung disease
120	0.05	Annual mean	100	Annual mean	Increased frequency and severity of respiratory diseases among school-children
115	0.04	Annual mean	160	Annual mean	Increased mortality from bronchitis and lung cancer

SOURCE: Data from Air Quality Criteria for Sulfur Oxides and for Particulates, *U.S. Public Health Serv. Publs.*, 1969.

oxidants in Table 5-17.   The goal for the air quality criteria is to arrive at a rational standard for the concentration of pollutants in the ambient air.   The original documents of the Air Quality Criteria series give the literature citations, the discussion of findings, and the criteria.   Health effects are a primary consideration, but other effects are included.

QUALITY OF COMMUNITY AIR   Certain toxicants, notorious as the causes of occupational diseases, are found in measurable concentrations in the community air supply, although well below the TLV for occupational exposure.   Four examples are lead, nitrogen dioxide, beryllium compounds, and asbestos particulates.   Each presents particular issues which further illustrate the intracacies of health effects of airborne contaminants.   Lead in the community air was subject to 3,400 air samples from 20 sites in Cincinnati, Los Angeles, and Philadelphia, along with blood samples on 2,300 people, and urine samples on 1,700 males for lead determination in a year-long study, June 1961 through May 1962 (Ref. 5-13).   Using the downtown and industrial area annual average of 3 μg/m^3 found in Los Angeles and Philadelphia and a daily air intake of 15 m^3/day, the lead intake of an individual would be about 0.05 mg/day.   At the highest monthly value of 6.4 μg/m^3 in Los Angeles in December 1961, the daily intake by inhalation would be about 0.1 mg.   For the United States, estimates for ingestion of lead with food range from 0.1 to 4 mg/day with an average of about 0.3 mg/day.   The contribution from water by ingestion adds from 0.01 to 0.09 mg/day, which provides a total ingested average of about 0.35 mg/day.   At low lead ingestions, only about 10 to 15 percent of the lead is absorbed into the body.   On inhalation of

Table 5-16   CARBOXYHEMOGLOBIN CONCENTRATIONS AND EFFECTS OF CERTAIN CARBON MONOXIDE EXPOSURES

Concentrations of carbon monoxide			Carboxyhemoglobin in nonsmokers	
mg/m^3	ppm	Exposure time	Percent	Effect anticipated
12–17	10–15	8 hours or more	2.0–2.5	Impaired time of interval discrimination
35	30	8 hours or more	5.0	Impaired performance on certain psychomotor tests
9–16	8–14	Weekly average		Increased fatality rates among hospitalized myocardial infarction patients associated with this exposure

SOURCE: Data from Air Quality Criteria for Carbon Monoxide, *U.S. Public Health Serv. Publ.* AP-62, 1970.

finely divided lead, from 20 to 50 percent has been reported as absorbed (Ref. 5-13, pp. 10–12).   Within these ranges, the total absorption would be from 0.05 to 0.1 mg/day.

R. A. Kehoe estimates that lead poisoning may develop in several weeks in adults at intakes of soluble lead of 6 to 10 mg/day (Ref. 5-13, p. 11).   Goldsmith notes that there have been no identifiable cases from lead as a community air pollutant (Ref. 5-9, vol. 1, p. 600).   Among the 2,300 individuals on whom lead determinations from blood samples were made during the urban air studies, only 11 were found with blood lead level equal to, or in excess of, 60 micrograms of lead per 100 grams of blood. These 11 were in occupations, among them 4 garage mechanics and 4 aircraft workers, in which there are opportunities for occupational exposure.   From 60 to 80 milligrams of lead per 100 grams of blood is generally viewed as an analytical sign of an undesirably high lead intake.   Evidence at hand does not indicate that the lead concentrations in our community air supply are risks to otherwise healthy people.

In six United States cities with stations of the Continuous Air Monitoring Program the observed concentrations of nitrogen dioxide were rarely above 0.2 ppm (about 350 μg/m^3), which is too low to produce irritation directly from nitrogen dioxide.   Even a recorded high of about 3 ppm (5 mg/m^3) in Los Angeles is below the concentration that causes nasal and eye irritation.   The importance of nitrogen dioxide and the other oxides of nitrogen is their role in photochemical smog rather than their possible direct irritant action in the respiratory system.

Beryllium and its inorganic compounds, particularly the oxides, pose two community air-contamination exposures.   The first is among people living within a mile or less of beryllium production plants.   In 1949 Eisenbud and associates reported on

Table 5-17   EFFECTS ASSOCIATED WITH CERTAIN OXIDANT CONCENTRATIONS IN PHOTOCHEMICAL SMOG

Concentrations of oxidant			
μg/m^3	ppm	Measured as	Effect anticipated
Exceeding 200	0.1	Peak values	Eye irritation, demonstrated by panel response
490	0.25	Max. daily value	Aggravation of respiratory diseases, asthma; such a peak expected with maximum hourly averages as low as 300 μg/m^3, or 0.15 ppm
Exceeding 130	0.07	1 hour	Impaired performance of student cross-country runners exposed for 1 hour before racing

SOURCE: Data from Air Quality Criteria for Photochemical Oxidants, *U.S. Public Health Serv. Publ. AP*-63, 1970.

cases of a chronic pulmonary disease with a fatality rate of over 35 percent among people living near an AEC contract plant producing beryllium.[1]   Fortunately, the case prevalence rate is low, 27 per 100,000 population.   The AEC set a community air standard of 0.01 $\mu g/m^3$, a very low level indeed.   Occupational cases were observed at about the same time involving low concentrations of finely divided beryllium oxide dust and possibly elemental beryllium.   The AEC adopted an occupational exposure limit for beryllium of 2 $\mu g/m^3$.   This remains the occupational TLV, expressed as 0.002 mg/m^3.   It is the lowest numerical value among some 400 listed substances. The second exposure is from test firing beryllium-fueled rocket engines.   The principal combustion product is beryllium oxide, but because of the high temperatures it is a "high-fired" form.   This form, which makes up 99 percent or more of the exhaust discharge materials, has been found to be toxicologically inert.

For at least 40 years the inhalation of asbestos fibers and dust in occupational uses has been recognized as dangerous.   Asbestos depositions produce a distinctive pneumoconiosis called *asbestosis*.   It is disabling, but among asbestos workers it has been observed that asbestosis "will not kill him because the lung cancer will get him first."   A rise in lung cancer among asbestos workers in various parts of the world and the increased observation of tumors in the lining of the pleural cavity and the abdominal cavity have renewed concern for exposure to asbestos particles.   The tumors are called *mesotheliomas* as they appear in the squamous cell layer, the mesothelium, of the lining, or epithelium.   These tumors are associated with asbestos inhalation.   From the early tumor observations in 1959 to 1965 it became evident that such tumors were not restricted to asbestos workers.   Asbestos bodies are found within the tumors.   These findings have raised the question of whether asbestos fibers in the community air are producing such mesotheliomas.   With a number of issues on occupational exposure to asbestos still uncertain, it is understandable that general population exposure to asbestos materials in the community air supply and damage from such exposure is far from a closed case.

The evidence cited in this section on health effects is not overwhelming.   Neither is it satisfying as a classical epidemiological cause-effect case.   Nor is it a decisive association.   There are too many variations in sources, in transport interactions, and in receptors.   Our measure of effect is that of sensed or observed damage.   The occurrence of acute episodes is generally convincing, although some of the New York City reported excesses of deaths during moderately heavy pollution have been suspected to be within long unexplained cycles of death rates.   Reviews of the totality of evidence on the health effects have a convincing impact, particularly when written from the human interest angle.[2]

[1] *J. Ind. Hyg. Toxicol.*, **31**:282 (1949).
[2] Edith Iglauer, The Ambient Air, *The New Yorker*, Apr. 13, 1968.

Effects on domestic animals and vegetation   At first blush it might be expected that there would be a plethora of evidence of air pollutant injury to domestic animals. The specific and scanty evidence is a reminder that animals depend on man to observe their condition.   Distressed animals do not call the health department, the veternarian, the complaint officer at air pollution control, or the ombudsman.   The evidence is from acute episodes, from notorious poisons ingested after settling on grazing lands, and from some isolated observations of known toxicants.   Table 5-18 summarizes the fate of animals during four acute air pollution episodes.   There are three notorious poisons that have affected cattle, sheep, and horses in particular areas for extended periods.   These are arsenic, lead, and fluoride compounds.   The instances of arsenic and lead injury have been among cattle, horses, and sheep grazing or on feed forage from land near large metal processing plants.   The relatively few occurrences are detailed in Ref. 5-14.

In comparison, exposure of domestic animals to fluoride is widespread.   Fluoride is a cumulative toxicant through ingestion, which reaches domestic animals over a few to several years of grazing in fallout areas.   Acute poisoning in domesticated mammals by ingestion or inhalation under field conditions has not been recognized, except by mishandling of organic fluoride rodenticides.   The grazing areas or feed-crop fields are contaminated by fluoride fallout from phosphate rock mills and fertilizer plants, from metallurgical processing of aluminum, iron, and steel, and oc-

Table 5-18   THE FATE OF ANIMALS DURING ACUTE AIR POLLUTION EVENTS

Event		Toxic agent	Animals, effects, and numbers
Meuse Valley, Belgium	1930	Sulfur dioxide and sulfuric acid mists strongly suspected	Cattle, many sickened, many slaughtered; those evacuated to high ground above the fog recovered.
Donora, Pa.	1948	Sulfur dioxide, smoke, and zinc compound particulates	Canaries, 20% affected; dogs, 15% affected; cattle, sheep, horses, and swine, not significantly affected.
Poza Rica, Mexico	1950	Hydrogen sulfide release for 25 min	Canaries, all died; chickens, cattle, pigs, geese, ducks, and dogs, unknown number died or ill.
London, England	1952	Sulfur dioxide, smoke, likely sulfuric acid mists	Of 351 cattle at Smithfield Cattle Show in London, 52 seriously ill, 5 died, 9 slaughtered; sheep and swine housed one floor above ground not affected; primates at London Zoo, increased bronchitis and pneumonia.

casionally from brick kilns.   The four major fluorosis areas in the United States are in Florida, Tennessee, Utah, and along the Washington-Oregon border.   Of domestic farm animals, cattle are the most susceptible and tolerate less fluorides in the feed than sheep and swine.   Horses are quite tolerant of high intakes.   Poultry are the least affected of domestic farm animals.   Tolerance levels in feeds in parts per million by weight for farm animals are for cattle, 30 to 50; sheep and swine, 70 to 100; broilers 150 to 300; hens, 300 to 400.   The behavior and distribution of several fluoride compounds in animals is well defined.   The soluble compounds are more readily absorbed.   To a limit, absorbed fluoride is eliminated by the kidneys.   Beyond the limit there is kidney damage.   A portion of absorbed fluoride is fixed in bone as apatite crystals.   Abnormal calcification results.   Animal teeth show fluorosis. Dairy cattle produce less milk.   There is weight loss, lameness, stiff posture, and rough coats.   In extreme cases there is gross thickening and shortening of leg bones.

The photographs compiled by Jacobson and Hill (Ref. 5-15) far surpass any words that can be said or written on air pollution injury to vegetation.   It is a pictorial atlas of brilliant color photographs for identifying and recognizing the damage patterns to particular species by particular pollutants.   The most obvious damage to vegetation is to the leaves, blades, or needles, the energy factories of plants.   The damage is described as chlorosis, in which the chlorophyll is bleached out in spots; as tip or edge burn, in which the extremities are burned to a yellow or brown; as flecking, in which the chlorophyll is removed in small spots or flecks on much of the exposed leaf area; or as necrosis, in which major and usually progressive cell damage results in distortion, curling, drying, and decay.   Few plant species are spared damage on exposure to one or more of the principal injurious air pollutants—the fluorides, sulfur dioxide, and the photochemical oxidants, which include ozone, peroxyacyl nitrate, and the nitrogen oxides.   There are variations in sensitivity among plant species to given pollutants.   While leaves with more exposed area are more evidently the place of damage, flowers and fruit also show injury.   Such injury is a greater economic loss in commercial flower gardens and orchards than superficial leaf markings.

Fluoride damage to vegetation was recognized in the nineteenth century but did not become widespread until the 1940s.   As in animal poisoning, fluoride injury to plants depends on accumulation in the tissue.   In plants it is in the leaf structure. Concentrations of 50 to 200 ppm by weight is the range of necrosis in sensitive plants such as gladiolas, tulips, and peach, apricot, and pine trees.   Resistant species such as asparagus, cotton, pear, strawberry, and tomato can accumulate as much as 500 ppm without injury appearing.   The gaseous forms of fluoride, hydrogen fluoride and silicon tetrafluoride, are mainly responsible for plant damage, as these are readily absorbed.   Insoluble particulate fluorides are washed off by rain.   Soluble forms are partly absorbed, depending on leaf surface moisture.   The cumulative mode of action means that relatively low air pollutant concentrations can be injurious in the lifetime of a plant (Ref. 5-15, sec. D).

In contrast, sulfur dioxide is a direct fumigant. It enters the leaf stomata as a gas. The leaf cells have a limited capacity to detoxify the sulfite that is formed by converting it to sulfate. Beyond that the cell is disrupted and chlorophyll is destroyed. Photosynthesis cannot be sustained. Sulfur dioxide damage occurs near the pollutant source. The major offenders have been large copper smelters. The one at Trail, British Columbia, Canada, gained international notoriety in the 1930s, as its sulfur dioxide discharges crossed the border into the United States and destroyed conifer forests. Fossil-fueled power plants burning sulfur-bearing coal or oil have emitted enough sulfur dioxide to fumigate the immediate surroundings. Time of exposure-concentration formulas have been worked out to predict sulfur dioxide injury, in the course of an enormous amount of work on this exposure. Similarly there are formulas for percentage of leaf damage before crop yields are diminished for small grains and alfalfa. Alfalfa is one of the most sensitive plants. It shows chlorophyll loss on exposure to sulfur dioxide of 0.5 ppm in the air (1.3 mg/m^3). Among trees, the conifers and eastern hardwoods are quite sensitive, along with pear and apple trees. Pumpkin and squash are the most sensitive of all plants and are used as markers of early signs of sulfur dioxide fumigation. Most of our table vegetables are relatively sensitive, including broccoli, carrots, lettuce, radishes, spinach, and sweet potatoes (Ref. 5-15, sec. C, and 5-9, vol. 1 pp. 408–409, 414–415).

The photochemical oxidants that include ozone and PAN (peroxyacylnitrate) are accompanied by nitrogen oxides. This complex group was recognized as damaging vegetation in the Los Angeles basin in 1944. Ozone was identified as a component in 1959, and PAN in 1961. Although these pollutants came on the scene late, the group causes more injury to plants than the fluorides and sulfur dioxides. Their action is no longer solely a Los Angeles phenomenom. Injurious concentrations are observed more than 70 miles from the urban centers. Ozone stipples grape leaves, flecks tobacco and spinach, and burns the tips of eastern white and ponderosa pines. Grain crops that are injured are barley, oats, corn, rye, and wheat. Chrysanthemum, carnation, lilac, and petunia are among the sensitive flowering plants injured by ozone. Geranium and gladiolus are comparatively resistant. PAN damages pinto beans, dahlias, lettuce, oats, and tomatoes readily at concentrations in the field as low as 0.01 to 0.05 ppm. A number of plants noted as sensitive to other pollutants are relatively resistant to PAN. These include broccoli, chrysanthemums, corn, cotton, and radishes. Total oxidant concentrations of 0.02 to 0.04 ppm injure sensitive species after 4 to 6 hours of contact. The role of the nitric oxides in plant damage is less certain. Nitrogen dioxide requires 2 to 10 ppm for several hours to cause acute effects. There may be a slowing of growth on exposure to nitrogen dioxide concentrations of about 0.5 ppm for 2 to 3 weeks. Yields have been reduced as much as 25 percent. (Ref. 5-15, secs. B and E, and 5-9, vol. 1, pp. 409–411, 415–417.)

Efforts to use plant damage as biological monitors of air pollutant distribution

have met with some success.   As it is cumulative in action, fluorides have been monitored by such sensitive plants as gladiolus and ponderosa pine seedlings.   Annual
bluegrass has been used in the Los Angeles basin to monitor photochemical oxidants.
Since the 1960s, as the Tennessee Valley Authority brought coal-burning generating
stations on the line, using high-sulfur-bearing fuel, areas in the stack-plume patterns
have been systematically monitored for vegetation change and damage.   Botanical
monitoring, including test plots, is a defense action used by potential polluters to have
evidence at hand to meet claims for air-pollutant damage.

Effects on urban weather and visibility   Table 5-14 indicates that urban areas have
less sunshine, less ultraviolet radiation, and more cloudiness and fog than rural areas.
Other differences are more rain and more frequent reductions in visibility.   Reduction
in visibility is due to light scattering.   Small particle sizes in the range of 0.2 to 2 μm
produce the strongest scattering.   The relations are those of particle diameter to
wavelength of light and the refractive index of the material.   For a unit mass, smaller
particles have a greater scattering effectiveness.   Water mists 0.8 μm in diameter have
a scattering effectiveness four times those of 2-μm diameter.   Substances which cause
visibility reductions are hygroscopic compounds such as ether-soluble organics and
sulfur trioxide combining with water vapor to form mists; opaque particulates of
carbon, tars, and metals; transparent crystals of iron, aluminum, silicon, and calcium
present in salt forms with sulfates, chlorides, nitrates, and fluorides; and the by-products
of photochemical interactions of the alkanes, and the oxides of nitrogen.   Nitrogen
dioxide has a further interesting property of absorbing visible light in the blue-green
end of the spectrum.   This results in giving the sky horizon viewed through nitrogen
dioxide pollution an unappealing yellow-brown color.

Relative humidity has a marked influence on the hygroscopic materials producing visibility reduction.   Figure 5-9 dramatically shows the effect of relative humidity on visibility at the Los Angeles International Airport.   In relating concentrations
of pollutants to visibility reduction, it is necessary to specify relative humidities.
Reduced visibility interferes with traffic movement in and out of airports, on highways, and in harbors, and increases the collision hazards of these facilities.   The
Airline Pilots Association has been an active supporter of air pollution control despite
the fact that jet planes add to pollution by engine smoke trails, certain fuel drainage
dumping, and vapor trails.   Early morning ground fogs along expressways have repeatedly been the scene of multivehicle, front-end to rear-end collision chains started
by tailgate drivers.   The approaches to New York City through the petrochemical
centers of Linden and Bayonne, New Jersey, are notorious for such events.

Reductions in solar radiation at the ground level of our cities deprive us of the
stimulus of bright sunlight, of a desirable level of ultraviolet radiation, of natural illumination, and possibly of air temperature changes sufficient to affect local convection

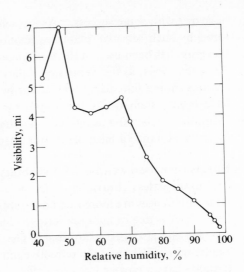

FIGURE 5-9
The loss of visibility with relative humidity increases at the Los Angeles International Airport. [*Source*: *M. Neiburger and M. G. Wurtele, Chem. Rev.*, **44**:321 1949. *The William and Wilkins Co., Baltimore, Md.*]

currents and outdoor comfort. Polluted urban air has been observed to reduce visible light by one-half and ultraviolet by two-thirds compared with clean air in the surrounding countryside. Measurements of losses of solar radiation at Pasadena, California, showed large drops as the heavy midday Los Angeles smog formed. The largest reductions are in the short wavelengths, including ultraviolet, by as much as 90 percent. Particulate concentrations of 100 to 150 $\mu g/m^3$ in persistent smoke cause reductions in direct sunlight at ground level of one-third in the summer and of two-thirds in the winter. The greater frequency and longer duration of fogs in cities than of fogs in rural environs is explained by the condensation nucleii accompanying air pollution. Condensation nucleii are particles smaller than 0.2 nm in diameter, termed *Aitken nucleii*. Formation begins at concentrations of 1,000 Aitken particles per milliliter, a quite clean air. Fog density increases rapidly with increased concentrations to 70,000 Aitken particles per milliliter, a moderately polluted air found even over small towns. Further increases of Aitken particle concentrations do not appear to increase fog density.

Effects on materials and property Table 5-19 shows the diversity of materials affected by air pollutants, from metals to paper. To these must be added the filth from the air that lands on our hair, neck, cars, draperies, windows, floors, streets, and building surfaces. All that mess adds up to a sizable cleaning task and bill. Note that sulfur dioxide and the acid gases are the principal offenders for six of the eight materials listed in Table 5-19. For many of these attacks, the chemical reactions are known. Carbonic acid, formed from carbon dioxide and water vapor, acts on limestone and marble to produce soluble calcium bicarbonate.   Sulfur dioxide acts on the same building stones and produces calcium sulfate.   Hydrogen sulfide produces the classical darkening of lead paints by forming lead sulfide from lead oxides.

These reactions and others involved in the damages enumerated in Table 5-19 are influenced by moisture, temperature, sunlight, and air movement.   Some damage is done by direct abrasion of particulates driven by the wind, blasting away at exposed surfaces.   Some actions are a bit indirect, as the absorbed sulfur dioxide in leather being converted to sulfuric acid with time, moisture, and oxygen to speed deterioration.

Ozone is a strong oxidizing agent and a very reactive substance.   It causes the cracking of rubber under tension at air concentrations of 20 to 40 $\mu g/m^3$ (0.01 to 0.02 ppm).   Ozone weakens fabric fibers in the following order of susceptibility: polyesters, nylon, acetate, and cotton.   Ozone and nitrogen oxides act on dyes, among which certain blue and green shades were easily faded by nitrogen dioxide.   The chemical industry has met rubber cracking by adding p-phenylenediamine derivatives at a cost of about 50 cents per tire.   Dyes have been modified or used selectively on fabrics to eliminate fading due to ozone and nitrogen dioxide at added cost to the consumer.   Nitrogen oxides damage nylon and cause yellowing of Spandex, a synthetic elastomeric fiber.   Particulate nitrates attack nickel-brass alloys and so cause troubles in telephone and computer systems.   Some pollutants for which quantitative data have been assembled are:

1   Particulates in the range of annual geometric means of 60 to 180 $\mu g/m^3$ in the presence of sulfur dioxide and moisture accelerate the corrosion of steel and zinc panels.

Table 5-19   EFFECTS OF AIR POLLUTANTS ON MATERIALS

Materials	Typical manifestation	Principal air pollutant
Metals	Spoilage of surface, loss of metal, tarnishing	SO_2, acid gases
Building materials	Discoloration, leaching	SO_2, acid gases, sticky particulates
Paint	Discoloration, softened finish	SO_2, H_2S, sticky particulates
Leather	Powdered surface, weakening	SO_2, acid gases
Paper	Embrittlement	SO_2, acid gases
Textiles	Reduced tensile strength, spotting	SO_2, acid gases
Dyes	Fading	NO_2, oxidants, SO_2
Rubber	Cracking, weakening	O_3, oxidants
Ceramics	Changed surface appearance	Acid gases

SOURCE: Modified from Ref. 5-9, vol. 1, p. 624.

2   Sulfur dioxide at 345 $\mu g/m^3$ (0.22 ppm) with high particulate levels increase the corrosion of steel panels by 50 percent.

3   In cities with annual average concentrations of nitrate particulates of about $3\mu g/m^3$, palladium-nickel electrical contacts suffer "creeping green." Green-corrosion products on the palladium keep the switches electrically open. The problem has appeared in telephone systems in Cincinnati, Cleveland, Detroit, Los Angeles, New York, and Philadelphia.

The economic costs of polluted air continue to defy accurate estimating. Fragments have been subject to study. Examples are:

1   Steubenville, Ohio, heavily polluted, and Uniontown, Pennsylvania, quite clean in the upper end of the Ohio River Valley, were paired for cleaning costs. The items included inside and outside house maintenance, laundry, dry cleaning, and hair and face care. Steubenville's annual per capita cost came out $84 more than Uniontown's.[1]

2   A St. Louis metal fabrication plant started processes emitting odoriferous and irritating gases in 1962 in a residential neighborhood. The nuisance continued unabated for the next 4 years. During that time, sellers suffered a $1,000 loss on their homes compared with a control area (Ref. 5-9, vol. 1, pp. 648–649).

3   The Committee on Air Pollution Report for the United Kingdom (H.M. Stationery Office, London, 1954) estimated direct costs of air pollution as £152.5 million. To this the committee added another £100 million for indirect costs resulting from losses in efficiency. No estimate was made for health impairment.

4   Estimates for the cost to the United States for dirty air have ranged from $2 to $16 billion per year. That is from $10 to $80 a person per year. A staff report for the Committee on Public Works of the United States Senate on air pollution in 1963 settled for an annual property damage estimate of $11 billion per year, based on $65 per capita.

5   The Pittsburgh, Pennsylvania, campaign to control smoke began intensively in the 1950s. The improvement has been estimated to save the community $27 million per year. A like effort in the 1960s in St. Louis was reported to save the hotels, alone, $154,000 per year in cleaning and redecorating costs.

The Measurement of Air Pollutants

The techniques of sampling and measuring the toxicants encountered in the occupational setting are applicable to a large extent in evaluating the quality of our community air supply. When our concern for air pollutants reached beyond smoke and settling

[1] I. Michaelson and B. Tourin, *Public Health Reps.* (*U.S.*) 81 and 505, June 1966.

particulates, the instrumentation of industrial hygiene provided the starting point.   It proved insufficient in meeting at least three needs.   As air pollutants are usually present in lower concentrations than the specific contaminants measured in occupational disease exposures, instruments with a greater sensitivity are needed.   As air pollutant concentrations have large variations in daily cycles and longer ones, instruments with recording responses or timed tape sampling are required.   While industrial-hygiene air sampling is most frequently directed to a single known or suspected contaminant, air pollutant sampling is often directed to multiple contaminant and pollutant components.   The air pollutant mixture presents issues of interferences among the constituents during sampling or during analysis.

The scientists and engineers who have become engaged in maintaining the quality of our community air have responded by developing continuous or intermittent sampling instruments with automated analytical systems and recording and readout devices.   For monitoring process sources, alarms and cutoffs can be provided.   Computer sort-out data make it possible to analyze and interpret a vast array of data into short peaks of 5 min or less, into daily highs and lows, monthly averages, and annual geometric means.   The development of such instruments has met the needs of communitywide air-quality surveillance networks by fixed and mobile stations.   For the most part air pollution control prior to the 1950s was "smoke chasing" and dust-fall detection.   The Ringelmann chart which had been introduced to the United States in 1897 was the device for spotting excessive smoke discharges from chimneys.   It still is a utilitarian method for rating smoke-plume opacity in a graded series from 0, all white, to 5, all black.   The numbers are in steps of 20 percent opacity.   A Ringelmann 2, frequently the greatest smoke-emission opacity permitted for periods of more than 5 min, is a 40 percent blackness.   Optical viewers for smoke plumes with comparison split images for direct transmittance are also used.   These are identified as Telesmoke, Umbrascope, and Smokescope.   The Ringelmann chart, despite difficulties with lighting conditions and nonblack smokes, has the advantage of having been accepted in the courts as evidence.   Ringelmann reading requires practice and skill.   Smoke generators producing variable plume opacities are necessary and useful training devices for preparing field personnel.

Settleable particulates in sizes above 10 μm can be estimated by using dust-fall jars.   These are widemouthed cylindrical vessels about 15 cm (6 in) in diameter, made of glass or polyethylene.   The collection of several days or more at various points in a city provides information for estimating the weight of particulates deposited in milligrams per square centimeter or tons per square mile, usually expressed per month.   Bird droppings, algal growths, freezing, and target-practicing marksmen are among the difficulties dust-fall jar users must face.

The tape sampler of the American Iron and Steel Institute (AISI) is an instrument for measuring and recording smoke and particulates.   Air is continuously pumped through a filter-paper strip collecting the suspended matter on a circular patch of the tape, usually of 1-in diameter.   At a preset time, from 10 min to $3\frac{1}{2}$ hours, the tape advances to expose a fresh clean patch to the sampling head.   The exposed patch is read by transmitted light to give an optical density reading.   This reading is frequently interpreted in "COHs per 1,000 lineal feet."   COH is an acronym for "coefficient of haze."   The 1,000 lineal ft is the base unit used to express the length of airstream drawn through the exposed patch.   The thousands of lineal feet passing can be calculated from the air quantity as a volumetric rate.   The patch area and flow rate must be known.   The usual sampling rate is 0.25 cfm (about 0.12 l/s).   One COH unit equals the quantity of light-scattering solids that produces an optical density of 0.01. The AISI tape sampler can be fitted with an automatic, simultaneous, optical readout and tape recorder.

A variant of the AISI sampler is built for hydrogen sulfide monitoring.   The tape is a paper impregnated with lead acetate, and the air is prefiltered to remove particulates.   The lead acetate darkens as the sulfide combines with the lead to form black lead sulfide.   At 0.25 cfm through a 1-hour sampling time, impregnated paper has a sensitivity of from 0.001 ppm (1.5 $\mu g/m^3$) to 0.04 ppm (60 $\mu g/m^3$) (Ref. 5-4, pp. B10-29–B10-40).   Some additional simple techniques for detection and approximation are the use of lead peroxide candles for sulfur dioxide; rubber strip cracking for ozone; lead acetate paper strips, without an AISI sampler, for hydrogen sulfides; plastic bags for large-volume grab samples; and the aerophyte, Spanish moss, for fluoride detection (Ref. 5-9, vol. 2, pp. 44–49).   These simpler means of sampling are emphasized as a starting point for community air monitoring in areas where elaborate instrumentation is not available and perhaps not even desirable or necessary.

The Control of Air Pollutants

A technology for the control of air pollutants can be outlined readily.   As in other facets of environmental management and protection, the deficiency is not a control technique.   The shortcoming is that of readiness to commit public and private capital for control.   This failure of readiness finally rests on a lack of conviction that the threats outweigh the benefits of the control effort.   In the national air pollution control program in the United States, four steps have been followed.

1 Data collection and analysis by the national air sampling network and the Continuous Air Monitoring Program have sketched the magnitude of air pollution.

2 Air quality criteria are defined to answer the question, How clean should our air be?   Several examples of information used to define air quality criteria have been cited in the section on effects.   Reference 5-12 gives the series, which covered particulates, sulfur oxides, carbon monoxide, photochemical oxidants, hydrocarbons, and oxides of nitrogen by 1971. The Air Quality Criteria series documents the quantities of contaminants and pollutants which we can breathe and which we can have in the air envelope that surrounds animal and plant life, our land, buildings, structures, and material goods without undue bad effects.

3   Air quality criteria are then translated into a set of air quality standards. These define permissible concentrations in the ambient air. To attain a desired ambient air quality, discharges from particular sources must be limited. The limitations on the quantities of pollutants that are discharged from a particular source are emission standards. This, in fact, is allocating our air envelope—with some imperfectly defined assimilative capacity for particular pollutants—to particular users of our air as a dump for their waste products.

4   Implementation of controls to bring particular emissions to levels prescribed by the emission standards is a continuing, complex step. It has been possible to apply certain emission limits on new motor vehicles at the point of manufacture. The manufacturer provides emission controls for all vehicles intended for sale in the United States without exception for locale of usual actual use. Very large stationary sources such as electricity generating stations, solid-waste incinerators, and metallurgical plants have characteristics of uniformity which makes nationwide control appear feasible. Beyond these are millions of sources of varied characteristics of size, processes used, cycles of operation, economic viability, and managerial skill. The Los Angeles control effort provides some pattern for approaches to varied sources.

Table 5-20 presents five alternatives for managing air pollutants. These are not mutually exclusive. In any practical effort all must be used. The first, using the dilution capacity of the local air envelope in accord with natural meteorological constraints, fits the concept of air quality standards. Public understanding that the dilution capacity is finite is necessary for preventive control measures. It provides a base for accepting a plan for the use of the local air resource for the dispersal of wastes to be airborne. Adherence to a plan requires restrictions on the freedom of use of property and likely the sacrifice of a short-term profit. The last example for control action *1* is not a restriction on land use, but on the use of the personal automobile. Such a restriction requires the availability of good public transportation to make the denial of personal driving convenience an acceptable sacrifice for reducing the downtown pollution loads. The relief of the concommitant burdens of traffic congestion, parking shortages, and increasing costs of personal driving make the choice more palatable.

The remaining four alternatives listed in Table 5-20 are directed at the point of generation of the pollutant. The second is elimination of the pollutant by substitution of materials or methods that do not produce the obnoxious pollutants. The third and fourth are the modification of combustion equipment and improvement in pollutant-emitting processes in use to reduce the quantities of pollutants emitted. The fifth is the capture and cleaning of the air or gas-stream carrying the pollutant. A general measure of air pollution control in manufacturing plants and materials handling depots is equipment maintenance, housekeeping, and cleanliness of all facilities and premises. Ducts, piping, valves, pumps, seals, and gaskets must be kept tight. Floors, decks, storage bins and silos, loading areas, and transfer conveyors and chutes must be kept clean. In like manner, pollution controls on motor vehicles must be maintained if any benefit is to come from the engineering effort and added cost.

Table 5-20 A RATIONALE AND ALTERNATIVES FOR MANAGING AIR POLLUTANTS

Control action	Required information	Examples of use
1 Define the assimilative capacity of the local air envelope to accept pollutants without impairing air quality	Extensive meterological data, detailed emissions inventories, knowledge of behavior of pollutants and of interactions in the air	Land use restrictions, control of industry location, control of transportation methods and their use
2 Prevent pollutants from forming at potential sources	Materials and their use, particularly fuels, raw process ingredients; disposal of waste products	Limits on sulfur content of oil and coal, modification of gasoline composition, prohibition of open burning, control of incineration, substitution of propane for gasoline
3 Reduce the quantity and types of pollutants formed in combustion in furnaces and engines	Optimum air-fuel ratios; combustion characteristics of furnaces, flues, and engines; maintenance effects; use-cycle effects	Improved firing of furnaces, reconstruction of flues and stacks, crankcase and exhaust emission controls on motor vehicles
4 Prevent or reduce the formation and emission of pollutants by changes in process or equipment	Recognition of the source, availability of an acceptable alternative	Vapor recovery systems in petrochemical processes; use of fully enclosed systems in such processes; use of floating covers on volatile-fluid storage tanks; replacement of cupolas with electric furnaces and reverberatory ovens in metallurgical operations; use of electric and steam power instead of gasoline engines, and of diesel locomotives instead of steam locomotives
5 Capture and remove pollutants at the point of generation	Identification of pollutant; design, construction, maintenance, and use of efficient air cleaning equipment	Removal of pollutant from the contained airstream by burning, masking, or collection

Cleaning Particulates from Dirty Air

The techniques of industrial ventilation hood and duct design described earlier in this chapter apply to the capture of any pollutant. Capturing and confining pollutants at the point of generation keeps the volume of air that must be moved and cleaned small, and prevents dispersion. The collected dirty airstream is then carried to an air cleaner. Table 5-21 lists several types of cleaners used to remove particulates. Particulate cleaners operate on one of four principles.

1 Mechanical removal is effected by reducing velocity to allow settling or by changing airstream direction. Five such devices are listed in Table 5-21, and four are shown in Fig. 5-10.
2 Water is added to improve collection by mechanical action or is used alone as in gravity countercurrent collectors. Examples are listed in Table 5-21, and shown in Fig. 5-11.
3 Filtration is provided by fabrics or fibrous mats. As in the case of a water filtration bed, an air filter acts by more than simple sieving. There are forces of inertial impaction, diffusion, and electrostatic attraction at work. A wide variety of fabrics fitted to temperature of the airstream and resistant to chemical action of the pollutants are in use. A frequent configuration for mounting fabric filters is the *baghouse* shown in Fig. 5-12. Fibrous mat filters are selected in accord with the particulate sizes that must be removed, ranging from coarse, as in a home air circulation system, to ultrafilters, as needed in "clean rooms."

Table 5-21   AIR CLEANERS FOR PARTICULATES

Operating principle	Types	Examples	Removal efficiencies, %
Mechanical collection operating dry	Settling chambers	Simple chamber	40–60
	Centrifugal separators	Cyclones	20–80
		Dynamic precipitators	60–90
	Inertial separators	Baffled chambers	50–70
		Impingement chambers	60–80
Wet collection, mechanical action and and wetting combined	Spray towers	Gravity countercurrent	
	Wet impingement	Wet dynamic separators	20–99
		Venturi scrubbers	30–99
Filtration	Fabric filters	Baghouses	90–99
	Fibrous mats	Coarse filters	65–80
		Ultrafilters	99+
Electrostatic precipitation	Electrostatic precipitators	Wire in tube	80–99+
		Wire in plate	80–99+

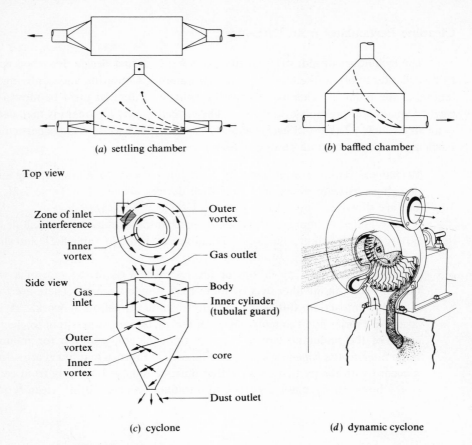

(a) settling chamber   (b) baffled chamber

FIGURE 5-10
Mechanical, dry, air cleaners: settling and baffled chambers, cyclone, and dynamic cyclone. [*Sources*: For chambers, *RATSEC Manual*, *PA-C-pm* 58-5-60; for cyclone, *Air Pollution Engineering Manual*, *U.S. Public Health Serv. Publ.* 999-*AP*-40; *for dynamic cyclone, American Air Filter, Inc., Louisville. Ky.*]

4 Electrostatic precipitation is the deposition of particulates on a grounded collecting surface by imposing a high voltage from a negative wire electrode across the charging field through which the airstream passes (see Fig. 5-13). The first successful commercial use of electrostatic precipitation was developed by F. G. Cottrell in 1907 for application at a Dupont sulfuric acid plant near Berkeley, California.[1]

[1] Smoke Problems in California, *Trans. Commonwealth Club, Calif.*, **8**(9):489 (September 1913).

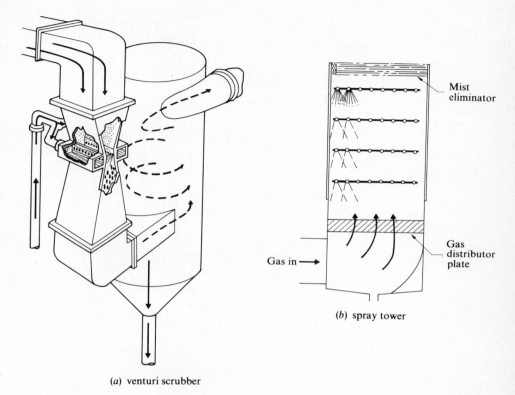

(a) venturi scrubber

(b) spray tower

FIGURE 5-11
Wet type of air cleaners for particulate removal: Venturi scrubber, spray tower.
[*Source*: *Control Techniques for Particulate Air Pollutants, U.S. Public Health Serv., Publ. AP*-51, *pp.* 59 *and* 55, 1969.]

  The ranges of percentage of removals by particulate air cleaners given in Table 5-21 are broad and approximate. The high-side percentages for mechanical collectors hold for large particulates over 20 to 40 μm in diameter. Wet collectors achieve a better removal than dry collectors on particles below 5 μm. Venturi scrubbers and wet dynamic separators provide as much as an 80 percent removal of particles of about 1 μm. Fabric and fibrous mat filters and electrostatic precipitators can be designed to remove over 99 percent of particles at 1 μm and as much as 80 percent of those of $\frac{1}{10}$ μm. Figure 5-14 shows the collection efficiency versus particle size for five types of air cleaners.

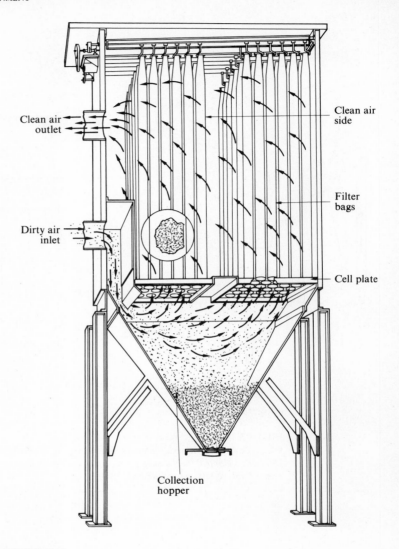

FIGURE 5-12
Fabric filter baghouse for dry particulates. [*Source: Control Techniques for Participate Air Pollutants, U.S. Public Health Serv., Publ. AP*-51, *p*. 103, 1969.]

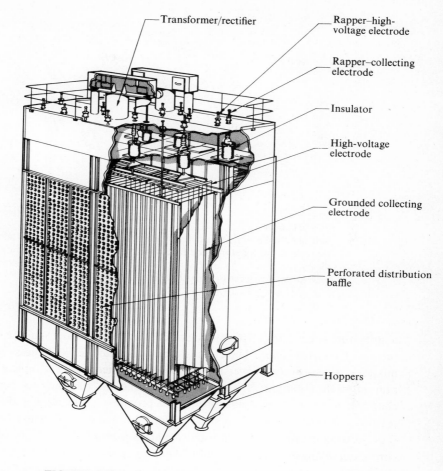

FIGURE 5-13
Electrostatic precipitator for dry particulates and mists. [*Source: Universal Oil Products, Air Correction Division, Darien, Conn.*]

Cleaning Gases and Vapors from Dirty Air

The four means of removing gases and vapors from air are listed in Table 5-22.   Types of units applying the four methods—absorption, combustion, adsorption, and condensation—are listed in the table and illustrated in Fig. 5-15.   Examples of application suggest limitations on the choices for dealing with specific pollutants.   Further comment on each method follows:

1 Combustion in an afterburner device is complete if the necessary combustion

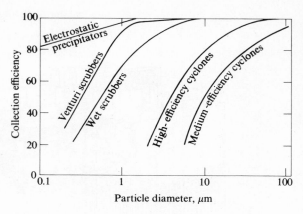

FIGURE 5-14
Particulate collection efficiencies by particle size for five types of air cleaners: electrostatic precipitator, Venturi scrubber, wet scrubber, and high- and medium-efficiency cyclones. [*Source*: *A. T. Rosano* (*ed.*), "*Air Pollution Control*," *p.* 143, *Environmental Science Service Division, E.R.A., Inc., New York, 1969.*]

temperature is reached.   This requires a correct fuel-air ratio, ignition temperature, and contact time.   Direct fired units can handle very messy pollutant mixtures.   Temperatures over 1200°F (650°C) are needed for complete combustion of such pollutants.   Therefore, supplemental fuel and a combustion chamber that allows good mixing must be provided.   In catalytic afterburners temperatures below 1200°F (650°C) achieve complete combustion because of the oxidizing catalyst.   This is usually platinum in alloys.   Oxides of copper, chromium, manganese, cobalt, and nickel also catalyze the oxidation of organic gases and vapors.   The catalyst is a porous, adsorptive surface on a supporting bed material.   The presence of particulates in the pollutant stream may damage the catalyst or bed.   Solid oxides and vapors of mercury, lead, arsenic, and zinc poison most catalysts.   Catalytic oxidation cannot be used if such materials are in the dirty air stream.   With correct location and sizing of inlets, combustible pollutants can be fed directly into furnace fireboxes.   The temperature, retention time, and turbulence in the firebox must be fitted to the burning characteristics of the pollutant.

2 Absorption of a gas is by solution into a solvent.   The examples given in Table 5-22 are all gases, some very soluble in water, as ammonia and hydrogen chloride, and others moderately soluble.   In air pollutant absorption, the usual solvent is water.   It may contain a neutralizer or reactant to change the chemical form of the pollutant both to increase absorption and to recover components.   An

example is the absorption of hydrogen sulfide in a sodium hydroxide solution to form sodium sulfide. Countercurrent flow towers packed with inert material to provide a large thin film surface of solvent are frequently used for absorption. The packing materials are in shapes to provide large surfaces and voids. Towers with horizontal, perforated plates and trays to retain the absorbent in combination with the rising gas stream or simple spray towers are used. Particulates which can clog the absorbent support beds must be removed before the air-gas stream enters the tower.

3 Adsorption is the phenomenon of contact and adherence of the molecules of materials in a fluid state to the surface of a solid. In air pollution control,

Table 5-22 AIR CLEANERS FOR GASES AND VAPORS

Operating principle	Types	Example of application
Combustion in afterburners	Direct fired units	Mixed dirty aerosols, gases, vapors; may contain some particulates and odors; emissions from smokehouses, rendering cookers, varnish cookers, paint-baking and foundry core ovens, coffee roasters, and flue-fed incinerators
	Catalytic combustion units	Solvent and organic vapors from industrial ovens such as fabric coating and backing, metal decorating and coating, binder baking, and wax burnout
	Feed to existing boiler furnaces	Visible emissions and odors from rendering and smokehouse processes and from oil refinery operations
Absorption	Packed towers, plate and tray towers, spray chambers	Gases free of particulates, such as sulfur dioxide, ammonia, oxides of nitrogen, hydrogen sulfide, hydrogen chloride, chlorine
Adsorption	Activated carbon	Organic solvent vapor recovery, odor removal
	Silica gel	Dry gases of organic and inorganic compounds
Condensation	Water-cooled units or air-cooled units in shell and tube or finned configurations for surface condensation	Organic vapor recovery in oil refineries, petrochemical processes, chemical manufacturing, degreasing operations, dry cleaning plants, and asphalt manufacturing

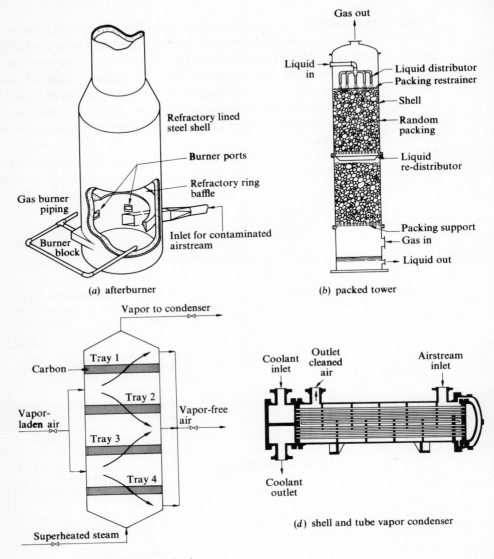

(a) afterburner

(b) packed tower

(c) activated carbon adsorber

(d) shell and tube vapor condenser

FIGURE 5-15
Air cleaners for gases and vapors: afterburners for combustibles, packed tower for soluble, activated carbon for adsorbables, and shell-and-tube condenser for vapors. [*Sources: U.S. Public Health Serv., Publ. 999-AP*-40, *pp. 142, 197, and* 203; for packed tower, "*Mass Transfer Operations,*" *R. E. Treybal, p. 16: 2d ed., McGraw-Hill Book Company, New York, 1968.*]

adsorption is used most frequently to remove organic vapors and odoriferous components by passing the gas air stream through a bed of activated carbon. The application that is most frequent and benefits any traveler is the bank of activated carbon cannisters in the air recirculation system in planes, buses, and railway passenger cars.   Body odors and stale tobacco smoke odors are adsorbed on the activated carbon.   The use of activated carbon to remove organic solvent vapors is attractive in industrial situations, as the adsorbed material can be recovered and the adsorbent regenerated.   In units such as that illustrated in Fig. 5-15, superheated steam drives off the adsorber vapor to a condenser and restores the activated carbon for reuse in place.

4 Condensation of a vapor can be accomplished by increasing pressure or extracting heat.   In air pollutant removal practice, the latter is used, with water the usual coolant.   A surface condenser is a device that has the coolant on one side of a separating barrier, as inside of a pipe, and exposes the outer cooled surface to the vapor to be condensed, as on a series of fins on the pipe.   Shell-and-tube units are more frequently used than finned units for surface condensers.   Figure 5-15 shows a line drawing of a shell and tube unit.   The coolant circulates within the tubes.   The air vapor stream circulates between the outer shell, or housing, with the vapor condensing on the cool surfaces of the tubes and dropping as a liquid to collectors at the bottom of the shell.   In many applications, the recovered condensate is a useful material for recycling or as a byproduct.

The four methods of cleaning gas and vapors from a waste airstream are sometimes used in conjunction with particulate removal systems and sometimes with one another.   The methods are often integrated into chemical processes, which eliminates pollutant discharges and conserves materials in the same unit operation.   Such satisfying solutions have been found to reduce emissions and losses in oil refineries and petrochemical plants.   Engineering design data on control equipment for gases and vapors are in Ref. 5-16 (pp. 171–232).

Exhaust Emissions from Gasoline-fueled Motor Vehicles in the United States

United States automobile use has been the source of 40 percent, by weight, of the total pollution load discharged to our national air supply.   The three pollutants from gasoline internal-combustion engines are carbon monoxide (CO), hydrocarbons (hereafter HC), and oxides of nitrogen (NO_x).   R. W. Hurn states that for each automobile, the exhaust gas average of HC is about 1,400 ppm; of CO, 31,000 ppm (or 3.1 percent); and of NO_x 850 ppm.   This holds for vehicles without any form of emission controls during routine stop-start driving at an average speed of 25 mi/h (40 km/h).   The HC emission

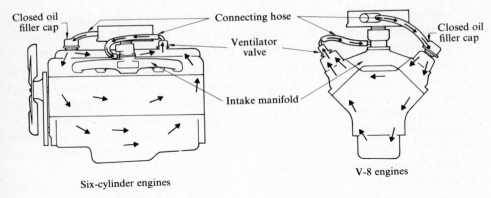

Closed oil filler cap · Connecting hose · Ventilator valve · Intake manifold · Closed oil filler cap

Six-cylinder engines

V-8 engines

FIGURE 5-16
Positive crankcase ventilation system. [*Source*: *Chrysler Motor Products Bulletin on PCV, p.* 3, *Detroit, Mich., March* 1966.]

equals 3.3 percent of the gasoline supplied to the engine (Ref. 5-9, vol. 3, p. 59). From the uncontrolled situation, the steps that have been taken nationally in the United States for control of automotive emissions since the federal Clean Air Act of 1967 have been:

1   Positive crankcase ventilation, Fig. 5-16, has been required on all gasoline-fueled cars built or imported since 1968 models. This requirement reduced HC emissions by 20 percent. (Model years used in this section refer to cars sold from September of the preceding year to August of the model year.)

2   Exhaust-gas emissions at the tail pipe for 1968 models were limited for CO to 1,500 ppm (1.5 percent) and for HC to 275 ppm, at the point of manufacture. Meeting the limits during a prescribed driving mode results in emission reductions of 50 percent for CO and about 65 percent for HC.

3   For 1971 models, the capture of evaporating gasoline from the car's gas tank and from its carburetor was required. This requirement and improvements in positive crankcase ventilation and engine modifications have reduced the emissions of CO by 70 percent and those of HC by more than 80 percent.

The next round poses much more stringent requirements and tougher problems for the proponents of the internal-combustion gasoline engine in a four-cycle piston-cylinder configuration. The requirements hinge on a clause in public law 91-604, the Clean Air Amendments of 1970, of the United States Congress. That public law states that CO and HC emissions on 1975 models shall be at least 90 percent less than the emissions allowable from 1970 automobiles. The 90 percent is not cumulative. It is a 90 percent reduction from the 1970 levels. The resulting cumulative percentages by years are shown in Fig. 5-17.   The numerical emission levels that must be met are in Table 5-23.   There are stated for HC, CO, and NO$_x$ in grams per mile through a

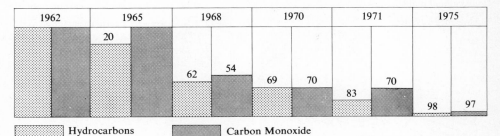

| 1962 | 1965 | 1968 | 1970 | 1971 | 1975 |

20

62   54   69   70   70   83   98   97

Hydrocarbons   Carbon Monoxide

Above reductions are compared to cars without emission controls (1962 and earlier), based on Federal requirements for new cars in the model years shown above. Similar reductions in effect on California cars one or two years earlier.

FIGURE 5-17
Percentage reduction in automobile emissions of hydrocarbons and carbon monoxide, for United States automobiles by model years 1962 to 1975.   [*Source: Ford Motor Co., Dearborn, Mich., September* 1971.]

Table 5-23   NATIONAL EMISSION STANDARDS FOR EXHAUST FROM AUTOMOBILES IN THE UNITED STATES, 1968 TO 1975

Model year	Hydrocarbons		Carbon monoxide		Oxides of nitrogen	
	Emission, g/m	Reduction from baseline, %	Emission, g/m	Reduction from baseline, %	Emission, g/m	Reduction from baseline, %
1968–71 baseline by federal test procedure	11.2	...	73.0	...	5.4	
1972 baseline by federal test procedure	17.0	...	124.0	...	3.0 proposed for 1973	
1968	3.4	70	35.1	52		
1970	2.2	80	23.0	68.5		
1972	3.4	80	39.0	68.5		
1975	0.41	97.5	3.4	97	0.4	87

Note: For hydrocarbons as hexane, 2.2 g/mi = 180 ppm by volume; for carbon monoxide, 23 g/mi = 1 % (or 10,000 ppm) by volume.

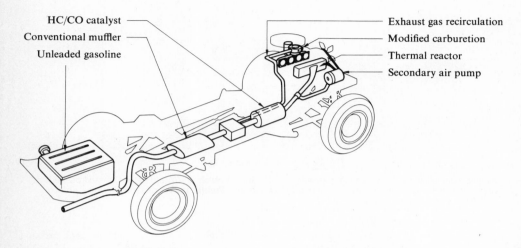

FIGURE 5-18
Three emission-control devices projected for 1975 model cars burning unleaded gasoline in the United States. [*Source*: *Environ. Sci. Technol.*, **5,6**: 495, *June 1971. Amer. Chem. Soc., Washington, D.C.*]

prescribed driving mode from a cold-engine start. The agreed-upon or directed testing, sampling, and analytical procedures make a large difference in compliance in such an evaluation. Hot-engine versus cold-engine starts alone produce large differences in unburned HC at the tail pipe. The requirement is, in law, binding on the regulatory agency in the same way that the Delaney clause on carcinogens is binding on the U.S. Food and Drug Administration.

The move to marketing unleaded and low-lead gasolines in the United States in 1971 was in anticipation of the necessity of making and distributing the large volumes of a changed gasoline by 1975. Present leaded gasolines contain about 3 g of tetraethyl lead (TEL) expressed as lead per gallon of gasoline. This concentration is equivalent to 3 ml of TEL in its liquid state per gallon, as 1 ml of TEL contains 1 g of lead. The lead residues in the exhaust gases poison the catalysts in afterburners, attack the ceramic linings in manifold reactors, and clog the tubes and orifices in exhaust-gas recirculators. All three components are now planned for 1975 models. Low-lead gasolines contain 0.5 g of lead per gallon. Even this reduced lead content causes rapid catalyst poisoning in afterburners.

The search for substitute additives has produced one or two compounds, as yet

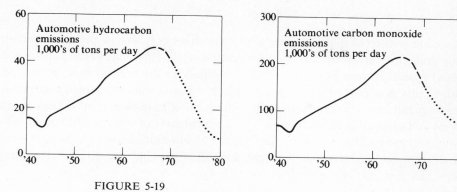

FIGURE 5-19
Effects of controls on automobile exhaust emissions in the United States from
1968 to 1970, and projections to 1980. [*Source*:   *General Motors Corp., Detroit,
Mich.*]

very costly, but promising candidates according to laboratory tests.   The manufacturers of TEL are working strenuously to perfect a durable, thermal exhaust-manifold
reactor that will make a catalytic oxidation afterburner unnecessary.   That would
permit continuing use of leaded gasolines.   It would solve, or at least simplify, the
complexities of multiple control devices on the same car.   The advertising in the fall
of 1971 by major manufacturers informed the public that 1975 models with all three
control systems, presumably along with existing devices, would meet the emission
standards.   Figure 5-18 schematically shows control equipment that would meet the
needs on unleaded gasoline.   The reductions in automobile emissions of HC and CO
that implementation of the 1975 standards will achieve are shown in Fig. 5-19.   This
graphic presentation is based on data presented to a Senate committee in 1970 by
federal officials.

Although development will improve methods and results, the results of 1971
tests by the Inter Industry Control program showed a 27 percent loss in fuel economy.
The test vehicle was equipped with a thermal or manifold reactor, a catalytic converter
operating at 1600°F (about 900°C), and an exhaust-gas recirculator.   The high temperatures under the hood and along the entire system posed many operating difficulties, including in proper braking.   The control equipment did bring emissions of
HC down to 0.28 g/mi, of CO to 3.4 g/mi, and of NO_x to 0.76 g/mi.   These results
compare with the announced 1975 standards of 0.41, 3.4, and 0.4 g/mi for HC, CO,
and NO_x, respectively.[1]

[1] *Environ. Sci. Technol.*, **5**(6): 495 (June 1971).

Some Warning Signs on Air Pollution

This section is directed to areas where alert concern seeks to initiate preventive action on air pollution before air quality deterioration is extreme, but where human and material resources must be allocated most carefully in the face of many economic, social, health, and environmental needs.   Such situations are encountered in major urbanizing and industrializing centers in countries that have been rural in their living patterns and agrarian in their economy.   The benchmarks of warning of an approaching difficulty are relatively simple.   The needed observations do not require elaborate field instrumentation or more than the support a capable quantitative analytical chemist can provide.   Here are four warning signs.

1   When dust-fall jars show that settleable solids approach 1.5 mg/(cm^2)(month) the air is dirty.   That value equals 42 tons/(mi^2)(month).   Control efforts can well begin at the level of 1 mg/cm^2.   Burning practices, furnace firing, street dust, and debris removal warrant attention.

2   When gasoline consumption exceeds 5,800 l/(km^2)(h) over a large area, the emissions are sufficient to produce photochemical smog if solar radiation is high and air movement is low.   An even lower value may be appropriate where many vehicles are powered by two-cycle engines.

3   Some of the usual effects of aggravated air pollution such as eye irritation, visibility reduction, odors, and vegetation damage can be expected when the following contaminants and pollutants in the ambient air reach or exceed the concentrations stated: carbon monoxide, 8 ppm by volume (or 9.2 mg/m^3); hydrocarbons as methane, 1 ppm by volume (or 655 μg/m^3); oxides of nitrogen as NO$_2$, 0.25 ppm by volume (or 470 μg/m^3); oxidants as ozone, 0.15 ppm by volume (or 294 μg/m^3.)   These values, except for carbon monoxide, are higher than those set in 1971 as national air quality standards in the United States.

4   When the total of uncontrolled emissions of gaseous and particulate pollutants is estimated to be 2 or more tons/(mi^2)(day), it is likely that there is a marked degree of air pollution.   In metric units, that value is about 1,700 kg/(km^2)(day). It can be rounded to 2,000 kg/(km^2)(day).   Among United States examples is Philadelphia, Pennsylvania, which with an estimated 5,000 tons of emissions on 125 mi^2, has an estimated pollutant emission rate of 4 tons/mi^2.   The Los Angeles area discharges an estimated 25,000 tons/day on an area of 1,200 mi^2 for a rate of just over 2 tons/(mi^2)(day).   Estimating total emissions requires skill and experience.   It can be done with the use of published emission rates for specific processes, such as prepared by Duprey.[1]

---

[1] Robert L. Duprey, Compilations of Air Pollutant Emission Factors, *U.S. Public Health Serv. Publ. AP*-42, 1968.

Those who are initiating air pollution studies will find valuable assistance and very likely strong support from meteorologists in their area. Meteorologists have long arrays of data—as a minimum, that from airport observation stations. These data can be examined and discussed to determine the likelihood of periods of air movement stagnation. Conditions that can be expected to worsen the dispersion of air pollutants occur when:

1 Surface winds are less than 9 mi/h (15 km/h).
2 Upper-level winds at about 18,000 ft (5,500 m) are less than 30 mi/h (about 50 km/h).
3 Subsidence inversion developing from a high pressure area is present below 14,000 ft (about 4,300 m).
4 The persistence of such inversion conditions is forecast to be more than 36 hours over a very large area.

Air Quality Criteria and National Air Quality Standards in the United States

The concepts and difficulties of the assignment of numerical values to air quality by criteria and standards and their attainment by defining emission rates, and also control equipment design and performance standards are examined meticulously and systematically by Stern (Ref. 5-9, vol. 3, pp. 601–718). The distinctions among the terms *air quality criteria*, *air quality standards*, and *allowable emission rates* have been noted in the section on control. These terms are to be used carefully and correctly to assure meaningful communication with others, including public discussions. Numerical values describing environmental quality have an unfortunate history of being used out of context and sometimes without consideration of the original intent of their declaration. They become magic numbers substituted for professional analysis and judgment. Table 5-24 is offered to make the data that are developed at length in the Air Quality Criteria series succinct and to show its relation to the 1971 statement on national air quality standards. The identity of the concentrations as annual arithmetic or geometric means, or as a maxima for certain time periods, should be noted and must be considered in any interpretations or comparisons. The numbers that are taken from the Air Quality Criteria series are those singled out in the résumé section of each of the publications (Ref. 5-12). All concentrations are in weight per cubic meter. The weight is in milligrams for carbon monoxide and in micrograms for all other pollutants. The conversion factors for each material to, or from, parts per million by volume are given in the original publications. A statement that is the identical last sentence in each of the résumés must be borne in mind in considering or discussing the relations between the criteria and the standards:

Table 5-24   NATIONAL AIR QUALITY CRITERIA AND NATIONAL AIR QUALITY STANDARDS IN THE UNITED STATES, 1971

Pollutant	Adverse health effects observed at these concentrations	Air quality standard, protective for health
Particulate matter	80 μg/m^3, annual mean.	75 μg/m^3, annual geometric mean. 260 μg/m^3, max. 24-h value may occur once each year.
Sulfur dioxide	115 μg/m^3, annual mean. 300 μg/m^3, 24-h av. for 3–4 days.	80 μg/m^3, annual arithmetic mean. 365 μg/m^3, max. 24-h value may occur once each year.
Carbon monoxide	12–17 mg/m^3 for 8 h produces concn. of 2–2.5% carboxyhemoglobin. 35 mg/m^3 for 8 h produces concn. of 5% carboxyhemoglobin.	10 mg/m^3, max. 8-h value may occur each year. 40 mg/m^3, max. 1-h value may occur once each year.
Photochemical oxidants	130 μg/m^3 hourly av. impaired performance of student athletes. 200 μg/m^3 instantaneous level increased eye irritation. 490 μg/m^3 peaks with 300 μg/m^3 hourly av. increased asthma attacks.	160 μg/m^3, max. 1-h value may occur once each year.
Hydrocarbons	With nonmethane hydrocarbon, 200 μg/m^3 in 3 h, 6–9 A.M., produced (2–4 h later) photochemical oxidant of up to 200 μg/m^3 that lasted 1 h. By extrapolation downward, conc. of HC of 100 μg/m^3 can produce lowest injurious level of photochemical oxidant.	160 μg/m^3, max. level that may occur 6–9 A.M. once each year.

Table 5-24   (Continued)

Pollutant	Adverse health effects observed at these concentrations	Air quality standard, protective for health
Oxides of nitrogen	$118–156$ $\mu g/m^3$, 24-h mean over 6 mo produced increase in acute bronchitis in infants and schoolchildren; this av. associated with a 24-h max. of 284 $\mu g/m^3$. $117–205$ $\mu g/m^3$, 24-h mean over 6 mo and mean suspended nitrate level of 3.8 $\mu g/m^3$ or more produced increased respiratory disease in family groups.	100 $\mu g/m^3$, annual arithmetic mean.

It is reasonable and prudent to conclude that when promulgating ambient-air quality standards, consideration should be given to requirements for margins of safety which would take into account long-term effects on health, vegetation, and materials, occurring below the [air quality criteria] levels.

The national air quality standards are ambient-air quality values carefully designated " protective for human health."   Their attainment may be beneficial in protecting vegetation, other animal life, and materials from the effects of air pollutants, and may limit visibility reductions and other undesirable local atmospheric effects.   Such gains will be bonus benefits to the prime objective of protecting human health.   The enormous and costly task of implementing control to attain the national air quality standards has already begun.   Actually the federal work began over 20 years ago with the study of the Donora episode by the Public Health Service, Division of Industrial Hygiene.   The steps to reduce automotive emissions are the first nationwide control of air pollution under law.   The second nationwide control move has been the promulgation of national emission standards for electricity generating stations.

CHANGES AND DEVELOPMENTS

Observations on changes and developments in controlling air quality are restricted to what are essentially technological matters, although it is evident that major developments will continue in the administrative realm at varying levels of government throughout the world and in the private sector.   In the management of toxic gases, vapors, dusts, and fumes, the strong demand for more refined toxicological data will require more elaborate and lengthy experimental and epidemiological studies. Such studies are faced with the complex interrelations of exposure to mixed agents in contrast to exposure to a single substance. The assessment of human factors of aging, nutrition, and life style must be made in evaluating on-the-job exposures. Some life-style issues are the use of lengthening leisure, or at least off-the-regular-job time, nutrition, smoking habits, use of alcohol, and drug abuse. The longer life expectancy and the development of illnesses after retirement are new factors in evaluating occupational disease. The pulmonary distress of old and retired coal miners is an example. For many years, the accumulations of coal dust in miner's lungs was regarded as benign and not recognized as causing disability, at least during a working life. Now "black lung" is a national political issue. For even less-clear reasons, byssinosis is being recognized among southern cotton textile workers. For many years, it was stated with certainty that such a lung disorder was unknown among that group. One explanation has been that mechanically harvested cotton contains large amounts of field debris from the plants and the soil. Occupational disease prevention and control is but one facet of a worker's health and well-being. The industrial hygienists' primary concern with environmental measures to control occupational diseases moves to broader concerns about the work environment and workers' behavior in it. There are some activities in ergonomics among those responsible for industrial hygiene.

Developments that are shared in common in managing dirty air in the occupational setting and in the community are improvements in devices and methods for air sampling, measurement, and cleaning. Improvements in all these will continue. Techniques of systems analysis and mathematical modeling are already in use in air pollution in meteorological work, in stack-diffusion predictions, and in cost-benefit analysis. Opportunities for their use in industrial hygiene are less evident, although the air supply in a large manufacturing plant constitutes a system of movement and of chemical and physical characteristics. The actions for air control by industrial hygienists on the one hand within the plant and those by air pollution officials on the other hand outside the plant are joined at the points of air cleaning and of providing makeup air. Where specific regulations include compliance with design and performance standards on air cleaning equipment and internal ventilation systems, there must be compatibility between industrial hygiene and air pollution control requirements.

Changes and developments in community air quality control in the United States are examined by the major sources: transportation, fuel combustion in stationary sources, industrial processes, and solid-waste disposal. The plan for control of automotive emissions to about 1980 is set. It is based on modifications of the gasoline-fueled four-cycle reciprocating engine and on control of the emissions by prescribing emission rates in grams per mile for CO, HC, and NO_x. Automotive engineers and gasoline producers have means in development to meet these. The present schemes may be altered to some degree and even replaced by devices not yet known or disclosed. Alternative power sources such as the rotary engine and battery-power and steam engines will continue to be explored. None of these is expected to replace the present engines in mass production by 1975 and probably not by 1980, either. More attractive mass transportation will reduce the rate of car-commuter increases. The only alternative that can be provided speedily is the use of express routes, including public street and highway lanes reserved exclusively for buses. Rail systems of any type require 5 to 10 years to construct in urban areas.

The control of sulfur dioxide from coal- and oil-fired furnaces in the United States has reached the point of establishing national emission-rate standards. As there is not a sufficient supply of naturally occurring low-sulfur coal or oil, the alternatives for the large users, the electricity generating stations, are to use nuclear fuel in new stations, to pay the added cost of desulfurized fuels, and to find an effective way to eliminate sulfur dioxide from the stack discharge. All three are being pursued. Each presents its difficulties. Nuclear reactor units have been required to meet restrictions on radioactive releases, on the handling of radioactive fuels and spent fuels, and on the dissipation of the thermal loads from the condenser water. Crude oils are being successfully desulfurized at a cost increase of about 30 to 40 percent a barrel. Improved technology and economy of scale is likely to reduce that percentage increase. Desulfurizing coal is still in early development. Some very complex multi-step processes for removing sulfur dioxide from stack gases are in use. Control alternatives do not stand in isolation. For example, if a substantial number of commuters used battery-powered vehicles, the power load to recharge the batteries would have to be met. The generating capacity might be sufficient if charging was on home circuits from 9 or 10 P.M. to 6 A.M., but whatever the fuel source at the generating station, the consequent emissions would be greater as a substantial number of the generators would be on the line around the clock.

The control of industrial manufacturing processes producing pollutants is more an administrative requirement than a technological one. A variety of air cleaners are available and in use. The task is to organize a control plan that can reach the multitude of sources and implement an equitable control program. One development that can be anticipated is that, faced with the costs of elaborate control systems based on capture and cleaning, industry will devote skill and time to find process changes that will eliminate the generation or the release of as many pollutants as possible. The outlook for the control of emissions from incinerators is poor. It becomes progressively worse in considering industrial solid-waste incinerators, municipal incinerators, and small incinerators serving apartment buildings. Industrial solid-waste incinerators are most likely to have a homogeneous feed for which combustion can be regulated and for which control devices can be designed with the assurance that the combustion products will not vary widely in composition and concentration. Municipal incinerators do not permit the assumptions of uniformity of feed materials. The combustion products are among the most difficult to remove consistently with high efficiencies by present air cleaning methods.   The costs and uncertainties of effectively controlling air pollutants was a major factor in the decision of New York City authorities to abandon plans in August 1971 for a superincinerator on the site of the old Brooklyn navy yard.   Their consternation on learning within weeks that their New Jersey upwind neighbors were planning a similar superincinerator to be located on the Jersey Meadows is understandable.   The experiences with undertaking control of apartment building incinerators has been so discouraging that air pollution control officers have been quoted as saying, "The best thing to do is to plug the flues and chutes with concrete and find another way to get rid of the refuse."

APPRAISAL

On the first level of control of toxic gases, vapors, dusts, and fumes to prevent direct health injury in the occupational setting, industrial hygiene has the necessary technology.   Certainly in the United States, industrial hygiene is being very incompletely applied.   The work environment of only a fraction of our total work force receives the benefit of industrial hygiene surveillance from the limited staffs of state and federal agencies.   Workers in large industrial plants and those exposed to recognized toxicants, such as free silica, lead, and beryllium, receive the largest share of the time of such agencies.   Large corporations and some of the labor unions have their own industrial hygienists.   The number of these is increasing.   In the United States the number of governmental industrial hygienists has not kept pace with the growth of industry or the multiplication of exposures.   Small plants, the service trades, and office worker environments are rarely provided any industrial hygiene service.   The National Occupational Safety and Health Act of 1970 is designed to expand these services.   It provides a definite statutory basis of occupational health responsibilities at the federal level.   It creates the National Institute of Occupational Safety and Health (NIOSH), within the Department of Health, Education, and Welfare.   This gives the occupational health activities of the U.S. Public Health Service, which have been the chief source of research and program development for 50 years, a strong administrative position. The NIOSH is responsible for research, development, and field studies.   The responsibility for day-to-day operations is in the U.S. Department of Labor.   The act provides mechanisms and incentives to expand and improve the organizations in the states.

In practice, industrial hygiene embraces the control of the physical energies of noise, radiations, and thermal stress as well as workplace ventilation. The control measures do more than prevent specific occupational diseases. There is a general improvement of the quality of the work environment, providing a more comfortable, cleaner, and more pleasing surrounding. To this extent, the second level of environmental betterment, for comfort and esthetic objectives, is reached. Industrial hygiene has no direct program objectives bearing on ecological balances. There are localized influences when highly toxic materials are eliminated to prevent worker exposure. The toxicant is then no longer a part of the plant water and air waste discharges.

The growth of the air pollution control program in the United States, spearheaded by federal initiative, during the last 10 years is unparalleled in any phase of environmental control. The activity has developed from a nucleus of men in the Public Health Service, mobilized at the start from industrial hygiene specialists. The scope of the present work, grounded in strong and specific federal legislation, is unprecedented in environmental control history anywhere on any facet of environmental quality. The first steps of control have been directed to two of our largest industries, the automobile manufacturers and the electric power companies. This control influences every one of us, as we depend on their products in our major and trivial daily activities. The two targets are the emissions from motor vehicles and from electricity generating stations. A fantastic amount of work has gone into preparing the foundations for the program that is well underway. There has been a prodigious effort not only of a technical nature but of a political nature in arousing public awareness and in gaining legislative support.

The control of air pollutants is directed to all three levels of environmental quality, to the factors with direct health effects, with comfort and esthetic effects, and with ecological balances. As the review of effects has indicated for man, the first two levels are interwoven. The benefit of control now evident in the cities of the United States and the United Kingdom is the reduction in settleable particulates and of visible smoke from chimneys. The change from coal to oil and gas in thousands of industrial, commercial, and domestic furnaces, plus specific controls, has worked. In parts of London it has been reported that certain species of birds have returned. The work of the Los Angeles Air Pollution Control District on stationary sources of air pollutants has at least kept that area inhabitable. The decisive phase of automotive emission control during the next 10 years, a responsibility of the state and national authorities, will improve the quality of Los Angeles air. It will mark a passing of the point of just managing to hold the line. Like efforts will produce like results elsewhere. The technology is at hand and will improve. Very difficult administrative issues must be met. Large amounts of public and private funds must be committed. Political and scientific leadership must be strong and steadfast to maintain public support.

REFERENCES

5-1   HEIMANN, HARRY: Air Pollution and Respiratory Disease, *U.S. Public Health Serv.*, *Publ.* 1257, 1964.

5-2   HENDERSON, YANDALL, and HOWARD HAGGARD: "Noxious Gases," Reinhold Publishing Corporation, New York, 1943.

5-3   Committee on Threshold Limit Values: Threshold Limit Values of Airborne Contaminants and Physical Agents with Intended Changes, *Am. Conf. Gov. Ind. Hyg.*, 1971 (issued annually).

5-4   "Air Sampling Instruments," 3d ed., *Am. Conf. Gov. Ind. Hyg.*, 1966.

5-5   HUNTER, DONALD: "The Diseases of Occupations," 4th ed., Little, Brown and Company, Boston, 1969.

5-6   Committee on Industrial Ventilation: "Industrial Ventilation," 11th ed., *Am. Conf. Gov. Ind. Hyg.*, 1970.

5-7   "Documentation of the Threshold Limit Values," 3d ed., *Am. Conf. Gov. Ind. Hyg.*, 1971.

5-8   Third Report of Secretary of Health, Education, and Welfare to Congress: Progress in Prevention and Control of Air Pollution, *Sen. Doc.* 91-64, March 1970.

5-9   STERN, ARTHUR C. (ed.): "Air Pollution," vols. 1–3, Academic Press, Inc., New York, 1968.

5-10 Air Quality Criteria for Particulate Matter—Summary and Conclusions, *U.S. Public Health Serv. Publ.*, February 1969.

5-11 ROUCHÉ, BERTON: "Eleven Blue Men," Medallion Books, Berkley Publishing Corporation, New York, 1965.

5-12 Air Quality Criteria: "For Particulates," *AP*-49, 1969; "For Sulfur Dioxide," *AP*-50, 1969; "For Carbon Monoxide," *AP*-62, 1970; "For Photochemical Oxidants," *AP*-63, 1970; "For Hydrocarbons," *AP*-64, 1970; all *U.S. Public Health Service Publs.* Also, "For Nitrogen Oxides," *U.S. Environmental Protection Agency, Publ.* AP-84, 1971.

5-13 Working Group on Lead Contamination: Survey of Lead in the Atmosphere of Three Urban Communities, *U.S. Public Health Serv., Publ.* 999-AP-12, 1965.

5-14 LILLIE, ROBERT J.: Air Pollutants Affecting the Performance of Domestic Animals, *U.S. Dep. Agr., Handbook* 380, 1970.

5-15 JACOBSON, JAY S., and A. CLYDE HILL: "Recognition of Air Pollution Injury to Vegetation: A Pictorial Atlas," *Air Pollut. Control Assoc.*, Pittsburgh, Pa., 1970.

5-16 DANIELSON, JOHN D. (ed.): Air Pollution Engineering Manual, Los Angeles Air Pollution Control District, *U.S. Public Health Serv., Publ.* 999-AP-40, 1967.

6

SOLID–WASTES MANAGEMENT

THE SOLID–WASTES ISSUES

Solid Wastes on Stage

Solid wastes have moved to the center of the environmental stage in the United States in the last 5 to 10 years in obedience to the exponential law of the P game, that is, growth and concentration of people, products, power, pollutants, and places. The discard of our consumption has outstripped the capacity of our customary methods of disposing of garbage, rubbish, trash, and obsolete hardware and furnishings. The discard of 8 million motor vehicles per year in the United States illustrates the issues and the intensification of these matters. Our space use and distribution of people make the old method of hide and forget of limited acceptance. The costs of collection and transportation of the junked vehicle have risen in the face of a decreasing value of scrap steel. Steel manufacture has switched from the open-hearth furnace, which could take 50 percent scrap of a messy sort, to the basic oxygen process, which can take not more than 25 percent of clean scrap. The scrap-steel price dropped from $40 per ton in 1950 to $15 per ton in 1970. The increased use of bonded plastics, rubber, and nonferrous alloys has made cleanup of the scrapped vehicle more difficult and costly.   The number of junked vehicles rose from 3 million in 1950 to 7 million in 1965.   The average life of cars has dropped from 10 to 6 years.

With the "hide it, forget it" option diminished, there are three others: burn it bury it, or transform it for reuse.   The constraints on the options are natural, technological, and economic.   The penalties of bad choices or bad use of the chosen method are esthetic offenses, nuisances, ecological upsets, and health hazards.   Each step—from an economy of farm-based producer-consumer, the subsistence farm family, to that of urban-suburban consumer increasingly removed from the producer —has intensified solid-waste production, removal, and disposal.   Concentrations of people in village, town, city, or metropolis magnify the task of solid-waste handling. The sole exception is the elimination of ashes as oil, gas, and electricity have been substituted for wood and coal for heating and cooking in homes and commercial, manufacturing, and public buildings.   The magnification is marked by increasing use of throwaway packaging materials; single-use containers, utensils, fabrics, and even wearing apparel; early obsolescence of a variety of domestic appliances and furnishings; and a decreased incentive for salvage and reuse of materials and goods. Fewer people live in homes and on sites that provide storage space for items of reduced usefulness, which speeds more material to waste and lessens the chance for subsequent repair and further use.   High-speed, partially automated manufacturing methods use electric welds, pressed seams, extruded metals and plastics, riveting, and thermal bonding.   The products are not readily repairable in the home when seams, joints, and connections fail.   Shop repair is frequently as costly as original manufacture. The "broke-down" item becomes solid waste.   Maintenance is increasingly a skill of component replacement rather than repair and restoration of the original materials. Each new kit, cartridge, and renewal component sends the discard to solid waste along with the new one's elaborate packaging materials.

Some Definitions, Origins, and Changes

If it is not capable of being fluid-borne in free flow in an airstream or liquid stream, a waste is a solid waste despite a high moisture content.   Its owner refuses it for further use; it is refuse.   A few classifications and comments on terms set a common word usage and may help communication.

Garbage is our food reject at any point from growing to final eating.   Garbage is putrescible, and it is still food for many insects, rodents, hogs, and a few less familiar scavengers.   Left to rot, it stinks.   Left accessible, it attracts a variety of flies, roaches, and rats for feeding and breeding.   As it rots, it adds pollutants to our air, our surface water, and our groundwater.   The developments of food production, processing, distribution, and use in this century in the United States, now being emulated elsewhere, have moved the garbage-generation point away from the home, the farm, and the store to the processing plant. Mechanical harvesting and fast transport have moved some of the mess from the farm to the processing plant. That is too bad, as the mess was readily handled at the farm by rotting where it was or by being plowed under. The cattle and hogs ate some.

The processing plant must handle the washings, the trimmings, the rejects, the peelings, the pittings, and the residues of its sweeteners, preservatives, additives, and its cleanup waters. The difficulties are:

1 Food processing plants are often seasonal operations resistant to capital investment for waste handling and treatment.
2 The wastes are formidable in quantity and in strength.
3 Plants are located in rural sites or near small towns where legal action is least likely and where technical skill is not readily available.
4 The wastes vary with seasonal harvest runs of early beans, corn, and late summer fruits to fall crops of potatoes, squash, and pumpkins.

The advantages are:

1 The wastes are concentrated in place and in time.
2 There is a chance for by-product conversion to plant and animal food.
3 There is a chance for process control and change to modify waste quantity and quality.
4 There can be an integrated industrywide approach with food technology and waste control joined.
5 The bill can be passed to the final buyer and consumer.

In the United States and urban centers in much of the world, food wastes in the home can be reduced to that left on our plates. Canned, frozen, dehydrated, and prepackaged foods have nearly eliminated the feathers, scales, entrails, peelings, leafy tops of beets, carrots, and turnips, and much of the bone, fat, and gristle of meats and poultry from our kitchen wastes. The extent of the elimination is roughly tied to economic status as pre-prepared foods are more expensive per unit of weight or volume. Public eating places continue to produce sizable amounts of garbage through serving gluttonous portions and poor menu planning. Such sources are frequently on the collection route of hog raisers.

Rubbish is the nonputrescible solid wastes generated in increasing per capita amounts. The combustibles include paper, cardboard, wood, cloth, rubber, leather, burnable plastics, grass and shrub clippings, leaves, and tree prunings. The noncombustibles are metals, glass, ceramics, nonburnable plastics which only melt, masonry waste, stone, inert dusts, grit, and sand.

Ashes have left the home scene except for the output from coal-fired home boilers and open fireplaces. There are prodigious amounts produced at coal-fired electricity generation plants, industrial boilers, and institutional central heating plants. In the United States, power plants burned 300 million tons of coal in 1969. Ash content of power-plant coal varies from lows of 5 to 7 percent to highs of 25 percent. At 10 percent ash, the power-plant residue would be 30 million tons/year. On-site refuse incineration in apartment and commercial buildings, and in manufacturing plants, has its end product of ashes. A part of this mountain of ashes is used in aggregates of masonry block and asphalt mix and some for land reclamation fill.

Debris from building construction, demolition, and major renovation is turning out to be a sizable quantity in cities where the air pollution control and fire departments are cracking down on on-site burning. Anyone who has lived or worked near the wrecking of a large building is quite aware that the dust produced is of itself a filthy mess of pulverized plaster, mortar, and brick. This can be reduced by wetting down. One-shot blasting for shell and frame destruction produces an initial great dust fall which subsequently can be wetted. Blasting reduces salvage which has not been economically attractive in the United States. In addition to prime construction materials of lumber, masonry, and plaster, the debris is wire, conduits, piping, roofing, insulation, vinyl and ceramic tile, floor covering, and plumbing fixtures. Uncorroded pipe, any copper, and lighting fixtures may be salvaged at a profitable market price.

Street and road litter—the mess in our streets—is painfully familiar and seemingly increasing. Information on quantities, characteristics, and behavior is virtually nil. The "whitewing" street sweeper left the scene about three decades after the horse whom he had served so well. Motorized sweepers of varying efficiency make periodic forays, well-announced by their noise. Street flushing is spasmodic in most communities, contributing to filling catch basins and where sewers combine street drainage and sanitary sewage, bringing the sewage treatment plant operator additional grit to handle. Street debris must contribute substantially to dust fall, raised by winds and traffic in daylight and resettling from midnight to dawn.

Oversized discards—cars for abandonment, kitchen stoves, refrigerators, washing machines, clothes driers, black-and-white TV units, the old mattress, bed, sofa, or easy chair, trees, stumps, and Christmas trees—are left by the no-longer-to-be owner to the public refuse collector, to the trade-in vendor, and to the private scavenger. Nobody in the United States wants it, because it is worthless. It requires manual labor to move and load. It is costly to transport. With a few exceptions, the salvage yard is too far from the source to make the trip profitable. It is scarcely welcome at the public refuse-disposal site, even if someone is willing to pay the haulage. No person or agency wants to foot the bill for collecting, transporting, and disposing of this class of solid waste. Clandestine abandonment is common. Some municipalities provide pickup on request with or without a fee. The answer is clear if distasteful—another tax, a disposal fee collected as a tax at purchase. The administration of the tax is certain to be as much of a headache as the present disposal system. At least, different people will have the headache. In other countries and cultures the disposal of durable goods is less troublesome, as salvage and restoration for second-hand use is still profitable.

Dead animals—pets, wild animals, and domesticated ones—must be collected and burned, buried, ground to sewage, or rendered for by-product value. Public repugnance to dead animals in streets and roads assures speedy removal even if by poorly equipped agencies with unrelated primary duties. Carcasses from teaching and research laboratories are handled by on-site cremation or contract removal promptly, quietly, and efficiently to avoid arousing the ire of the antivivisectionists.

Wastewater treatment plants end with an assortment of untreatables or no-further-treatables. Screenings and grit, grease and digested sludge are the items. Burial or burning or disposal at sea are used. Digested dried sludge is land-spread when sites are near at hand. The quantities are increasing as wastewater treatment is more widely provided, and as home, restaurant, and food-processing-plant garbage is ground at the source for sewer transport to wastewater treatment plants, where it adds to the settleable solids load in settling tanks, sludge digesters, and drying facilities.

Industrial solid wastes from the whole spectrum of manufacturing and process-ing operations are estimated at 110 million tons/year in the United States. There is a lot of salvage and reuse as the wastes can be separated at the point of generation, as these are uniform in character, and as these are predictable in quantity, such as metal trimmings, paper cuttings, even collected dusts and ashes. Some wastes go to by-products on-site, as milk wastes to casein glues, and fats to soaps at large meat plants. Some can be readily recovered and recycled as pulp screenings, the gate metal from brass, bronze, and iron castings, and recovery of foundry sand and blasting sand or steel shot. Industrial solid wastes are a management responsibility and not a public charge or service except for special fees. How industry handles these wastes is a public concern, as some of the more casual methods of dump, pile, or burn no longer are accepted as innocuous by new near neighbors or tolerable to the pressures of land use and values. An intense case is that of hog, cattle, and sheep manure which has moved from farms to the concentration of feeding lots in or close to urban and suburban zones. One-half of the total animal manure produced in the United States comes from the animal concentrations in cattle feeding lots, hog pens, and confinement poultry houses. The country's total quantity of manure production is estimated at 2 billion tons/year.

Mineral extraction and processing wastes are a new focus of the attention of people pressed closer to what used to be remote and inaccessible sites. The few who worried and lived close to the mines and refining mills are now supplemented by travelers, vacationers, weekend home seekers, and conservationists. The supplements are less tolerant of the mountain of tailings or of the smoldering " gob " piles and are generally more articulate politically. The annual United States output of mineral wastes is estimated as over 10 times that of other industrial solid wastes and over 4 times that of all urban domestic and commercial solid wastes. It is 1.1 billion tons/year. Such a stupendous quantity is understandable as copper ores mined in the country have no more than a 1 percent copper yield, and relatively rich Minnesota taconite ores have about a 30 percent yield of iron. What is new is that a whole new group of people feel that their interests are unfavorably affected by haphazard handling of such mineral wastes. Changes in strip-mining practices have come directly from the concern and demand of these people.

The Costs, the Quantities, and the Quality

Table 6-1 is based on the U.S. national survey of community solid wastes which secured data from over 6,000 communities in 33 states representing nearly one-half of the country's population (Ref. 6-1). Note that Table 6-1 details wastes generated, with an annual total of 4.0 billion tons/year. Most of the last three entries are wastes that are not collected or moved very far. Data on the 6 to 7 lb/(capita)(day) which are collected and disposed from household, commercial, and municipal sources, including street cleaning and 3 lb/(capita)(day) from industry activities, show that their handling costs $4.5 billion per year, that is, for storing, moving, and getting rid of 360 million tons of solid wastes per year at $15 per ton. An urban dweller generates about a ton per year. The $15 cost may be surprising or shocking. But very few are asking to do the job for themselves, although they all already do part of it by in-home handling, garbage grinding, on-site burning where still permitted, and providing containers. The three components of the $4.5 billion are expenditures by municipal services,

Table 6-1 SOLID WASTES GENERATED IN THE UNITED STATES, 1968 ESTIMATES, BY ORIGIN IN TOTAL WEIGHTS PER YEAR AND PER CAPITA PER DAY

Origin	Millions of tons per year	Pounds per capita per day	Percentage collected by public or contract service
Household, commercial, and municipal	250	7	85–90
Industrial	110	3	60–70
Agricultural and crop residues	550		
Animal manure	2,000		
Mining and refining	1,100		
Total	4,010		

SOURCE: National Survey of Community Solid Wastes, U.S. Public Health Serv., 1968, and agricultural engineering sources.

$1.7 billion; expenditures by private contractor services, $1.8 billion; expenditures by individual families and industries transporting and disposing of their own wastes, $1.0 billion.

The most readily identified cost is that budgeted for municipal services. The 1968 survey gives $5.40 per person per year for collection and $1.40 for disposal. In any community, a $7 per person per year service is a leading budget item, second only to education which is now funded in the United States from some combination of local, state, and federal taxes. That $7 per capita per year of public money keeps about 175,000 workers on local government solid-waste payrolls; it further keeps 44,000 packer trucks and 36,000 other vehicles collecting, hauling, and handling a part of our solid wastes. The part is the 56 percent of household wastes, 25 percent of commercial wastes, and 13 percent of industrial solid wastes which are moved by public collection. Except for periodic slum-area neglect and increasingly frequent collector strikes, collection service is quite good. The quality is regulated by taxpayer power and response registered by telephone calls to the mayor and city manager. Note that 80 percent of the per capita cost goes to collection; 20 percent goes for disposal.

The 20 percent that goes for disposal buys a very poor service. Open dumps, uncontrolled burning, and overloaded, badly operated incinerators abound. The national survey found that 94 percent of existing land disposal operations and 75 percent of our public incinerator facilities are inadequate. As there are only 300 municipally owned and operated incinerators in the country, the deficiencies that are greatest in number are the thousands of land disposal sites that range from crude open dumps to well-managed sanitary landfills. The 20 percent of the total public cost for solid-wastes handling does not mean that disposal is a low-cost phase of the handling. It reflects the negligent way in which the job is being done, a surrender to the cheapest expedient so long as the people tolerate it. It is the remnant of the " hide and forget" method. Figures 6-1 and 6-2 are from a report prepared in 1964 by the Surgeon General's Advisory Committee on Urban Health Affairs of the U.S. Public Health Service. The exponential character of the total-refuse-production curve is being maintained. The straight-line projection of the per capita refuse-production curve is optimistically low. Besides providing useful data, the committee's report helped to convince our Congress to enact public law 89-272, the Solid Waste Disposal Act in 1965.

Health Matters

The literature fails to supply data which would permit a quantitative estimate of any solid waste/disease relationship. The circumstantial and epidemiologic information presented does support a conclusion that, to some diseases, solid wastes bear a definite, if not well defined, etiologic relationship. The diseases so implicated are infectious in

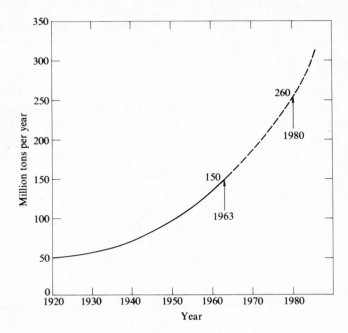

FIGURE 6-1
Total refuse production, United States, 1970 to 1985. [*Source*: *Solid Waste Handling in Metropolitan Areas, U.S. Public Health Serv. Publ.* 1554 (*reprinted*), 1968.]

nature; no relationship can be substantiated for noncommunicable disease agents associated with solid wastes, not because of negating data, but because of lack of data. (An exception to this statement may exist in the instance of methemoglobinemia of infants in which nitrates of excretory origin may play a part.)

The communicable diseases most incriminated are those whose agents are found in fecal wastes—particularly human fecal wastes. Where these wastes are not disposed of in a sanitary manner, the morbidity and mortality rates from fecal-borne diseases in the population are high. Despite the fact that other factors are known to contribute to some reduction of these rates, the inescapable conclusion is *that the continued presence in the environment of the wastes themselves is the basic causative factor.* Therefore transmission—whether by direct contact, vector transfer, or indirect contact—is due to environmental contamination by these wastes.

These carefully chosen words open the summary of Solid Wastes/Disease Relationships by Thrift G. Hanks, a literature survey of 1,236 items (Ref. 6-2). Note the words "quantitative estimate" in the first sentence. Specific disease outbreaks are not in the evidence. Changes in prevalence of intestinal infections are well documented as fly populations rise and fall by natural cycles or man-manipulated control. In the second sentence, note " definite, if not well defined, etiologic relationship," and finally

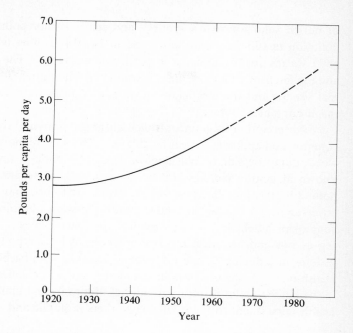

FIGURE 6-2
Per capita refuse production, United States, 1920 to 1985. [*Source: Solid Waste Handling in Metropolitan Areas, U.S. Public Health Serv. Publ.* 1554 (*reprinted*), 1968.]

that "The diseases...are infectious." The garbage component of solid wastes provides the maternity wards and free-lunch counters of flies and rats. The rubbish and trash provide the housing. This goes on from home holding for collection, through filthy collection containers, vehicles, and transfer stations, to disposal sites and facilities. In warm climates exposed garbage has been found to produce as many as 70,000 flies per cubic foot in a week. Home refuse cans with accumulated residues and loose garbage have produced over 1,000 fly larvae per week, with one champion can providing over 20,000 larvae in 1 week. These larvae seed the dumps and complete their cycle there. Some leave the cans through corroded bottoms and split seams. Disease transmission by flies and rats is in the chapter on vector control.

Some culex mosquitoes are wastewater breeders and will breed in dirty water pools in dumps. *Aedes aegypti* is a fastidious clean-water breeder. On dumps she can use rainwater accumulations in cans, bottles, and tires. With a short flight range, such discarded or stored items in backyards are more likely sources of this highly domesticated mosquito which transmits yellow fever and dengue. The implications of buried solid wastes for ground- and surface-water pollution are documented by pollution in Illinois groundwater and in North Carolina tributary streams. Buried solid wastes are troublesome in particular instances. The extent of such pollution and the intensity of it are miniscule compared with untreated and undertreated municipal sewage and the prodigious quantities of industrial and agricultural wastes that reach our water sources.

Air pollution from uncontrolled burning dumps and overloaded incinerators are common and apparent to near neighbors. The most reknowned has been the Kennilworth dump outside of Washington, D.C. Its smoky, stinking pall has made itself known in motion pictures, TV broadcasts, and the Congressional Record. An air pollution emissions inventory in St. Louis, Missouri, and six surrounding counties covering over 3,500 mi^2 in 1966 showed solid-wastes burning of all types to be major sources of aldehydes, benzo-α-pyrene, and particulates. In the case of open burning dumps and backyard incinerators, control for air pollution provides the added benefits of reducing fly and rat feeding, breeding, and harborage. A rather different health matter is the toll of injuries among solid-waste collectors and handlers, which in the United States is second to injuries of loggers and lumbermen. That is a severe health impairment to these 350,000 workers in public and private refuse work.

Esthetics and Resource Conservation

The esthetics of "managed" open dumps are negative and most offensive to near neighbors. The clandestine dumps along rural roads, at dead-end streets, along drainage canals, streams, railroad embankments, and at bridge abutments and highway culverts number at least 100 per county in the southeastern United States. These have regular patrons who generate the 12 percent of individual household wastes for which there is no collection service, public or private. At a home production of 3 lb per person per day this one-eighth of the United States' 200 million people must find a place for something like 37,000 tons of refuse each day. About one-half of that is burned on the homesite, which reduces the volume by 60 to 70 percent. A little goes to the home gardener's compost pile. Farmers usually burn and dump on site in some gully or off in the woods or brush. Some gets to roadside collection cans.

More offensive is the litter dropped at the point of no further use on our streets, roads, beaches, parks, drive-ins, hallways, public rooms, and gathering places of every sort except churches, synagogues, and mosques. Careless convenience prevails. The answer to the radio-TV blurb, "Litter makes you sick. Are you sick enough to stop?" is a large, silent, "No." The annual cost of picking up our own public mess in urban areas is about $1 per citizen per year—New York City, $1.12; Philadelphia, $1; Lincoln, Nebraska, $1.30; Washington, D.C., $1.75—as the locals pay for the patriotic tourists' leavings. Each year pickup along state highways alone costs Florida

$850,000; Maine $200,000; Massachusetts $750,000; Missouri $484,000; Oregon $600,000; Texas $1,500,000. These 1970 figures have been rising 10 percent per year. The national bill for litter pickup is estimated at one-half billion dollars a year.

The resource conservation view of solid wastes presents the paradox of wanting to conserve the natural resource materials, as ores, pulpwood, and rubber, by recycling, yet of opposing the use of natural sites for disposal from a desire to preserve wildlife and to reduce the risk of residues changing water, air, and soil characteristics. Composting is one of the few disposal methods that gets strong conservationist support. The economics of salvage and recycling materials is a larger paradox in the United States. It would appear that the salvage of the 180 million motor vehicle tires and of the 11 billion bottles discarded each year would be readily profitable. Such has not been the case in this country. Development efforts on tire salvage by two major manufacturers began in 1970. Firestone is at the pilot plant stage for recovering chemicals and raw materials from used tires. Goodyear has a process for converting the rubber to carbon black required in new tires. If all manufacturers used it, 60 million tires, one-third of the annual discard, could be processed to carbon black. No use has been found for the rubber-coated wire and fabric that is a waste from the rubber recovery. The nonreturnable bottle has been a prime target of antilitter efforts. In 1970 the Glass Container Manufacturers Institute started bottle redemption centers and had 100 operating in 25 states. Remelt requires sorting according to types of glass, coloring agents, and additives to provide specific qualities. Before such efforts can be part of the whole technology, the initial product will have to be designed and fabricated to facilitate recovery and reprocessing. The costs of labor, materials, manufacture, and transportation have been driving technology toward single-use throwaway products. Only raw-material price increases, disposal taxes, penalties, or subsidies for recycling can reverse the trend in the next decade. In the next several decades recycling will become a necessity as reprocessing becomes less costly than getting the raw materials from increasingly distant and inaccessible places and from high labor cost sources. Five hundred years of colonialistic development of areas which western men called frontiers—yielding raw materials easily and cheaply, and accepting manufactured goods in a controlled market—is nearing an end. Only the polar regions and ocean beds can provide a renewal at a much greater capital investment and possibly with environmental controls imposed on extraction methods.

Since World War II, salvaging has been on the decline in three European countries where it had been practiced assiduously and profitably: the United Kingdom, the Netherlands, and West Germany. C. A. Rogus[1] states the reasons:

1 The manual sorting to get the salvables is prohibitively costly and insanitary.
2 Paper reuse has declined with the use of synthetics.

[1] *Public Works*, **93**:162 (1962).

3 Ink buildup in recycled newsprint requires de-inking.
4 Recovery of dirty, oily textiles has become unprofitable.
5 Recycling scrap metal has had an adverse effect on the properties of steel.

The salvage of cloth wastes has dropped in the United States as the valuable part was natural fibers, i.e., cotton, wool, and linen.   These are now woven with synthetics such as dacron, rayon, the acetates, and nylon, which makes recovery difficult, costly, and unprofitable.

PHASES AND CHOICES

Handling at the Source and Storage

Changes from the kitchen can and yard can for pickup are under-the-sink garbage grinders and treated-paper or plastic-film bags for pickup storage.   Garbage grinders handle food wastes only, not cans, paper, plastics, or glass.   These require the usual storage and holding for other handling.   It is a serious limitation.   Two community-wide installations of home grinders have been Jasper, Indiana, and the Short Hills development outside of Chicago.   The Jasper use was planned with a new sewage treatment plant sized to handle the added settleable solids and increased BOD (bio-chemical oxygen demand).   The Jasper use has been satisfactory despite the necessity to increase the frequency of collection for other household rubbish, which was planned to be monthly.   The accumulations were too great, and fly and rat infestation increased.   Weekly collections suffice.

Since 1963, plastic film bags of high tensile strength have become widely marketed. Santa Clara, California, has coupled plastic-bag use to its collection system.   It is the reduced collection handling that effects a savings, particularly when the home occupant must place the bags at curbside.   As early as 1965, one-half of Sweden's municipalities were using paper bags for holding their solid wastes.   The cost of the bags ranges from 8 to 12 cents.

The handling of solid wastes in apartment buildings continues to be awkward, messy, and costly.   New York tenement houses of 60 to 100 units of the first third of this century had dumbwaiters to move occupants' cans to the basement for transfer of the contents to collection cans.   The second third of the century brought larger and higher apartments with flue-chute incinerators in each vertical grouping.   Even without a thought for the air pollution from poor combustion, such incinerators have stoppages and filthy accumulations on side walls and joints, and they leave the poorly burned combustibles and noncombustibles for removal and collection.

One immediate alternative is to use the flues as simple transfer chutes of bagged rubbish. In high-rent units, garbage grinders take the putrescibles to the sanitary sewer. On-site compactors with detachable containers for transfer pickup are coming into use in the garden type of apartment developments. These provide a volume reduction of about 2 or 3 to 1. Special pickup vehicles are required. Smaller compactors for volume reduction before can or bag filling are available for basement use. The limit is the weight and size of the container a man must move and lift to get it into the collector truck.

Shopping centers, retail stores, and other buildings produce large quantities of bulky paper and plastic wastes. Transfer to large storage containers for pickup and replacement or for transfer by special loaders, such as the Dempster Dumpster system, have provided neat deposit and storage facilities. Regular cleaning is a necessity. The squirt of deodorant disinfectant provided from the transfer pickup truck unit is a palliative, not a substitute for hose-down and steam cleaning. The frequency required depends on the amount of food wastes and wet wastes deposited. Fly and rat attraction cannot be dismissed, as doors are left open or become poor-fitting with careless handling. The bulk of the wastes, mechanical transfer, and advantage of increasing the weight of hauled material has resulted in stationary packers and transfer containers, as already noted for garden-apartment areas. The packers apply up to 30 lb/in^2 to crush bulky waste and to compact most components to one-third of original volume. The transfer containers can either be picked up and replaced, or the contents tipped into a compactor-hauler truck. Stationary packer units make the rubbish inaccessible to desultory scavengers by sealed doors and the compaction provided. Loose litter is reduced.

Stationary packer units are useful in hospitals, which have solid wastes with particular characteristics and hazards. Any infectious matter must be separated for disinfection or complete burning. Any radioactive wastes require carefully controlled handling under supervision of a radiological health specialist. Even with care for these, there are numerous single-use ampules, syringe-needle packets, glass and plastic containers with traces of every variety of pharmaceutical material, endless throwaway paper products, dressings, bandages, and cast discards.[1]

The food wastes from restaurants and institutional feeding facilities are usually attractive and profitable for separate collection and cooking for hog feeding. Scrupulous cleaning of containers and handling areas is a necessity during storage and pickup. Garbage grinding and sewer disposal is the alternative. There is less cleaning, but there is loss of the food-waste use. The growing use of plastic eating ware and molded compartment trays in institutions is reducing uneaten-food recovery, as the entire unit goes to waste without plate scraping or machine washing.

[1] Environmental Aspects of the Hospital, vol. 2: Supportive Departments, *Public Health Serv. Publ.* 930-C-16, 1967, pp. 20–28.

Collection and Transportation

Table 6-2 shows the magnitude of solid-waste collection in the United States, and some of the significant issues of collection. The fact that 64 percent of our population is provided with some form of collection service means that our urban and suburban areas are covered. The 36 percent unserved remainder is about the same as our rural farm and rural nonfarm population, which in the 1970 census was 31 percent of our people. The distribution percentage among public, private, and self-collection service makes clear that the private operations are very large even in the household service. The self-service among householders and commercial waste producers is too large for assurance of sanitary handling, as these are rarely equipped to do a satisfactory job.

It is surprising that one-third of our population is still required to separate their wastes into such components as food wastes and containers, paper, and ashes. Many such regulations date to the early 1900s when municipalities tried food recovery for hogs, paper for salvage, and ashes for fill. The present composition and market make separation at the household antiquated, unnecessary, and ridiculous. In fact, collectors in municipalities requiring separation have been seen placing all the " carefully " separated wastes in the same packer truck, dutifully pressing it into one mass for transport to the land disposal site.

With 48 percent of the people served already by a once per week collection, the frequency of collection is going down. Less putrescible matter, packer trucks, higher

Table 6-2 **CHARACTERISTICS OF COLLECTION OF SOLID WASTES IN THE UNITED STATES FOR THE 64 PERCENT OF ITS POPULATION HAVING COLLECTION SERVICE**

Collection of solid wastes	By public service	By private contract	By self-service
From households	56%	32%	12%
From commercial sources	25%	65%	10%
From industry	13%	57%	30%
Refuse components for collection	Are separated 33%	Are combined 56%	Use both means 11%
Frequency of collection	Once/week 48%	Twice/week 32%	Other 20%
Number of vehicles	Compactor type 93,000	Other 179,000 (This number includes 80,000 used for street cleaning)	
Population per vehicle	2,100	1,100	

SOURCE: National Survey of Community Solid Wastes, *U.S. Public Health Serv.*, 1968.

labor costs, longer hauls to disposal sites or transfer stations, and better management analysis are reasons for less frequent collections of household wastes. There have been major studies on collection by simulated mathematical models and systems approaches. In Simulation and Analyses of a Refuse Collection System,[1] J. E. Quon, A. Charnes, and S. J. Werson use nine parameters in preparing graphs, equations, and flow sheets to plan and analyze collection patterns. In a Johns Hopkins study completed in 1968, M. M. Truitt, J. C. Liebman, and C. W. Kruse developed and tested three models for Baltimore. The differences in cost with frequency changes are predictable for various quadrants of the city. C. G. Golueke and P. H. McGauhey examine all facets of solid wastes from the standpoint of systems analysis (Ref. 6-3).

Three innovations in collection which are aimed at lowering costs and getting the most ton-miles from high-cost packer trucks are collection trains, scooter pickups, and packers manned by a single person who drives and collects. The first two cover assigned areas and rendezvous with a packer manned solely by a driver. Packer trucks designed for one-man handling include dual drives, left and right or front and rear controls, operation from standing position, low side-feeder points, and sizing to routes. Experiences with the "one-man crew" are reported by Ralph Stone and Company, Los Angeles.[2]

The exhaustion of close-in land disposal sites and the failure to acquire sites before either rising land costs or near-neighbor resistance to solid-waste disposal in their territory has lengthened the haul from collection routes to disposal. Rising labor costs and capital cost of packer trucks have caused a look for an alternative to the special-purpose vehicle and a three to five man crew enroute to and from the disposal site for an hour or more per trip. The response is transfer stations where collectors dump their loads into bins. These loads are transferred, with or without additional or second compaction, to trailer units from 35 to 60 yd^3 capacity for towing to the distant disposal point. Route compaction achieves about 300 lb/yd^3. With more powerful transfer-station equipment, 700 lb/yd^3 is gained. Further advantage can be gained by pulverizing and baling. This combination can produce solid wastes for transfer at over 1,500 lb/yd^3. That is at least a tenfold compaction of mixed solid wastes at their origin. It opens new options of rail transport for final disposal at sites such as mine pits, exhausted quarries, and possibly stacking in a desert. Transfer stations require a high quality of supervision to get a maximum return on the capital cost of the equipment and site, and from the crew manning the station. Cleanliness is a necessity to prevent neighbor objections to mess, odor, rats, and flies. This is not only important for present stations, but to prevent objections to proposed locations for new stations. Good maintenance of all equipment including vehicles reduces

[1] *J. Sanit. Eng. Div., Am. Soc. Civil Engrs.*, **91**:17 (1965).
[2] A Study of Solid Waste Collection Systems Comparing One-Man with Multi-Man Crews, *U.S. Public Health Serv. Publ. 1892, 1969.*

objectionable noise.   Site design with minimum grades and shielding shrubbery and banks along with the selection of sound-deadening materials reduces noise.   Limited data show that the total cost of capitalizing and operating a transfer station in 1970 is from $2 to $3 per ton with full use of capacity and effective management.

Rail transportation from transfer stations to disposal sites has been more fancy than fact to 1970.   Los Angeles has moved some of its wastes by rail for many years. Proposals have been examined in detail with contract offers exchanged among public officials, railroad management, and contract haulers in Denver, Milwaukee, Philadelphia, and San Francisco.   The transportation contracts carry the hauling cost to cents per ton with proposals of $4.61 per ton to Denver and to Milwaukee of $6.23 per ton.   For the latter, a countywide service, eliminating several small town incinerators, could use rail transport at a cost of $2 per ton less than a modern nonpolluting central incinerator.   Philadelphia has transfer-station buildings which fit into a rail transport plan.

First-stage Disposal

The modifier *first* replaces the word *final* in the usual refuse-handling lexicon.   The eight methods listed in Table 6-3 with their advantages and disadvantages are no longer final in communities where land use, water use, and air use have been intensified by the concentration of people and places, and by an increased sensitivity and demand for less casual and careless use of our environmental assets.   Each method in Table 6-3 produces new residuals which claim and must find some bit of the assimilative capacity of our environment for man-made wastes.

Efforts to get compliance with requirements for cooking food wastes before feeding to hogs for the purpose of trichinosis control were nil until the 1960s.   The only beneficiary would have been man, in the view of the hog raisers.   That would not have been worth the added cost.   Then vesicular exanthema (VE) hit the United States hog population in a swift epizootic.   It became clear that food-waste feeding of pork scraps was a factor in the VE transmission cycle back to hogs.   Control of VE and of hog cholera are supported by cooking man's food wastes before feeding to hogs. Equipment and operational control requirements for cooking have resulted in a fewer number of larger organizations in the business of recycling man's food wastes to new fresh food.

Air pollution emissions, high maintenance costs, often residential growth out to, and around, the incinerator, outstripping the design capacity, and uncertain results due to wide variations of combustibles are factors which spelled the doom of the incinerators built in the United States before World War II.   Many had been built during a nationwide public works expansion in the late 1930s.   As interest in the

Table 6-3 FIRST–STAGE DISPOSAL METHODS OF SOLID WASTES

Methods	Advantages	Disadvantages
Hog feeding	Revenue from contract or from hog sale. Salvage and conservation.	Trichinosis transmission. Fly and rat feeding and breeding. Separate disposal of rubbish. Necessity of supervising contractor. Hog diseases must be controlled.
Incineration	Combustion of breeding materials. Takes combined garbage and rubbish. Can be very efficient and run 24 h/day in large cities.	Final ash residue, cans, and bottles remain. High capital investment. High operational and maintenance cost. Particulates and odors from poor operation. Often requires addition of combustibles.
Open dumps	Hauling is only cost. Combined collection.	Optimum for rat and fly breeding. Neighborhood depreciation. Mosquito breeding. Air pollution from dump fires. Water pollution from leaching.
Dumping at sea	Combined collection.	Cost of tugs, barges, and operation. Float back to beaches and shores. Possible toxicity to fish and flora.
Grinding and adding to sewage	Gives garbage same handling as excreta. For home units, collection phase of food wastes is eliminated.	Takes only garbage. Requires proper sewer design if home units are used. Requires added sewage plant facilities for central grinding and treatment. Rats appear in sewers. Digested solids must be handled.
Sanitary landfill	Combined collection. Low capital investment. Moderate operational cost. Land reclamation for restricted use. Adapted to small towns.	Land requirement may result in long hauls in the future. Requires selected soil for cover. Requires standby fire control. Leaching adds pollutants to ground- and surface-water sources.
Composting	Conserves and recylces wastes. Provides humus for soil. Decomposition heat controls flies. Aerobic action free of odors. Sewage sludge can be combined.	Requires presorting and grinding and turning. High capital equipment and maintenance cost. Requires assured market for compost. Requires disposal of noncompostables. Requires carbon : nitrogen ratio of about 30 : 1.
Salvage	Recovery of usable and salable material. Conservation of resources. Defrays cost of waste handling.	Limited to special wastes and selected materials. At mercy of market.

incinerator option is again strong, incinerator designers and builders face three questions:

1 Can the air pollutants be controlled?
2 Can the new combinations of solid wastes be burned without producing combustion products that damage the grates, fire brick, breeching, and pollution control units?
3 How much will still be left, including the air pollutants trapped, filtered, or washed from the gas stream?

The incinerator issues are capsulated in this quotation from George J. Kupchik.[1]

> Does this indicate apathy, indifference or incompetence in our planning and engineering personnel? Not at all. Several are suffering from chronic frustration bordering on psychosis. Our primary problem has been local community resistance to any sanitation facility, be it garage, transfer station, salt shed, sanitary landfill or incinerator site. And the politicians who determine the priorities for expenditure of city funds have postponed, vitiated, studied and outrightly rejected projects that might be unpopular with a segment of the voting population, however small.
>
> Finally though, in August 1968, after 10 years of debate and indecision a site was approved for our first superincinerator, a 3,200 ton per day waste heat recovery plant. Preliminary designs which have just been completed indicate a capital outlay of $72 million for this installation. We have also managed to get a small piece of the old Brooklyn Navy Yard as a site for another superincinerator, a 6,000 ton per day steam generating plant. Although only in early preliminary design, the estimated cost is more than $120 million. We know we will need at least three additional superincinerators at 5,000 tons per day capacity, and are exploring sites in remote locations where there will be a minimum of flack from residents. After selection of a site, time required for construction of an incinerator is approximately 5 to 6 years.

Despite formidable design, operational, and capital cost factors, large cities in the United States and Western Europe again are resorting to incinerators, complete with air pollution controls and, it is to be hoped, with some heat recovery. Another quotation from George Kupchik's paper in the American Journal of Public Health states the case very well from the firing line. He was Assistant Commissioner of Sanitation in New York City at that time.

> Now, what about our operating problems? As I mentioned before, because of new air pollution regulations we have closed three of our four batch-fed pre-World War II incinerators. For the seven modern traveling grate installations we must provide control devices to reduce particulate emissions to less than 26 lbs. per 20,000 lbs. of refuse charged per hour. Because we could find no device that had been applied to our type of incinerator, and because of the extreme urgency, we contracted to spend $1.6 million to build three prototype devices, a wet scrubber, a Research-Cotrell electrostatic precipitator and a Wheelabrator (Lurgi) electrostatic precipitator. These have only recently been put "on line" and emissions have yet to be tested. After six

[1] *Am. J. Public Health*, **61**:359 (1971).

months of operating experience, the most effective device will be installed at all 24 additional furnaces, at a cost approximating $20 million.

Our incinerator grates have been deteriorating ("burning out") at a very rapid rate. Perhaps this is due to heats of extremely high intensity developed by burning plastics or aluminum. We are sponsoring a study to determine the causes and possible preventive measures. We are constantly involved in restoring furnace grates and refractory walls, replacing cooling jackets, air-conditioning crane cabs, etc.

A conventional incinerator fueled by the wastes reaches temperatures of 1300 to 1500°F. Metals and glass are scorched, not melted or burned. The unburned materials and ash are 20 percent by volume of the original and must be handled further. The super, high-temperature incinerators use supplemental fuels, oil or pulverized coal, to reach 3000°F. The end solid product is a fine ash. Metal and glass have been oxidized, melted, vaporized, and recondensed to a fine frit. This has by-product use as first-class fill and cover, masonry aggregate, and road subgrade material. Liquid wastes from incinerators include drainings from the stored wastes, quench waters from ash channels and pits, and wastewaters from wet scrubbers used to clean the gas stream for air cleaning.

Open dumps have no place in the theory or rhetoric of solid-waste technology. These have an abundant frequency in practice, including those under municipal and private contractor auspices along with the millions of clandestine roadside dumps. In the United States, 30 percent of land disposal is reported as "open dumps." The thing that recommends their existence is no cost after dumping. There are some euphemisms, for example, "controlled dumps" and "controlled dump burning." These translate to: "When the complaints become threats, some palliative action is taken to cover partly and to contain the spread of the mess." The most damaging consequence of partially controlled dumps has been that these have been passed off as sanitary landfills. The municipal officials have their day of reckoning on the next round of land acquisition for what is declared to be a new sanitary landfill site. The new, more articulate neighbors fight the proposed acquisition to a standstill with photographs and visits to the ones long standing as monuments of bad practice. Their evidence is rats, smoke, stinks, and loose, light paper and plastic film dispersed by the winds.

The practice of dumping at sea is no longer a means to dispose of collected mixed bulk refuse from oceanside cities and towns by barging to over-shore points for dumping. Bitter complaints through the summer from beach users and resort owners and from surf fishermen throughout the year paid off as marine hauling costs mounted and hauls extended farther to sea. Our oceans continue to get large quantities of raw sewage sludge barged to sea and dumped. Some of New York's sewage treatment plants have no alternatives, given their present sites, processes, and equipment. Indeed there may have to be more of selective ocean disposal, despite good and pious intentions to keep the ocean waters pristine. Some disposal under planned procedures can be beneficial.   The reef of automobile bodies dumped off Long Island at Sheepshead Bay has provided much needed protection for fish to spawn and grow.   The reuse of our solid wastes as food and harborage for marine life is worth studying.

Addition to sewage of the garbage fraction of solid wastes is provided for the food wastes of homes equipped with under-the-sink grinders and for those few cities which grind the collected garbage fraction at the sewage treatment plant.   In the 1950s the marketing of home grinders prompted several studies of the effects of these added solids on sewage treatment processes.   The largest single community installation was 900 home units, 75 percent of the homes, in 1952 in Jasper, Indiana.   That choice was triggered by an outbreak of hog cholera among garbage-fed hogs which reduced the number of contractors for the town's garbage to zero.   The sewage treatment plant in design at the time was provided with a 50 percent increase in aeration and 60 percent increase in sludge digesting and drying capacities.   These added capacities have been adequate.   K. S. Watson and C. M. Clark reported that Aurora, Colorado, where 65 percent of the homes have garbage grinders, had a 30 percent increased loading on its digesters at its sewage treatment plant.[1]   The number of grinders in Aurora was nearly 10 times the 900 originally installed in Jasper in 1952.   As grinders have come down in cost from about $150 to $200 in 1960 to between $25 and $85 in 1970, the number of installations are increasing despite the reduction in food-waste quantities in United States homes.   Sewage treatment processes can handle the added load and are being designed to do so.   Home septic tank systems with added tank volume and subsurface absorption line capacity can handle the added loads from home-ground garbage.   Watson found water use up 1 to 2 percent, suspended solids up 26 percent, BOD up 17 percent, and grease up 35 percent.[2]

A disagreeable and potentially hazardous result of transporting the home-ground-food wastes in public sewers is the increased number of rats in sewers attracted and fed by the fluid conveyor-belt "cafeteria."   Cleveland and Philadelphia have added regular rat killing to their sewer maintenance, using special baits and poisons suspended through manholes.   Commercial vendors of rat poisons have responded to the needs with paraffin-impregnated briquettes and handy holders.   Another consideration is the added pollution of the waterways when grinders are used in homes on combined sewer systems.   Such systems sometimes discharge without treatment.   In areas of New York City where combined sewers continue in use, garbage grinders are illegal.

Grinding of the municipal garbage collection for combination with a town's sewage at the treatment plant was first tried in Southampton, England, in 1885.   In the 1940s and 1950s, the process was reported in favorable use in Goshen, England, and Richmond, Indiana, and in experimental use at Lansing, Michigan.   The operat-

[1] *Public Works*, **93**:105 (1962).
[2] *J. Water Pollution Control Federation*, **39**:2039 (1967).

ing ratios of ground garbage to sewage sludge and their changes vary considerably. A doubling of solids, an increase in BOD of 15 to 30 percent, and a lower methane and higher carbon dioxide percentage in the sludge gas can be expected.   The green garbage adds to organic acid production during digestion.   Careful control to prevent a pH drop below 6.8 is required to protect the methane-generating bacteria from extinction. More scum and grease separates in the digester.   The digester supernatant liquor is viler.

In 1934, rough land in Fresno, California, was reclaimed for farming by filling with the city's refuse, compacting it with a crawler tractor, and covering it with 30 in of soil.   Sanitary landfill had begun.   Since then, this most widely used, controlled method has changed only in site preparation, a constant effort to get greater compaction to conserve area, a much thinner cover, and a variety of after uses as parks, sporting fields, light-aircraft fields, and highly selective, limited building sites.   The United States Army adopted the method for its proliferation of World War II training camps.   The U.S. Public Health Service studied the military practice and recommended it for civilian adoption.   After World War II, cities and towns welcomed it as a change from overloaded incinerators that had received little maintenance during the war because of shortages of men and material.   The method thrives despite two continuing struggles:

1 Keeping the landfill sanitary
2 Acquiring low-cost new sites within economical hauling distances from collection or transfer points.

Figures 6-3, 6-4, and 6-5 show the method in its three most usual techniques. The figures and captions illustrate the essential needs of space in which to dump the wastes, a heavy vehicle to compact the mess, and earth to cover and seal the packed wastes at the end of each day.   The trench method is used on level areas in which the final grade will be 6 to 8 ft above the original elevation.   The trench cut provides the space and cover material.   It most readily provides separation into cells by leaving undisturbed strips between parallel trenches.   The ramp method can be used across varied terrain, moving forward in a series of sloped cells.   The area method pushes fill forward onto land and often requires bringing the earth to cover it from other sites or from cutting down nearby high ground.   The continuous compaction of the refuse and daily cover with well-compacted earth keeps out rats and flies.   With optimal loamy clay, fly larvae cannot emerge through as little as 2 in of well-compacted cover. Figures 6-6 and 6-7 show the types of equipment in use.

Landfills should not penetrate groundwater strata which are actual or potential sources of domestic or irrigation waters.   Landfills should not drain to surface waters for which beneficial use does not permit a high of dissolved solids content and contamination with organic acids.   California State Water Pollution Control Board

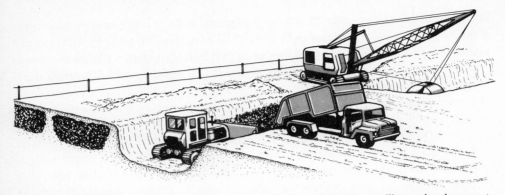

The waste collection truck deposits its load into the trench where the bulldozer will spread and compact it. At the end of the day, the dragline will excavate soil from the future trench, and this soil will be used as the daily cover material. Trenches can also be excavated with a front-end loader, bulldozer, or scraper.

FIGURE 6-3
Trench method of sanitary landfill. [*Source: Sanitary Landfill Facts*, *U.S. Public Health Serv. Publ.* 1792, 1968, *p.* 6.]

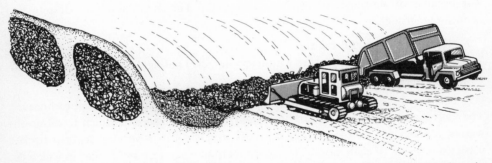

The solid wastes are being spread and compacted on a slope. The daily cell may be covered with earth scraped from the base of the ramp. This variation is used with either the area or trench method.

FIGURE 6-4
Ramp method of sanitary landfill.　[*Source: Sanitary Landfill Facts*, *U.S. Public Health Serv. Publ.* 1792, 1968, *p.* 6.]

Publication number 1954 reported that continuous leaching from each acre-foot of a sanitary landfill will extract 1.5 tons of Na and K, 1 ton of Ca and Mg, 0.9 ton of Cl^-, 0.2 ton of SO_4^{--}, and 3.9 tons of HCO_3^- in a year or less.　It is the CO_2 from the decomposing waste which forms the solvent, dilute carbonic acid.　The acid extracts these components from waste and soil to be carried to the groundwater. Dissolved-mineral concentrations were observed to increase twentyfold in groundwater in contact with landfills, and ammonia nitrogen to 10,000 times the baseline values.

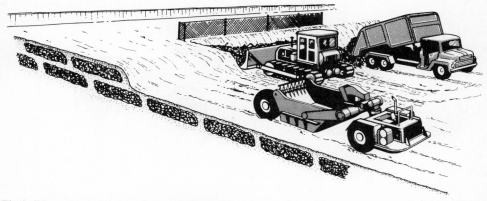

The bulldozer is spreading and compacting a load of solid wastes. The scraper (foreground) is used to haul the cover material at the end of the day's operations. Note the portable fence that catches any blowing debris; these are used with any landfill method, whenever necessary.

FIGURE 6-5
Area method of sanitary landfill. [*Source*: *Sanitary Landfill Facts*, *U.S. Public Health Serv. Publ.* 1792, 1968, p. 6.]

Increased BOD also comes from fills.   Fills to reclaim swamp lands, tidal flats, and flood plains will add to the pollutant loads on the waters which the fill drains to or contacts.   As such waters are often of little or low beneficial use, the added pollution is accepted in exchange for the beneficial use of the reclaimed land.

There is limited and quite variable information on the decomposition processes in the thousands of sanitary landfills, some in being for 30 years. Settlement is variable, with some showing only slight settlement and others as much as 1.5 ft in the first 2 to 3 years.   The emissions of methane, carbon dioxide, and ammonia nitrogen indicate that the anaerobic bacterial processes dominate. The production of these discharges accelerates slowly for the first 1 to 2 years and then shows a most variable sort of equilibrium.   Landfills should be well marked and recorded with land-survey precision to avoid unknowing penetration or use and to pinpoint the sites when the investigation of air and water pollution sources requires it.

Composting solid wastes depends on the same action as the home gardener's leaf compost pile or the farmer's manure pile.   It is an aerobic decomposition by bacteria and fungi.   With a favorable ratio of carbon to nitrogen of about 30 : 1 to ensure the nitrogen supply for the bacteria, and with turning to provide aeration, a prepared municipal waste is stabilized under ideal conditions to a dark humus in 20 to 30 days with a minimum of fly attraction, no fly breeding, and without odors.   The product is about one-half the weight or volume of the original placed in the compost pile.   It is not a balanced plant food, as it is deficient in phosphorous and potassium.   In some

Standard landfill equipment

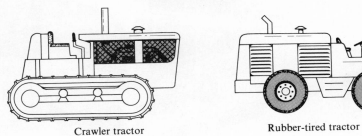

Crawler tractor   Rubber-tired tractor

Front end accessories

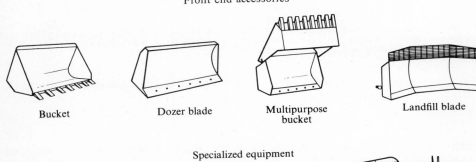

Bucket   Dozer blade   Multipurpose   Landfill blade
                                        bucket

Specialized equipment

Scraper

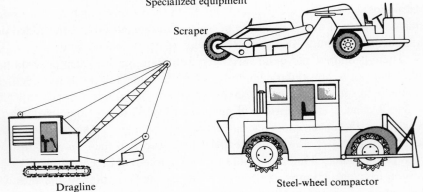

Dragline   Steel-wheel compactor

FIGURE 6-6
Equipment for sanitary landfill operation. [*Source*: *Sanitary Landfill Facts,*
U.S. Public Health Serv. Publ. 1792, 1968, *p.* 16.]

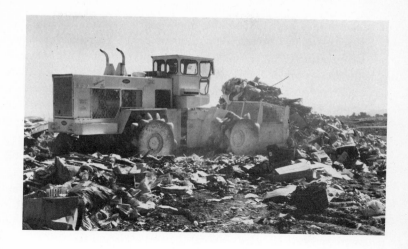

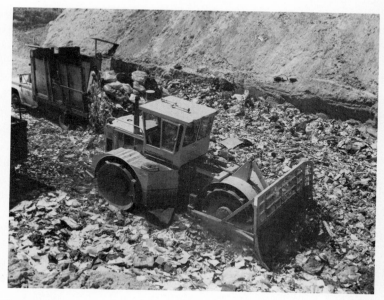

FIGURE 6-7
Specialized trash compactor for sanitary landfill in operation. [*Source: American Hoist and Derrick Company, St. Paul, Minn., and Rex Chainbelt Inc., Milwaukee, Wis.*]

instances it may have undesirable traces of toxic metals and residues of pesticides and weedicides.   It will be free of pathogens as the decomposition heat raises the inner pile temperature to 140°F (60°C) or more and sustains it for several days.   These facts plus the entries under composting, advantages, in Table 6-3 are the reasons the process has continued to attract interest, effort, and capital over the years around the world, in Japan, Thailand, South Africa, Israel, Switzerland, West Germany, Holland, England, Scotland, France, and among the adventurous and hopeful in the United States.

For the last 50 years there have been several mechanical devices to accelerate the decomposition process by continuous stirring and turning in one way or another. These seek to reduce the time from 3 weeks for natural turned-windrow stabilization to 3 to 5 days.   The methods carry the names of their inventors such as Dano, Fairfield-Hardy, Frazer-Eweson, Riker, and for the exception, the Indore process patented by Lord Howard.   What then has stymied the success of this disposal technique?   The disadvantages listed in Table 6-3 put the case succinctly.   Additionally, until the last couple of years the method has been advanced as a money-maker, profit from refuse.   A public mixed solid-waste collection must be sorted, shredded, rasped, or ground, the compostables stabilized, the rejects rehandled, the stable compost screened, and all taken to their final use or stored until demanded.   The sorting step carries a high labor cost and a salvage return dependent on the local price of recovered bottles and cans.   The plastics are wholly a liability.   These have been the major deterrent to an expansion of an excellent composting plant in Bangkok, Thailand. The present techniques of composting require a reduction in size of the organics to gain surface contact area, to aerate thoroughly, and to mix.   No wholly satisfactory equipment for shredding, rasping, or grinding has been built.   The Dutch have the nearest thing to it in power, capacity, metallurgical resistance, and mechanical reliability.   A Dorr-Oliver rasper performs well if the plastic film is removed at the sorting belt.   The noise around any of these units is horrendous.

After composting, whether by the 20 to 30 day "natural" windrow system or by one of the mechanically accelerated processes, the material must be screened to remove noncompostable residues and to form a granulated compost.   A profitable market for the compost has been a hypothesis of composting advocates.   It has rarely been a reality.   Two exceptions are the product from a plant in Israel, where the compost goes to a desert reclamation project, and a series of plants in West Germany, where the compost is used to retain the soil quality of the steep sloped vineyards which produce prized grapes for wine.   Even the tight land economy of Holland, which until 1965 had 25 to 30 percent of the country's solid wastes composted, has not prevented the retreat to incineration for the mounting quantities of wastes from its major cities, mainly because of the mounting costs of composting and hauling.   The fate of composting plants in the United States is given in Table 6-4.   It has been estimated that

with an acceptable pricing and distribution procedure, all land requirements for compost use in the United States would only require the composting of 1 to 2 percent of
the country's total solid waste.   Even if this estimate is off by a factor of 5, composting
cannot be regarded as a major means of first-stage disposal for the rest of this century.

Table 6-3 fairly presents the advantages and disadvantages of salvage as a phase
of waste handling.   Its use in the United States for public mixed collections is limited
to metal salvage from the grate droppings after incineration.   The statements do not
suggest the magnitude and extent of salvage of metals and animal products in the
United States.   The total salvage value is $5 to $7 billion per year.   The greatest part
is in four nonferrous metals: copper, lead, zinc, and aluminum.   Recovered copper
provides 40 percent of the total annual United States requirement and is equal to
80 percent of our new domestically mined output.   Recovered aluminum makes up
25 percent of our total annual requirement.   This recovery is 1 billion tons of copper,
$\frac{1}{2}$ billion tons of lead, and $\frac{1}{4}$ billion tons of zinc per year.   Much of this is scrap from
fabrication shops, building demolition, and for the lead, from dead storage batteries.
If the material has a high market price, is quite accessible, and can be readily processed
from waste to reuse form, it will be salvaged.

For countries which must import pulp and paper, recycling of paper wastes is an
item in the balance of imports and exports.   Japan recovers 46 percent of its waste
paper, and West Germany 33 percent.   In the United Kingdom, the largest importer
of pulp and finished paper products, there has been a drive to increase its recycled
percentage from the 27 percent level.   That percentage is low for a heavy importer, as

Table 6-4   MUNICIPAL SOLID–WASTE COMPOSTING PLANTS IN THE UNITED STATES

Location	Process	Capacity, tons/day	Began operation	1965 status
Altoona, Pa.	Fairfield-Hardy	45	1961	Operating
Largo, Fla.	Peninsular Organics	50	1963*	Operating
Norman, Okla.	Naturizer	35	1959	Closed 1964
Phoenix, Ariz.	Dano	300†	1963	Closed 1963‡
Sacramento Co., Calif.	Dano	40	1956	Closed 1963
San Fernando, Calif.	Naturizer	70	1963§	Closed 1964
Springfield, Mass.	Frazer-Eweson	20	1954¶	Closed 1962
Williamston, Mich.	Riker	4	1955	Closed 1962
Wilmington, Ohio	Windrow	20	1963	Operating

* Date of initial operation of the original Hardy plant is unknown; plant rebuilt in 1963.
† According to European Dano practice, the plant capacity is about 175 tons/day.
‡ Reported to be back in limited operation, March 1965.
§ Date of initial operation is unknown; continuous operation began in July 1963.
¶ Partially burned in 1958; rebuilt in 1961.
(SOURCE: *Compost Science*, Summer 1965, p. 7.)

the United States recycles 25 percent of its raw material requirement.   That 25 percent is 10 million tons of paper stock which would have required the cutting and pulping of the trees from 13 million acres (over 20,000 mi^2) of forest and woodland.   That is an area greater than Vermont and New Hampshire.

Handling the Residues and Emissions

The review of the alternatives of first-stage disposal has cited the residues and emissions from incineration, sanitary landfill, and composting.   Salvage has its residues.   The printed page must be de-inked and that waste handled.   Copper wire must be stripped of its insulation, cans of their labels, and cars of their paint, upholstery, and under-coating.   Up to 20 percent by weight of a car must be stripped before its iron and steel are bared for return to the furnace.

Incinerators produce ashes and the stack waste of gases and particulates.   The stack gas cleaners produce particulates and if wet scrubbers or spray chambers are used, a polluted wastewater.   Quenching channels and pits for the ashes add to the incinerator wastewater.   Ash makes up the largest weight fraction and in a conventional incinerator equals 20 percent of the input by weight.   After magnetic separation of ferrous metals, the ash must be moved for use as fill or cover.   The wastewater goes to the sanitary sewer, presumably to the wastewater treatment plant.

For the first 25 years of their use, the leachate and gaseous discharges from sanitary landfills escaped notice, except in a few overt gassing problems and fill fires. As other land uses have moved out to surround the fills, and as water pollution sensitivity has increased, landfills are being examined suspiciously as water and air pollution sources.   The gas releases have produced toxic and explosive concentrations in buildings placed above completed fills, and also vilely odorous conditions in basements and crawl spaces.   The only general air pollution from a landfill is smoke when fires are allowed to go unchecked.   Our handling of wastes can only translocate and transform them to the least noxious state, or prepare them for reuse.   Even when buried well out of sight, the matter remains for change to new forms of matter or energy on nature's terms.

Costs of First-stage Disposal

Table 6-5 covers the ranges of capital and operating costs for the disposal of public mixed solid-wastes collections by sanitary landfill, incineration, and composting. Only the first two are in appreciable use in the United States, and at that, there were only 300 municipal incinerators operating in 1970.   The broad ranges reflect the economics of scale and the lack of uniformity in what is included in estimating such costs.   The range of costs is also determined by real differences in hourly rates for labor and the means and costs of financing capital works.   The data are sufficient to mark the high cost of the public service of solid-waste handling.   It requires only 400 people to generate a ton of wastes per day.   These disposal costs are in addition to the annual $8 to $10 per capita to collect the refuse.

AN AGRICULTURAL WASTE—ANIMAL MANURE

Two billion tons of animal manure are produced in the United States each year.   At a round figure of 200 million population, that is annually 10 tons per person.   Put on a BOD population equivalent, farm animal wastes are tenfold the BOD of human population.   Or, 1 dairy cow's daily manure has a BOD equivalent of from 12 to 16 people; 1 beef steer = 3 to 4 people; 1 hog = 2 people; 7 chickens = 1 person's BOD equivalent.   Fortunately about one-half of our manure production and most of these animals are still on the farm.   Two happenings are changing the relation between man and manure.   Suburban development moves urbanites close to and around farms.   In their nostalgia for the country life, these people have forgotten the grimier side of farm life: hog-pen drainage, chicken-coop stinks, and cow-manure flies. People are moving animals closer to and, in some cases, into the cities.   These are cattle feedlots, chicken egg-laying plants, and some broiler breeding houses.   Similarly, specialized production of animal protein on the farm concentrates thousands of animals in small areas.   Confinement chicken housing units accommodate as many as 100,000 chickens.   Confinement facilities are able to produce from 3,000 to 10,000 hogs per year in a single large installation.   Cattle feedlots prepare steers for specification steaks by selective nutrition.   In their last weeks of life the steers get the job done in areas of only 100 ft^2 per animal.   A single feedlot can bring from 3,000 to 6,000 steers a year to market readiness, lean, tender, and free of disease.   Cattle feedlots are already under state registration in Texas, Kansas, Iowa, Nebraska, and Colorado.

Table 6-5   CAPITAL AND OPERATING COSTS IN THE UNITED STATES FOR FIRST–STAGE DISPOSAL BY SANITARY LANDFILL, INCINERATION, AND COMPOSTING

Method	Capital cost for capacity/(ton)(day)	Operating cost per ton disposed
Sanitary landfill	$1,000–$2,000 (land cost not included)	$1.25–$2.25
Incineration	3,500– 7,000	3.50– 5.00
Composting	1,500– 10,000	2.00– 7.00

SOURCE: Waste Management and Control, Publication 1400, Committee of Pollution, National Academy of Sciences–National Research Council, Washington, D.C., 1966, p. 196.

Restoring the Quality of Our Environment (Ref. 1-5, pp. 170–171) recognized the magnitude of the manure disposal from our changing animal husbandry practices with this comment:

> Despite a modest amount of research, there is yet no single method generally satisfactory for the treatment and disposal of animal manure originating in confinement livestock operations.   Field spreading, composting, anaerobic digestion, incineration, lagooning, dehydration and other procedures have been attempted or proposed as possible disposal methods.   Some of the procedures have been successful in certain regions, but none is widely applicable.   Manure has often been disposed of by distribution to gardeners and greenhouse operators, but at the present time there is no market for the large volumes of manure produced annually.   The classical method of field spreading is often effective in preventing accumulation of the wastes, but the frequent scarcity or unavailability of land often eliminates this as a feasible means of disposal. Composting has often been successfully exploited by private companies for short periods of time, but these operations usually have been short-lived; moreover, the supply of manure far exceeds the demand for compost.   Each of the methods devised or suggested has its advantages, but each has distinct limitations, and more information is required before these procedures can be widely employed.

Characteristics and Effects

As the population equivalents indicate and as anyone's cursory experience reinforces, compared with the diluted form of human excreta in water-carried domestic sewage, animal manure is quite concentrated.   It has a low-moisture content and a high volatile solids value.   Cattle manure on a feedlot has a 25 to 30 percent solids content. After a nominal dilution by rainfall, the runoff waters of cattle feedlots have BODs of 2,000 to 9,000 mg/l.   Bacteria counts are prodigious.   Direct microscopic counts which include dead cells from rumen work are from 250 million to 2 billion/g.   Cultures for "total" counts show 20 to 40 million/g.   Coliform counts on eosin methylene-blue agar range from 350,000 to 600,000/g with 95 percent typical *Escherichia coli*.

Pathogenic bacteria are in animal excreta.   To survive, these need to get into dilution waters.   Leptospira were isolated from an Iowa river swimming site that produced 15 cases of leptospirosis.   Cattle carrying *Leptospira pomona* were on pasture and feeding areas in the drainage basin.   Duck farm drainage is a contributor of salmonella to natural waters with pollution of recreational areas recorded on Long Island and of oyster growing beds in Virginia.   Salmonella infections by fecal transfer trouble hog herds.   Salmonella are common in chickens, appearing in eggs and egg products and in the tissue of dressed birds.   The organisms are being recycled in feeds made of various animals' wastes to recover the high proteins.   Careless processing contaminates the feed.   Chicken manure has been the source of organisms causing human respiratory disease, including the fungus *Histoplasma capsulatum*, and variants of mycobacteria.   These are airborne from dry friable chicken droppings.   Chicken manure also contains As, Mn, and Zn which can locally contaminate surface waters and shallow groundwaters.   The high nitrate content of animal manure definitely raises the nitrate content of surface waters and local groundwaters.   Feedlot runoff has from 400 to 1,200 milligrams of nitrogen per liter.   One study showed ground-water to increase in N from 2 to 15 mg/l as it flowed under a barnyard.[1]

Stored animal manure in decomposition produces gases that are both malodorous and toxic to man and animals.   Enclosed storage areas become low in oxygen by dis-placement and depletion.   These conditions and hazards also are met in animal hous-ing that has slotted floors with manure storage below.   The casualties have been animals in their confinement area above the manure storage pits and unwary men going down into the storage areas.   The cases are precipitated by the unusual: venti-lating fan failure, mechanical aerator breakdown, water level not covering the dropped manure, natural ventilation blocked owing to extreme weather.   The chemical identity of the gases collected in a building housing hogs immediately signals the obvious stinks and treacherous hazards.   Analysis shows amines, amides, alcohols, sulfides, disulfides, carbonyls, and mercaptans.[2]

The changes to confinement housing of livestock have magnified two long-stand-ing by-products of manure accumulations: odors and flies.   The increase in fly popula-tions in California is ascribed to livestock concentrations that have moved nearer the cities and also to residential expansions toward the farms with their new livestock practices.   Manure is another source of soluble phosphates so threatening the eutro-phication of low-circulation ponds and lakes.   In frozen soil areas, the daily spread freezes in place until spring thaws and rains return.   Field studies have shown that this sudden natural release sends a surge of phosphates to streams and lakes.   Measure-ments in Wisconsin indicated that 75 percent of the phosphates from manure are released from the frozen winter-spread manure, and that 45 percent of the phosphates in Wisconsin lakes comes in with rural land runoff.   The more immediate effect of exhausting a stream's oxygen by heavy slugs of high-BOD wastes has been observed from cattle feedlot runoff.   The Kansas State Water Resources Board reported that in 1964, of the 27 fish kills, 15 were caused primarily by runoff slugs from commercial livestock feeding lots.   High ammonia nitrogen and low oxygen conditions in the streams result from runoff slugs.

Options for Management and Treatment

Table 6-6 outlines the options for handling animal manure.   After the choice of wet or dry handling there are options of storage method and of later disposal.   Wet handling is the more usual for cattle and hog manure, as these have a high moisture

---

[1] *J. Water Pollution Control Federation*, **41**:1752 (1969).
[2] *Trans. Amer. Soc. Agr. Eng.*, **12**(3):310 (1969).

content and considerable urine.   Dry handling is better fitted to chicken droppings. Cattle manure handled by composting is done from an as-is moisture content permitting or requiring the addition of other drier solid wastes.   Farm disposal is by field spreading with different methods suited to the manure condition, the volumes, and the land use.   Wet materials are placed by gravity spraying from tankers much like street flushers, or by pumping from storage to ridge and furrow irrigation.   Pumping to spray-nozzle irrigation lines has been unsatisfactory because of nozzle stoppage by particulates.   One option on the farm is to go directly from wet collection to an oxidation pond.   This has been quite successful in the Midwest on large hog farms. Some hog farms have used a combination of an anaerobic and an aerobic pond.

Wet handling of animal manure from confinement facilities includes bio-oxidation treatment.   Trickling filters have been satisfactory for treating cattle feedlot wastes, designed for high-BOD loads.   Oxidation ponds are in use, with mechanical or tube aeration when odors threaten.   Oxidation ditches, or more properly channels, are in increasing use in Europe for animal manure and other types of liquid wastes (Ref. 4-4, p. 170).   Manure handled dry from the outset and the inevitable settled solids from any bio-oxidation treatment except oxidation ponds offer the recovery of high-nutrient organic material.   The necessities are dewatering, dehydrating, grinding, and pulverizing.   Chicken droppings processed along with other chicken-dressings wastes, sometimes including feathers and dead birds and rejects, are going into animal feeds.   Such use requires a sterilizing treatment and care not to mix the raw and finished materials even inadvertently by mixed use of carts, portable conveyors, front-end loaders, and shovels.   The remaining choices of burial or burning substantially wastes the materials with a minimum recovery except by nature's long cycles.

Table 6-6   ANIMAL MANURE–MANAGEMENT OPTIONS

| Method | At the origin | Storage | Disposal | |
			On the farm	From confinement facilities
Wet handling	Flushing or slotted-floor drop to wet storage	Water-covered in tanks or pits with or without agitation and aeration	Field spread	Bio-oxidation, settled-solids handling, and dilution
Dry handling	Manual or mechanical removal	Dewater, dehydrate, or compost	Field spread	Process to animal feed or to fertilizer; incinerate

IMPROVEMENTS AND DEVELOPMENTS

Immediate Trends and Changes

In handling at the source, the following patterns will accelerate:

1   More use of stationary compactor units in commercial areas, shopping centers, hospitals, schools, and apartments.
2   More home garbage grinders, with less to grind, as these are a cheap sale-rental attraction for medium to high income buyers and renters. For apartments, grinders reduce the nuisances from putrescibles.
3   More use of plastic bags with a drop in can use for home storage. This will be accelerated as curbside collection replaces yard pickup to hold down collection costs.

In collection, the changes will come as:

1   One man as driver-collector becomes widely used in suburban low-density residential areas, with curb placement by the occupant required. Plastic bags facilitate the work of occupant and collector.
2   Transfer stations increase in number, with pulverizing to get up to 10 : 1 compaction and with baling for the maximum use of the secondary hauling vehicles.
3   Fees for collection at actual cost are required for certain classes of service such as commercial wastes, institutional wastes, and low-density residential area wastes. Hempstead Township, New York, found that collection costs varied from $77 to $168 per acre, dependent on density and length of the haul.

In first-stage disposal, the trends which will continue are:

1   Open dumps will decrease under the antipollution sentiment and pressure for real cause.
2   Incinerators will stage a return.   These will be larger, equipped with air cleaners, and provided with preshredders and separators.   The units with a capacity of 1,000 to 1,500 tons/day will have the benefit of the economics of scale and be equipped for heat recovery.
3   Sanitary landfills will require greater utilization of area now made possible by preshredding and high compaction to 1,000 to 1,500 lb/yd^3.   Sites will be carefully selected and managed to minimize pollution from the fill.
4   Salvage will be used more extensively by manufacturers and processors to offset the increased costs of pollution control and wastes management.   Salvage will

be facilitated as products are designed and fabricated to make recovery cheaper. An end-use disposal charge on the initial cost will accelerate the response between salvage and design.

Longer-range Developments, Real and Fancied

Two methods are in use in Europe for apartments to move home wastes to central storage and collection points.   The Garchey system, in limited use in the United Kingdom, starts with an under-the-sink receiver which takes food, bottles, cans, and packaging.   The receiver is manually discharged through a water-carrier tube to a main collection chamber serving a number of "flats."   The main chamber is emptied weekly by a collector truck, which pumps the solid wastes and carrier water for transport to its first-stage disposal.   The method has been in development for 10 years and has yet to gain wide acceptance.   The AB Centralsug system is in use in Stockholm, Sweden, serving 3,000 apartment units and is proposed for the Martin Luther King Memorial Hospital, Watts section, Los Angeles.   Transport is by air under high vacuum from receiving bins through ducts of diameters up to 24 in.   Users drop their wastes into valved chutes which sequentially discharge to the duct system and on to central bins.   The Stockholm system has a maximum run of 1.5 mi to the central collection station.

Two United States proposals for home grinding and macerating of all organics, including paper, for injection into separate, pressure, waste transport lines of 2 to 3 in in diameter to be hung in existing sewers, and for sewer carriage with flow sustained by recirculating sewage, have been under feasibility and comparative-cost studies.   Technical Memorandum 10 of the American Society of Civil Engineers, February 1969, examines vacuum and pressurized sewer transport of solid wastes as a phase of new sanitary sewers to end sanitary sewage discharge with storm water in combined sewers.   The ideas of I. Zandi on pressurized lines and of Liljendahl on vacuum systems are covered.   More fanciful proposals have been a Franklin Institute staff member's intense study of a waste pipeline from Philadelphia across New Jersey to discharge beyond the continental shelf into the Atlantic Ocean.[1]

In making comparisons with such distribution-collection systems as water, gas, electricity, sewage, telephone communication, natural flow systems of streams and growing trees, and home delivery of milk, mail, and parcels, C. G. Golueke and P. H. McGauhey (Ref. 6-3) observe, " Furthermore, it [refuse collection] takes on an aspect of improbability which makes questionable its long-term survival."   A major part of the report of the same investigators at the University of California is on possible future options of disposal, plans to investigate these, and results of initial field and laboratory studies (Ref. 6-3).   The possibilities are grouped as:

[1] *Ind. Res.*, **11:**28 (January 1969).

1 Improvements in existing technology for incineration, composting, landfill, and salvage

2 Adaptation of the anaerobic digestion of sewage sludge to garbage and as much organic solid waste as can be digested

3 Application of two processes used in chemical engineering, wet oxidation and biological fractionation, to solid wastes by developing the necessary technology

AN APPRAISAL

Operation and Policy Needs

The needs for solid-waste handling, disposal, and control in operations and in policy which must be recognized are:

1 A more effective management of present procedures required to keep these economical and acceptable to the people.

2 Finding realistic means of financing solid-waste collection and disposal. Dependence on general tax receipts at the local level must give way to fees for services, disposal charges added to the initial price of the product to provide an ultimate disposal fund, and the realization that waste salvage can only rarely be profitable.

3 Dedicating land and sea sinks for waste disposal for short and long times. These must be used within their assimilative capacities, staying within hygienic, ecological, and esthetic bounds with a sensitive concern for fish, wildlife, and plant life.

4 A recognition that our wastes are residues of resources which we value too little to use or lack technology to use productively, costs and markets weighed.

5 A realization that the design, fabrication, and assembly of products and of packaging must consider the end point of discard to facilitate recovery and disposal.

6 The necessity to take another look at our manufacturing methods and materials selection which result in early obsolescence, to determine whether mankind's increasing numbers and rising demand for consumer goods can so be imposed on the world's resources without long-term threats to much of life and certainly to the quality of life for man.

Effects and Consequences

The health effects of the mismanagement of solid wastes are indirect, but these are not inconsequential. Given the present means of insect and rodent control, no method of solid-wastes handling which favors the breeding, feeding, and harborage of flies, mosquitoes, or rodents is hygienically acceptable. The epidemiological evidence of human disease and death from present poor practices is weak. The best that can be advanced is the fly populations emerging from solid wastes in the littoral regions of the Mediterranean Sea and the incidence of trachoma. The principal responsible solid-waste component in these regions is the manure of animals housed intimately with the family. The new and growing concentrations of people and product wastes in urban settings in the tropical and subtropical areas of the world must be viewed skeptically. Unless the putrescible organic content, attractive to flies and rats, of the solid wastes of these concentrations of people is extremely low, the disease propagation from open dumps and uncollected solid wastes will be greater than in the temperate regions. The present methods of landfill and incineration are facing the indictments of being sources of contamination and pollution of water and air detrimental to man's health.

The esthetic responses of people plague the managers of solid-waste collection, transport, and disposal more than all health and ecological concerns severalfold. These are what the professional practitioners call the nuisance complaints. These are the smells, sights, and noise of solid-waste handling or mishandling which irritate people to the point of midnight phone calls to mayors, city managers, and health officials. The stinks come from open dumps, insanitary landfills, filthy hog feeding-lots, and overloaded incinerators. The unsightly conditions are uncollected, spilled, and carelessly dropped refuse; windblown debris from dumps, landfills, and inciner-ators; street and road litter, including killed animals. The noise is from packer trucks enroute too early or too late for sleeping residents, and from the roar of heavy equip-ment on landfills and at transfer stations. The complaint list is as long as the sorry, inadequate practices.

The ecological effects of our solid-wastes practices are viewed as bad. Some must be beneficial in fact and some in prospect. The bad effects are cited as filling in tidal flats and swampy areas. Certainly that changes the plant and animal life of those immediate areas. Many such areas are not at all attractive and produce their share of mosquitoes, stinks, and water quality deterioration. Many immediate eco-logical changes are benefits or detriments dependent on point of view. Whatever our means of solid-waste disposal except burning, the material is food for some life forms, bacteria, fungi, beetles, flies, rats, and in time, plants. Nonfloating junk pushed over-board forms shelter for marine life and has been made so purposefully in areas being depleted of fish. Fish pursuing boats to eat the discarded wastes suggest that if we are willing to bear the costs of composting and of hauling to sea, there would be an immediate demand for the product. That is equally the case for using compost to restore vegetation on eroded land and bare, road embankments. On balance, our solid-waste practices have done less ecological damage than our liquid and airborne wastes. One reason is that the processes are slower and give time to establish new regimes. There are surely means to use our solid wastes with ecologic benefits.

REFERENCES

6-1 The National Solid Wastes Survey—An Interim Report, *U.S. Public Health Serv.*, 1968.

6-2 Solid Wastes/Disease Relationships, *U.S. Public Health Serv. Publ. 999-UIH*-6, 1967.

6-3 Comprehensive Studies of Solid Waste Management, *U.S. Public Health Serv. Publ.* 2039, 1970, pp. 7–61.

6-4 Solid Wastes Management—Abstracts and Excerpts from the Literature, *U.S. Public Health Serv. Publ.* 2038, 1970.

7

VECTOR CONTROL

Mosquitoes, flies, fleas, lice, roaches, rats, mice, and snails have provoked man to loathe and to kill them for four reasons.

1 Pathogenic organisms have become participants in the symbiosis with man. Man is not the only victim in some of these pathogenic intrusions. *Pasteurella pestis*, a bacterium which produces plague, is an example of very poor parasitism in cycling among rats, fleas, and man. It kills the rat, the flea, and the man. The microscopic size and fantastic pathways of many of the pathogens made the chain of transmission obscure and baffling to man for centuries. Working in China in 1878, Sir Patrick Manson confirmed suspicions about insects, man, and disease by observing *Wuchereria bancrofti* in a mosquito, *Culex fatigans*. This nematode, a worm, causes filariasis and, in some responses to the pathogen, elephantiasis in man. Manson's was the first laboratory proof of insect participation in man's sickness and death. Other triumphs in the unraveling of the mysteries of vectors, hosts, and pathogens are those over malaria, plague, and yellow fever between 1880 and 1900; and those over dengue, African sleeping sickness, sandfly fever, and Chagas' disease between 1900 and 1910.

2 Bites ranging from annoying to painful from several species of insects and occasionally from rats rarely accepted by man without protest and are an attempt to

kill the offender.   Insect species biting man are few among the 700,000 to 1 million identified species of all insects.

3   Economic losses they cause by eating and spoiling food, by structurally damaging buildings, and by making resort and recreational sites unlivable during periodic invasions are most difficult to estimate.   The U.S. Department of Agriculture estimated that 14.7 percent of the total potential yield of all cereals in the United States valued at $14.4 million was lost in 1965 to insects and that 5 percent of the world's wheat crop is lost annually to insects.   L. Ling (Ref. 7-1, p. 10) summarizes world estimates of 33 million tons of bread grains and rice lost to rodents each year.   This is 3.55 percent of total production.   He states that all losses of foodstuffs due to pests and disease, from planting to the dinner table, is 20 percent.

4   Esthetics and comfort influence our regard for rodents and insects.   Insect parts and rat hairs in our bread and cereals are no longer acceptable in the United States despite knowledge and assurances that these have been cooked or roasted and are pathogen free.   Cockroaches are usually not suffered despite the fact that epidemiological evidence of disease transmission rests more on pathogen recovery from roaches than on human cases of illness.   A single buzzing mosquito turns a bedroom into a hunting ground.

Biologists and chemists have provided the knowledge to make man's warfare against what he regards as his uninvited guests increasingly effective in selected spots and time periods against chosen targets.   Three things cloud the horizon of conquest and control.

1   Man's own need for food, shelter, water, and recreation have created conditions more favorable for some species.   Examples are structural methods which build out the Norway rat have favored the roof rat in some geographical areas; irrigation methods that allow the breeding of the snail hosts of the schistosomes; water storage projects which favor some mosquito species; piped water to towns without adequate wastewater disposal which creates breeding places for the vectors of encephalitis and filariasis; recreational penetration of sylvatic plague zones.

2   The variations of responses of insects and rodents to efforts to kill them have not been foreseen and have been underestimated.   Unsuspected reservoirs of infective organisms have come to light as control advanced against the recognized reservoirs.   Examples of vector response to man's control efforts are insect resistance to the synthesized organic insecticides; rat resistance to anticoagulant poisons in the United Kingdom, the Netherlands, and Denmark; and the discovery of monkey reservoirs of yellow fever in Brazil after *Aedes aegypti* control around human reservoirs was achieved.   What have appeared to be sure control

techniques have met adaptable adversaries when the full strength of the enemies was engaged on all battlegrounds available to them.

3 An uneasiness and some evidence that the specific attacks against identified enemies are buckshot volleys which kill beneficial and desirable wildlife and which create marked disturbances in existing population and habitat adjustments. The mission-oriented public health pest controller and his even more active agricultural counterpart have not had a broad ecological view in foresight (Ref. 7-2). Corollary to this are the persistent pesticide residues circulating through plant and animal pathways long after their usefulness to man in killing very specific insects.

THE RATIONALE OF CONTROL

Four steps lead to control action against vectors and hosts of pathogens. These are also applicable against pests declared undesirable for reasons of economic damage, comfort, or esthetics.

1 The responsible species must be found. This was first accomplished for filariasis, malaria, plague, and yellow fever. The work goes on against diseases less violent in their disabling power and killing, but widespread, such as hemorrhagic fever and scrub typhus.

2 The ecology of the species must be determined, at least in its crude outlines. Breeding places, breeding cycles, feeding preferences, resting and harborage, development times, and range of movement must be known. Disappointments and failures in control have required more sophisticated and detailed information on hibernation, behavior changes, and on genetic and metabolic processes. The knowledge of mating habits is making the release of sterile males a possible means of control which has been dramatically successful against the monogamous screwworm in Florida and Curaçao.

3 Ecological information provides the basis for determining vulnerability of the target species to attack. In the case of insects, there are choices of killing larvae or adults, of killing indoors or outdoors, of attacking during seasons of highest or lowest population densities, and of confining the attack to well-defined flight ranges. The development of residual contact insecticides seemed to simplify some of these choices and even to make them unnecessary. Insecticidal resistance has changed that, with a return to the elimination of breeding places and food attractants in the case of houseflies. In the case of plague and endemic typhus, the flea and rat must be attacked simultaneously. Indeed, flea control should precede rat killing.

4 An attack plan must be developed which is sure, safe, and economical and which is fitted to the objective.   The goal may be limiting the prevalence of the disease transmitted as in the case of endemic murine typhus control; limiting the number of insects present as in the seasonal control of salt-marsh mosquitoes in coastal beach resorts; so reducing the number of insects that transmission of disease in man is stopped as in the case of malaria eradication; or eliminating the vector species as in the case of *Aedes aegypti* eradication in Central and South America. The goals and results are not always as anticipated.   The work against rats and fleas in the southeast United States was to control murine typhus.   The disease disappeared!   Urban yellow fever outbreaks have been reported twice in the western Hemisphere in the last 30 years.

Malaria was thought to have been reduced to extremely low levels in Ceylon in 1963 with only three or four cases reported in that year.   Yet it resurged in 1967 to 1969 with nearly a million confirmed cases, and with the estimated number six times that. The account against *Anopheles gambiae* in northeast Brazil and in Upper Egypt is more heartening and final for those disastrous invasions.   The attack must be economical, as except in a few cases it is paid for by public funds which are usually scanty for environmental hygiene and preventive medicine.   When poisons are used they must be safe for the field staff itself, for the people protected, for their domestic and pet animals, and for wildlife.   Despite the toxicity of pesticides, there have been relatively few instances of human poisoning.

A CLASSIFICATION OF CONTROL METHODS

Permanent Control

Permanent control of vectors and hosts is the term applied to measures which alter the physical environment enough for reproduction and survival to become so low that the target population is kept low or disappears.   In simple words, it requires closing the maternity wards, closing the free-lunch counters, and forcing an enduring housing shortage for the unwanted guests.   Commensalism ends.   Inhospitality begins and continues.   Man has done a lot of this without design or intent.   Land drainage to increase cropland started malaria on a long, slow decline in the United States.   Most Midwesterners are mildly incredulous that their great grandfathers dreaded the annual malarial season.   The slow rise of the level of personal hygiene and home sanitation in the western countries has made rats very rare in our homes.   This benefit has been approximately proportionate to expendable income.   Rats are still numerous in the ghettos.   Examples of planned action are ratproofing ships, draining and filling mosquito breeding sites, eliminating uncovered refuse dumps which welcome rats and flies, making graineries, flour mills, bakeries, food processing plants, food storage depots, and markets quite vermin proof and more readily cleanable.

Temporary Control

Temporary control is the term applied to the periodic and seasonal kill of the vectors, hosts, and pests.   It is permanent for the individual targets.   But the intensity of the attack is not planned to get each and every one.   It is abatement for relief.   A sufficient number survive to restablish breeding and will do so to the limit of available breeding places, shelter, and food supply.

Species Eradication

Species eradication is the term applied to an intensity of vector killing that Dr. Fred Soper described as killing the last blood-filled, "pregnant" *Anopheles gambiae* which descended from the invaders of northeast Brazil.   There have been five planned species-eradication efforts.   Three succeeded.   Two were campaigns launched against *Anopheles gambiae* in northeast Brazil in 1939 to 1941 and in Upper Egypt in 1943 to 1945.   These were areas in which the species was a new invader.   The Sardinia project was an experiment to determine whether a level of killing intensity could be reached and sustained to eradicate *Anopheles labranchiae*, a mosquito which was as indigenous and at home as the people on the island.   The heroic measures from 1947 to 1949 are reported in John Logan's book (Ref. 7-3).   The level necessary for eradication could not be attained.   *Anopheles labranchiae* survived.   Malaria transmission stopped when the vector numbers were greatly reduced.   Malaria eradication was achieved and has been sustained in Sardinia.   The campaign in Cyprus against two well-established anopheline vectors had the same results as the Sardinia project.   Malaria was eradicated. The mosquito vectors persist.   A third success was against a well-established vector, *Anopheles sergentii*, in 1946 to 1947 at the Dakhla and Kharga Oases, Egypt.   Positive blood tests for malaria dropped from 12 percent in 1945 to less than 0.1 percent in 1949.

Naturalistic Control

Naturalistic control is the term applied to measures in which natural predators or infection are introduced or their presence is intensified among the target population. Examples are putting gambusia fish and top-feeding minnows in mosquito breeding

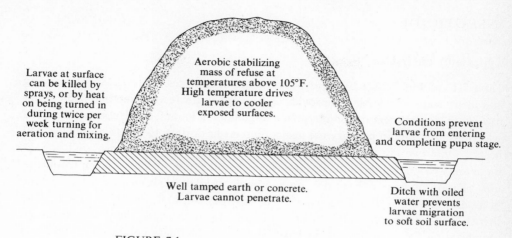

Larvae at surface can be killed by sprays, or by heat on being turned in during twice per week turning for aeration and mixing.

Aerobic stabilizing mass of refuse at temperatures above 105°F. High temperature drives larvae to cooler exposed surfaces.

Conditions prevent larvae from entering and completing pupa stage.

Well tamped earth or concrete. Larvae cannot penetrate.

Ditch with oiled water prevents larvae migration to soft soil surface.

FIGURE 7-1
The management of fly breeding in horse-manure piles, a case of control fitted to ecological vulnerability.

waters to eat the larvae; bringing cats, terriers, and ferrets into rat-infested places to hunt and kill the rats; the procedure of dubious safety of introducing *Salmonella enteritidis* bacteria among rats to infect, sicken, and kill them; putting chickens on a manure pile to eat fly larvae.   Naturalistic control measures have been quite successful in the agricultural field and considerable credit is given to gambusia for the control of malaria in Spain and Iran.   Satisfactory naturalistic control of human disease vectors is difficult to document.   Unfortunately, the introduction of biological control agents has generally not been followed carefully enough.   The World Health Organization is presently making a considerable effort to evaluate several biological and environmental control measures.   It may be necessary to utilize the biological control agents as one does chemicals, by introducing them at intervals when required.   There have been recent successes in mosquito larvae control in California by constant introductions of large numbers of fish into the mosquito breeding waters.   Another group of measures which are naturalistic is altering the quality of breeding places so that oviposition or maturation do not occur.   Examples are exposing mosquito breeding waters to sun or to shade in opposition to natural preference, or altering salinity.   An example of an effective procedure is the management of fly breeding in horse manure piles adopted by the U.S. Army when it had horseborne cavalry.   Figure 7-1 illustrates the procedure, which capitalizes on the vulnerability of the ecology of fly larvae.   Solid-waste compost piles manage fly breeding by similar means.

INSECTICIDES

Types and Their Use

Table 7-1 and Fig. 7-2 are brief introductions to insecticides.   The chemical grouping and identification in Table 7-1 provides a framework for recognition and some order to a chaotic assortment of compound names, common names, and trade names.   The selections are those in primary use against insects hazardous to health and household pests.   Only two chemicals which are primarily agricultural pesticides are listed, as these are well known, give the group firmer identification, and have given trouble in use.   Parathion is quite hazardous in handling.   Aldrin has been a persistent residue in foods and water.   It degrades in the free environment to its analog, dieldrin.   The British Standards Institute, the American Entomological Society, and the International Organization for Standardization have worked to eliminate confusion in pesticide nomenclature for the basic chemicals.   Formulations under proprietary names must be identified by labeling which has become closely regulated, or from the formulator's specifications.   The specifications for Pesticides Used in Public Health, published by The World Health Organization (Ref. 7-4) provides information on identifying names, composition, chemical and physical property requirements to ensure the quality of the material, and means of testing and analyzing for compliance.   The Organization recommends that these specifications be used for procuring pesticides for use in public health vector control programs.

Naturally occurring insecticides are not included in Table 7-1, although these are the oldest and still in use.   A species of chrysanthemum was centuries ago recognized by the Persians to yield extracts which killed insects.   The flower is *Pyrethrum cinerariaefolium*.   The active derivatives are pyrethrins and cinerins.   These have immediate knockdown action against flying insects.   They or synthesized analogs are ingredients in commercial sprays and aerosols for knockdown with the final killing power provided by one or more residual contact agents.   Another natural insecticide is rotenone derived from the roots of derris and cube.   These are widely used dusts for flower gardens.   To intensify the knockdown power of the pyrethrin group, synergists are added.   Sesame oil has this effect, and sesamin is the refined component in the oil.   Piperonyl butoxide, which is a derivative of a methylenedioxyphenol compound, is a synthesized synergist found in many aerosol insecticidal "bomb" formulations with a Freon as the propellant.

In 1793 the *American Daily Advertiser* of Philadelphia advised its readers that "common oil," probably whale oil, added to rainwater casks and cisterns would stop mosquito breeding in these.   The search goes on, for one phase of a field study by the *Aedes* research unit of the World Health Organization in Bangkok, Thailand, is to find the most effective, most economical, and least toxic agent to add to rainwater

Table 7-1 A CHEMICAL GROUPING AND IDENTIFICATION OF SELECTED INSECTICIDES, THEIR ROUTE OF PENETRATION, AND PRINCIPAL USES

Common name	Further identification	Route of penetration	Principal use
Inorganic compounds:			
Arsenic	As_2O_3	Stomach	Vs. ants and roaches
Sodium arsenite	Na_3AsO_3 and/or $NaAsO_2$	Stomach	Vs. ants and roaches
Sodium fluoride	NaF	Stomach	Vs. roaches
Paris green	Complex of copper metaarsenite and copper acetate	Stomach	As mosquito larvicide
Chlorinated hydrocarbons:			
DDT	Dichlorodiphenyltrichloroethane	Contact	Applied for residual contact vs. larvae and adults
BHC or HCH	Benzene hexachloride	Contact	Vs. a variety of insects
Gamma-BHC	99% isomer content, lindane	Contact	
Methoxychlor	A DDT analog, malate	Contact	
PDB	Paradichlorobenzene	Respiratory	Fumigant vs. moths
Chlorocyclodienes:			
Aldrin	Made by Diels-Alder type of reaction	Contact	Vs. agricultural pests
Chlordane	Chlorinated pine oil, octochlor	Contact	As residual vs. adult insects
Dieldrin	Analog of aldrin, by Diels-Alder type of reaction	Contact	Vs. mosquitoes and flies resistant to DDT; use increasingly restricted
Heptachlor	Related to chlordane	Contact	Vs. termites by soil treatment
Carbamates:			
Propoxur	Baygon, Bayer 39007, arprocarb, OMS-33	Contact	As residual vs. adult insects
Carbaryl	Sevin	Contact	Vs. household and agricultural pests
Organophosphorous compounds:			
Abate	A phosphorothionate	Contact	Vs. mosquito larvae
Diazinon	A phosphorothionate	Contact	Vs. DDT-resistant household insects
Dichlorvos	DDVP, Vapona	Fumigant	Vs. flying insects indoors, and in impregnated collars of pets vs. fleas
Fenchlorvos	Korlan, ronnel, Trolene	Contact	Vs. roaches, houseflies
Fenthion	Baytex, Bayer 29493	Contact	Vs. polluted-water breeders
Fenotrithion	Folithion, a phosphorothionate	Contact	Vs. mosquito larvae and adults
Malathion	A phosphorothionate	Contact	Vs. DDT-resistant flies
Parathion	A phosphorothionate	Contact	Vs. agricultural pests
Trichlorfon	Dipterex	Stomach	In fly and roach baits

(*Source: WHO, Tech. Rep. Ser. No.* 443, 1970. "Insecticide Resistance and Vector Control.")

(*a*) A chlorinated hydrocarbon

Common name : DDT
Generic name   : Dichlorodiphenyltrichloroethane
Chemical name : 1,1,1,-trichloro-2,2-bis (p-chlorophenyl)
                ethane

Structural formula

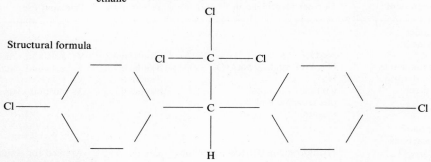

(*b*) A chlorocyclodiene

Common name : Dieldrin
Generic name   :
Chemical name : 1,2,3,4,10,10-hexachloro-6,7-epoxy-1,4,4a
                5,6,7,8,8a-octahydro-1,4,5,8-endo-exo-dimethano
                naphthalene

(c) An organophosphorous compound

Common name: Malathion
Generic name :
Chemical name: 0,0, dimethyl dithiophosphate of
                diethyl mercapto succinate

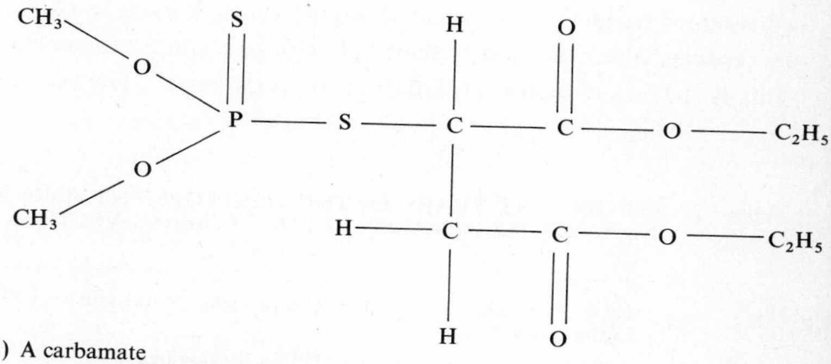

(d) A carbamate

Common name: Baygon
Generic name : Propoxur
Chemical name: o-iso propoxy-phenyl methyl carbamate

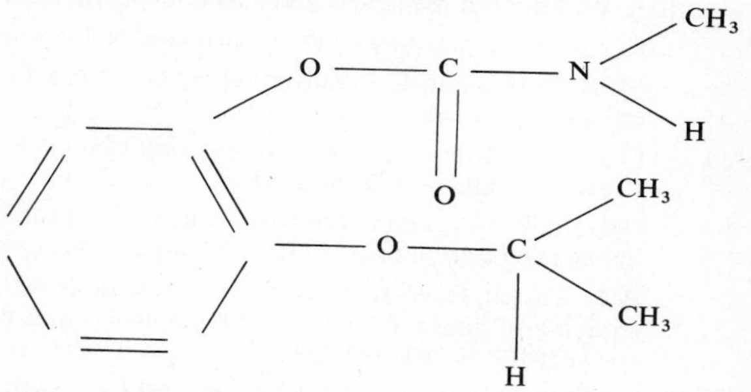

FIGURE 7-2

Examples of the structural formulas and chemical names of each of the four major types of man-made insecticides: (a) a chlorinated hydrocarbon, (b) a chlorocyclodiene, (c) an organophosphorous compound, (d) a carbamate.

catchment jars as a residual larvicide. Such an agent is needed in *Aedes aegypti* eradication for the same purpose. A few highlights of man's long search are listed in Table 7-2. The chemical names and structural formulas of one representative of each of the groups in Table 7-1 are given in Fig. 7-2.

Insect Resistance

Insect resistance to toxicants is one reason why pesticide research continues. The Italians began to use DDT in their malaria eradication in 1946. In 1947 they reported that domestic flies and culex mosquitoes were no longer being killed by the DDT residues on walls. Fortunately, the anopheline vector of malaria continued to be killed by the DDT. Earlier, in 1946, housefly resistance to DDT had been observed in Sweden. The first thought was that the formulation or spraying technique was faulty. The second was that the flies were not resting as they once had on the nearest convenient surface. The latter thought is now known to explain the resistance of a few species which do modify their behavior in response to repeated chemical contact. This is the behavioristic explanation for resistance. The second is the physiological

Table 7-2 SIGNIFICANT YEARS IN THE DEVELOPMENT AND APPLICATION OF INSECTICIDES AGAINST HUMAN DISEASE VECTORS

1867	L. O. Howard observes the mosquito larvicidal effect of illuminating oil, kerosene, in the United States.
1874	Othmar Zeidler synthesizes DDT in Strasbourg.
1911	G. Giemsa and P. Muhlens use pyrethrum in alcohol as a spray against mosquitoes in Germany.
1916	B. W. Marston uses Paris green as a mosquito larvicide in New Orleans.
1919	Kerosene extracts of pyrethrum are used as household sprays in the United States.
1921	M. A. Barber and T. B. Hayne report on comprehensive studies of Paris green as a mosquito larvicide.
1930–1931	G. A. Park Ross uses pyrethrum spraying of houses during malaria epidemics in Natal Province, Zululand, South Africa.
1934	G. Schrader of I. G. Farben begins the synthesis of 300 organophosphorous compounds in Nazi German war gas project, and finds some toxic to aphids. Nothing is published.
1936	P. F. Russell, F. W. Knipe, and T. R. Rao demonstrate the effectiveness of pyrethrum spraying of houses in India, and recommend it as economical at 10 cents per capita per year for malaria control.
1939	Paul Herman Müller of J. R. Geigy and Co., Switzerland, resynthesizes DDT and discovers its insecticidal potency in a search for a clothes-moth killer.
1942	DDT is used in Switzerland vs. potato beetles as Gesarol and vs. lice as Neocid. Major A. R. W. Jonge, U.S. military attaché in Berne learns of these uses and sends samples to the U.S. and U.K.
1942–1943	Schrader patents TEPP, an organophosphorous compound, in Germany, 1942, and in the U.S., 1943.
1943	The British Ministry of Supply coins the name *DDT*. Production begins in U.S. with 9.5×10^6 lb in 1944, and rises to 47×10^6 lb in 1947. In 1963, U.S. production reached 179×10^6 lb.
1944	G. Schrader discovers the insecticidal properties of parathion. Nothing is published.
1946	H. Martin and H. Shaw publish B.I.O.S. Final Report 1095 on the organophosphorus work of the Nazis before and during World War II.
1947	J. R. Geigy and Co. of Switzerland develop carbamate types of insecticides, dimetan, pyrolan, isolan.
1951	G. Schrader publishes his work on insecticides based on organofluorine and phosphorous compounds as Monograph 62, *Versl. Chem. GMBH*, Weinheim, Germany.

explanation. Some individual insect variants have a capacity to metabolize the absorbed insecticide rapidly to an innocuous compound before toxic action is well under way. These individuals survive and produce resistant descendants. Genetic selection is at work. The resistance of *Musca domestica*, the common housefly, to DDT has been pinpointed to a single gene. The detoxification mechanism has been described as dehydrochlorinating DDT or its analogs by a single enzyme. The resistance factors of other insect species are continuing to be investigated as they are not completely defined. A third explanation for insects' surviving supposedly lethal contacts is variations in dose tolerance and in vigor among individuals in a population. The strong live on to reproduce descendants with the same characteristics. This has been termed *vigor tolerance* as distinct from resistance.

The number of species of public health concern demonstrating resistance to man-made insecticides has risen from 1 in 1946, to 13 in 1951, to 37 in 1955, to 71 in 1961, to 97 in 1967, and to 102 in 1968. Among the insects of public health concern, only two genera have not shown insecticidal resistance, *Phlebotomus*, the sand flies, and *Glossina*, the tsetse flies. The blackflies, *Simulium*, were among the susceptibles until some species of *Simulium* recently showed resistance. Among those insects having resistance are 38 species of anophelines including such well-known malaria vectors as *A. labranchiae, gambiae, sergentii, stephensi, sacharovia*, and *quadrimaculatus;* six species of *Culex* including *quinquefasciatus, pipiens*, and *tarsalis;* 11 species of *Aedes* including *aegypti, sollicitans*, and *albopictus;* 21 species of flies with *Musca domestica* leading the list by resisting chlorinated hydrocarbon, the cyclodienes, and the organophosphates; three species of cockroach, the German roach, *Periplaneta brunnea*, a wood-eating roach, and the oriental roach. The German cockroach shares the housefly's ability to resist all three of the major chemical groups of insecticides. Additionally there are five species of lice, five of fleas, two of bedbugs, and three of ticks found resistant to the chlorinated hydrocarbon or the cyclodienes or both. Fuller discussion of vector resistance to pesticides is in Ref. 7-5.

Choice of Insecticides and Their Use

The choices of insecticides and means of application that are in use are given in Annex 18, Chemical Methods for the Control of Vectors and Pests of Public Health Importance of Ref. 7-5. Alternative chemicals for use against DDT-resistant species, and in turn, to supplement chlorinated hydrocarbon compounds, are stated. The usual pattern had been that when the DDT of compound failed, the dieldrin type (the cyclodienes) was used. In the face of the rising tide of concern for the organochloride persistence in the environment, DDT and dieldrin are used only when these are clearly the necessary choice. In preference, the organophosphates, such as malathion, are applied. In the face of organophosphates resistance or because of clear advantages, the carbamate, propoxur or arprocarb (Baygon, Bayer 39007, OMS-33) is in increasing use.   Annex 18 of Ref. 7-5 indicates the choice of technique against the species listed for most effective and economical results.   Concentrations to be used in sprays or dusts, rates of application, and doses to treated areas are stated.   For United States procedures, the latest annual spring issue on *Public Health Pesticides*, prepared by the vector control group of the Department of Health, Education, and Welfare at the Center for Disease Control, Public Health Service, Atlanta, Georgia, should be consulted.   It contains recommendations on pesticides of choice and the means to use these effectively.   Up-to-date information on reports of resistance and of safeguards required is given, plus recommended changes in formulations, rates, and doses resulting from field and laboratory studies.   The item of equipment needed for vector control, specifications for it, and techniques of using, testing, calibrating, and maintaining it are set forth in detail in a practical manner in a World Health Organization publication (Ref. 7-6).

The unique properties of DDT and the families of organic pesticides which followed are that they are stable when sprayed on surfaces, adhere well, are absorbed slowly into the surface, and volatilize slowly.   These characteristics result in an extended activity against pests which contact the treated surfaces by resting or moving on them.   The recommended formulations and rates of application produce residual concentrations which provide lethal absorption within habitual contact times for periods of 3 to 6 months.   Table 7-3 gives the cost in United States dollars per metric ton, the duration of effectiveness, the required number of applications per 6 months, and the cost per $100 \, m^2$ treated for DDT malathion and propoxur to interrupt malaria transmission. The economic advantage of DDT is obvious by any measure, and clear in the ratios in the far right-hand column.   The advantages of long intervals between sprayings are not only lower costs but less frequent disruption of households by spraying crews. The primary means of malaria eradication is the residual from spraying at the longest

Table 7-3   COMPARATIVE COST OF INSECTICIDES USED FOR RESIDUAL SPRAYING OF HOUSES FOR INTERRUPTING MALARIA TRANSMISSION

Insecticide	Cost/metric ton, U.S. $	Effective duration, 2 g/m²	No. of applications per 6 months	Cost/100 m², U.S. $	Comparative cost
DDT	500	6 months	1	0.13	1
Malathion	870	3–4 months	2	0.70*	5.3
Propoxur	3,400	3–4 months	2	2.72*	20.4

* Additional expenditures accrue when malathion or propoxur are used.   The cost of operational personnel doubles because two applications are required instead of one each 6 months.   When propoxur is used, it is desirable to provide some basic protective clothing, which is an additional cost.
SOURCE: Data provided by Roy Fritz, scientist-entomologist, Geneva, Switzerland, 1971.

effective intervals on the interior walls and ceilings of dwellings and usually the underside of furniture. The residual attribute of the organic pesticides also makes possible long intervals between larvicidal sprayings of breeding waters of mosquitoes when the insecticide is in emulsion form and is used in high application rates. The choice of insecticides for such use is restricted. No persistent organochloride may be applied to general-use waters, as this produces long-term contamination of the biosphere. A larvicidal method which utilizes the stability of the organic insecticides is the distribution of granules or briquettes of clays impregnated with Abate. These are spread or placed in the breeding waters. Sand granules coated with Abate have been effective in controlling mosquito breeding in water storage containers. Concentrations as low as 0.1 mg/l have been effective for 70 days without risk in drinking the water. Impregnated briquettes have been tested in rice fields in Southeast Asia with promising results.

Other means of securing residual effectiveness of the organic pesticides are the use of impregnated cords which are choice resting places for flies; the slow release of dichlorvos (Vapona) from suspended plastic strips or on plastic pet collars, which provides a long-term fumigant action; the slow volatilization of propoxur (Baygon) from residually sprayed surfaces, which provides a fumigant action against anophelines that do not rest on the walls but on hanging clothing and cobwebs, such as *Anopheles d'thali*, or that are semidomestic, as *A. sergentii* in Israel and Jordan; and against nonflying pests, the use of surface dusting, ground impregnation, and poisoned baits on runways and on resting and nesting places. Insecticidal aerosols dispersed by Freon bombs, fine nozzle sprayers, and fogging machines act by immediate contact in resting places or in flight. No residual effect is sought in such space spraying whether indoors or outside. The relief of the reduced density is quite temporary. As long as food attractants and harborage are provided, the insect population will be speedily reestablished by migration and reproduction.

VECTORS AND HOSTS, AND THE MECHANISMS OF TRANSMISSION

Figures 7-3 and 7-4 show the means by which insect vectors are involved in disease transmission among men, and by which rodents serve as the host or reservoir of the pathogens which fleas or occasionally other ectoparasites transmit to man.

Mechanical Transmission

Mechanical transmission is the simple transport of pathogens on the feet, body surface, and proboscis of the insect. A further means is a pass through the gastrointestinal tract, the pathogen being in the food intake of the insect and leaving in its feces or by (*a*) Mechanical transport by flies and cockroaches.

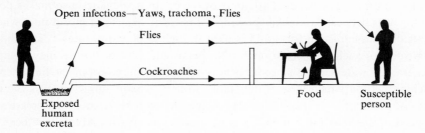

Laboratory proof of transmission of 30 diseases by the housefly and related flies principally pathogenic bacteria and intestinal helminths, and recovery of pathogens from cockroaches are the bill of indictment.

(*b*) Biological transmission by bloodsucking insects taking blood meal from person in infective stage

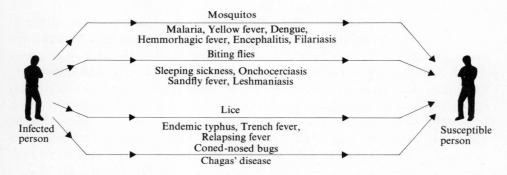

FIGURE 7-3
Vector roles in disease transmission to man: (*a*) mechanical transport by flies and cockroaches, (*b*) biological transmission by bloodsucking insects' taking a blood meal from person in infective stage.

regurgitation by some flies.   There is no biological cycle of development of the pathogen in or on the insect.   As shown in Fig. 7-3*a*, there must be insect contact with the infective human discharges and transport to an entry to a susceptible person.   The open sores of yaws, the fluids on infected eyes from trachoma, and acute purulent conjunctivitis are accessible to flies for transport to the exposed tissues of susceptibles. Exposed human excreta allows transportation to our food by pests for gastrointestinal pathogens ranging from viruses to helminths.   Field recoveries and laboratory experiments have shown houseflies and cockroaches carrying organisms of some 30 diseases.

(a) Plague

From domestic rats

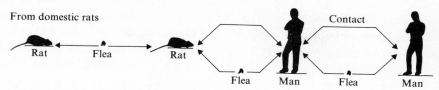

<u>Pasteurella pestis</u> bacteria infect, sicken, and kill the rat, the flea, and the man. Man-to-man by fleas and by contact. Flea regurgitates <u>P. pestis</u> and transmits mechanically while biting for its blood meal.

For wild rodents

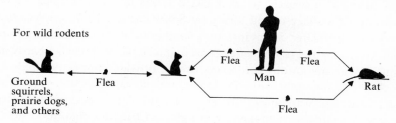

Among wild rodents, wild rodent-to-man, wild rodents-to-domestic rats-to-man.

(b) Endemic typhus fever

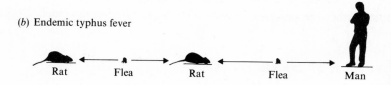

<u>Rickettsia typhi</u> infects the rat, the flea, and man. It sickens the man. Flea passes the rickettsia in its feces while on man. Rickettsia penetrates abraded skin.

FIGURE 7-4
Vector roles in disease transmission to man from a second animal host or reservoir: (a) plague, (b) endemic typhus fever.

One reported outbreak attributed to cockroaches was the transmission of *Salmonella typhimurium* in a children's ward of a Brussels' hospital.[1] Cockroaches have been observed feeding on excreta of cholera patients and on the sputum of tuberculosis cases. They make privy pits and drains their habitat. The explanation for the absence of much epidemiological evidence by outbreaks and cases in spite of the cockroach's filthy habits and clear evidence of pathogens on their bodies is their very limited range of movement. Where safe harborage, water, food, and warmth are provided, the

[1] M. Grafar and S. Mertens, *Ann. Inst. Pasteur*, **79**:654 (1950).

cockroach's nightly forage will be within the food storage room or kitchen cabinet-work, and limited to 20 ft or less from its harborage.   This, fortunately, reduces opportunities for contact with infective organisms and their successful transport and penetration of new hosts.   Exceptions have been observed.   With population increases, the American cockroach has been found to migrate readily out of sewer manhole covers for 50 ft with extremes up to 475 ft.   Table 7-4 presents characteristics of the species of cockroach most usually in domestic commensalism.   Their geographic identification does imply such restricted distribution.   At best these are alleged points of origin.   The Australian cockroach, for example, is found in a wide tropical to sub-tropical belt around the world, crossing Africa, the South Pacific Islands, the Americas, the southern edge of the United States including southern California, and, to be sure, Australia.   The longevity and reproductive capacity make the cockroach a hardy and persistent visitor.   The ubiquitous cardboard carton provides protective folds and spaces for cockroaches to move with the goods, and in carton reuse, from food processing plants through warehouses to the storeroom of the local market to our homes.   Cockroaches fair poorly in the face of tight construction, tight food-storage methods, and good and thorough housekeeping.   The adjuncts of insecticidal control are in Ref. 7-5.

The role of the housefly, *Musca domestica*, and other flies close to man has been observed and studied since the sixteenth century when Soares de Souza associated flies

Table 7-4   CHARACTERISTICS OF COCKROACHES

Species	Common names	Color	Adult size, in	Life span, days	Egg cases per life No. produced	No. fertile
Blatella germanica	German or brown roach, croton bug	Yellow brown	$\frac{1}{2}$	260	6, 30–48 eggs/case	4 or 5
Blatta orientalis	Oriental, water bug	Chocolate brown	1	140	8, 16 eggs/case	5
Periplaneta americana	American, Bombay canary	Reddish brown	$1\frac{1}{2}$	440	50–60, 14–16 eggs/case	30
Periplaneta australasiae	Australian roach	Reddish brown	$1\frac{1}{2}$	?	? 24 eggs/case	?
Supella supellectilium	Brown banded roach	Light brown with 2 light bands	$\frac{1}{2}$	?	14, 18 eggs/case	?

and yaws. Military operations in Cuba in 1899, and later in Greece and Turkey, reported correlations between heavy fly populations and widespread diarrhea among soldiers. In 1932 F. Ara and U. Marengo isolated typhoid fever bacteria from 44 percent of the flies trapped in the rooms of typhoid fever patients and found the organisms viable in the fly's intestinal tract for 6 days. In 1951 L. S. West showed laboratory proof of transmission of 10 bacterial infections, 2 viral pathogens, 5 protozoans, the ova of 8 helminths, 1 flagellate, and the organisms of yaws and hydatid cysts. The initial effectiveness of DDT against flies gave great promise for fly control and the reduction of fly-borne diseases. Both were accomplished until DDT resistance developed. There are well-documented studies by J. Watt and D. R. Lindsay in Hidalgo County, Texas, 1946 to 1948; by D. R. Lindsay, W. Stewart, and J. Watt in Thomas County, Georgia, 1949 to 1951 and by A. Missiorli in Italy, reported in 1948. The incidence of shigellosis was strongly affected by strict fly control. In Hidalgo County, a high-morbidity area, the incidence of shigellosis and the death rates among children under 2 shifted down in areas of fly control. When control was applied to the "normal" areas and stopped in the insecticided towns, the death rates and shigellosis incidence reversed accordingly.[1]   In Thomas County towns the results were less dramatic as it was a moderate-morbidity area. There were consistent drops in diarrhea cases and positive rectal swabs for *Shigella* bacteria in children under 10 in accord with control and fly densities, until flies became resistant to DDT, dieldrin, and chlordane.[2] J. M. Weir observed that reductions in acute conjunctivitis obtained by larviciding against flies in Egyptian villages were lost after 1950 when *Musca vicina* developed lindane and chlordane resistance.[3]   The reduction in acute eye diseases in the villages with fly control was accompanied by lower rates of dysentry and infant mortality. In these Egyptian towns, fly breeding was very heavy as animals were quartered and their manure stored integrally with homes. A diurnal fly movement in accord with temperature changes produced heavy invasions of living quarters when breeding was not controlled or controllable. Fly transmission was so large a factor in these circumstances that the partial benefits of improved water supply, human-excreta disposal, and refuse collection in villages selected for observing the effects were overwhelmed.

Biological Transmission

Biological transmission by bloodsucking insects propagates diseases which have determined the economic and political development of the world, and which have influenced major military campaigns. Two or three species of tsetse flies transmitting sleeping sickness among men and among cattle and horses limited the white man's domain in

[1] J. Watt et al., *Public Health Rep.* (*U.S.*), **63**:1319 (1948).
[2] D. R. Lindsay et al., *Public Health Rep.* (*U.S.*), **68**:361 (1953).
[3] J. M. Weir et al., *J. Egypt. Public Health Assoc.*, **27**:55 (1952).

Africa.   Malaria has affected military operations from Napoleon's time to McArthur's. In 1809 the British Walcheren Expeditionary Force against Napoleon was reduced from 40,000 to 24,000 by malaria.   In the South Pacific theater of World War II from 1942 to 1945, McArthur had to accept and plan around the tolls of 546,320 cases of malaria and 107,853 cases of dengue.   He had 4,407 officers and enlisted men on anti-malaria work.   During the Sicilian action of World War II, several thousand Allied soldiers were put out of action by the bites of the *Phlebotomus* fly's transmitting sand-fly fever (Ref. 7-7).   Figure 7-3 shows four insect groups, mosquitoes, biting flies, lice, and the cone-nosed bugs, and the principal diseases transmitted with their blood meals from infected persons.   The pathogens taken with man's blood have a cycle of development in the insect.   Some of these cycles are very intricate, as for the plasmodia of malaria; that is, intricate in the sense of development stages in specific sites in the female anopheline for defined time periods.   In comparison, the virus of yellow fever in the *Aedes aegypti* appears simple.   When more is known of the biochemistry of virus multiplication, the accommodation between the mosquito and virus is likely to be as remarkable as the classical parasitic cycles of malaria, filariasis, and onchocerciasis.   The record of the masterpieces of microbiological and epidemiological observations on malaria are given in a stimulating and moving account by P. Russell (Ref. 7-8). The difficulties were not solely scientific and environmental, but at times administrative.   Sir Ronald Ross's work was interrupted when a superior, deeming his search for Laveran's parasite in mosquitoes a waste of time, ordered him to do bedside care of the sick.   President Theodore Roosevelt's intervention was necessary to prevent the chief engineer of the Panama Canal Commission from sacking Colonel Gorgas and curtailing mosquito control in 1904.   That chief stated, "A dollar spent on sanitation is like throwing it in the bay."   In August 1905, a successor, J. F. Stevens, appeared, who supported Gorgas.   At the end of the job, Stevens reported that from 1904 to 1914 the cost of prevention of disease was less than 2 percent of the cost of the canal and that the annual malaria case admission rate dropped from 821/1,000 in 1906 to 76/1,000 in 1913.   In 1906, more than 4 out of 5 had to be admitted to a hospital for malaria.   In 1913, the number was less than 4 in 50, a tenfold reduction.

Insects vary greatly in their participation in disease transmission.   Of about 300 species of anophelines making up the genus, 11 or 12 are the principal vectors of malaria, although 60 have been recognized as vectors.   In some areas *Aedes aegypti* transmits filariasis although usually it does not.   The several species of tsetse flies differ greatly in the transmission of sleeping sickness in man.   *Glossina palpalis* is involved in human cases, while *Glossina morsitans* transmits another trypanosome causing nagana among cattle and horses.   Among the factors which influence the vectorial capacity of insects are the female's preference for man for her blood meal, adaptation to man's dwellings and its surroundings for resting, adaptation to breeding places within easy flight range of man, a life span long enough to allow the parasite to complete its cycle in the insect and reach its infective stage for man, and the ease with which a species can maintain high population densities in the environment provided. These are fairly straightforward factors. In their specifics, they do not hold for the same species in all parts of the world. The breeding places of choice for *Aedes aegypti* are very intimate with man's urban environment in the Western Hemisphere. It is vastly different in Central Africa, where its choice is in the forests. Taxonomic identities do not guarantee ecological identities.

There are less evident factors at work. *Anopheles gambiae*, recognized and dreaded for its vectorial capacity, has been found to develop a very high number of oocysts of plasmodia in its stomach walls and has a correspondingly high number of sporozoite forms of the plasmodium in its salivary glands ready for injection into the human bloodstream with the bite. In comparison, *Anopheles albimanus* of moderate vectorial capacity has a low number of oocysts and sporozoites at the corresponding points of parasite development. However, *A. albimanus* usually occurs in vast numbers. The resultant high density makes it an important vector. Laboratory studies of *Aedes aegypti's* ability to transmit the filaria worm indicate a single gene which makes the difference. Among the *Glossina*, one species prefers wild animals for its blood meal, but has turned to man as the number of easily accessible wild animals was reduced by man's hunting and destruction of their habitat. Thus in the factors influencing vectorial capacity there are some that man has recognized and manipulates to his advantage, some that he unwittingly creates to his disadvantage, and some that he is exploring, which may provide highly effective new control methods.

Transmission from an Animal Host

Figure 7-4 diagrams the relations among fleas, rats, and men in plague; among wild rodents, fleas, man, and rats in sylvatic or campestral plague; and among rats, fleas, and man in endemic murine typhus fever. The movement of *Pasteurella pestis* in plague is a dead end for all participants, as bacterial infection kills the fleas, the rats, and until the use of antibiotics, about 80 percent of human cases. There is some evidence that there are species of rodents relatively immune to plague. These rodents maintain the infection between outbreaks. For centuries man recognized that an increase of sickly and dead rats in his dwelling, neighborhood, and town was a certain precursor to plague. Those that could took speedy escape action. Now it is known that what followed was fleas turning to man for their blood meal as the rats died. It is not that fleas remain attached to a single rat and depart upon its death. Fleas continuously move from rat to rat in their nests and burrows, and along their runways. This characteristic makes insecticidal dusting of these locations extremely effective in controlling plague and murine typhus fever. When plague becomes well established in man, man-to-man transmission is completed by fleas or by intimate respiratory contact.

Sylvatic plague is worldwide.   Its history in the United States is well defined. Plague entered San Francisco from overseas in 1900.   The human cases numbered 121 in the next 4 years, with 118 deaths.   In 1904 the city was declared free of plague. In the interim, plague moved from rats to ground squirrels, with three human cases after squirrel contact reported in Contra Costa County across the bay in 1903.   The cycle of rats, fleas, and man was not wholly accepted at that time, although vigorous rat killing and ratproofing of buildings were pursued in San Francisco in 1902 and 1903.   If it did not get a firm hold in wild rodents then, plague did move to squirrels during the second San Francisco epidemic of 1907 to 1908.   Rat-borne plague spread to Oakland in 1907 and produced human cases until 1911.   In 1908 the disease was detected in Contra Costa County with human deaths, squirrel deaths, and plague-positive squirrels.   From there on it slowly spread eastward.   It took over 25 years to extend beyond California to Oregon, Nevada, and Montana.   In another 35 years sylvatic plague in ground squirrels, prairie dogs, and other wild rodents reached an eastern line, north to south, approximately through the centers of the Dakotas, Nebraska, Kansas, Oklahoma, and Texas.   Plague is imbedded in our literature, art, and history.   It has never ceased to exist in pockets of human misery and has reappeared with the extension of misery, as it did in San Francisco in 1907 following the earthquake and fire, and in South Vietnam with over 5,000 confirmed and suspected human cases in 1967.

Thomas. G Hull (Ref. 7-9) catalogs 199 diseases which are known to pass from animals to man.   Most of these are rare transmissions of familiar diseases such as measles.   He singles out 20 diseases or conditions in which domestic animals and birds are the usual hosts, and 19 in which rodents and wild animals are the usual hosts. There is an insect vector in only a fraction of the biological parasitic panorama among man, animals, and microorganisms.   Table 7-5 gives a selection of the major diseases and disease groups in which an insect provides transmission from an animal host to man.   These diseases are widespread, ranging from rickettsial pox, discovered in apartment dwellings in New York City by a fascinating bit of epidemiological detective work by Dr. Morris Greenberg and his city health department staff, to tsutsugamushi disease, or scrub typhus, which harassed Allied Forces in Southeast Asia during World War II and has been endemic there, in the Japanese Islands, Korea, and northern Australia for many years.   The classical pattern of tsutsugamushi was worked out by Japanese scientists in the early 1900s.

There are many varieties of the hemorrhagic and tick fevers in which there is a virus transmission from animal hosts to man by ticks.   Not all these patterns are well defined, as virus manipulation is difficult work.   The transmission of these fevers varies considerably.   The dengue hemorrhagic fevers are mosquito-transmitted. Table 7-5 lists only those encephalitis types generally occurring in the United States.

Another four or five types of encephalitis could be added, of which Japanese B is well known.   Some of the encephalitides are transmitted by tick bites, rather than mosquito bites, such as Powassan and Russian spring-summer encephalitis.   Tick-borne encephalitis is not listed in Table 7-5.   The animals implicated as hosts of the insect-borne diseases are varied and numerous.   Table 7-5 cites those animals most frequently involved.   For example, R. Pollitzer (Ref. 7-10) states that 200 species and subspecies of wild rodents have been implicated as reservoirs of sylvatic plague, but only 8 are principally involved.   Veterinarians and wildlife biologists are needed in study and control of these disease transmission processes.   The ecology of the animal host may be as important as that of the insect vector in achieving and maintaining control.

Table 7-5 SELECTED DISEASES TRANSMITTED FROM ANIMALS TO MAN
BY INSECTS

Disease	Animals	Insect and its action
Plague:		
Bubonic	Rat: roof, Norway	Flea regurgitates on biting.
Sylvatic	Squirrel, bandicoot, prairie dog, other wild rodents	Flea regurgitates on biting.
Typhus:		
Endemic, murine	Rat: roof, Norway	Flea defecates during biting.
Encephalitis:		
Equine	Horse, cow, rabbit, ground squirrel	Mosquito bite.
St. Louis	Wild birds, domestic hen	Mosquito bite.
Western	Wild birds, domestic hen, horse, deer, squirrel	Mosquito bite.
Eastern	Small wild birds, duck, turkey, pheasant	Mosquito bite.
Hemorrhagic fevers:		
Some types	Wild rodents	Tick bite.
Leishmaniasis:		
Three types	Dog, other canines, wild rodents	Sand-fly bite.
Rickettsial pox	House mouse, wild rodents	Mite bite.
Tick fevers:		
Several types	Small wild rodents	Tick bite.
Trypanosomiasis:		
African	Cow, sheep, horse, hog, antelope	Tsetse fly bite.
American or Chagas' disease	Dog, cat, monkey, bat, opossum, armadillo, squirrel, other rodents	Fecal material of triatomid bug.
Tsutsugamushi, or scrub typhus	Field rats and mice, voles, swamp birds, parrot, monkey, bush hen	Mite bite.

MALARIA ERADICATION—A GLOBAL CAMPAIGN

Figure 7-5 shows the status of antimalaria activities and malaria eradication in the world, June 1969.   This vast effort seeks to apply the knowledge of malaria gained primarily in the last 75 years to achieve global control of a mosquito-borne disease which has limited human productivity and economic development for centuries.   The rationale, the costs, the successes, the benefits, and the risks of this effort must be examined, as it is a major commitment to manage the quality of our environment. Malaria eradication is extending many lives to the reproductive ages, and is thus adding to population increases.   It is also adding to man's productivity and to that of the land he uses.

In 1955, the Eighth World Health Assembly resolved that the World Health Organization should take the initiative in providing technical advice and coordinating resources for a campaign to eradicate malaria from the world.   The WHO Expert Committee on Malaria defines eradication as "ending the transmission of malaria and the elimination of the reservoir of infected cases in a campaign limited in time and carried out to such a degree of perfection that, when it comes to an end, there is no resumption of transmission."   The objective is to take the parasite out of circulation by antianopheline measures, and in the consolidation phase of the campaign, by the treatment of residual human infections that make up endemic foci.   The campaign area may be an entire county or its malarious areas.   The attack need not be simultaneous throughout the campaign area.

Figure 7-6 diagrams the sequence of operations of malaria eradication.   The preparatory phase is for epidemiological and geographical reconnaissance, training of personnel, and organization of administrative, logistic, and operational services. During the attack phase the essential measure is the complete, systematic, sustained residual spraying of dwellings and accessible resting places in the attack area. This reduces the number of female anophelines to such a low level that parasite transmission is interrupted and stays that way for about 3 years.   At this point, wide-area systematic spraying is stopped.   The consolidation phase starts.   Remaining human infections are eliminated with chemotherapy.   Intensive case finding goes on to ensure that malaria has been eradicated.   The maintenance phase continues from there on in a given country or in its malarious areas.   It will have to be continued as long as malaria cases appear in one part of the world or another, for these hold the risk of reintroducing the parasite.   It must be the responsibility of a well-organized public health service carrying on a broad range of activities of which eradication maintenance is one.

Three things led to the concept of malaria eradication.   One was the demonstration of its feasibility over large areas by the campaigns in Italy, the United States, and Venezuela in the late 1940s.   A second was the development of insecticidal resistance

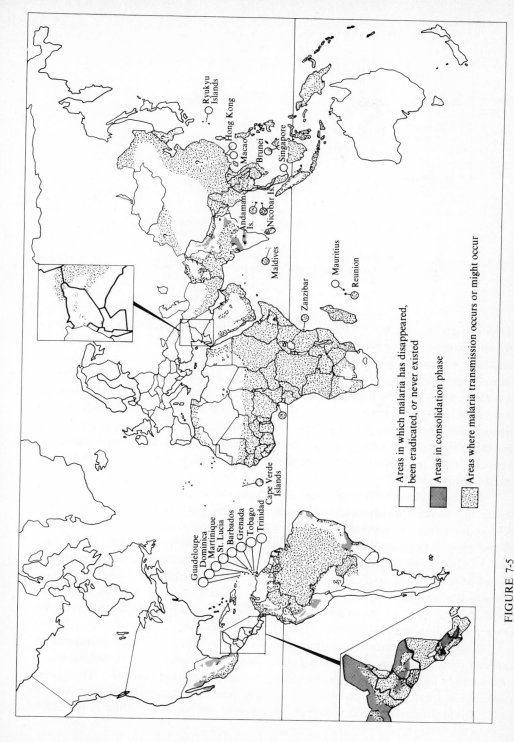

FIGURE 7-5

Malaria situation in the world, June 30, 1969. [*Source: WHO Chron.,* **24**:398 (1970).]

Ryukyu
Islands

Hong Kong

Macao
Brunei
Singapore
Andaman
Is.
Nicobar Is.

Maldives

Mauritius
Reunion

Zanzibar

Cape Verde
Islands

Guadeloupe
Dominica
Martinique
St. Lucia
Barbados
Grenada
Tobago
Trinidad

☐ Areas in which malaria has disappeared,
been eradicated, or never existed

▨ Areas in consolidation phase

▧ Areas where malaria transmission occurs or might occur

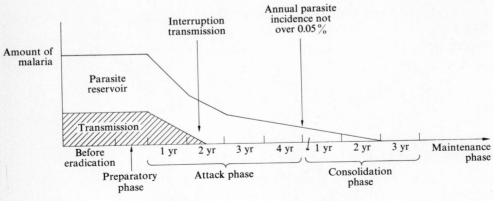

FIGURE 7-6
Phases of a malaria eradication campaign.   [*Source*: *WHO Drawing* 4438.]

of the malaria mosquitoes over a period of years of low-intensity control.   An intensive and extensive antimosquito effort holds the promise of malaria eradication before resistance becomes widespread in a particular malarious area.   The third was the comparative costs of an apparently endless annual control effort to hold down the number of malaria cases and the high annual cost of a malaria eradication campaign limited to 8 years.   Of these, the resistance issue was paramount.   The effectiveness of the organic insecticides against anophelines must be utilized before these species acquire resistance by exposure during annual control efforts of a partial nature.   Table 7-6 compares three levels of malaria management, control, eradication, and anopheline species eradication.

There are 171 million people, equal to 85 percent of the population of the United States, in countries which have now completed malaria eradication which have been held malaria free for several years, and which therefore qualify for entry on the World Health Organization's official register of complete eradication.   There are now 1 billion people who have the protection of the maintenance and consolidation phases of the malaria eradication campaign.   That is one-third of the world's population.   It is two-thirds of those living in malarious areas.   Only slightly more than one-fifth of those of the malarious areas are still outside the plans of eradication.   Of these 210 million are in Africa and 45 million in Indonesia.

The risk in malaria eradication is the reintroduction of a sufficient number of infected persons among immigrants, transients, or repatriates from malarious areas, and possibly by isolated long-term relapses, to reestablish transmission.   The consequences are great as the population is largely without any acquired immunity and an active anopheline population is present to transmit the parasite.   Malaria has reappeared in Ceylon twice.   The eradication, started in 1948, was relaxed too soon in 1953. It had to be renewed in 1958.   By 1963 there were only three or four cases a year among 7.7 million people in formerly malarious areas.   The further sequence has been:

Year	1964	1965	1966	1967	1968*	1969
Confirmed cases	126	276	207	3,465	425,937	552,234

There have been few deaths, but it is believed that there are about six cases for each confirmed one in the present epidemic.   Although it has the advantage of an island geography, Ceylon faces the hazard of importation of the disease, and of relaxation

Table 7-6   A COMPARISON OF THREE LEVELS OF MALARIA MANAGEMENT—MALARIA CONTROL, MALARIA ERADICATION, AND SPECIES ERADICATION

Comparative points	Malaria control	Malaria eradication	Anopheline species eradication
Objective	Hold down incidence to 10 cases/10,000 people	Eliminate the reservoir of infective cases in man	Eliminate the species down to the last female
Time span	Continuous	3–5 years for attack phase, and 3 years for consolidation phase; then maintenance phase for indefinite period	Determined by geographical spread and intensity of effort
Area of control	Selective in accord with disease incidence	Complete coverage of all malarious areas	Complete coverage wherever vector appears
Costs	Constantly recur	High; definable for period of campaign	Very high; not definable, as determined by vector behavior
Vector	Continues to be present	" Man-mosquito contact is greatly reduced but may return to original levels after insecticide pressure and reservoir of infection is gone without risk of renewed malaria transmission "†	Eliminated
Imported cases	Of no importance	Must be controlled, as vector and susceptibles present.	Of no importance as there is no vector
Surveillance required	Of disease incidence only and to keep it manageable	Of human case recurrence, and ability to control immediately	Of reintroduction of the vector, and ability to control immediately

* *WHO, Wkly. Epidemiolog. Rec.*, **44**: 489 (1969).
† Ennilio Rampana, "A Textbook of Malaria Eradication" p.1, Oxford University Press, London, 1963.

in the apparent absence of the disease.   The necessity of vigilance in the face of a few scattered cases per year is difficult to sustain among the people who must bring their cases to official attention, among appropriating bodies and budget officers, and among the health staff itself.   As is the case of waterborne diseases, malaria is more readily buried in the literature than in biological reality.   Taiwan presents another island situation.   Since 1965 it has been on the official register of the World Health Organization.   A few scattered cases have been reported yearly.   These must have prompt and zealous attention to maintain eradication.   The issue is one of administration and management.

RODENT ACTION AND MAN'S COUNTERACTION

For man, rodents produce disease, damage, and discomfiture.   Of all rodents, the two species of rats, *Rattus norvegicus* and *Rattus rattus*, which live most intimately with man, cause all three.   Other rats which make their habitat away from man's dwelling and buildings, such as the Polynesian rat, *Rattus exulans*, in the Hawaiian sugar cane fields and the fruit rat, *Rattus frugivorous*, in the Florida orchards, are principally economic liabilities, although there is a disease transmission potential.   The house mouse, *Mus musculus*, has a poorly recognized role in disease transmission, contributes substantially to the cost of damage, but has done these without earning the dislike and disgust directed to rats.   Estimates of the number of urban rats in the temperate zones in ratio to man have been moving downward in this century from 1:1 to 0.5:1 or less.   The disappearance of horses and backyard animal raising in the cities, which provided common housing and food for the domestic animals and the rats; the changes in building techniques and materials; the centralized processing and distribution of food with more care in tighter buildings; the improved collection and disposal of wastes; and direct control measures have together made rat survival more competitive.   On farms the ratio of rats to man is estimated to be 2:1 around the outbuildings.   Field rodents, dependent on man's crops, and wild rodents, avoiding man and living off natural vegetation, are reported to be very static in population, often in deep burrows providing quite constant temperature and humidity throughout the year. However, the numbers may be large in ratio to man.   A Pasteur Institute study in villages in India calculated a ratio of 5:1 for domestic rodents and ratio of 100:1 for field rodents.   The static populations of field rodents occasionally experience eruptions.   One in the Philippines during 1952 to 1954 produced from 200 to 2,000 rats per hectare, about 2.5 acres, and caused losses of 90 percent of the rice, 50 percent of the sugar cane, and from 20 to 80 percent of the corn.   Population ratios of rodent to man are based on observations in small areas, a single farm, or a number of dwellings in a city block.   Extrapolation to large areas and different ecological settings produces illusions, not data.

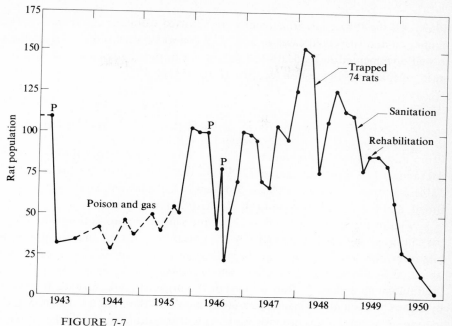

FIGURE 7-7

Changes in numbers of rats in a Baltimore block, 1943 to 1950. (*Source: P. E. Sartwell*, "*Maxcy-Rosenau Preventive Medicine and Public Health*," *9th ed., p. 476, Appleton-Century-Crofts, Inc., New York*, 1965.)

Any population in an area—rodent, mosquito, or man— is the resultant of three forces, birth, death, and migration. The magnitude of the forces is determined by fertility, ease of access to habitat, predation and disease, and the intensity of competition for food, shelter, and mates. Population observations of rodents in small areas can be extended to larger ones where the environmental factors are similar. This may be for a number of blocks of an urban slum, the farms of a Midwest county, or a number of villages in a district in India. Census methods for rodents are direct counts, estimates from counts of signs of infestation or from measurements of food consumption, or observations from trapping procedures. Figure 7-7 shows the response of rats in a block of dwellings in Baltimore to poisoning, trapping, sanitation, and, finally, building rehabilitation, from 1943 to 1950.

Rodents and Disease

The interaction of rats, fleas, and man in plague and endemic typhus, and the relation of rats, wild rodents, and man in sylvatic plague have been stated. Table 7-7 shows that plague cases continue where man lives in squalor and misery, and in the social shambles of war. Note the fourfold increase in the world's total cases from 1965 to

1967.   Of the 1967 cases 80 percent were reported from South Vietnam.   The 5,999 confirmed and suspected cases of 1967 in the world caused only 308 deaths.   Plague is well documented in its death toll before use of antibiotics came to save lives.   A series of epidemics in London recorded (Ref. 7-11, p. 53):

Year	1563	1593	1603	1625	1636	1665
Deaths	20,163	10,662	33,347	41,213	10,400	68,596

From mid-1834 to the dry summer heat of 1835, plague moved through Egypt from Alexandria to Cairo and caused 32,000 deaths.   Of the 850 plague cases shown in Table 7-7 for 1965 in the Americas, 574 were in Equador and Peru, 268 in Bolivia and Brazil, and 8 of sylvatic origin in the United States.

Figure 1-5 shows the course of endemic murine typhus in the United States and the southeastern states.   Appendix A gives brief information on leptospirosis and rat-bite fever, for which rats harbor the pathogens.   The role of rats in salmonellosis is obscured by the variety of means by which *Salmonella* can be moved from excreta to food intake by humans.   Rats do harbor the organism, are sickened by it, are killed by some species and strains, and certainly pass it in their feces.   Their fecal contamination of human food is grounds for barring that food from the market in the United States.   Until 1966 such contaminated food could be converted to animal feed without treatment that would kill *Salmonella* or any other pathogen which might be present. In that year the Federal Food and Drug Administration required the heat treatment of such food to kill *Salmonella*.   The reason was the steady increase of reported human cases of salmonellosis in the United States from 504 in 1942 to 15,390 in 1963.   Poultry fed on the contaminated converted food showed *Salmonella* in eggs and on the tissue after killing and cutting.   As some means of preparing chicken and the use of eggs do

Table 7-7   CASES OF HUMAN PLAGUE REPORTED TO THE WORLD HEALTH ORGANIZATION, 1961 TO 1965 AND 1967, BY CONTINENTS*

Area	1961	1962	1963	1964	1965	1966	1967
World total	781	1,443	861	1,604	1,326	...	1,023 confirmed 4,976 suspected
Africa	24	121	50	539	49	...	18
The Americas	308	527	431	659	850	...	223
Asia	449	794	380	406	427	...	782 confirmed 4,976 suspected
Europe		1					

* No reports are received from mainland China.
SOURCE: International Quarantine Office, WHO.

not require high heat and long cooking, *Salmonella* survival does occur.   Trichinosis is listed among rat-related infectious diseases, as the organism is adapted to rats.   The chain of events to hogs, the source of infection for man, takes place in insanitary garbage feeding to hogs.   Hogs eating infected rats are part of the filthy cycle.

A wide variety of organisms pathogenic to man have been identified in wild rodents.   These include the organisms of such diseases as taeniasis, echinococcosis, Chagas' disease, toxoplasmosis, glanders, tularemia, brucellosis, sand-fly fever, and the encephalitides.   All these have reservoirs in animals much closer to man, such as cattle, horses, dogs, commensal rodents, and domestic insects.   Transmission from wild rodents is rare, as it is dependent on the frequency and extent of contact.   The possibility is a reason for caution in handling wild rodents found injured, sick, or dead.

The house mouse is responsible for transmitting *Rickettsia akari*, which causes rickettsial pox in man with symptoms like chicken pox.   A bloodsucking mite moves the rickettsia from mice to man.   A skin condition, called *favus*, can be caused by a fungus, *Achorion quinckeanum*, which has been traced to mice.   A virus from the discharges of mice contaminates dust which causes lymphocytic choriomeningitis in man.   Mice can be the source of leptospirosis.   In Hawaii, H. P. Minette found mice to be the major carrier, surpassing rats, which are usually the principal reservoir of the spirochete causing leptospirosis.[1]   Mice can be the source of the tapeworms, *Hymenolepis nana* and *dimunuta*.   On occasions mice have been found to carry the pathogens of plague, murine typhus, and tularemia, but with minor responsibility as a reservoir of these for man.   House mice are frequently infected with *Salmonella* and can contaminate man's food with their feces.

Economic Losses and Discomfiture

Data on economic losses from specific situations are more reliable than statements extrapolated to a whole country.   An examination of crop losses to *Rattus exulans* on 25 sugar plantations totaling 231,000 acres in Hawaii showed an annual loss of $4.5 million plus an expenditure of $300,000 for control work.   In India, there are records of rodent burrows' weakening dikes, which failed and resulted in thousands of acres' being flooded near Delhi; of burrows' undermining railway embankments and causing derailments; and of burrows' damaging irrigation systems so that water leakage and loss of control resulted in crop yields 10 percent below norms.   The study of areas in India has shown crop damage to vary from 10 to 35 percent.   The Philippine loss of rice is estimated at 1.3 million tons/year with a value of $125 million.   Losses in storage are not great in terms of the actual rodent consumption, but are large because of contamination by feces and urine and destruction of sacks and other containers.   A

[1] *Amer. J. Trop. Med. Hyg.*, **13**:826 (1964).

mouse may eat only 70 to 100 wheat grains in a day, but it puts out 50 droppings which are spread about in 5 lb of formerly clean wheat.   Studying rats in England, S. A. Barnett[1] found that 10 to 26 rats with access to 1 ton of sacked wheat in a period of 3 to 7 months used 4 to 5 percent of it, fouled 70 percent, and caused a loss of nearly 20 percent of the original value of the wheat and sacks.

The frequently cited figures of $10 of damage per rat per year in the United States with a population of 100 million rats were stated by E. M. Mills in 1953[2].   Thirteen years later Mills conceded a 10 percent reduction in rats.   Such generalized data requires caution with the risk of having to prove their applicability to a locality.   The risk of an appropriation for control equal to the board bill is nil.   In 1968 the House of Representatives of the United States refused $40 million for rat control in urban slums until a journalistically aroused people expressed their indignation and discomfiture with rats in terms the members of Congress understood.   Subsequently, $20 million was appropriated.

The Bad Actors among Rodents

The zoologists have placed names on 570 species and subspecies of the genus *Rattus*. Table 7-8 gives the characteristics of the two species that have fully domesticated in man's dwellings, urban, rural, and suburban.   These two plus a few other species identified with heavy crop losses are the target of control.   Each of the two have aliases derived from alleged origins, color, or occasional habitat.   *Rattus norvegicus* did not originate in Norway.   It is called the *brown rat, sewer rat,* or *Norway rat*. *Rattus rattus* includes some subspecies and is variously known as *roof, ship, grey, black, Alexandrian,* and *English rat*.   When food and harborage are generously available, Norway and roof rats are found in the same buildings.   Under competitive con-

Table 7-8   DISTINGUISHING CHARACTERISTICS OF THE TWO PRINCIPAL SPECIES OF DOMESTIC RATS

Species	Body and head	Ears	Tail/body ratio	Climbing ability	Nesting and harborage
Rattus norvegicus, Norway rat	Heavy, thick; blunt muzzle	Small, close set	Shorter than body	Very limited	Shallow burrows usual
Rattus rattus, Roof rat	Slender pointed muzzle	Large, stand out	Longer than body	Agile and able	Within and under secure spaces in buildings

[1] *J. Hyg.,* **49**:22 (1951).
[2] *U.S. Fish. Wildlife Serv., Circ.* 22, 1953.

ditions the Norway rat drives out the roof rat with the latter's taking refuge in attics and upper stories.   Without having to use burrows for nesting, the roof rat is closer to man and uses its climbing ability to gain access to dead spaces in walls, between floors and ceilings, and in roof structures.

Table 7-9 provides dismaying and comforting information.   Rats are prolific in breeding, but mortality is high.   D. E. Davis found that in a year, between two and three older and juvenile adult rats die for each one surviving in the rat population. Among weanling rats nine die each year for each one living out a year.   The average life of a weaned Norway rat in the wild is estimated to be about 6 months.   With high rates of reproduction, rat populations are at saturation for the available food and housing.   The short home range is a reminder that the rats you see about your dwelling and buildings are your own, or at least have their nests or burrows close at hand.

When rats are seen during the day, large numbers are about, as rats seek their food by night, warily avoiding man and any predators.   When infestations are moderate or heavy, rat signs are readily evident.   These include droppings, gnawing, despoiled food, damaged containers, and loss of material that is used for nests, rat runways, rat burrows of the Norway rats, nests of roof rats, rat "swings," the marking of roof rats as they swing under floor joists in a trip across a main beam, and urine stains which fluoresce under ultraviolet light.   Such signs are used to estimate populations and to measure the progress of control measures.

Control Methods

All three techniques of control, permanent, temporary, and naturalistic, are in use against rodents.   Permanent control is the only means which can produce a lasting reduction in commensal rodent numbers.   Temporary measures are necessary in the face of disease outbreaks, population eruptions, and an aroused public demand for immediate action when the people perceive a real or fancied threat.   Naturalistic

Table 7-9   REPRODUCTIVITY, LONGEVITY, AND RANGE OF THE NORWAY AND THE ROOF RAT

Species of rat	Reproductivity*			Average life span	Home range, ft
	Litters/year	Number/litter	Number/year		
Norway	4.3	8.7	37.4	6 months	100–150
Roof	5.4	6.4	35.6	?	Up to 200

* Data from D. E. Davis, The Characteristics of Rat Populations, *Quart. Rev. Biol.*, **28**:373 (1953).

methods continue to reveal our ecological ignorance, continue to have a few enthusiastic supporters, and have shown a backlash in some applications.

Enough is known about the movement, nesting, and food sources of rats to apply permanent control to our homes; to buildings for food processing, storage, and handling; to ships, planes, trucks, and railway cars; and to the management of solid wastes. These measures are not as effective against mice because of the size of mice and their ease in penetrating openings less than $\frac{1}{2}$ in. The measures are more difficult to apply to farm buildings because of our customary ways of building these and the liberty of rodents to move from field to buildings with season and food availability. Permanent control requires structural materials, structural design, and careful workmanship which produce a building or a food storage or transport container to keep rodents out, to deny them nesting and harborage, and to minimize access to food and water. *Rat proofing*, as these measures are called, are wholly compatible with sound design and careful workmanship. Maintenance is necessary to hold the line. Attention to alterations which require a pass through outside walls such as for pipes, conduits, wires, and air ducts is necessary. The access opening must be sealed tightly about the new line and collared. A frank open space or a gnawing edge is the starting point for rat entry. Closure of rat openings to old buildings requires careful examination and repairs around windows and doors and vent, pipe, and wire pass-throughs; pointings up of old brickwork; and replacement of broken glass. There is a need to have architects, contractors, and building repair people aware of rat proofing. There is a rat control benefit from the enforcement of minimum housing quality by local health, building, and housing authorities.

The history and development of rodent killing duplicates that of killing insects. The first poisons were natural alkaloids such as red squill and strychnine. These are still useful. Inorganic compounds came into use such as arsenicals, barium carbonate, zinc phosphide, and thallium sulfate. In part, these continue to have effective applications. In the 1940s organic compounds entered with alpha-napthylthiourea (ANTU), sodium fluoroacetate (1080), and the anticoagulants of which warfarin, or WARF-42, was the first. As with DDT and its residual killing power for insects, WARF-42 was greeted as the agent that would rid man of rats. Its safety, its ease of application, and its effectiveness appeared to put the permanent (continual) control methods on the shelf. It took Swedish and Italian houseflies only 2 years to dispel the DDT miracle. It has taken the rats of the United Kingdom the best of 20 years to show resistance to the anticoagulants. The rats of Denmark and The Netherlands have matched the the English rats in presenting the rodent control specialists with the dilemma of resistance and are restoring permanent control measures to grace (Ref. 7-5, pp. 18, 241).

Table 7-10 gives the characteristics of the anticoagulant type of rodenticides. Reference 7-12 (pp. 18–19) provides detailed data on the natural alkaloids and inorganic, single-dose rodenticides, and additional data on the anticoagulant, multiple-dose types.

A choice of rodenticides requires facts about the rodents, the immediate locale, the people, the pets and animals of value in the area, the work force, and the objective of the effort, its duration, its finances, and its relation to permanent measures of control. The range of circumstances is from a weekend volunteer effort in a United States suburban area where two or three rats have been sighted, to a sustained effort in an English urban area with a disciplined, trained crew working under professionals utilizing the full armamentarium of rat control methods backed by laboratory service.   In either case the objective is to kill rats, but in the first one it is for a temporary decrease.   In the second one, the objective may be attempted eradication by intensive and varied use of poison, selected in accord with each locale and premises, and scheduled block by block.   In the first case, safety against misuse of the poison must depend upon the choice of the one with the least risk to the workers, the families, and exposed pets.   In the second case, safety can rest on the skill and knowledge of the workers, the matching of poison to premises, and on accurate records of time, place and means of distribution.   In the first case, the plan is one round of coverage.   The second can plan a dogged campaign matching tactics to rat response.   The first is restricted to a choice of red squill or possibly zinc phosphide.   The second can select the poison fitted to the task as it unfolds.   The use of 1080, an organic fluoride (sodium fluoroacetate), is possible in locked, unoccupied warehouses overnight and weekends, with quantities and placement recorded and indexed.   Anticoagulants can be used

Table 7-10   MULTIPLE–DOSE RODENTICIDES OFFERED IN BAITS THAT KILL BY BLOOD ANTICOAGULANT ACTION

Generic name	Trade or other name	Concentration in baits, mg/kg	Bait mixtures and preferences	Hazard to man and other animals
Coumafuryl	Fumarin	250–500	Anticoagulant rodenticides are used with foods attractive to rodents. These are meat, fish, grains, nuts, fruits, sweets, and vegetables; yellow cornmeal is readily accepted and cheap; Norway rats prefer meat and fish mixes.	Slight
Diphacinone	Diphacin, PID	50–250 highs for mice		Slight
Pindone	Pival, Pivalyn, Pivalyn Valone	250–500		Slight
Warfarin	WARF-42	250–500 except 50–250 for Norway rats		Slight

with bait mixes varied with observed changes in preference and quantities consumed. Signs of tolerance and resistance can be studied in the laboratory.

With the exception of the water-soluble organic fluorides and the anticoagulants rodenticide use assumes a single feeding of enough poison, mixed in an attractive bait, to be lethal.   Prebaiting of unfamiliar habitats is used to determine bait preferences and quantities taken.   The organic fluorides are offered in rat drinking water.   Likely the rat takes more than one drink to get a lethal dose, which is as low as 2 to 5 mg/kg of rat weight.   The anticoagulants require repeated feeding for several days to build up the internal hemorrhaging which kills the rat as its blood system loses its coagulant properties.   This mean that baits must be attractive and mold resistant, and they must be put out repeatedly, placed in a bait box or station to limit access for other animals, and monitored for condition and refill.   By well-planned and managed work, 100 percent control of rats by anticoagulants has been achieved in English and German towns.   This continued success is threatened by the survival and reproduction of rats with the genetic attribute of withstanding the anticoagulants in use.

The hazard to man and other animals puts severe restrictions on rodenticide choice and use.   Those with a high risk and poor kill should not be used at all. Arsenic trioxide, barium carbonate, and yellow phosphorus give erratic results.   Their high toxicity does not warrant the risk, with other more effective poisons available. Sodium fluoroacetate (1080), fluoroacetamide (1081), strychnine, and thallium sulfate are very effective against rats, but have a high risk in use.   This requires regulated use. In the United States, the regulation extends to banning the household use of thallium sulfate under the federal Insecticide, Fungicide, and Rodenticide Act.   Both 1080 and 1081 are restricted to use by those trained in their application and then only on premises with controlled access for man and animals, with careful placing, recording, and collecting of the poison-water containers.   Formula 1080 kills rats better than any other poison, but unfortunately kills other animals better than it kills rats.   "Better" means at lower milligram per killogram doses.   Three questions are considered in a choice of risks:

1   What is the margin between lethal dose to rats and that to the protected species? For the latter, consider the weight of poisoned bait that must be consumed.
2   Is an emetic effect produced either naturally as by red squill or by adding tartar emetic to the poisoned bait?   Effectiveness against rodents is not changed as they do not have a vomiting response.
3   Is there an antidote, and is it available to cope with an accidental ingestion?

Attempts to intensify natural predation among rodents have been disappointing and have had undesirable consequences in some instances.   Cats and rat terriers have a firm place in folklore which cannot be documented.   An occasional kill is not sufficient intensity.   The mongoose was introduced from Jamaica to some of the Hawaiian and Fijian Islands to kill rats. It showed a preference for fruit, poultry, and other birds. On Puerto Rico, the mongoose, introduced to kill rats, became a rabies reservoir. Varanid lizards and the Japanese weasel have been nominated and tried on Pacific and Japanese islands. The local abundance of food alternatives and ease of preying on animals other than rats determines the success of introduced predators. As varanid lizards had reduced the rat damage to the coconut crop on one Pacific island, a preintroduction study was made on another, otherwise similar island by a consultant of the World Health Organization. He found that the crab population was far more attractive to the new lizard than the rats. The crabs were easier to catch and soon showed reduced numbers from the new predation pressure. The Japanese weasel was recommended as it has been an effective rat killer on a few small Japanese islands.

The first suggestion to kill rats by introducing bacterial infections is attributed to Pasteur. The idea is to trigger an epizootic among rats by putting out rich cultures of pathogenic bacteria. Since the 1890s *Salmonella typhimurium* and *enteritidis var. danysz* have been used. As both are pathogenic to man, the extension to man is a real risk and has occurred in the United States, Denmark, and Germany. After World War II, a rat irruption in eastern Poland was curbed by the use of 50 tons of *Salmonella enteritidis var. danysz* cultures. The exposed human population was immunized during the rat campaign. As the enthusiasts for these agents have often used poisons in combination with the biological agent, a clear advantage over other methods with more manageable risks is not established. The World Health Organization considers the use of *Salmonella* organisms for the control of rats unsafe.

SCHISTOSOMIASIS

The Dynamics of Transmission

An estimated 200 million people are infected by one of the three trematode worms, or blood flukes, the schistosomes. These people are almost wholly among the world's vast number of subsistence agrarian families. The most severe infections are among male adolescents and adults to their midtwenties. Those hosting *Schistosoma mansoni* are in Africa, South America, and the Caribbean islands. Those hosting *Schistosoma japonicum* are in China, the Philippines, the Celebes, Japan, and in other localized areas of Southeast Asia. Finally, large numbers of people are infected with *Schistosoma haematobium*. Most of these are in Africa along the Nile River and spreading westward north and south of the Sahara, with some in areas near Bombay, India. The disease is debilitating in its acute phase with dysentery, fever, and cystitis.

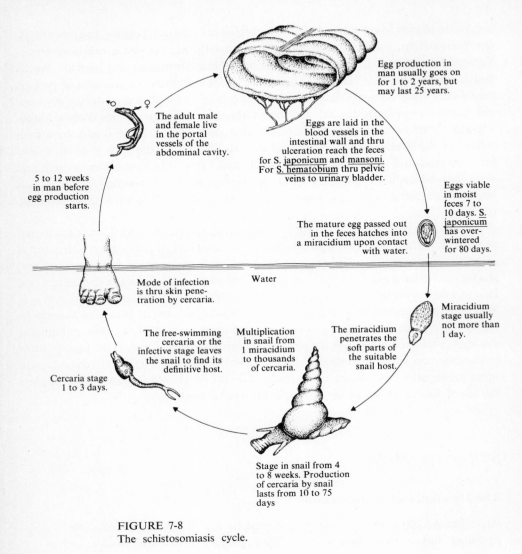

Egg production in man usually goes on for 1 to 2 years, but may last 25 years.

The adult male and female live in the portal vessels of the abdominal cavity.

Eggs are laid in the blood vessels in the intestinal wall and thru ulceration reach the feces for S. japonicum and mansoni. For S. hematobium thru pelvic veins to urinary bladder.

5 to 12 weeks in man before egg production starts.

Eggs viable in moist feces 7 to 10 days. S. japonicum has over-wintered for 80 days.

The mature egg passed out in the feces hatches into a miracidium upon contact with water.

Mode of infection is thru skin pene-tration by cercaria.

Water

Miracidium stage usually not more than 1 day.

The free-swimming cercaria or the infective stage leaves the snail to find its definitive host.

Multiplication in snail from 1 miracidium to thousands of cercaria.

The miracidium penetrates the soft parts of the suitable snail host.

Cercaria stage 1 to 3 days.

Stage in snail from 4 to 8 weeks. Production of cercaria by snail lasts from 10 to 75 days

FIGURE 7-8
The schistosomiasis cycle.

It is not a dramatic killer. It wastes the nutritional resources of its victims. In its chronic phase there is liver damage, pulmonary complications, spleen enlargement, and intestinal or urogenital effects depending on the species. There are no epidemic flare-ups. It is difficult to control. So it has been endured with considerable apathy to the detriment of the development of individuals, families, and communities. The mummified dead of Egypt show the infection. In Egypt about 1850, Theodor Bilharz found the worm, now *S. haematobium*, in the blood vessels of the bladder, and identified it as the cause of the common bloody urine of young males who worked the irrigated fields along the Nile.   The disease is also called bilharziasis and in Africa is better known by that name.   As aquatic or amphibian snails are needed for the parasite cycle, occurrence goes with water use and land development.   The prevalence of the disease is increasing, as efforts to increase food production require more irrigation, more cattle wateringholes, more fishponds, more migration to sparsely populated areas (Refs. 7-13 and 7-14).

Figure 7-8 shows the cycle from man's feces and urine to water, to snail, to water, and back into man.   Time and numbers are stated.   These are formidable factors. Each egg produces one miracidium to seek a snail.   Each miracidium produces thousands of cercaria which try for skin penetration to reenter man.   The age and sex distribution of human cases reflects frequency of water contact which gives the cercaria their chance.   Animals close to man are reservoirs for man's schistosomes.   *S. japonicum* has been found in dogs, cats, rats, mice, cattle, water buffalo, pigs, horses, sheep, and goats.   These animals are proved reservoirs of human infection.   *S. mansoni* is found naturally in many animals in Africa and South America, especially in monkeys, cattle, and several rodents.   *S. haematobium* has been observed only sporadically as natural infections in animals.   The snail hosts are *Biomphalaria* for *S. mansoni*, *Oncomelania* for *S. japonicum* and *Bulinus* for *S. haematobium*.

The Control of Schistosomiasis

The environmental conditions required for transmission are:

1   The discharge of feces and urine so that these reach bodies of fresh water
2   Water characteristics which permit egg survival and production of miracidia
3   An aquatic environment which supports snails
4   Production of cercaria in snails and cercaria survival in the water
5   Human contact in the water for cercaria penetration through the skin

Ecological study to date has not revealed any definitively manageable physical or chemical characteristic of water which would prevent schistosome egg development, or miracidia or cercaria survival.   Table 7-11 highlights the action required and the outlook for success of control measures aimed at items *1*, *3*, and *5*.   The use of molluscicides to kill the snails has the great attraction of not having to change the existing aquatic environment or the peoples' habits.   Table 7-11 lists four widely used molluscicides. Additional "candidate" molluscicides are discussed in Ref 7-14.   A low-cost molluscicide effective against all snail species which host schistosomes and which can be easily used in a variety of aquatic conditions is not available.   The chemicals that are most convenient to use are Bayluscide and Frescon.   A sustained and concerted campaign against schistosomiasis requires a combination of all the actions noted in Table 7-11. For long-term success such a campaign must be a part of the socioeconomic rise of agrarian communities.   This has been observed in Puerto Rico, where schistosomiasis has decreased as the economy developed.   In the Philippines a decrease has come in areas where there have been control measures in conjunction with changes in farming methods.

Table 7-12 summarizes information on ecological factors recognized as adverse or favorable for snail hosts and the schistosomes.   The information is gross and not sufficient to suggest a control mechanism or to explain the selective adaptation or preferences which snails reveal by their ability to populate some water sites without successfully colonizing others in the same locale.   Relatively few people care about

Table 7-11   ENVIRONMENTAL CONTROL POINTS FOR BLOCKING SCHISTOSOME TRANSMISSION

Vulnerable point	Required action	Means available	Outlook for success
Keep urine and feces from water.	High degree of excreta control.	Privies, individual discipline for disposal in fields.	Good in and around villages, poor for control in irrigated fields, education and motivation necessary.
Human contact with infected water.	Restrict and control water use, provide special-use water sites.	Water for bathing and laundry isolated from other uses; fence water holes, and pipe water out to use points; fill clandestine waterholes.	Good for bathing and laundering facilities convenient to villages; waterhole fencing and filling require maintenance and discipline.
Snail host.	Prevent production by changing environment.	On irrigation canals, cyclic drying, edge cleaning, and weed control. In waterlogged areas, drainage, channeling, filling, and grading reduce snail numbers; deepening areas to create fishponds reduced snails in Philippines.	Good where it is part of irrigation system design and management; reduction in snails requires sustained effort.
	Snail killed by chemical dose to water.	Copper sulfate, Frescon, niclosamide (Bayluscide), sodium pentachlorophenate.	Good if sustained; cost is high; dosage must be repeated frequently; careful field tests required.

schistosomiasis, including, unhappily, those infected. Emile A. Malek states, "Schistosomiasis is a waterborne disease, and cultural habits which encourage pollution of the water and bring a population into contact with infested waters propagate the disease. This cultural element is a fundamental factor in the control of schistosomiasis, differentiating it from malaria, with which it is often compared." (Ref. 7-13, p. 262.)

CHANGES AND DEVELOPMENTS IN CONTROLLING ANIMAL VECTORS

Three Restraints on New Chemical Usage

When DDT came into production and use, the insect killers applied it widely against many insects. No questions were raised. That freedom of action in applying any new compounds is now restrained. Three restraints emerged from the experiences in using DDT and subsequent compounds.

Table 7-12 ENVIRONMENTAL EFFECTS ON SNAILS AND SCHISTOSOMES

Environmental elements	Favorable for snails	Adverse for snails	Favorable for schistosomes	Adverse for schistosomes
Temperature °C	22–26	Below 0, above 40	25–30	Below 20, above 35
Light	Moderate sun, microflora growth	Darkness	Phototropic, active in daylight hours	Darkness
Seasons	Rainy for breeding, growth, and transport to new colonies	Dry	Rainy for excreta transport and snail contact	Dry for egg survival and hatching
Water movement	Slow current and gentle waves	Swift and violent		
Turbidity	Low to moderately rich in organics	High, silty		
Salinity	*Biomphalaria* can tolerate gradual increases	Above 1,000–2,500 mg/l for *Bulinus*	....	No hatching over 5,000 mg/l
Dissolved oxygen	Necessary	....	Necessary	Less than 6.5 mg/l
pH	6–8	Below 5, above 10	5–8	Below 5, above 8

1   Target-insect resistance
2   Effects on nontarget species, such as beneficial bees
3   Long-term contamination of the free environment and cumulative transfers in plant and animal feeding cycles by very stable compounds with lifetime genetic effects unknown.

The World Health Organization has been following a seven-step protocol for new insecticide evaluation and testing, in which manufacturers participate.   There are three screening stages in the United States laboratories, with concurrent toxicity studies in England.   The successful candidates go on first to small-scale field tests; then to operational evaluation in active control areas of 20,000 to 30,000 people; and finally for chemicals which can be used in malaria eradication evaluation in a control area of 250,000 people.   The laws of many nations now require extensive testing of new compounds, registration of formulations, and accurate labeling before release for public use.   Wildlife observers have a new awareness and sensitivity to localized species "wipe-outs."   A systematic environmental surveillance has not begun.   The result is a higher cost for new insecticide development, a more effective marketed product, and a larger view of the responsibilities and consequences of sustained attacks on undesirable animal species with chemicals.

Genetics and Reproductivity

The genetic base of most insect, and now rat, resistance to man's chemicals has stimulated research on the genetics of insects and on insect control by genetic manipulation. Ionizing radiation and chemosterilants are a means of producing sterile male insects for release to produce nonreproductive matings.   The study of genetic distinctions among single mosquito species has shown that certain crosses do not carry reproduction to success.   Male *Culex fatigans* of exceptional vigor, produced by a cross of a Fresno, California, strain, and a Paris strain, were released in a Burmese village.   Eggs were laid, but a cytoplasmic incompatibility prevents complete fertilization.   In a 3-month trial *Culex fatigans* was eliminated from the village.   Genetic differences among *Anopheles gambiae* are the basis for a study by the World Health Organization on introducing nonfertile crosses in Upper Volta, Africa (Ref. 7-5, pp. 36–42).   The possibility of hormone use for insect control is being investigated.

The Ecological Gap

The three restraints on the use of new poisons against animal vectors has underscored the gaps in our ecological information on these vectors.   The application and study of genetic controls require more ecological information.   More precise knowledge of vectorial capacity is needed to use mathematical models such as G. MacDonald has proposed.   Data on vector characteristics such as biting preferences, habitat, breeding cycles, range, longevity in the free state, fertility, reproduction, and survival are acceptably complete for the rough and ready control in general use.   The rigorous application of cost-benefit analysis and a prior selection of alternative methods with predictions of success require infinitely more detailed data.   The ability of the vectors to adapt to man's measures is recognized.   The continued assessment of these adaptations requires more known biology of animal vectors.

In the use of the physical environment during the past century, man, without a thought about disease control, has taken some actions in which animal vectors have been placed in highly disadvantageous relations.   The recession of malaria from the north-central United States is cited.   He is also continuing to take actions which favor the animal vectors, again without thought about disease transmission.   The extension of schistosomiasis to south Brazil when infected humans migrated from the endemic areas of Northeast Brazil to newly opened farm lands, where the snail host already existed in the local waters, is an example.   The requirement is a holistic concept of man's management and use of the physical environment.   Many inputs are needed to achieve such management.   The ecology of animal vectors is one.

AN APPRAISAL OF MAN'S CONTROL OF INSECTS AND RODENTS

The First Level—The Prevention of Disease Transmission

With accurate information on the transmission of malaria, yellow fever, and plague less than 100 years old, public health organizations have developed and deployed control methods with extraordinary effectiveness.   In the case of endemic typhus in the southeastern United States, the time between K. F. Maxcy's analysis of the epidemiology of the disease in 1926 and its disappearance through intense communitywide rat control was less than 25 years.   Yellow fever has been controlled in the Western Hemisphere.   One billion people, two thirds of all the world's population, living in malarious areas have been protected from malaria.   Plague outbreaks have been speedily contained except where the community structure is racked by war, as in the case of the South Vietnam outbreaks in 1967 and 1968.

From the standpoint of techniques, malaria eradication is not in doubt except for Africa south of the Sahara.   There the habits of the mosquitoes and the people require more analysis for the design of effective campaigns.   There, too, the financial and human resources for such an effort are thin, and are required to meet many social and economic needs of recently created nations.   The global strategy of malaria eradication is being reexamined by the World Health Organization for three reasons.

1   As campaigns approach success or achieve it, the urgency of malaria recedes and appropriating bodies become reluctant to continue the necessary funds.   Their demands for economic proof of the developmental return cannot be met with complete and accurate data.

2   The task of carrying eradication through its last stages is costly and tedious, with a heavy drain on organizational morale and zeal.

3   Eradication is difficult to maintain where infected persons can move from malarious areas.

Malaria eradication is achieving its goal and has done so with an economic benefit which has been easier to demonstrate in developed areas.   The reexamination will provide more complete socioeconomic data, a careful analysis of effective organizational patterns, and directions for technical adjustments.   All this will be beneficial to eradication planning in underdeveloped areas, where the costs are high relative to financial and manpower resources.

The emergence of mosquito-borne viral disease in Southeast Asia has been met with field and laboratory studies of the disease and the vector.   When sufficiently complete data is at hand, effective control measures can be devised.   Some control measures taken from Western Hemisphere *Aedes aegypti* campaigns are already in use.   The spread of schistosomiasis goes with people and the opening of land for farming with and without irrigation.   Economic, effective, and easily applicable control methods are not developed.   Sylvatic plague has slowly extended across the western third of the United States.   An eradication effort would be costly and on a heroic scale.   The United States *Aedes aegypti* eradication was going forward on a scale fitted to the funds the Congress has been willing to appropriate, and that with a view to our international posture rather than health benefits to the people of the southeast and south-central states, until the work was terminated in the fall of 1968.   Each of these disease-vector situations culminate in the question, Is control by present methods worth the cost?   In the past, public health practitioners met this question with emotion-ladened statements on epidemics and threats of epidemics.   The present and the future require more objective analysis of costs and benefits.

The Second Level—Comfort, Convenience, and Esthetics

The elimination of pestiferous insects and obnoxious rodents can be achieved in any target area.   Again the issue is the cost of the sustained effort.   Salt-marsh mosquito abatement adjacent to seaside resort areas is an example.   The control of flies, rats, and roaches around high-cost suburban dwellings in the United States is another example and also marks a second point.   That is, control of insects and rodents for these second-level benefits is directly related to socioeconomic status.   Some is the result of the ability of those in better socioeconomic conditions to demand and to get more community services of solid-waste collection, sewerage, area drainage, and water supply.   These families are able to utilize these services more fully by providing the complementary facilities in and about their homes.   Their homes are newer, better built, better maintained, and usually more distant from breeding and harborage provided by dumps, swamps, run-down warehouses, insanitary stockyards, and filthy food processing plants.   Those in better socioeconomic conditions have more knowledge or at least awareness, and they have the means to make the changes to control the insects and rodents they deem undesirable.   An analysis of the geographical origin of a couple of hundred cases of children bitten by rats for any large city in the United States will support the relation of poverty and rat infestation.

The Third Level—Safeguarding the Ecological Balance

The presence of DDT and its analogs in the free environment and in all animal cycles precipitated Rachel Carson's *Silent Spring*.   Her observations produced a thoughtful appraisal of man's use of pesticides for his sole and immediate benefit.   These have brought changes in practice, are influencing development of new pesticides, and have improved evaluation before use.   The President's Committee report (Ref. 7-15) is a conscientious assessment of the issue.   The 1969 report of a special study commission appointed by the Secretary of the Department of Health, Education, and Welfare is lengthy and detailed.   It provides the best that concerted expertise could bring to the issues.   It recommends mechanisms for the specific exception of DDT and DDD from restrictions for uses " essential to the preservation of human health and welfare " (Ref. 7-16, p. 8).   Use of pesticides for public health purposes is small compared with agricultural use.   Nevertheless, public health users have responded.   Their required response is compatible with the resistance of vectors to the pesticides.   The requirement is better knowledge of the ecology of their target species and of species incidentally affected by prescribed procedures.   The issue arises in evaluating molluscicides, as damage to fish life and aquatic plants and effects on water quality for drinking, cooking, bathing, laundering, and irrigation must be considered.   No major dilemma has had to be confronted.   If the choice of using a toxic chemical to curb an epidemic had to be made in the face of demonstrable evidence that there would be damage to other animal species, the toxic chemical would be used.   In the face of an endemic situation, the use of such a chemical would be withheld.   Dependence would be placed on less efficient controls with efforts continued to find better means without damage to other plant and animal species.

Changes in the physical environment for the control of disease vectors have eliminated other species.   Drainage for mosquito control modifies an existing aquatic environment which sacrifices a variety of plant and animal forms.   These areas have been small and are not known to have eliminated any species, rare or treasured by wildlife people. Such projects are smaller in scope than man's demands on existing land status and use for agriculture, roads, airports, harbors, and building sites. When a valued species or site is at stake, a careful analysis of the choices should produce alternative control procedures or modifications of the project to serve public health needs and to attain conservation objectives.

REFERENCES

7-1 Vector Control, *Semin. Rodents and Rodent Ectoparasites*, *WHO*, 1966, p. 217.
7-2 CLARK, L. R., P. W. GEIR, R. D. HUGHES, and R. F. MORRIS: "The Ecology of Insect Populations in Theory and Practice," Methuen & Co., Ltd., London, 1967.
7-3 LOGAN, JOHN: "The Sardinian Project," The Johns Hopkins Press, Baltimore, 1958.
7-4 "Specifications for Pesticides Used in Public Health," 3d ed., *WHO*, 1967.
7-5 Seventeenth Report of World Health Organization's Expert Committee on Insecticides: Insecticide Resistance and Vector Control, *WHO*, *Tech. Rep. Ser.* 443, 1970.
7-6 "Equipment for Vector Control," *WHO*, 1964.
7-7 CUSHING, E. J.: History of Entomology in World War II, *Smithsonian Inst.*, *Publ.* 4294, 1957.
7-8 RUSSELL, PAUL: "Man's Mastery of Malaria," Oxford University Press, London, 1955.
7-9 HULL, THOMAS G. (ed.): "Diseases Transmitted from Animals to Man," 5th ed., Charles C Thomas, Publishers, Springfield, Ill., 1963.
7-10 POLLITZER, R.: "Plague," *WHO*, 1954.
7-11 HIRST, L. F.: "The Conquest of Plague," Clarendon Press, Oxford, 1953.
7-12 BJORNSON, B. F., H. D. PRATT, and K. S. LITTIG: "Control of Domestic Rats and Mice," *U.S. Public Health Serv. Publ.* 563, 1969.
7-13 MALEK, EMILE A.: The Ecology of Schistosomiasis, in JACQUES M. MAY (ed.), "The Ecology of Human Disease," vol. 2, chap. 10, Hafner Publishing Company, Inc., New York, 1961.
7-14 Epidemiology and Control of Schistosomiasis, *WHO*, *Tech. Rep. Ser.* 372, 1967.
7-15 President's Science Advisory Committee: "Use of Pesticides," The White House, 1963.
7-16 "Pesticides and Their Relationship to Environmental Health," *Comm. to Secr.*, *U.S. Health, Education, and Welfare Rep.*, Department of Health, Education, and Welfare, 1969.

8

FOOD PROTECTION FROM SOURCE TO USE

COMPATIBILITIES AND CONTRASTS BETWEEN CULTURAL PATTERNS AND FOOD PROTECTION GOALS

Men, mice, and elephants take an inspecting look, a suspecting sniff, and expecting taste before loading in the first mouthful of any food new to their experience or from a new hand or new source. To this innate safeguard, shared with other animals, man adds a fascinating collection of culturally conditioned preferences. The reasons and goals of food preferences are remarkably like those for food protection. In the main, the order is reversed. The culturally based choices made within the tradition of a society have been directed to:

1 Achieve abundance
2 Make the food palatable and attractive in the local frame of values
3 Keep the nutrient value as high as possible
4 Handle it in storage to reduce losses
5 Keep it free of filth and of objectionable additions
6 Keep it free of poisons, by rejecting naturally poisonous foods, removing poisonous parts, and processing to inactivate poisons, and avoid knowingly adding materials in quantities which cause poisoning
7 Keep it free of pathogenic biological agents.

The application of hygiene for food protection requires that the rank order of seven goals be reversed:

1 Free of pathogens
2 Free of toxic chemicals
3 Free of adulterants
4 Effective protection in storage
5 Nutrients intact
6 Palatable and attractive
7 Abundant

In practice, the goals are mixed and overlapped. This holds whether the actions of a sanitarian visiting a local drive-in or the decisions of a Joint Expert Committee of the United Nations are examined.

THREE PRIMARY TARGETS OF FOOD PROTECTION

Pathogenic Biological Agents

Pathogenic biological agents are the top priority target of actions to protect our food. The organisms have been quite adaptive to changes in food technology. A gap ensues as scientific study catches up with the organisms. A longer gap follows before field practice adjusts to apply the new understanding of the organisms' new behavior. An example is the salmonella bacteria. Much restaurant sanitation effort goes into sanitary toilet facilities, handwashing, cleaning work surfaces, utensils, and equipment to curb the salmonella of human origin. Salmonellas are present in these environments in small numbers except when a frank human case is in the preparation line. These measures are helpful in reducing the risks from symptomless human carriers of salmonellas. That approach was more productive in the days when the restaurant food supply was of local origin and the menu fitted to the growing seasons. Food technology has developed low-cost frozen eggs, dried milk, and mass produced, handled, transported, and processed chickens, pigs, and ducks. The salmonellas joined in the procession of change, appearing in the eggs and the dried milk, moving from the intestines of the animals to the tissue during the physiologically stressful truck and train trips to the assembly-line slaughtering plants, and appearing in chickens fed on partially processed animal wastes. Sanitary technology has caught up with the behavior and is being applied through egg pasteurization, better disinfection of the milk drying equipment, improved handling of livestock, effective sanitation at meat and poultry processing plants, and pasteurization of reprocessed animal wastes. It has reduced salmonella in these foods, but has not wholly eliminated the contaminants. The safeguard is in reducing the mass of the dose.

In this review the biological agents are grouped by morphological type with the bacteria divided according to their mode of physiological attack.   The principal actors are cited with their main roles and their favorite stages noted.   The full cast is long and varied with many "bitplayers" making rare, short appearances in special scenes. Appendix A notes some of the lesser role players, which use food occasionally to reach man.   Such organisms reach man more frequently, and with more success, by direct contact, by insect vectors, and by water.   Table 8-1 presents the reported outbreaks and cases of food-borne illnesses caused by eight types of bacteria, one virus, and two parasites in the United States for the years 1967, 1968, and 1969.

Toxin-producing Bacteria

Staphylococci usually lead as a cause of acute food poisonings in the United States. These multiply in pastries, custards, creamy salads and salad dressings, sliced meat, and meat products held for 2 or more hours at temperatures over 40°F (4.4°C) and under 120°F (49°C).   In growth, enterotoxins that are stable at 212°F (100°C) are produced. Their ingestion causes nausea, vomiting, cramps, diarrhea, and prostration in 1 to 6

Table 8-1   OUTBREAKS AND CASES OF FOOD-BORNE ILLNESSES BY SPECIFIC ETIOLOGY REPORTED IN THE UNITED STATES IN THE YEARS 1967, 1968, and 1969

Agents	1967		1968		1969	
	Outbreaks	Cases	Outbreaks	Cases	Outbreaks	Cases
Bacterial						
Staphylococcus	55	1,914	82	4,419	94	3,481
Clostridium perfringens	29	3,493	56	5,966	65	18,527
C. botulinum	3	6	9	10	10	17
Salmonella	35	12,836	42	1,287	49	1,892
S. typhosa	5	54	Not summarized separately			
Shigella	7	587	6	407	10	1,444
Brucella	22	23	4	12	None reported	
Streptococcus	5	51	15	1,282	4	37
Viral						
Hepatitis	9	196	6	238	9	116
Parasite						
Trichinella spiralis	42	47	9	82	11	35
Entamoeba histolytica	1	5	Not included in summaries			

hours in accord with the dose and individual susceptibility. Food handlers with infected cuts, abscesses, and nasal secretions and "shedders" from apparently normal skin provide the inoculum. Outbreaks have been traced to staphylococci of bovine origin via milk and milk products, including dried milk. Reheating the food is of no use as the toxins are thermostable. This alone makes the storage rule, "Keep it hot; keep it cool; or don't keep it," a sound food protection doctrine. Among 68,301 reported cases of food-borne illness from 1967 to 1969 in the United States, 9,814 were staphyloccal cases (see Table 8-1). Deaths are rare.

Clostridium perfringens (*welchii*) is found in the feces of man, cattle, pigs, and rodents, all being animals that frequent kitchens alive or butchered. The nonhemolytic *type A* produces an exotoxin and is heat resistant. Meats held at serving temperatures for long periods, or not cooled promptly between servings, provide the incubation. Stews, large cuts of beef, meat pies, and salt-risen bread have been vehicles of incubation and poisoning. The effects, sudden abdominal colic followed by diarrhea, appear in about 10 to 12 hours, last a day or so, and are not severe. The number of reported cases in the United States is increasing, being more than the salmonella cases in 1968 and 1969 (see Table 8-1). Control rests on prompt refrigeration of meats between servings and high holding temperatures during extended serving times. The popularity of rare roast beef sandwiches of slices from large beef quarters held at serving temperatures for 3 hours or so coincides with the case rise. The coincidence merits a bacteriological look. Until the mid-1960s, *C. perfringens* poisoning had been a unique claim of the British. At least they were the only ones identifying and enumerating cases of it.

C. botulinum elaborates a powerful neurotoxin which causes botulism. In the whole panorama of man's ills and injuries, botulism is rare. It is dramatic. It is preventable. A case of botulism requires a sequence of four events:

1 Food contamination by *C. botulinum* spores. As the spores are widespread on the soil, in vegetation, and for *type E*, in water, such contamination of raw foods is frequent.
2 Food is heat-treated sufficiently to kill the normal microflora but not enough to kill the spores. Sporicidal combinations of time and temperature are plotted in Fig. 8-4 (shown later).
3 Food must provide a substrate which is anaerobic with pH over 5 and very high moisture content. Temperature is not critical as *types A* and *B* grow at temperatures down to 50°F (10°C), and *type E* down to 37°F (2.8°C). The occurrence in long-stored canned foods means that ample time is required to produce a sickening dose of toxin, although the *type E* fish cases have had relatively short growth times, that is, days or a week or two, not months as canned foods are meant to provide before use.

4 The food must be eaten without boiling or substantial reheating after being taken from the can, jar, or vacuum package.   The toxin is thermolabile.

Symptoms appear in 12 to 36 hours as the toxin attacks the central nervous system.   A change of voice, double-vision, dizziness, headache, and nerve paralysis set in.   Constipation occurs, but vomiting and diarrhea are not usual.   Hence a food association is not a first thought.

Massive Bacterial Ingestions

The *Salmonellae* group grow in such massive numbers that eating the contaminated food is such a speedy and violent assault that the victim groans, " I've been poisoned," usually from 12 to 24 hours after eating.   The shear number of salmonellas arriving in full phalanx in the gastrointestinal tract of man overwhelms him.   The most susceptible are the very young, birth to preschool, and the old.   Then comes the traveler, exposing his psychological and physiological "set" to new stimuli.   The internationalist's vocabulary includes "Delhi belly," "Montezuma's revenge," and "tropical trots" to describe the diarrhea.

Salmonellosis does not have a single etiological species.   The group *Salmonellae* has worldwide distribution and has its reservoir in the intestines of domestic and wild animals and in man as an active case, as a convalescent, and as a short-term carrier for a few days to 6 months.   From animal hosts, it finds its way via eggs, milk, meat, poultry, and fish.   Rodents defecate on exposed foods as they eat.   Man has kept the animal cycle going by processing animal slaughter and fish kill wastes to animal feed without pasteurizing times and temperatures.   Man gives the cattle, pigs, and poultry a rough trip to slaughter.   Under stress, the animals do not contain the salmonellas to their intestines.   General tissue invasion occurs.   The principal species in the United States is *S. typhimurium*, accounting for 40 percent of cases. *S. heidelberg*, *S. newport*, *S. infantis*, and *S. enteritidis* rank after it with 8 to 4 percent of the cases from each.   Other species occurring in the United States and elsewhere are *S. choler-aesuis*, *S. montevideo*, *S. derby*, *S. oranienburg*, *S. saint-paul*, and *S. manhattan*. Unfortunately, salmonella infections confer no lasting immunity.   Some type-specific immunity for a time has been observed.   The bacteria that cause typhoid and paratyphoid fevers are *Salmonellae*.   These are primary infections in man and are not in the group causing salmonellosis.   See Table 8-1 for the reported occurrence of salmonellosis in the United States for 1967 to 1969.   The reported numbers of salmonellosis and other food-borne illness, excepting botulism, are estimated to be only 1 in 100 to 1 in 200 of actual occurrence, as severity is mild and therapy nonspecific.

Bacterial Infections Requiring Incubation Time in Man

Several bacterial species, such as the typhoid bacteria, require time in the body to produce disease. Their normal course of infection is for a substantial number of organisms to enter the body. These then find their way to a preferred site, colonize and multiply. For bacteria making their entrance through food, the time to set up shop, the incubation time, is from 1 to 3 weeks, with 2 weeks a working hypothesis for tracing the origin of the infection. The list of bacterial species that trouble man by this pattern through the food or water route includes species which enter more effectively by inhalation and broken or abraded skin penetration. The size of the initial invasion can be kept manageable by good personal hygiene and environmental sanitation. The success of the invasion can be blunted by a well-nourished, well-rested body in healthy physiological rhythm. Small wonder that the occurrence is high among the poor, the ignorant, the ill-fed, ill-housed, and among society's rejects in prisons, orphanages, asylums, and reservations.

Four groups of the *Shigella* bacteria, *S. dysenteriae*, *S. flexneri*, *S. boydii*, and *S. sonnei*, account for most of the outbreaks and cases of shigellosis, bacillary dysentery. Man is the reservoir and his feces the vehicle, assisted by transfer by hands, work surfaces, utensils, and flies to food and water. Incubation time is less than a week. Infection is repeated, as immunity, if any, is brief and type-specific. Among the children of the wretched, bacillary dysentery repeats three to four times a year to age 5. By that time about half of the children are gone, with the fittest achieving a kind of survival. Poor nutrition in such children is their greatest handicap in combating the infection. A high quality of hospital care provided for the affluent keeps the fatality rate under 1 percent for them. No immunization exists. For the principal-target populations, the only effective approach is basic sanitation, much improved nutrition, and continued efforts to raise their quality of life by education.

Typhoid and paratyphoid fevers *A*, *B*, and *C* have yielded to preventive medicine, sanitation, and a rising standard of life in the United States. About 400 to 500 cases of typhoid continue to occur annually, mainly in rural areas, as sporadic cases in well-confined outbreaks traced to carriers often already known. Reported para-typhoid cases are few. Some go unreported. More are not recognized. Food, including milk and shellfish, has been the mode of transmission in historic outbreaks. Food is more likely to be the mode for the paratyphoids than for typhoid, for which water predominates. Occurrence is worldwide, but reporting is too uncertain to provide quotable data, let alone to make distinctions among waterborne, food-borne and contact-carrier outbreaks. Action against these infections is the model of public health practice. In the developing countries it has been feasible to implement communitywide environmental action. Often this is accepted without full under-standing of the health benefits, but well supported for the convenience advantages to the people.   Examples are hygienic water service, to a lesser extent excreta disposal changes, to a still lesser extent milk pasteurization and some facets of food protection such as improved abattoirs and central markets, and animal disease control.

A part of animal disease control which has reduced human disease is the work against bovine tuberculosis and brucellosis, Bang's disease.   Both of these diseases are transmissible to man by the milk and meat products.   Eradication of tuberculosis in cattle and the pasteurization of milk have made the bovine form of the disease in children rare in countries applying these measures.   In 1921, when milk pasteurization was in very limited use, there were 1,100 deaths from bovine tuberculosis among children under 5 in England and Wales.   In 1953 with 80 percent of the milk pasteurized, these deaths dropped to 12.[1]   Similar and greater gains have been made against bovine tuberculosis in the United States, Canada, the Scandanavian countries, The Netherlands, Switzerland, France, and Germany.   Brucellosis cases reported in the United States are less than 300 a year.   These are almost wholly from occupational contact with infected animals, their discharges, and their aborted fetuses.   Eating milk and meat from infected cattle, pigs, sheep, goats, and horses will infect, but it has always caused a minority of total human cases.   This is readily disclosed by a review of the age, sex, and occupational distribution of 300 or more cases.

Streptococcal serological groupings are an intricate bacteriological pattern of streptococci producing a varied pathology in man and a mammary organ infection in cows, mastitis (Ref. 8-1, pp. 161–172).   The means of transmission are equally varied. Food has a dramatic, minor role in the serious streptococcal consequences of sore throat, scarlet fever, erysipelas, nephritis, rheumatic fever, and endocarditis.   Mastitis is a bacterial infection of the cow's udder, or one or more quarters of it.   It is a persistent infection reducing milk production, and a threat to the herd.   Solely for economic reasons, a dairyman must control it.   Streptococci are among the bacteria that cause it.   *Streptococcus pyogenes* is the species that passes back and forth between man and cow and produces infection in both unless interrupted by milk pasteurization and good dairy farm procedures.   Other organisms causing and obscuring the mastitis syndrome are *S. agalactiae, Staphylococcus aureus, Mycobacterium tuberculosis, Corynebacterium pyogenes*, and the *Brucellae* group.   In the absence of control, the bacteria of mastitis occasionally produce infection in milk drinkers and cow handlers. Given other food substrate, such as custard cream pastries, and the time and temperature in which these can thrive, streptococci from human nasal secretions grow to large infective doses.   Fortunately, streptococci are not toxin producers.   A reheat to the equivalent of pasteurization will kill the streptococci and end the threat of infection.   In exceptional circumstances cholera may be food-borne, but in outbreaks

---

[1] W. A. Lethem, *Monthly Bull.*, *British Ministry Health Lab. Ser.*, **14**:144 (1955).

the water route is overwhelming. Secondary cases during epidemics and endemic cases from in-family carriers get their infection by direct contact and by contaminated food handled by the carrier.

Rickettsia and Viruses in Foods

These organisms are too cell-tissue dependent to venture into and survive the vagaries of man's food supply. Their preferences outside of man are insect vectors. Among the rickettsia, solely *Coxiella burnetii* (*Rickettsia burnetii*) is food-borne and that limited to raw milk. Milk is a minor means of transmission for *C. burnetii*. It much more frequently is disseminated by direct contact and air-dust-borne in stockyards, stables, feedlots, meat packing and rendering plants, wool processing plants, and diagnostic laboratories where infected cattle, sheep, and goats and parts and products of them are handled. Milk pasteurization at 145°F (62.5°C) for 30 min or at 161°F (72.5°C) for 15 s inactivates *C. burnetii*. Immunization exists for animals and for man. The organisms are in many species of ticks and small wild animals, but these have not been frequent sources of human infections. The disease produced is Q fever. The rickettsia was identified nearly simultaneously during 1937 to 1938 in ticks in Montana and in human cases in Australia. The "Q" has been assigned both to query fever and to Queensland fever.

Animals included in man's food supply carry many viruses. Fortunately, none of these viruses are infective to man through food from the infected animals, not even foot and mouth disease so dreaded in livestock. The virus of infectious hepatitis is believed to have made its way to man in 80 cases by raw oysters taken from polluted waters in officially "closed" growing areas on the Gulf coast of Mississippi and Alabama in 1961. The cases, reported over a 3-month period, were among adults.[1] About that time, several hundred adult cases of infectious hepatitis were attributed to eating raw clams from the Raritan Bay, New Jersey. With the bay at the end of a densely populated and industrialized drainage area, it is remarkable that the clams were there at all, but no surprise that the virus was, as it is discharged in human feces and appears to be more hardy than similar viruses. The two episodes revived strict adherence to shellfish sanitation. The viruses of poliomyelitis and of some tick-borne encephalitis have been found in milk of cows, sheep, and goats. For poliomyelitis such occurrences must be regarded as rare and insignificant in light of the epidemiological patterns of the disease. However, the transmission of the tick-borne encephalitis in goat milk has been increasingly reported in central and northern Europe and in parts of Asia (Ref. 8-2, p. 51). The enteroviruses are common

---

[1] J. O. Mason and W. A. McLean, *Am. J. Hyg.*, **75**:90 (1962).

in the human intestine and leave with our feces, but these have not yet found their way back through our food or water in sufficient numbers to be infective or to produce disease frequently and severely enough to be recognized.

Parasitic Worms and Flukes, and the "Hitchhikers"

To manage the diversity of biological life that is the concern of the parasitologist, those organisms which get to man through his food intake are reviewed under three groupings:

1 The worms, cestodes and nematodes, in meats and fish of occidental diets
2 The flukes, trematodes, in crustaceans and fish of oriental diets
3 Those which are casually in the food as hitchhikers from other sources.

The taeniae, or meat tapeworms, *Diphyllobothrium latum* (also called *Dibothrio-cephalus latus*), a fish tapeworm, and *Trichinella*, in pork, are parasites with essential phases of their intricate life cycles in the food animal.   With two exceptions, reasonably well nourished people can sustain moderate infestations with these parasites without serious effects.   The first exception is an infection with the eggs of *Taenia solium*, the pork tapeworm, producing a distinct and dangerous illness, cysticercosis. The second exception is a massive infection with trichinellae from a single large feeding as from fresh nearly raw pork sausage.   With the exception of trichinellae, the eggs of the parasites in this grouping leave in man's feces and make their way to the flesh of cattle, pigs, and fish by ingestion.   The fish tapeworm also infects bears, foxes, wolves, and mink, whose feces in turn contaminate the water to recycle the parasite. With the exception of cysticercosis, thorough cooking of beef, pork, and fish is certain protection.   A tissue temperature of 130 to 135°F (54.5 to 57.5°C) kills the cysticerci.   The exception arises as a human case of pork tapeworm can add fecal contamination containing the *T. solium* eggs directly to food already cooked for direct infection of the eater.   The fish tapeworm, *Diphyllobothrium latum*, thrives in the fish of cold freshwaters of the Northern Hemisphere.   Geographic groups which depend on fish as a protein source and which use it raw or undercooked have high infestation rates.   The Eskimo of western Alaska and local populations of the Baltic reach nearly 100 percent positives.   Twenty percent of all Finns carry *D. latum*.   Other high incidence regions are parts of Siberia, Manchuria, Japan, around the Great Lakes of North America, and eastern Canada.

Trichinella spiralis, a nematode, stakes its parasitic existence on carnivorous man and animals, as it moves by a flesh to flesh cycle without a stage in the free environment or in a vector.   Man is a dead end for *T. spiralis*.   The life cycle was worked out between 1835 and 1865, and raw garbage feeding to hogs was recognized as contributing to transmission in 1888.   Control measures have not been accepted and implemented vigorously, for the disease is still with us. The United States seems to have two or three times as much trichinosis as the rest of the world. This must be due to preference for rare cooking of meat, except in the South, and some continuance of raw garbage feeding to hogs. However, the disease is declining in the United States, as autopsy positives 25 years ago were 1 in 6 compared with 1 in 20 recently. The disease is declining among man and pigs in Germany. In 1954, only 37 German pigs in over 14 million examined were reported to be infected. Trichinosis was never common in France, where hogs are kept herbivorous, or in Italy, Denmark, The Netherlands, or Switzerland. High areas continue in Poland, Greece, and Rumania. Cooking customs and religious proscriptions keep trichinosis low in the East Asian and Latin American countries. Animal protein is in short supply in those areas so that little, if any, muscle tissue is allowed to become garbage for hog feeding.

Two flukes, trematodes, parasitize a large number of Asian people whose protein diet is long on crustaceans and freshwater fish. *Clonorchis sinensis*, the oriental, or Chinese, liver fluke, produces a virtually lifelong infection of the bile duct, clonorchiasis, among those eating the cysts in freshwater fish which have been eaten fresh, dried, salted, pickled, or only partly cooked. The eggs leave man via feces. Cats, dogs, pigs, and wild fish-eating mammals are also parasitized and put out eggs in their feces. *Paragonimus westermani*, the oriental lung-fluke, produces an equally lengthy infection of the human lung and a few other lesser sites such as intestines, lymph glands, genitourinary tract, and the brain. The infection starts by eating the infective larvae already in freshwater crabs and crayfish that are raw or only partly cooked. The eggs leave with human spit and feces. Dogs, cats, pigs, and wild animals eating crustaceans and crayfish are also parasitized and act as reservoirs. Both flukes have a lengthy cycle much like the schistosomes. There are stages in freshwater and in specific snail species, and a cercaria stage from the snail to the intermediate host which infects when it becomes a part of man's diet. This cycle is at least 3 months. Another month or two are required to go from eaten food to maturity at the final site in man. That is home for the next 15 to 20 years, if the host lives that long.

The hitchhikers that must be included in covering parasites that can get to man in his food are the protozoan *Entamoeba histolytica* and another tapeworm, *Hymeno-lepis nana*. These two are hitchhiking parasites on man's food as the food is solely a mechanical transfer from one parasitized host to a susceptible. The two require nothing more than a ride on the food from the feces of a parasitized host, man in the case of *E. histolutica*, and man or murine rodents for *H. nana*. Neither has a bio-logical multiplication or life-cycle change on the food. Each contaminates the food in the same form in which it enters the mouth of the food eater. Each poses varia-tions of behavior in the host or host-to-host transfers which have been confusing to expert parasitologists.   Understandably then, the practitioners of environmental hygiene have placed undue emphasis on single environmental factors in the control of these diseases.   Examples are the role of water in *E. histolytica*, and the arguments on whether murine rodent feces are the principal contaminant of food carrying *H. nana* or whether human feces from fingers to food are the mode of transmission.

It is the form of amebiasis with acute dysentery that has come from the notorious waterborne outbreaks in the United States.   It is also this type that hits a few of the newcomers that come to live in endemic clinical areas.   The waterborne outbreaks have been caused by massive doses in water heavily contaminated by fresh sewage. These are best exemplified by the two Chicago outbreaks; that from the 3-day stockyard fire studied by Hardy and Spector in 1935, and that during the 1933 Century of Progress World's Fair among the guests of three downtown hotels with common plumbing.   In both of these, massive quantities of fresh sewage were added to the drinking water by gravity dripping to open tanks or by hydraulic forces within interconnected and cross-connected supply and waste pipes, or by both.   The attack rate for recognized clinical amebiasis in the Chicago hotels by length of stay was:

Days in hotels	Clinical cases/1,000 guests
1	3
7	11
8–14	13
30–90	111

These data underscore experimental results with animals and human volunteers that large numbers of organisms are required to start an infection, and likely additional predisposing conditions to produce a clinical case.   Environmental hygiene practitioners who view amebic cysts found loose in food or in water as a relation of one cyst–one case of acute amebic dysentery are at variance with epidemiological evidence and with parasitological behavior (Refs. 8-1, pp. 250–257).

Hymenolepis nana is a tapeworm which does not require an intermediate host as do *Taenia saginata*, *T. solium*, and the fish tapeworms.   The eggs of *H. nana* go from man to man by the feces-food route, or from murine rodent to man by the rodent droppings to man's food route.   The eggs can adapt and make a pass through fleas or grain beetles, go into a cysticercoid stage, and then infect man or rodents that eat the insects along with their food.   *H. nana* is found worldwide with greater prevalence in warm climates.   Young children show the severest symptoms of systemic toxemia, with heavy infections.   Leading parasitologists state that it is the most common tapeworm of man.   The evidence is that man is the principal source of his own *H. nana* infections (Ref. 8-1, p. 376).

Toxic Substances in Food

Defining hazardous poisons in our food is quite clear-cut on identity and dose when the result is an acute effect from a single feeding or short-time regimen. The cause and effect are quite decisive. The issue becomes increasingly difficult and, in short order, is impossible to define when the results of intakes are only suspicions of possible chronic effects, of long-delayed effects, or of biochemical evidence of tissue accumulations or excretions without functional impairment. Suspected hazards from such intakes may be a low-level chronic poisoning from lead or arsenic, a cardiovascular change related to sodium or saturated fats, a higher risk of cancer due to a recognized carcinogen in the diet as 3,4-alpha-benzo-pyrene in heavily smoked fish or meat, and finally, alleged genetic effects laid at the doorstep of mutagenic substances in our food. As the concentrations become lower, the time span of intake longer, the interval between dose and effect longer, and the effect less and less specific, the task of defining the hazard becomes impossible. For example, there is some evidence on which to set a limit for a lifetime intake of silver. However, if laboratory tests show a new synthetic organic coloring agent to shorten the life span of a particular strain of mice, there is a dilemma. For the illustration, the question can be answered by noting that there is a sufficient number of safe coloring agents at hand. Therefore, why incur any risk at all by adding another with a dubious characteristic? Indeed, technological productivity is so great in variety of products and methods that the question, Do we need to use this at all? must be asked more often. Safe or safer alternatives are at hand or can be developed. Toxicants in our foods are presented in four groupings:

1 Present in the food as a consequence of natural event
2 Result from excessive use or from unauthorized use of intentionally applied additives during processing
3 Result from residues of known hazardous materials used in growing or in processing that carry over into the consumer product
4 Result from container and packaging contact or reuse, from gross blunders, and from accidents.

Toxicants Occurring Naturally

Poisons present in our food as a consequence of natural events are examined in fascinating detail in Ref. 8-3. Table 8-2 summarizes information on seven examples of these phenomena. Man does not get caught in this snare very often. He has learned to be very selective of wild plants and to avoid certain fish. He rarely eats insects and little of aquatic plants. The examples in Table 8-2 illustrate the mechanisms by which poisons get into our food. Some toxicants are inherently a part of the food tissue: anthraquinones in some leafy stemmed vegetables, the cyanogenic glycosides in several plants, and the mushroom poisons.   Some require a transfer, as tremetol from the white snakeroot to man through milk from a cow that eats the weed and is poisoned, too.   A second mechanism is concentrating the toxicant from the growth environment, as selenium from the soil and arsenic from water.   A third is for the food to be parasitized by a mold which produces a toxin for man. This has produced the most dramatic and, at times, communitywide poisonings.   As recently as 1951, a French town found itself back in the Middle Ages, hit by the poison that causes St. Anthony's fire.   In 6 to 48 hours after the bakery of *Pont St.-Esprit* used a rye flour contaminated with ergot from *Claviceps purpurea*, about 150 people experienced varying digestive symptoms of nausea, vomiting, diarrhea, burning pain

Table 8-2   SOME TOXICANTS OCCURRING NATURALLY IN OUR FOODS WITH USUAL FOOD SOURCE AND ORIGIN OF TOXICANT INDICATED

Toxicant	Food source	Origin	Comment
Alphatoxins	Grains, peanut butter, cottonseed oil, milk	Growth product of some varieties of the mold, *Aspergillus flavus*	Occasional varieties of *Aspergillus flavus* produce the toxin; reaches milk from grass eaten.
Ergot	Rye principally, wheat, oats, barley, and products of these	Growth product of the mold *Claviceps purpurea*	Acute attacks in 2 forms: *1* Blood vessel constriction, St. Anthony's fire, gangrene *2* Convulsions
Hydrogen cyanide	Cassava, tapioca, rarely lima beans	Cyanogenetic glycosides in plant tissues	HCN released by hydrolysis; cyanogenetic compounds inactivated by heating the food.
Anthraquinones	Rhubarb leaves, fresh, early summer	Inherent in plant tissue	Earlier work suggested oxalates as the toxicant.
Phalloidine, Muscarine	Mushroom, *Amanita phalloides* Mushroom, *A. muscaria*	Inherent in plant tissue	Amanita found in U.S.; muscaria found in Europe.
Safrole	Root beer, cinnamon, nutmeg	In oil of sassafras, inherent in plant tissue	A weak hepatic carcinogen in rats and dogs; oil of sassafras discontinued in root beer in U.S.
Selenium	Grains	Absorbed during growth on soils high in selenium	Localized high-selenium soils in central plains of U.S.

from stomach to anus, chills and fever, and insomnia for several days. About 25 cases became severely delirious, with muscle spasms, hallucinations, cramps, anguish, and fainting. Four died, two old and sick men, one woman with a history of low thyroid function, and one 25-year-old man in good health.[1]

Toxicity of Additives

Toxic effects from the excessive or unauthorized use of additives to foods during processing and distributing are calling forth a major speciality in food science and technology. In a society such as the United States, which has an eccentric sensitivity about its food, the effects may be real, potential, or alleged. Additives are a key to mass processing, distributing, and retailing foods which are premixed, precooked, frozen, in dried form for reconstitution, of guaranteed nutrient content, and of specified hygienic quality. There are additives for nutritive value: iodine to salt; vitamin A to margarine, iron, calcium, and B vitamins to flour, rice, and cornmeal; vitamin D to milk; and vitamin C to fruit drinks. There are additives to enhance or provide flavor, both taste and aroma; to hold color, texture, palatability, and wholesomeness by antioxidants, bactericides, bacteriostats, fungicides, and antibiotics. There are additives to provide and to keep consistency, such as emulsifiers in ice cream, candies, salad dressings; stabilizers in frozen desserts and jellies; and flavor oils in mixes for cake, gelatin, and puddings. There are additives for acidity-alkalinity control, for bleaching and maturing bananas, cheeses, and flour. There are humectants, sequestrants, solvents, sweeteners, and agents for firming, curing, and anticaking, and also for foaming or inhibiting foam. Some of these needs can be met by natural substances such as fruit pectin for gels and vegetable dyes for color. Versatility, uniformity in control, and economy have given the synthetic chemicals a wide edge over the natural ones in the varieties and quantities used.

Each additive must be examined for toxicity in the form, quantity, and combination in which it is used. A formidable task for acute toxicity evaluation, the task for judging long-term risks of the imposing lists of compounds, is a heroic undertaking. It is the responsibility in the United States of the Food and Drug Administration. Presently there are 600 substances on the GRAS (generally recognized as safe) list and 2,400 on the non-GRAS list. The non-GRAS list is of substances which may be approved upon petition from a manufacturer or user to the Food and Drug Administration. The petition provides data which shows clearly that the chemical is safe in the intended food use at the intended concentrations. Since the 1958 Food Additives Amendment to the federal Food, Drug, and Cosmetic Act, the burden of proof rests with the proposer. The test protocols have become elaborate, particu-

---

[1] A. Gabbai et al., *Brit. Med. J.*, 2:650 (1951).

larly to comply with the Delaney clause of the 1958 amendment.   The Delaney, or cancer, clause states that no additive may be in any food if at any concentration it produces cancer when fed to man or animals, or if it can be shown to be a carcinogen by an appropriate test.

Table 8-3 gives a few examples of the 600 materials on the GRAS list grouped as preservatives, including antioxidants, and as sequestrants, emulsifiers, stabilizers, and nutrients.   Of the 16 examples, 12 are materials found naturally in foods or derived directly from natural components of food.   This ratio would not hold for the entire 600.   It is characteristic, however, to favor the use of additives that are made from accepted foods.   Among coloring agents, natural source materials such as beet juice, carrot oil, chlorophyll, and paprika are more readily accepted than newly synthesized organics.   Table 8-4 gives a few examples of the 2,400 non-GRAS list entries.   Most of these are familiar and can be found in the small print on the label of many packaged food items under "Ingredients."

The task of control of food additives requires four steps:

1   First uses must be approved with the burden of proof now on the proposer.
2   Tolerances or limits must be set for some substances and for particular proposed uses.
3   Adherence to the uses and tolerances must be checked by field inspection and laboratory analysis of samples.
4   New information requires a review of previous judgments, tolerances, and usage.

Table 8-3   EXAMPLES OF SUBSTANCES GENERALLY RECOGNIZED AS SAFE BY THE FOOD AND DRUG ADMINISTRATION, THE GRAS LIST

Intended purpose	Substances	Illustrative Applications
Preservatives	Calcium propionate	Mold inhibitor in bread and cake
	Sorbic acid	Mold inhibitor in cheeses
	Tocopherols	An antioxidant, a component of vitamin E
	Ascorbic acid	An antioxidant, a component of vitamin C
Sequestrants	Citric acid	To sequester or chelate trace metals in foods,
	Calcium gluconate	such as copper and iron to prevent catalysis
	Sodium polyphosphates	of oxidation and off-color formation
Emulsifiers	Tartaric acid esters	Must be made from edible fats and oils
	Mono- and diglycerides	Must be made from edible fats and oils
	Propylene glycol	
Stabilizers	Agar-agar	Ice cream and frozen dessert mixes
	Carrageenin	Gravies and pie fillings
	Carab gum	Derived from locust bean gum
Nutrients	Ferric phosphate	For iron supplement in cereals
	Riboflavin	Vitamin B supplement in breads
	Ascorbic acid	Vitamin C supplement in juices

Toxicants from Residues of Growing and Processing Chemicals

Pesticides, weedicides, disinfectants, detergents, hormonal growth regulators, and antibiotics are used at one or more phases of the cycle of food production from seed, plant, or animal, to the moment the morsel or sip reaches the mouth of the eater. The very usefulness of these materials depends on their chemical, biological, and physiologial effects. The effects sought are permanent, as death of insects, and they are complex, as influencing the anterior pituitary gland of a steer. With some exceptions, these materials are known to be hazardous to the men using them occupationally and known to require great care over the amounts and for the points in the food cycle at which they are applied. Whether there will be injury or even absorption into the body's system is dependent, as for all toxicants, on:

1 The mode of exposure: inhalation, ingestion, or contact
2 The quantity taken
3 The time span of intake, including the intervals between intakes, which are critical for excretion and for recovery
4 The physiological and emotional status of the individual, and the sum of his assets and deficits which determines his ability to cope with the toxicant
5 Synergistic or potentiating effects of other substances taken in concurrently.

Table 8-4 EXAMPLES OF SUBSTANCES WHICH THE FOOD AND DRUG ADMINISTRATION HAS APPROVED ON PETITION, THE NON-GRAS LIST

Substance	Illustrative applications	Tolerance
Benzoic acid	Tomato ketchup preservative	0.1%
Butylated hydroxyanisole (BHA)	Antioxidant in potato chips, cereals, salted nuts	0.02% of total fat or oil content of food makeup
Caffeine	Flavoring in cola types of soft drinks	0.02%
Calcium silicate	Anticaking agent in baking powder	5%
Ethyl formate	Fumigant in cashew nuts	0.0015%
Ox-bile extract	Emulsifier in dried egg whites	0.1%
Potassium iodide	Dietary iodine in table salt	0.01%
Sulfur dioxide	Preservative for dried fruits, apricots, peaches	Not for use with meats or foods that are a source of vitamin B_1

The materials in this grouping pose two additional toxicological problems:

1 The prediction and management of exposure of the whole general population to residues in the food when eaten
2 The prediction and management of the contamination of the whole world as residues escape to the free environment of air, water, and soil, during the use in food production.

Requirements for the management of these materials are:

1 The need to know the fate of the chemical in the immediate circumstances of use, as a weedicide sprayed on the soil, or a pesticide sprayed from a low-flying plane. What is the effective persistence time? Are there soil absorption, hydrolysis, evaporation, humidity effects? What are the physiological pathways of these substances in both the primary target and the secondary contacts? As a minimum, it is necessary to know the time, between the last application and first use of the food product, that is required for natural action to eliminate the material used to a nondetectable level or to a well-established safe level in the food.
2 If natural actions do not provide the required elimination, there is a need to know the fate of the chemical after the crop has been harvested, or the animal slaughtered. Can surface residues be washed off? Are there concentrations in certain parts of the plant, in the stem, the roots; or in parts of the animal, in the fat, the liver, the bone? What becomes of the substances in the usual processes such as blanching, pasteurizing, refrigerating, pressure cooking? Are there supplementary processes which reduce the residues? Are there time extensions of present processes, particularly storage, which reduce the residues?

Comprehensive information has been developed on a few widely used materials with great gaps on physiological mechanisms and biological pathways. No attempt has been made to mobilize our scientific abilities to gather such information before use or even after introduction of these materials. Information is sought in response to threats of injury and of liability, and in response to promises of benefits of more economical use. Governmental and industrial research in these matters is on a need-to-know basis. The hydrolysis time of parathion is investigated when drift from cottonfield spraying contaminates a crop of strawberries. The residues of amino-triazole on cranberries are investigated when the chemical is found to be a carcinogen in experimental animals. Rarely is there enough information, and more rarely is it at hand when needed. If discussions and decisions on the use of such materials are to be rational and minimally emotional, it is necessary to define and to keep clear the risk against which protection is sought. Distinctions must be recognized among:

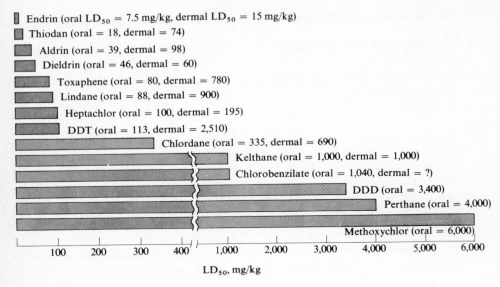

FIGURE 8-1
Acute oral and dermal toxicity of some chlorinated hydrocarbon pesticides as LD_{50} for laboratory rats, in milligrams per kilogram. [*Source: Bureau of Occupational Health, State of California Department of Public Health.*]

1 Occupational exposure in chemical manufacture and in formulation
2 Occupational exposure in application
3 Residues in food crops, including the point in processing at which the residue is a risk
4 Residues entering the free environment to become a component of all chemical, biological, and physical cycles in nature
5 Intakes, excretions, and accumulations in man and their effects in a few hours to a few weeks, in an individual's life span, or in all generations foreseeable

As a straightaway task of sampling, analysis, and interpretation, the complexity of the task escalates from point *1* through *5*. If the facts of *5* are required not only for man, but all surviving plant and animal species, an unparalleled scientific mobilization is on order.

No single measure of toxicity is sufficient to characterize the risk of pesticide residues in food. Acute oral and dermal doses to produce death in 50 percent of a test species, the LD_{50} (median lethal dose, for 50%), are relatively easy first steps. As the concern at this point is ingestion of residues in our foods, such data are only a starting point. Figures 8-1 and 8-2 are graphic scalings of acute oral LD_{50} in

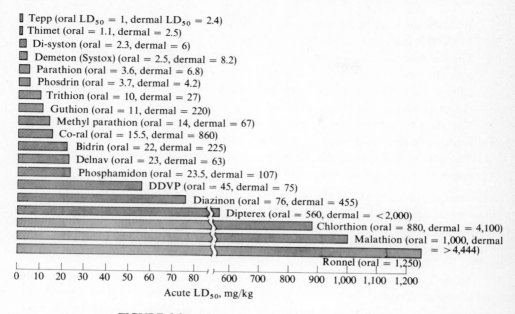

FIGURE 8-2
Acute oral and dermal toxicity of some organic phosphate pesticides as LD_{50} for laboratory rats, in milligrams per kilogram. [*Source: Bureau of Occupational Health, State of California Department of Public Health.*]

milligrams per kilogram for laboratory rats tested with the chlorinated hydrocarbons and with the phosphate ester compounds.   These data originate from the laboratory of the Office of Pesticides, Public Health Service, Atlanta, and are comparable with those in D. E. Frear's 1965 "Pesticide Index," College Science Publishers, State College, Pennsylvania.   In each figure, three groupings can be made.   In Fig. 8-1, among the chlorinated hydrocarbons, endrin, thiodan, aldrin, and dieldrin have oral LD_{50}'s under 50 mg/kg; toxaphene, lindane, heptachlor, and DDT have from 80 to 113; the last five have from 1,000 for Kelthane to 6,000 for methoxychlor.   Chlordane stands alone at 335 mg/kg between the up-to-100 and above-1,000 groups.   In Fig. 8-2 covering the phosphate ester pesticides, the first six from TEPP to Phosdrin have oral LD_{50} values under 5 mg/kg; the next seven range from 10 to 23.5; DDVP, also known as dichlorvos and Vapona, and diazonin are 56 and 76, respectively; the remainder, including the widely used malathion, are from 560 to 1,250 mg/kg for the oral LD_{50} on laboratory rats.

The difficulties of interpreting toxicological data are apparent from the following observations about these data on acute oral LD_{50}'s for laboratory rats.

1 What factor shall be applied to set a safety factor for man? An allowance of 1 in 100 is accepted as feasible and defensible.

2 The data reveal nothing on long-term behavior of small fractionated intakes over the years with respect to excretion, storage, organ concentration, cellular effects, decomposition products in human metabolism, and influences on chromosomes and genes.

3 The data reveal nothing on effects of inhalation and contact, which are the routes of entry for those occupationally exposed.

4 The data reveal nothing on the behavior in solvents, dispersants, and extenders required as carriers in sprays and dusts.

Nevertheless, the data are a starting point and provide a range of relative toxicity. Those pesticides which have been the really bad actors for exposure in use, as residues, and in being immediately toxic in the free environment are in the top ranks of each of the classes of compounds. These are the first four chlorinated hydrocarbons and the first six phosphate esters in Figs. 8-1 and 8-2.

In the United States, the following actions have developed to cope with agricultural chemical hazards. Instruction on use, including time spacing before harvesting; registration of use; clear labeling; crop, soil, and water sampling for residues; changes in raw-food crop washing to remove residues; tolerances, sampling, and analysis of specific foods for specific chemicals; diet sampling; human bioassays for specific chemicals; continued and extended toxicological studies; extensive public discourse. The results of some of this are in Tables 8-5, 8-6, and 8-7, which give some indication of the magnitudes of concentrations encountered.

Note in Table 8-5 and others that the unit is milligrams per kilogram, or parts per million by weight for ingestion. The United States tolerances are as large or

Table 8-5   SOME MAXIMUM TOLERANCES FOR THE SEVEN INSECTICIDE RESIDUES IN FRESH FOODSTUFFS IN FOUR COUNTRIES

Insecticide chemical (common name)	Maximum tolerance, mg/kg			
	Switzerland	The Netherlands	U.S.	U.S.S.R.
Aldrin	0.1	0.1	0.25	0.0
Arsenic-containing	1.0	0.7	2.3	0.0
DDT	4.0	5.0	7	1.0
Diazinon	0.75	1	0.75	
Methyl parathion	0.75	0.5	1	
Parathion	0.75	0.5	1	5.0*

* The purified compound only; the "impure" compound is restricted to 0.0 ppm.

larger than those of the other three countries. The ranges for three are similar, with the U.S.S.R. the exception. In this particular exposure and in all environmental limit statements the U.S.S.R. values are usually only one-hundredth to one-thousandth of United States values and frequently are 0. This arises from including behavior parameters in experimental animals in assessing toxicity, not solely clinical pathology of cells, organs, and gross physiology. The U.S.S.R. parathion value of 5 in Table 8-5 immediately seems to contradict that tenet. However, there is a caveat. See the footnote beneath the table. To have some feel of Table 8-5 tolerances, which are maxima, take DDT in broccoli. The United States permits 7 mg/kg. The acute oral LD_{50} for rats is 113 mg/kg. A $\frac{1}{2}$-kg rat is a sizable animal. Its LD_{50} would be 56 mg of DDT. To get such an acute dose from the tolerance level of broccoli, the rat would have to ingest and retain 8 kilos, or 16 times its weight in broccoli. If we

Table 8-6   CONCENTRATION OF INSECTICIDES IN TOTAL DIET, UNITED STATES, 1962

Insecticide	No. of samples	Concentration, ppm		
		Min.	Mean	Max.
DDT	23	0.008	0.020	0.041
Dieldrin	6	0.003	0.027	0.075
Heptachlor epoxide	5	0.010	0.017	0.025
Lindane	18	0.002	0.005	0.010
Other	7	0.010	0.030	0.060

SOURCE: J. E. Campbell et al., Insecticide Residues in the Human Diet, *Arch. Environ. Health*, **10**:831 (1965).

Table 8-7   CONCENTRATION OF DDT AND DDE IN THE FAT OF PEOPLE BEFORE AND AFTER DDT'S INTRODUCTION AND BY TYPES OF EXPOSURE IN THE UNITED STATES

Exposure group	DDT, mg/kg	DDE, mg/kg
1. Died before DDT	0	0
2. Abstain from meat	2.3	3.2
3. General population	4.9	6.1
4. Environmental exposure	6.0	8.6
5. Agricultural applicators	17.1	22.3

SOURCE: Adapted from W. J. Hayes et al., Storage of DDT and DDE in People with Different Degrees of Exposure to DDT, *Arch. Ind. Health*, **18**:398 (1958).

allow man 1 mg of DDT per kilogram for a single oral dose, a 65-kg man (143 lb) may ingest 65 mg of DDT. To get such a dose from tolerance level broccoli, he would have to eat over 9 kg of the greens.

Table 8-6 shows the range of four specific chlorinated hydrocarbons in total diets in the United States. The data are the results of 36 market-basket survey samples made by the Food and Drug Administration.[1] The DDT values are only about 50 percent of those reported by K. C. Walker in 1954 and by W. J. Hayes in 1956. The DDT intake per person per day has been cited as 0.15 to 0.175 mg by J. E. Campbell.[2]

Within these ranges of intakes, the storage of DDT and its metabolic decomposition products, DDE, occurs in fat of all animals; DDE is dichlorodiphenyldichloro-ethylene. Table 8-7 presents Hayes' data for DDT and DDE in the fat of people in five groups, from those who had no DDT exposure, as they died before its insecticidal use, to those who work with it. These are United States data. The same phenomenon is reported in other countries, with lower amounts in the general population of Canada, Germany, England, and France, with comparable amounts among those samples in Hungary and in India except around Delhi. In that area and in Israel the observed storage loads are as high or higher than the local highs in the United States. Delhi reported 26 mg/kg in 1965; Israel 19 in 1965 compared with United States highs in 1956 of 20 in Tallahassee, Florida, and 16 in Atlanta, Georgia. There are two very remarkable things about this storage. First, it has not yet been found to produce any clinical effects in man. The highest storage reported in the United States has been 648 mg/kg of DDT and 483 mg/kg of DDE in the fat of a healthy formulator. Volunteers on 35 mg/day intakes for 11 months and 21.5 months reached 234 and 281 mg/kg of DDT in their fat without detectable impairment. This dose is 200 times the estimate of 0.175 mg/day as an average for the general population in the United States. It is recognized that these volunteers and DDT workers are able-bodied adult males. These are not infants on high butterfat diets, not women in gestation, not the chronically ill, nor the aged. The factor of 200 is reassuring. The second remarkable observation is that DDT-derived material in the body fat reaches a cumulative limit and that urinary excretion of the metabolites strikes a balance with intake. M. F. Ortelee showed the excretion-intake balance explicitly among a group of DDT workers.[3]

Campbell and associates sum up the case in this meaningful and sensitive statement.[2]

Although the biological significance of pesticide residues in the diet is of considerable interest, no reliable evidence even suggests that current levels of pesticide exposure in the general population are harmful when judged by traditional toxic manifestations

[1] *Natl. Agric. Chem. News*, no. 22 (February 1962).
[2] Insecticide Residues in the Human Diet, *Arch. Environ. Health*, **10**:831 (1965).
[3] Study of Men with Prolonged Exposure to DDT, *Arch. Ind. Health*, **18**:433 (1958).

observed in occupationally exposed individuals, accident and suicide cases, and in animal toxicity studies.

Tolerances for pesticide residues in foods incorporate a safety factor of at least 100 below the no-effect level observed in chronically exposed experimental animals and obviously provide a reasonable degree of safety from excessive exposure.   On the other hand, the possibility of almost universal contact with pesticides through foods, as is clearly the case with DDT, calls for a more critical evaluation of possible biological effects than is now being made.   In addition to strengthening current activities, particularly those concerned with occupational exposure, a comprehensive surveillance program is needed to determine the kinds and levels of pesticide residues in all segments of the population and in their environment, and particularly in food.   Additional research is also needed on the biological effects of pesticides and on methods to determine the total body burden based on the concentration of the pesticide or its metabolites in blood or urine.   Such a technique is needed to generate data on the large population groups that have had either relatively high or low exposure.   These data are required for epidemiological studies to determine whether pesticides have any predisposing influence on the incidence of disease or impairment in man that is not obviously related to excessive exposure.

In 1881 Charles Darwin reported on the photoresponses of canary-grass seedlings, in *The Power Movement of Plants*.   He observed that while the tip of the first tubelike leaf "perceived" the light, the curvature occurred at the base.   He concluded that some "influence" was transmitted from the stimulated tip to the responsive base of that leaf.   The existence of growth regulation by phytohormones had been recorded. By the 1930s, indole-3-acetic acid (IAA) was isolated from plants and confirmed to be a major plant growth regulator.   As a selective weed killer, 2,4-D was tested in 1942, and by 1952 the United States was producing 26 million lb/year for weed killing. Table 8-8 shows the proliferation in five major chemical groups of the principal weed killers used on fields growing food crops.   Details of chemical nomenclature and structure of the compounds in the table are in Dr. A. J. Vlitos' chapter in Ref. 8-4.

With two exceptions, the weed killers have not posed the serious toxicity questions of the pesticides.   The reasons are that:

1 The plant growth regulators must be selective so that the fields are not barren.
2 The applied doses and the timing of application must not impair crop production.
3 The compounds are very costly, 2,4-D and 2,4,5-T concentrates cost from $5 to $7 per gallon, and therefore are used sparingly.
4 The compounds metabolize in plants, with resistant species detoxifying the active agent, fortunately without producing a metabolite toxic to man.
5 The weedicides in use are not persistent, but decompose by hydrolysis and oxidation and by microbial action in the soil.
6 The compounds are of low to moderate toxicity as measured by the acute oral LD_{50} for laboratory rats.   Those in Table 8-8 range from 300 mg/kg to 14,000 mg/kg.   That comfort is shaken to the roots by the very compound with the highest value in the table, amitrole, of cranberry notoriety.

By any scale of adjectives, the acute oral LD_{50} of amitrole indicates a very low order of toxicity.   However, extended animal feeding tests of amitrole showed an enlargement of glands in experimental animals.   This observation resulted in the Food and Drug Administration's placing a 0.15 mg/kg tolerance for amitrole in cranberries in November 1959.   A second exception to the safe position of the weedicides is a peculiar, natural action sequence among 2,4-D, nitrates, forage grass, the rumen of cattle, and the animals' hemoglobin.   The 2,4-D accelerates forage grass metabolism.   Nitrates accumulate in the plants to unusual highs.   In the rumen, the nitrates are reduced to nitrites.   The nitrites combine with hemoglobin in cattle to

Table 8-8 WEEDICIDES USED ON FOOD CROPS, BY CHEMICAL GROUPS

Chemical group	Compounds in use	Acute oral LD_{50} for rats, mg/kg	Weed killer in food crops of:	Comment
Chlorophenoxy compounds	2,4-D	375	Wheat, oats, corn	Dosage 1–2 lb/acre
	2,4,5-T	300–500	Barley, sugar cane	Hydrolyze to acid forms and on to CO_2; no residuals in milk
Substituted ureas	Monuron	3,700	Sugar cane,	All of low solubility
	Diuron	3,400	citrus,	in water; all
	Fenuron	7,500	pineapple,	oxidized by soil
	Neburon	11,000+	avocado, asparagus	bacteria, particularly *Pseudomonas*
Symmetrical triazines	Simazine	5,000	Corn,	Corn withstands
	Atrazine	3,080	sugar cane	8 lb/acre; cane, 16 lb/acre; degrade in plants in 1 week
Carbamates	IPC	1,000	Spinach,	Release vapor in soil
	EPTAM	3,160	mustard, sugar beets, beets, beans, broccoli	to kill weed seeds
	Vegadex	850	Corn, soybeans, sugar beets, peanuts	
Substituted benzoic acids	TBA	700–1,500	Tomatoes,	Persistent in clay
	Dinoben	3,500	pumpkins,	soils and under
	Amiben	3,500	corn, carrots, peppers, soybeans	heavy rains; highly selective in kill
Aminotriazole	Amitrol or amitrole	14,000	Strawberries, cranberries, citrus fruits	Degrades in plants to amino acids in 1–3 weeks; tolerance in cranberries, 0.15 mg/kg

form methemoglobin.   The result is the same as among infants on feeding formulations made up with high-nitrate water.   The cattle lose the blood's oxygen-transport capacity, with deaths reported.

The use of plant growth regulators for weed killing is only a first application of these essential hormones.   Plant physiologists already have extensive test results for (1) control of preharvest fruit drop; (2) control of rooting and flowering; (3) promoting the set of seedless tomatoes and figs; (4) promoting the abscission of leaves, flowers, and fruit; (5) prolonging the dormancy of potatoes and onions; (6) extending the storage life of apples and citrus fruits; (7) increasing the size of pineapples, seedless grapes, apricots, strawberries, and figs; and (8) controlling the chemical composition and production of plants such as sucrose content of cane, oil in peppermint plants, and latex flow of rubber trees.   The application of phytohormones directly to our food crops will require and will produce more information on man's response to these substances.   Man has met the natural hormone IAA in many plant foods.   An indole growth regulator, IAA is detoxified.   The parallel use of animal growth regulators to manage the food product is already a part of animal husbandry on the farm and the feedlot.   The substances in use are antibiotics, a synthetic hormone, and arsenicals.   The power of these materials to determine the chemical composition and growth time of the food animal results from research in the past 30 years.   J. Kastelic's chapter in Ref. 8-4 is a concise appraisal of animal growth regulator use.

The modes of action of the antibiotics, of the synthetic hormone diethylstilbestrol (DES), and of the arsenicals are manipulations of the natural synthesis of proteins and fats and of the animal's nutritive system.   The action of the antibiotics is less profound, as much of it is an effect on the third-party participation of the intestinal flora by suppressing nutrient-consuming parasitic populations, by promoting microbial synthesis of vitamins, and by favorable effects on nutrient releases and transport through the intestinal wall.   It is curious that traces of arsenic appear to do such things in animals and that slight increases of arsenic in the diet are favorable for nutrition and growth.   Man contains about 0.3 mg/kg of arsenic.   The synthetic DES has more profound actions, as it changes hormone production.   As now used, the results are increased protein production, changes in fat deposition with increases in poultry and decreases in cattle, and an increase of calcium and phosphate retention. Animals on DES show changes in these glands: anterior pituitary, adrenal, ovaries, and thyroid.   Dosages are critical, and species responses differ.

Carryovers to man as a consumer have not occurred except from carelessness or uses difficult to control.   The antibiotics decompose on cooking.   A stop in arsenic and DES supplements before animal slaughter provides elimination time, 6 days for arsenic, 3 days for DES.   The maximum DES derivatives found in cattle and lambs taken off DES 48 hours before slaughter has been 10 μg/kg, that is, 10 parts per billion.   The use of DES implants in poultry was stopped by the Food and Drug Administration when the method was found difficult to manage, with residues localized in eatable tissue.   Despite apparent reassurances that scarcely detectable amounts are in our meat foods, DES is closely supervised.

Other Adulterants in Food

The third primary target of food protection is that the food contain what the buyer and eater believes it should by custom, by sellers' statements, and by accepted standards and definitions for foods.   Under the Food, Drug, and Cosmetic Acts of the United States, a food is adulterated by legal definition if it contains any of the pathogenic biological agents or any of the toxicological agents that have been discussed as the first and second primary targets of food protection.   That includes any excesses of authorized additives above tolerance levels, as happened with amitrole in the cranberries.   Additionally there are six other practices:

1 Misbranding
2 Falsification of contents
3 Falsification of condition
4 Unidentified or unlawful use of substitutes or additives
5 Putrid, filthy, or decomposed contents in whole or in part
6 Production under insanitary conditions or on insanitary premises.

Aside from the last, these additional practices or conditions are usually not issues of health impairment.   These are sharp practices to benefit the seller by cheating and duping the buyer and consumer.   It is a part of food protection which has an economic return for the consumer, and which safeguards his comfort, convenience, and esthetics.

ACHIEVING FOOD PROTECTION IN GROWING, PROCESSING, STORING, TRANSPORTING, AND RETAILING

The goals of food protection must be pursued at each step of production.   The three primary targets of freedom from biological pathogens, toxic chemicals, and adulterants cannot be compromised.   The fourth, effective protection in storage, is a necessity of having a marketable, eatable product.   There are some compromises of goals 5 and 6, keeping nutrients intact and keeping the food palatable and attractive.   Processing and handling do produce changes in these.   Nutrients can be restored by additives as vitamin C to fruit drinks after heating, which destroys the natural vitamin C.   The use of antioxidants, coloring and flavoring compounds, and firming and bleaching agents is to keep the food palatable and attractive through such processes as canning, freezing, and long storage.   The final goal, abundance, is supported by all the others through increasing productivity and keeping quality, and through cutting losses from spoilage, insect damage, and nutritional deterioration.

Food Protection during Growing and Producing

Milk, meat, and marine foods must come from healthy animals to be free of biological pathogens and in some instances from toxic substances.   Cows infected with tuberculosis, mastitis, Q fever, or brucellosis discharge the pathogens in their milk.   Cattle with these diseases have the organisms in their tissues at slaughter.   Similarly, parasites of trichinosis are in pork, the tapeworms in pork, beef, and fish.   The salmonellas break out of the intestines of poultry to invade and contaminate the eatable tissue during rough transport and careless dressing.   Shellfish grown in fecally contaminated water concentrate the pathogens in their tissue, which is eaten in its entirety and frequently raw.   *Type E Clostridium botulinum* begins its ride in fish from the growing waters.

The application of sound animal husbandry and veterinary medical science prevents animal diseases and enhances the quality of the animal food product.   Selective and wise use of antibiotics has been helpful.   Wise use includes accurate dosage and timing to avoid antibiotic residuals in animal tissue and in milk.   Antibiotics in milk result from excessive dosage and from marketing milk from cows recently treated for mastitis.   A 3 to 4 day interval is needed for the udder to clear a therapeutic dose to nondetectable levels in the milk.   Antibiotic residues in farm produced milk are monitored for three reasons:

1   Concentrations may be sufficient to set off reactions in sensitized persons drinking the milk.   Ten percent of the United States population is believed to be penicillin-sensitized from therapeutic use in man.
2   The residues interfere with culturing such milk products as yogurts and cheeses.
3   To curb the temptation to use penicillin to clean up contaminated milk with high bacterial counts.

Pre- and postmortem inspection of animals at slaughter gives productive and necessary stimuli for good practices throughout the cycle of meat production.   The experienced observer detects sick suspects by their behavior in feeding lots and holding pens.   Gross macroscopic examination of critical tissue at evisceration and dressing reveals infections.   Samples for laboratory and microscopic examination are useful for some conditions, such as trichinellae in the diaphragm.   Reactor tests for tuberculosis and brucellosis are most productive when done on the farm or range as part of the eradication of these diseases.

Sanitary maintenance of barns, stables, pens, lots, and yards is basic prevention. It requires clean water and feed, removal of wastes and filth, control of vectors, adequate drainage and ventilation, enough space for each animal. Healthy animals cannot be produced in animal slums—filthy, stinking, crowded, and uncleanable. Growing waters for marine foods have analogous requirements, with bacterial contamination and chemical pollution most evidently prejudicial to the quality of the eatable product. The increasing development of "marine food farms," such as for fish and shrimp, makes the need urgent for information on a healthy environment for the species grown. A minimum is needed to keep the farm going. Concentrations of a single species in a small space, animal or plant, is an invitation for parasitism, disease, waste accumulations, and unanticipated toxic exposures to reek havoc with devastating losses. The target population is assembled as neatly and unwittingly as Hiroshima's was for the first nuclear bomb. Whether it is shrimp, sheep, or man, the safety margins for the successful biochemistry of the species can be overrun by crowding the living-set, physically, chemically, and biologically.

The management of agricultural chemicals at the point of use is in the hands of the farmer and the agricultural pesticide operator. Their occupations require a high level of technical skill and judgment. The rate of introduction of new products has been so fast that even if they have followed the directions on the package and the instructions of the agricultural specialist, these men have been unknowing accomplices in spreading DDT to the arctic and antarctic zones and in adding nitrates and phosphates to our waterways. Biological, chemical, and physical agents are brought into use with only the first round of direct effects known. Carryovers into food have come to light later. For the farm user this means more new learning. To keep the chemical residues of pesticides, weedicides, animal growth regulators, and animal pharmaceuticals out of the raw food material, or at least to manageable minima, growers must confine specific materials to specific crops, must apply these at times in the growth cycle when they neither damage the crop nor carry over into the harvest. Doses must be applied accurately. Some of these potent chemicals are applied in fractions of a pound to an acre and in feed in amounts of 50 to 100 lb/ton. Such work requires good equipment for measuring, mixing, spraying, and dusting and a very knowledgeable operator. In the United States there are organizations and people for teaching correct methods. Agricultural extension and home demonstration agents at the county level have won the confidence of farmers by over 50 years of effective help backed by research laboratories, experiment stations, and demonstration farms in every state.

Minimizing contamination by handlers, insects, and rodents is another farm producer responsibility. Milk is the food which has received the greatest effort to prevent contamination at the point of production. It has been a recognized vehicle of communicable disease since the late nineteenth century, with the victims being the heavy milk users, children.   It is a balanced food for animals, including bacteria of both pathogenic and spoilage types which grow prolifically in it.   The question is regularly raised, "Why bother about bacteria in milk at the farm?   Won't you kill them at the pasteurization plant anyway?"   The answers are:

1 The pathogenic organisms will be killed.   Where staphylococci are the contaminants, thermostable enterotoxins already formed will be unchanged by pasteurization.
2 There are bacterial types in heavily contaminated milk which survive pasteurization.
3 Nonpathogenic bacteria with souring and spoiling effects produce changes during growth.   If these are unlimited in number and in reproduction before pasteurization, changes in taste, keeping characteristics, odor, and chemical composition during the raw state carry over in the pasteurized milk.

"Sorry" raw milk before pasteurization makes sorry pasteurized milk.   That holds for milk products such as butter, cultured milks, and cheeses.   Shakespeare's admonition to pursemakers applies to dairy product manufacturers.

The management of contamination of foods from handlers rests on two things:

1 Clean hands and control of infectious discharges from nose, mouth, and any skin breaks that are infected, most certainly those forming pus
2 Handlers free of intestinal and respiratory infections who are either in the diseased state or are carriers

These two requirements apply to all handlers throughout the food cycle from horny-handed milkers at the farm to the cute blonde assembling the "submarine" or "poor boy" at the local drive-in.   The first requirement can only be met by training, by supervision, by employee rules, and by providing facilities at work for personal cleanliness.   Compliance requires paid sick leave and medical care for those who are infectious.   Whether or not the second requirement can be met by periodic medical examinations of food handlers must be tested by two criteria.

1 Is the prevalence of the diseases and carrier states against which protection is sought sufficiently high among food handlers to make the examination productive?
2 Is the examination sufficiently rigorous and frequent to find the cases among food handlers?

The diseases reported among food-borne outbreaks in the United States in the present are not those preventable by a routine physical examination.   These will not be detected or suspected at examination time if the food handler is free of excessive respiratory excretions, pustulating skin breaks, and diarrhea.   When community health

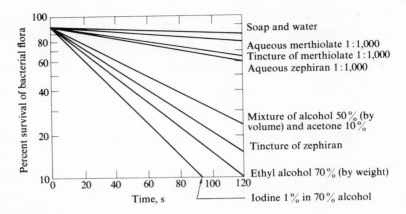

FIGURE 8-3
Comparative effects of various antiseptics on the resident flora on the hands and arms. [*Source: Carl A. Lawrence and S. Block, " Disinfection, Sterilization and Preservation," p. 538, Lea and Febiger, Philadelphia* 1968.]

levels of food-borne and environmentally communicable diseases are high, food-handler medical examinations are productive for direct control and are part of the whole community effort. A succinct statement on these issues is made by W. C. Cockburn in a chapter on health control of dairy workers in Ref. 8-6 (p. 531).

Handwashing is not in controversy as a practice. It is universally urged on all food handlers after excreting and during work as soil accumulates. Very often it is required of food handlers "after toilet use" by regulations and occasionally by law. What is at controversy is what handwashing technique is necessary to reduce bacterial numbers on skin surfaces. To get those numbers down by 95 percent or better requires a surgical scrub to loosen and kill the bacteria. Figure 8-3 shows the percentage reduction of bacteria on the skin of hands by seven disinfectants. There have been reports of touch contact tests with agar plates demonstrating that dry unwashed fingers release fewer bacteria than wetted washed fingers. The conclusion must be not that handwashing be given up, but that different means are needed. Warm water, a full lather, thorough rinsing in the absence of any satisfactory residual bactericide on the skin, and drying do remove gross filth and soil.

Food Protection by Processing

Within hours after collection, harvesting, killing, or catching, raw foods change rapidly. The four causes of change are microorganism growth, enzymatic action, oxidation, and dehydration. Time, temperature, humidity, air contact, and access for microorganisms, insects, and rodents influence the rate of change. With a few exotic exceptions, the changes make the food unattractive, unpalatable, uneatable, and sometimes infectious or intoxicating. Man does two things to manage these changes. He processes the raw food, using means that may alter the food considerably, as fermenting cabbage to sauerkraut. Without, or after, processing, he maintains storage conditions that regulate further changes in the food. Food processing slows down the activities of the change mechanisms or eliminates one or more of the causes entirely. The reasons for processing are to extend shelf and storage life, to provide abundance, to protect against hazards of biological and chemical contamination, and to provide variety by altering the raw material. Examples of the latter are the processing of milk to numerous cheeses, forms of butter, and cultured milks, and the processing of bland cucumbers to pickles—sweet, sour, and dill.

The methods of food processing are (1) dehydrating, (2) heat treatment, (3) freezing, (4) fermenting and similar inhibitions of microbial growth, (5) irradiating with gamma rays or high-energy electrons. The use of any processing technique poses the issues of how much change will there be in appearance, taste, odor, texture, and nutritive value, of how these changes will affect preparation for eating, and of how these changes will affect consumer acceptance. A major issue on new techniques is whether the process results in any deleterious substances or introduces contaminants hazardous in eating. Processing by ionizing radiation is hung up on that right now. The processor seeks compromises which achieve his objectives, which raise the minimum of resistance in consumers, and which add minimally or not at all to the burden of biological and chemical risks all along the line.

Three things apply to all equipment used in food processing.

1   The equipment must apply the process uniformly and effectively to the food. An example is heating and holding every bit of the milk to the pasteurizing temperature of 161°F (72°C) for 15 s in a high-temperature, short-time pasteurizer. In a pressure-pack canning unit, the food at the center of each can is raised to the temperature and held for the time needed to destroy the spores of *Clostridium botulinum* in that type of food.
2   The equipment must be designed and constructed so that it wholly prevents contamination of the product, both in process and thereafter. Such devices as drip shields, leak-protector valves, lipped covers, and pipe lines under pressure from process unit to filler unit are used.
3   The equipment should be made of materials and in shapes that are easily cleanable. It should be formed so that it is easily dissembled and easily accessible for cleaning. Stainless steel alloys, coved corners, clamped joints, wide openings, single-service gaskets are used.
4   The equipment should be fool-proof and tamper-proof in assembly for parts

vital to the process and the protection of the product. Examples are leak-protector valves that cannot be put together backwards; sealed controllers on variable-speed pumps, timers, and temperature devices; raw-product lines that cannot be at pressures higher than for the processed product.

Accomplishing such design and fabrication has been a remarkable cooperative effort in the United States. For milk processing equipment, the Public Health Service, the International Association of Milk, Food, and Environmental Sanitarians, and the Dairy Industry Committee have prepared detailed specifications of equipment in a continuing series called the 3-*A Standards*. For restaurant and retail equipment, the National Sanitation Foundation, a cooperative effort of manufacturers, buyers, and regulatory agencies within the framework of the School of Public Health of the University of Michigan develops, tests, and approves equipment. The National Canners Association has been the means by which the canning companies of the United States pool their resources for process and equipment development. Similarly those concerned with food vending machines have concerted their efforts through the National Automatic Merchandising Association to develop designs and to certify the manufacture of equipment that delivers a high quality product.

Dehydration

Dehydration removes moisture, the major component by weight of all foods, to make the growth of microorganisms and of fungi impossible and to inactivate the enzymes. The food is drastically altered. It cannot be rehydrated to its original forms, with the near exception of freeze-dried products. Sun and air drying are the oldest methods and still in use for fish, meat, and fruits. Salting and sugaring draw the water from the tissue and produce conditions unfavorable for biological growth. Smoking does the job by itself or as an aid to air, salt, and sugar treatment. Dried foods are having a great revival and extension as ready-to-heat-and-eat mixes. Chemical additives make these possible, providing stabilizers, emulsifiers, antioxidants, coloring, and flavoring. Another boost to drying is the freeze-dry method in wide use for coffee and applicable to such delicate structures as strawberries. The process is to quick freeze the product and then to dry it while in the frozen state. This means that the control of heat input for drying must be so balanced that the water in the frozen product sublimates; that is, the water is energized from the frozen solid state to the vapor state without liquifying. The dewatered voids do not collapse, as the walls are rigidly frozen. Hence with packaging to keep out air and moisture, a freeze-dried strawberry is very much like a field berry. The process works for shrimp, diced chicken, sliced mushrooms, and meat cuts.

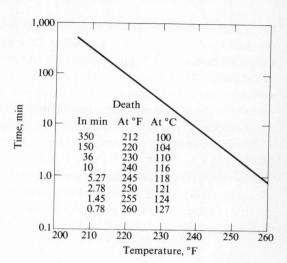

| \multicolumn{3}{c}{Death} | | |
In min	At °F	At °C
350	212	100
150	220	104
36	230	110
10	240	116
5.27	245	118
2.78	250	121
1.45	255	124
0.78	260	127

FIGURE 8-4
Thermal death curve for *Clostridium botulinum*.

Heat Treatment—Canning Foods

From his first cooking, man tried to get a little stretch-out of keeping time by storing cooked meats, fish, fruits, and vegetables.   N. Appert is credited with adding the exclusion of air from the food after cooking in a sealed container.   Lazzaro Spallanzani, who dissolved the myth of spontaneous generation with his microscope, fermentation vessels, and his heater, briefly experimented with heating foods in sealed containers in 1765.   Appert, an unschooled French food confectioner, did practical tests from 1795 to 1810.   In 1809 he won a 12,000-franc prize that had been a standing offer of the French governments since 1795 for a method on food preservation. The dangerous trades of going to sea and to war were the best customers and stimulators of early canning.   Appert's treatise on canning was in English by 1811. William Underwood opened canning operations in Boston in 1819, and Thomas Kensett in New York in 1820.   By 1853, Gail Borden had canned condensed milk on the market.

Bacteriological studies of canning began in 1895, and a chemical laboratory was started by the American Can Company in 1906.   In the 1920s, canning procedures were put on a scientific base and equipment engineered for efficient output.   Elemental to the procedure was establishing thermal survival curves for the pathogenic bacteria and spoilage organisms.   That had been well started for milk pasteurization by M. J. Rosenau in 1908.   Figure 8-4 shows the combinations of time and temperature required to kill *Clostridium botulinum*.   Subsequently two nonpathogenic spore formers were developed as test organisms, Putrefactive Anaerobe 3679 and *Bacillus stereothermophilus*, FS 1518, both more thermally resistant than *C. botulinum*.   These organisms provided the data for a series of tables, graphs, formulas, and standardized nomenclature for pressure packing over 300 products in several sizes of cans. For low-acid foods above pH 4.5, a factor of 12 is used to multiply the minimum time for killing 90 percent of the population of a test organism at the temperature best fitted to the food. There is a limit to heating, as the food has to be recognizable, acceptable, and palatable. For foods with a pH below 4.5, a factor of 5 to multiply the minimum period for the 90 percent kill is satisfactory. The operating temperatures are in the steep section of the survival curve, as can be noted in Fig. 8-4. A pure culture of *C. botulinum* in a low-acid food survives 0.78 min at 260°F (127°C) and 2.78 min at 240°F (116°C). That is 3.5 times as long at the lower temperature. The canned product from these processes is termed *commercially sterile*. A few resistant bacterial spores survive. These do not multiply during an expected 2-year shelf life of canned goods. Texture and flavor do change slowly from chemical actions, not from micro-organism growth (Ref. 8-5).

Heat Treatment—Pasteurizing Milk and Other Foods

Figure 8-5 lacks arithmetic precision, but has graphic clarity in displaying that those pasteurizing milk are between a lower millstone and an upper one. Pasteurization is a selective heating to kill specific microorganisms or to inactivate certain enzymes without changes that consumers notice to the point of objecting and rejecting. The lower millstone is the necessity to kill the pathogens of milk-borne diseases. Rosenau determined the thermal survival of the organisms when he was working at the Laboratory of Hygiene of the U.S. Public Health Service in 1908. Gail Borden began heating whole milk for the bottled market in New York in 1898. His product had objectionable qualities. The cream did not float up in full volume so the customers felt cheated on butterfat content. Often there was a distinct, unpleasant cooked flavor and sometimes a caramelized color.

Charles North collaborated with Rosenau in determining the temperatures and times which minimize such changes. In 1912, the results were graphically put down in North's chart which is shown in Fig. 8-5. More recent and detailed thermal death points of pathogens in milk are given in Ref. 8-6. Any combination of time and temperature in the "neutral zone" on North's chart will kill the pathogens with the minimum change in other quality factors. The low and irregular vitamin C content in milk is lost. It was known early that certain enzymes were destroyed, some in the "neutral zone." This was first a curse. Antipasteurization forces claimed that with these enzymes went all the life-giving power that nature had carefully placed in "natural cow milk." Later, in the mid-1930s, the blessing appeared. H. Scharer completed his search for a rapid, accurate, and sensitive test for one of the enzymes which was thermolabile at the time and temperature of milk pasteurization. The enzyme is phosphatase. The test is usually called the *phosphatase test*, sometimes

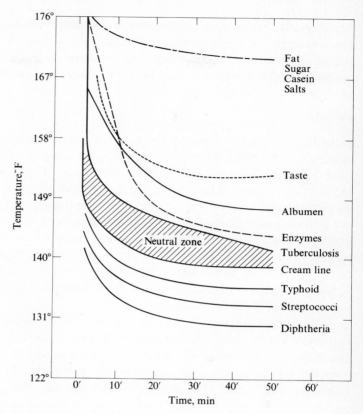

FIGURE 8-5
North's chart on bacterial kills and other changes in the heating and holding of milk to pasteurize it.   [*Source*: *U.S. Public Health Serv. Bull.* 147, 1925.]

the Scharer test.   Another enzyme, lipase, is destroyed with beneficial results.   If not inactivated, lipase quickly causes milk fats to go rancid.   It is a tribute to the work of Rosenau and North that the time and temperature for milk pasteurization in the United States remained unchanged from the 1920s until the late 1940s when, to inactivate *Rickettsia burnetii*, the etiological agent of Q fever, temperatures were increased to 145°F (63°C) for 30 min and 161°F (72°C) for 15 s.   A higher temperature of 175°F (80°C) is required for high-butterfat products.

Other beverages which are pasteurized are beer, fruit juices, cider, and the growing line of synthetic beverages replicating citrus juices and even milk itself.   In all applications pasteurization is the selection of a time-temperature heat treatment which kills certain undesirable microorganisms or enzymes, or both, without a heat intensity that alters other constituents with undesirable effects on flavor, appearance, and total nutritive value. It is not cooking. It is not sterilization. It is proving a safeguard against salmonellas in shelled, frozen eggs by using 143°F (61.5°C) for 3.5 to 4 min in equipment identical with that used for HTST pasteurization of milk.

Freezing

In the United States, fish and poultry were frozen in natural ice on a commercial scale as early as the 1860s. Mechanical refrigeration using ammonia began in 1875. In 1910, berries were frozen in the Pacific Northwest. The forward spurt came in the 1920s when Clarence Birdseye successfully applied his quick-freeze method to fish. By 1927 the quick-freeze was satisfactory for vegetables. At present 700 food items can provide a completely frozen menu including single servings packaged as a "TV dinner." The freezing of completely cooked items for simple heating developed in the last 15 years and continues to find new applications. These have great appeal for ease of preparation, zero waste other than the packaging, and choice of portion size. A recent addition to the variety is the "boil in the bag" single portions of chicken, turkey, or beef slices in seasoned gravies.

The actual freezing is done by one of the three basic methods, air freezing, indirect contact freezing, and immersion freezing. The technique used and the time and temperatures of exposure are quite specific for particular fruits and vegetables and even for growth strains of a single species (Ref. 8-5). The faster the freezing is completed, the better. The ideal is to have the least disruption of structure and texture. A rate of freezing penetration of $\frac{1}{2}$ in/h meets the needs. Immersion freezing achieves that rate readily. Plate contact methods meet the rate requirement. Air-blast methods have to cope with food dehydration and coil frosting, and the need for air velocities of 200 to 300 fpm at temperatures of $-20°F$ ($-29°C$) to $-50°F$ ($-45.5°C$).

Table 8-9 EFFECT OF THAWING METHODS AND TIMES ON THE MICROBIAL COUNTS OF FROZEN WHOLE-EGG MEATS

Method	Hours required	Increase in microbial count during thawing, %
In air, 80°F (27°C)	23	1,000
In air, 70°F (21°C)	36	750
In air, 45°F (7°C)	63	225
In running water, 60°F (16°C)	15	250
In running water, 70°F (21°C)	12	300
In agitated water, 60°F (16°C)	9	40
Dielectric heat	15 min	Negligible

SOURCE: Ref. 8–11, p. 103.

Air-blast methods have been made continuous processes with fluidized beds, with humidification during prechilling, and with propylene glycol sprays as defrosting agents.

Thawing frozen foods for use must be as fast as facilities can do it to keep the food attributes desired and expected, and to hold down bacterial growth. Table 8-9 states the case for fast thawing, using the percentage increase of microbial counts of frozen whole-egg meats. Between the 23 hours required to thaw in air at 80°F (27°C) and the 9 hours to thaw the eggs in agitated water at 60°F (16°C), the percentage of microbial count increased 25-fold.

Fermentation

This process has been used by many peoples, some who do not even have a recorded history. Milk to cheese is a fermentation. Plant sugars to alcohols are fermentation. It is the action of selected or self-selected microorganisms on the nutrients, providing desirable and acceptable changes which are valued for the new characteristics or which provide a storage method for a substantial portion of the bulk and of the nutrients for eating out of season. A fermentation requires a microbial population on a usable substrate, a means to confine the growth to the selected organisms, and a means to stop the action at the point of desired change. All fermentations proceed rapidly to pH levels below 4.5, which shuts off the growth of *Clostridium botulinum* and its toxin production. Fermentation lowers the caloric value of foods, as sugar converts to alcohol and on to acid in most cases. In some instances vitamin content increases by the elaboration of riboflavin and precursors of vitamin C. Mold action on grains and seeds releases nutrients that are indigestible before the fermentation. Enzymatic splitting during fermentation converts cellulose substances to simpler sugars which man and domestic animals can use. Some typical actions are those in wine making, where the yeast, *Saccharomyces*, ferments the fruit sugars to alcohol and CO_2; in fermenting apple cider to vinegar, where in a second stage, the acetobacters convert the cider alcohol and O_2 to acetic acid and H_2O; and in curdling milk, where the species *Streptococcus lactis* acts on the milk sugar to form lactic acid.

Irradiating with Gamma Rays and Accelerated Electrons

The world's food needs and losses are too large to pass by the potential benefits of irradiation. The issues are how much effort and risk shall be taken to have the benefits, and can the high cost of developing the methods be justified. Table 8-10 indicates the benefits, the means of attaining them, the foods which are targets, and the dose ranges. The benefits group into:

1 Inhibit sprouting of potatoes and onions to extend storage time
2 Extend storage, transportation, and shelf life of fish, meat, and poultry
3 Reduce and slow down spoilage loss and quality deterioration of fresh fruits and vegetables, and thus extend transportation and storage time
4 Kill or prevent reproduction of insects infesting grains, cereals, and dried foods
5 Kill pathogenic organisms

Table 8-10 APPLICATION OF IONIZING RADIATION TO FOODS, IN RANK ORDER OF DOSE FROM 6 MILLION TO 5,000 RADS, SHOWING PURPOSE, FOOD, AND MECHANISM

Dosage, Mrads	Food	Main objective	Means of attaining objective
1 4–6	Meat, poultry, fish, and many other highly perishable foods	Safe long-term preservation without refrigerated storage	Destruction of spoilage organisms and any pathogens present, particularly *Clostridium botulinum*
2 1–3	Spices and other special food ingredients	To minimize contamination of food to which the ingredients are added	Reduction of population of microbes in the special ingredient
3 0.3–1.0	Frozen meat, poultry, eggs, and other foods liable to contamination with pathogens	Prevention of food poisoning	Destruction of salmonellas
4 0.05–1.0	Meat, poultry, fish, and many other highly perishable foods	Extension of refrigerated storage below 3°C	Reduction of population of microorganisms capable of growth at these temperatures
5 0.1–0.5	Fruit and certain vegetables	Improvement of keeping properties	Reduction of population of molds and yeasts, and in some instances delay of maturation
6 0.01–0.05	Cereals, flour, fresh and dried fruit, and other products liable to infestation	Prevention of loss of stored food or spread of pests	Killing or sexual sterilization of insects
7 0.01–0.03	Meat and other foods carrying pathogenic parasites	Prevention of parasitic disease transmitted through food	Destruction of parasites such as *Trichinella spiralis* and *Taenia saginata*
8 0.005–0.015	Tubers (e.g., potatoes), bulbs (e.g., onions), and other underground organs of plants	Extension of storage life	Inhibition of sprouting

SOURCE: Modified from The Technical Basis for Legislation on Irradiated Food, *FAO Atomic Energy Ser.* 6, 1965, p. 8.

6   Kill all organisms and alter enzymes so that storage is very long and requires only special packaging, not controlled temperature and humidity

The levels of dose are fantastically high.   The range in Table 8-10 is from 5,000 to 6 million rads.   As a reference value, 400 to 600 rads of *x* or gamma radiation with whole-body exposure will cause death for 50 percent of humans within 30 days. The construction and operation of irradiators used in food work are formidable in safety and dosimetry requirements.   Gamma emissions from ^{60}Co (cobalt) and ^{137}Cs (cesium) and linear acceleration which bring electrons to energy levels of 10 MeV (megaelectronvolts) are in use.   Among the 10 food irradiators supported by the Atomic Energy Commission (AEC), there are the Hawaii development irradiator containing 225,000 Ci (curies) of ^{60}Co, and the portable cesium irradiator containing 170,000 Ci of ^{137}Cs.   The curie is the unit of the rate of radioactive decay.   One gram of radium has one curie of radioactivity.   The Hawaii irradiator applies a pasteurizing dose of gamma to tropical fruits, papaya, mango, and pineapple, at a throughput of 2 tons/h.   The objective is to control overripening rates so that low-cost sea freight can be used to reach stateside markets.   The portable cesium irradiator has been used for demonstration testing in 12 states by 75 companies processing fruits and vegetables to verify spoilage and ripening control under field conditions.   In food irradiation, doses used for benefits *3* through *8* are termed *low-level* or *pasteurizing doses*.   From 5,000 to 1 million rads are applied; 1 million rads is 1 megarad, Mrad. For complete sterilization of the entire food tissue and partial stoppage of enzyme action, benefit *1*, doses of 4 to 6 Mrads are required.   These are termed *high-level* or *sterilizing doses*.

The elemental event of ionizing radiations' encounter with matter is energy transfer.   In food irradiation, the benefits are secure when the energy transfer kills or inactivates organisms that cause spoilage or disease, inactivates enzymes that keep the ripening processes going, or kills or prevents reproduction of insects infesting the food at one or another of the insect stages, egg, larva, pupa, or adult.   The energy transfer is also made to the food constituents, the fat, proteins, carbohydrates, vitamins, and trace elements.   The dosimetry requirement is that the radiation adsorbed dose accomplish the desired objectives with the absolute minimum of other changes.   This means unaltered flavor and aroma.   Some early U.S. Army beef products were described as "wet dog."   Appearance and texture must be nearly unchanged.   Nutrient value must be retained.   No toxic substances must be formed.   The last requirement has raised controversy in the United States with the Food and Drug Administration on one side and the Atomic Energy Commission and U.S. Army on the other (Ref. 8-7).

Gamma irradiation does not make the food itself radioactive.   There is no induced radioactivity by gamma rays.   Electron bombardment by linear accelerators induces radioactivity only if the electron's energy is above 10 MeV.   The high-energy transfer at such high values alters atomic structure to the point that the unstable forms in turn release ionizing radiation. This is readily avoided by not exceeding 10 MeV as the energy of the bombarding electrons. In the issue of public understanding, it is most important to differentiate clearly between food irradiation and the contamination of food by radioactive compounds from fallout and careless radioactive-waste disposal. Irradiation has demonstrated its usefulness as a method of reducing spoilage and insect losses. In India, up to 50 percent of the fruit and vegetable production is lost each year. In Africa, up to 50 percent of the dried fish is lost through insect infestation. Africa's grain loss to pests is enough to feed 80 million people for a year. In Latin America nearly one-third of the harvests spoil before reaching the consumer. A variety of techniques of food science must be applied to cut these losses. Food irradiation has attributes which warrant continued support for its development. Answers to the immediate doubts raised by the Food and Drug Administration are being sought in 3-year animal-feeding studies.

Food Protection during Storage, Transportation, and Retailing

The time-temperature and humidity during storage, transportation, retailing, and final preparation of food determine the success of the control of spoilage by enzyme action and biological growth, of food-borne diseases due to pathogen growth, and of damage by freezing raw fruits and vegetables. As soon as he moved from the tropical regions, where he eats today what grows today, man had to answer the question, How long will it keep? His ability to colonize the temperate regions, where the intervals between growing-harvesting seasons lengthen and his consumption during no growing and poor hunting must continue, was and is determined by his capacity as a food technologist. A competent farmer from the fertile valley north of Bangkok in Thailand would not survive a seasonal cycle in the high plateau of Afghanistan without a lot of help. The cycle of production, storage, and use of food is entirely different.

Table 8-11 shows the differences of temperature ranges for storage of foods faced by the Thai and the high-plateau Afghan. The Thai farmer, producer, and user faces the 72 to 100°F (22 to 38°C) range. Those foods which he cannot market and eat in a day or two at most, must be dried. He must store his rice so that it is dry and not too accessible to insects, rodents, and birds. He polishes the rice to remove the oily coating that becomes rancid. The Afghan on the central plateau around Kabul is in the 32 to 72°F (0 to 22°C) range with a predictable seasonal variation. He uses a lot of dried foods to facilitate transport and marketing and to carry through a hard winter. He must protect his fall fruit and vegetables against freezing. But he has a fairly generous storage life for his meat, fish, and poultry and can fit his kill and catch to the time and distance of his marketing and transport. Table 8-12 shows the response of bacteria in milk to a favorable temperature, given 1 to 4 days. Growth is exponential. There are upper and lower temperature and humidity bounds for the storage of fruit and vegetables (Ref. 8-5, p. 134). Storage of fruits and vegetables outside the optimal ranges cause such unmarketable defects as internal browning of apples and avocados; pitting in snap beans, eggplant; unacceptable colors of bananas, okra, and pineapples; and internal discoloration of lemons, mangoes, and olives.

In people's thinking, frozen foods carry more of a halo of good bacterial behavior than is supported by laboratory observations. Table 8-13 is a reminder that bacteria survive for the storage life of frozen foods. A few bacterial types, the psychrophiles, multiply slowly at freezing and lower temperatures. The vast majority die away slowly. At extremely low temperatures below 0°F (-18°C), bacteria are in a stasis, but resume rapid growth as the food is thawed. As indicated in Table 8-13, surviving bacteria resume multiplication very rapidly. Only in the case of fruits frozen in sugar syrups is there a check on the zooming populations.

Table 8-11 STORAGE LIFE OF PLANT AND ANIMAL FOODS AT 32, 72, AND 100°F

Food	Generalized average useful storage life, in days at °F (or °C)		
	32°F (0°C)	72°F (22°C)	100°F (38°C)
Animal flesh	6–10	1	less than 1
Fish	2–7	1	less than 1
Poultry	5–18	1	less than 1
Dry meats and fish	1,000 and more	350 and more	100 and more
Fruits	2–180	1–20	1–7
Dry fruits	1,000 and more	350 and more	100 and more
Leafy vegetables	3–20	1–7	1–3
Root crops	90–300	7–50	2–20
Dry seeds	1,000 and more	350 and more	100 and more

SOURCE: N. W. Desrosier, "Attack on Starvation," Avi Publishing Co. Inc., Westport, Conn., 1961.

Table 8-12 THE INCREASE OF BACTERIA IN MILK AT ROOM TEMPERATURE AT 24-HOUR INTERVALS FROM 0 TO 96 HOURS

Storage hours	Bacterial count per ml
0	137,000
24	24,674,000
48	639,885,000
72	2,407,083,000
96	5,346,667,000

SOURCE: B. W. Hammer and F. J. Babel, "Dairy Bacteriology," 4th Ed., John Wiley and Sons, Inc., New York, 1957.

ACHIEVING FOOD PROTECTION IN FINAL PREPARATION AND SERVING

In all the steps of growing, processing, storing, and transporting food, the basic needs are:

1 Foods of high quality in all characteristics
2 Time and temperature controls fitted to specific foods and to the purposes of the processing or holding
3 The design and construction of equipment that works well and that facilitates cleaning
4 Construction and maintenance of buildings, vehicles, and vessels that prevent insect and rodent entrance and harborage
5 Personnel who apply hygiene and sanitation as part of their on-the-job work habits

These same needs are mandatory in final preparation and serving in public and private restaurants, dining halls, and cafeterias. These apply to home food handling in the family kitchen. These apply to automatic food-vending machines. In final preparation there are additionally particular temperatures that must be maintained to control bacterial growth particularly of pathogens during the cycle of cooking, serving, holding, and for frozen foods during thawing.

Table 8-13 BACTERIAL COUNTS IN SELECTED FROZEN FOODS IN STORAGE FOR 12 MONTHS AND AFTER 24 HOURS OF THAWING AT 70°F

	Bacteria per gram	
Product	Frozen	After 24 h at 70°F
Beef stew	390	1,400,000
Beef steak	390	1,400,000
Carrots, scalded	3,000	5,800,000
Eggs, in tin	190,000	70,000,000
Green beans, scalded	1,000	40,000,000
Haddock	38,000	770,000
Oysters	22,000	320,000,000
Peaches, with sugar 3:1	60	700
Peas, scalded	1,000	24,000,000
Pork chops	1,300	8,700,000
Raspberries, with sugar 3:1	3,000	8,000
Strawberries, with sugar 3:1	200	20,000
Sweet corn, scalded	1,500	60,000,000

SOURCE: Ref. 8–11, p. 104.

What does it take to kill them? What lets them grow? Table 8-14 states the thermal resistance of two groups of bacteria notorious for food-borne illness from the eating of two foods that nourish the bacteria very well, custard and chicken à la king. Note that at 130°F (54°C), the time spread to kill is from $\frac{1}{2}$ to 10 hours depending on the species and the food. At 150°F (66°C), the kill time is cut to a range of $\frac{1}{2}$ to about 12 min. Higher temperatures would do the job faster, but again an upper limit is imposed. The food has to be attractive and acceptable. Excessive drying, caking, protein coagulation, sugar caramelizing, and the loss of flavorful volatiles impose the limits. Heating meats, fish, and poultry during cooking to internal temperatures of 160 to 170°F (71 to 77°C) accomplishes the kill. The rare-beef and rare-pork fanciers indulge their tastes at some risk of beef tapeworm and trichinellas, and of surface contamination by pathogens of handler or animal origin in rolled meat and poultry preparations. Figure 8-6 shows the growth or decline of salmonellas and staphylococci in chicken à la king on a steam table. Steam tables are used for holding foods until or during serving in mass-feeding installations such as cafeterias, mess halls, and large institutional kitchens. Note how critical the temperature is for growth or decline. A shift of 2°F determines bacterial growth or decrease. The temperatures are food readings. The time scale is in hours.

The growth range for bacteria which cause food-borne outbreaks is from 40 to 120°F (4 to 49°C). For holding food, temperatures of 115 to 120°F (46 to 49°C) stop incubation. The holding time is limited to about 3 hours because of undesirable drying and slow overcooking in the range of 115 to 120°F (46 to 49°C). Longer

Table 8-14 TIME FOR THE KILL OF SALMONELLAS AND STAPHYLOCOCCI IN CUSTARD AND CHICKEN À LA KING

Exposure temperature °F	°C	Minutes required to kill 1×10^7 organisms per gram*					
		Staphylococcus aureus 196 E		*Salmonella senftenberg* 775 W		*Salmonella manhattan*	
		Custard	Chicken à la king	Custard	Chicken à la king	Custard	Chicken à la king
130	54	540	425	530	620	100	35.5
135	56	180	140	205	220	44	10.5
140	60	59	47	78	81.5	19	3.0
145	62	19.5	15.5	29.5	28.5	8.1	<1.0†
150	66	6.6	5.2	11.5	10.0	3.5	<0.3†

* Average value from duplicate experiments, 10 million organisms per gram.
† Extrapolated and rounded.
SOURCE: From M. J. Foter, Time-Temperature Relationships in Food Sanitation, *RATSEC-U.S. Public Health Serv.*, 1961.

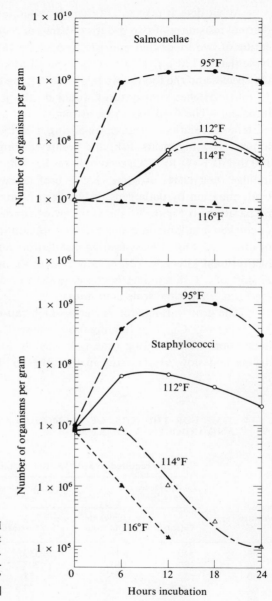

FIGURE 8-6
Growth or decline of salmonellae and staphylococci in chicken à la king at various temperatures on a steam table. [*Source*: *M. J. Foter, "Time Temperature Relationships in Food Sanitation," RATSEC, U.S. Public Health Serv.*, 1964.]

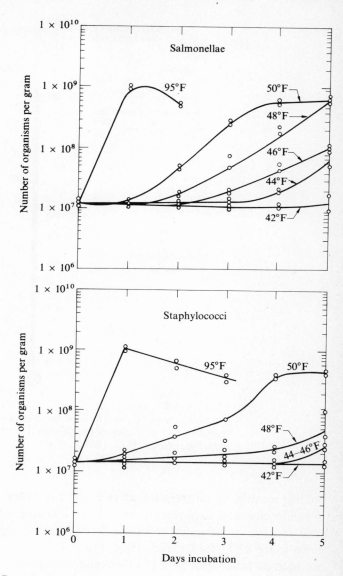

FIGURE 8-7
Growth of salmonellae and of staphylococci at 42 to 95°F on chicken à la king.
[*Source*: M. J. Foter, "*Time Temperature Relationships in Food Sanitation*,"
RATSEC, U.S. Public Health Serv., 1964.]

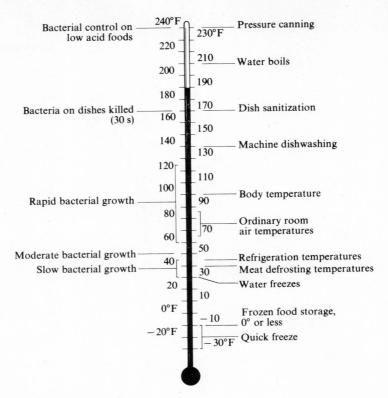

FIGURE 8-8
Temperatures in °F used in food processing and handling, and the bacterial responses. [*Source*: *School Food Service Sanitation*, *N. C. State Board of Health*, *Publ.* 500, Raleigh, N.C., 1966, *p.* 17.]

holding must be by refrigeration at 40°F (4°C) or lower. Figure 8-7 shows the fate of salmonellas and staphylococci on chicken à la king during storage, with the time scale in days. Mechanical refrigeration or liquid-nitrogen release is needed to get down to the 42°F (5.6°C) level, which Fig. 8-7 shows, to stop incubation. Iceboxes can hold no lower than 50°F (10°C) at summer ambient temperatures of 85 to 95°F (29 to 35°C). Just as fast thawing limits bacterial increases, fast cooling prevents a buildup of the bacteria. The practice of letting hot foods cool off to room temperature before placing them in the refrigerator guarantees high bacterial counts. In quite simple form, Fig. 8-8 shows the temperature responses of bacteria from 70 to 240°F (21 to 116°C) and associates the temperatures with familiar circumstances. Adherence to these temperatures in food handling will reduce bacterial contamination, food-borne illness, and food spoilage.

WASHING AND SANITIZING FOOD-PROCESSING EQUIPMENT AND FOOD-HANDLING UTENSILS

Disease prevention and product-quality protection require a thorough washing and efficient bactericidal treatment of equipment and utensils which contact the food and also of the premises to hold down insect and rodent attraction and fungus growths. A good washing job requires plenty of hot water and a detergent fitted to the filth, the food residues, and the metals and plastics. A good bactericidal treatment requires that the surfaces be clean and that a compatible bactericidal agent be applied at the effective concentration or intensity for the time needed to kill the target organisms.

Detergents

A detergent is a mixture of compounds which loosens filth from surfaces, gets the loosened material into the carrying water, keeps it suspended there, and finally aids in rinsing. The loosening is done by a wetting agent and is facilitated by a softening agent if the water is hard. The removal is done by the combined actions of an emulsifying agent acting on fats and a deflocculating agent acting on precipitated, coagulated food filth such as proteins. The suspension is done by dissolving and dispersing agents which reduce the size and change the aggregate states of the particles removed from the surface. Rinsing aid is a recent added task for detergents. It can be provided by chlorine and perborates. Plain old farmyard soap (saponified fat) with lye (sodium hydroxide), soda ash (sodium carbonate) if the water is hard, and finely ground pumice or fine sand will produce the mix to do the job. In turn, each is a wetting agent and emulsifier, a dissolving and deflocculating agent, a water conditioner and dispersant, and an abrasive and polisher. These are well fitted to hand methods, to cast iron surfaces, and to stainless steel if the abrasive is used lightly. To meet the needs of high-speed cleaning with pressure sprays, motorized brushes, clean-in-place pipelines, metal alloys, and plastic-coated surfaces which must be protected against corrosion, scratching, and peeling, and for a minimum of manual labor in the process, the chemical industry has developed a dozen or more compounds for each of the purposes, which can be blended or formulated into hundreds of mixes fitted, it is hoped, to special needs, including the local water characteristics. The greatest variety of basic materials are the wetting agents. Their inclusion in the mix led to the term *syndets*, synthetic detergents. Presumably, soap has been around so long that it is not regarded as synthetic, and probably not thought of as a wetting agent either. It is both.

Table 8-15 lists the types of materials which make up a detergent. Examples of mixes are:

1 General-purpose detergent   Trisodium phosphate, 60 percent; tetrasodium pyro-phosphate, 35 percent; sulfated alcohol, 5 percent.

2 A liquid detergent (patented product)   Tetrapotassium pyrophosphate, 13 percent; sulfonated lauric amide, 5 percent; alkyl aryl sulfonate, 2 percent; sodium xylene sulfonate, 4.5 percent; sodium lauryl sulfate, 2 percent; water, 73.5 percent.

Manufacturers, distributors, and agents provide technical data on their products. For practical and concise information on detergents and sanitizers, see Ref. 8-8.   For structural formulas of soaps and syndets and the distinctions among anionic, cationic, and nonionic wetting agents, see Ref. 8-9 (pp. 147–150).

Bactericidal Agents

The grouping of bactericidal agents in Table 8-16 is physical and chemical.   Only those in general use are given.   Ultrasonic vibration, gaseous chlorine, elemental iodine, and ionic silver are omitted, as these are rarely used for routine disinfection of

Table 8-15   EXAMPLES OF COMPONENTS OF DETERGENTS BY TYPES, WITH TRADE OR COMMON NAMES AND ACTION

Group	Compounds	Trade or common name	Action
Syndets	Sulfated fatty alcohols	Dreft, Duponol	Wetting agent
	Alkyl aryl sulfonates	The ABS Compounds	Wetting agent
	Linear alkyl sulfonates	The LAS Compounds	Wetting agent
	Ethylene oxide condensates	Antarox, nonionic compounds	Wetting agent
Carbonates	Sodium carbonate	Soda ash	Softener, mild general detergent
	Sodium bicarbonate	Bicarb	Useful buffer
Phosphates	Trisodium phosphate	TSP	Emulsifier, deflocculator
	Tripolyphosphate		Softener, dispersant, builder
	Sodium hexametaphosphate	Calgon	Softener, sequestrant, dispersant
Others	Sodium hydroxide	Lye, caustic soda	Saponifies fats, dissolves and hydrolyzes proteins; most corrosive
	Sodium metasilicate		Most widely used, multipurpose silicate; not corrosive to aluminum or tin coatings
	Borax	20 Mule Team	Mild alkali, good buffer

food equipment and utensils.   Heat is extremely effective.   Note that cabinet or chamber application of steam and of dry hot air requires 15 and 20 min, respectively. Such use is satisfactory for batch operations of cleanup or at the end of a run, as in shellfish-shucking plants of modest size.   The details on specifications on automatic spray dishwashing machines, in very wide use in United States restaurants and cafeterias, are stated in National Sanitation Foundation Standard 3 on spray types of dishwashers.   These specifications cover wash temperatures, time in travel, detergent use, nozzle pressure, and rates of spray, plus bactericidal rinse temperatures and times.

The effect of pH on the disinfectant power of chlorine was recognized in the nineteenth century.   The brief data in Table 8-16 indicate that as pH decreases, the bactericidal effectiveness increases.   Chlorine compounds kill bacteria by the formation of hypochlorous acid, HOCl, which speedily penetrates bacterial cell walls and inactivates enzymes.   A low pH, that is, a high hydrogen-ion concentration, increases the formation of the un-ionized hypochlorous acid.   This fact has made the use of chlorine compounds in conjunction with alkaline cleaning compounds difficult.   In

Table 8-16   BACTERICIDAL AGENTS IN COMMON USE FOR FOOD PROCESSING AND HANDLING EQUIPMENT

	Physical agents
Hot water	At 212°F, instantaneous after rise time: Automatic spray dishwashers, 180°F for 10 s. Immersion at 170°F for 30 s.
Steam cabinets	200°F for 5 min, 170°F for 15 min.
Steam jets	At ejection temperature for 1 min.
Dry, hot-air cabinets	At 180°F for 20 min.
	Chemical agents
Inorganic chlorine	Chloride of lime or high-test hypochlorite: 50 ppm for 1 min at 75°F. For each 18°F drop below 75°F, double the exposure time.
Organic chlorine	Chloramine T: 50 ppm for 1 min at pH 6.4. 100 ppm for 1 min at pH 6.8. 200 ppm for 1 min. at pH 7.2. Chlorinated hydantoin: 50 ppm for 1 min at pH 7 or less. Chlorinated isocyanoauric acid: 50 ppm for 1 min at pH 9.5 or less.
Quaternary ammonium	Specific QACs must be tested for compatibility with hard waters. Effective at 200 ppm in 1 min at 75°F or higher, and at pH 5 or higher.
Iodophors	At 12.5 ppm for 1 min at low pH's and at temperatures up to 120°F; verify by test.

sequential use, thorough rinsing is necessary.   Additionally, the rinse clears the surface of oxidizable residues, which dissipate the chlorine so needed for bacterial kill.   This is another case of chlorine demand.   Only a few of many quaternary ammonium compounds, QACs, are bactericidal under operating conditions.   The bactericidal effectiveness of a particular QAC is determined by its composition and concentration and by the aqueous solution in which it acts.   The factors are pH, temperature, and the interfering action of the chloride, sulfate, and bicarbonate salts of calcium and magnesium.   The concentration of these ions is expressed as hardness.   A few QACs disinfect in hardness concentrations up to 1,000 mg/l.   Others are formulated with sodium tripolyphosphate to sequester the Ca and Mg.   The QACs which are bactericidal have a limiting hardness.   This should be known before purchase and use in hard waters.

Manufacturers of two other halogens, bromine and iodine, have sought to get a share of the chlorine market in sanitation uses.   Strong nominees for food sanitation use are the iodophors.   The word is a compound of two Greek words, *iodo* for iodine and *phor* meaning to carry.   In an iodophor, the carrier is a nonionic syndet, or synonymously a nonionic surfactant.   All nonionic syndets are polymers of ethylene oxide, a simply structured organic which readily accepts new bonding arrangements. Compared with free iodine, the iodophors have increased stability in aqueous solution, do not stain surfaces, and are not irritating to the eyes or skin.   These compounds are effective bactericides and fungicides, show sporicidal and viricidal properties, and continue bacterial kill in the face of hardness, organic matter, and low temperatures.

Detergent Sanitizers

Detergent sanitizers are a single formulation which cleans and kills bacteria in a single step.   These are used in hand-cleaning operations to save a step and to reduce rinsing. The QAC and chlorine compounds are used with a nonionic syndet plus the materials to condition water, remove soil, emulsify fat, and sequester metallic ions.   An example of the QAC type is a mix of:

26 percent   sodium carbonate, water conditioner and mild alkali
7 percent   triton X-100, a nonionic syndet, as wetting agent
7 percent   hyamine 1622, the QAC to disinfect
30 percent   trisodium phosphate, alkali builder to remove soil and emulsify fat
30 percent   tetrasodium pyrophosphate, sequestering agent

The sequestering agent is needed to prevent Ca and Mg from interfering with the QAC disinfection.   The two sequestrants widely used in detergents, sodium hexametaphosphate and tetraphosphate, are incompatible with QAC.   For the chlorine type of detergent sanitizers, both inorganic and organic chlorine compounds are used.

Needs for Efficient Cleaning

Six things are needed for an economical, fast, and effective washup.

1 The washup area floor must be impervious and skid-proof, and sloped to ample drains. Walls and ceilings are treated to withstand splash and condensation. The space is well ventilated.

2 The water supply, hot and cold, should be abundant with hose connections convenient. A reliable boiler pressure is needed if steam jets or a steam-water mix is used. Thermostatically controlled mixing valves are desirable.

3 Sinks and vats in sufficient number and size for containers, valves, and pipe lengths should be available. Portable "roll-abouts" are useful.

4 Spray heads, nozzles, and brushes are needed to reach all food-contact surfaces.

5 Detergents and bactericides should be formulated to fit the filth and the water, and used in effective concentrations for the necessary contact times.

6 The men who supervise and who do the job need to be well trained, have the "know-how," and be well paid.

TESTS AND INSPECTIONS FOR FOOD PROTECTION

Food protection practices in the United States utilize more tests and inspections than any other phase of environmental control. It is common to have laws and codes requiring state and local health departments to inspect each restaurant, cafeteria, and drive-in four times a year. The U.S. Public Health Service *Food Service Manual*, 1962, recommends two a year. The Department of Agriculture inspects over 100 million pigs, sheep, cattle, and poultry birds a year at the point of slaughter, covering all meat products in nearly 2,000 plants which ship across state borders. This inspection service covers 85 percent of all marketed meat. Most of these plants require full-time resident inspectors. The processors pay for this service under a fee system. The cost appears in the price to the buyer. The Food and Drug Administration depends primarily upon sampling and testing to verify compliance with food standards, additive use, filth content, and packaging requirements, cooperating with state food and drug staffs. Fish products are inspected by the Bureau of Commercial Fisheries of the Department of the Interior. The U.S. Public Health Service has provided model laws, codes, and inspection procedures for milk, shellfish, and public eating places. The Service gives a tremendous amount of technical assistance in field and administrative work. All this is widely used by the state and local agencies. These consultant and educational methods of the U.S. Public Health Service are reinforced by a plan of certification of interstate shippers of milk and shellfish, and by legal powers over the food service on planes, ships, trains, and buses in interstate and foreign travel.   In 1969 the Public Health Service functions were transferred to the Food and Drug Administration.

Milk receives the most intensive coverage by tests and inspections.   The requirements are extremely detailed and explicit.   As in the past, the 1965 form of the U.S. Public Health Service milk ordinance and code, entitled *Grade A Pasteurized Milk Ordinance*, is a fine handbook not only on milk sanitation but on water supply, excreta disposal, and fly control.   The ordinance specifies the type and number of inspections and samples.   It specifies the tests to be run on each type of sample and the limits on the test results.   The sanitary supervision of milk accelerated the concentration of our milk supply system in larger and larger farm producers with centralized processors collecting milk in a radius of 100 miles or more and distributing the finished products across even wider areas.

Specific bacterial limits for other foods have neither been agreed upon nor adopted, with a few exceptions.   These exceptions are:

1   Coliform content of shellfish, recommended by the U.S. Public Health Service
2   Numerous and widely varying, total undifferentiated bacterial counts on ice cream, depending on geography and flavor
3   Coverage of a few foods by New York City and the Commonwealth of Massachusetts health regulations.

The reasons for the hesitancy in setting bacterial limits on other foods are:

1   Uncertainty of a cause and effect between easily verifiable bacterial content and the nature and risk of a health hazard
2   Lack of consistency, for a wide range of foods, in correlation between the bacterial content and the conditions of food production and handling, unless a myriad of limits are set for particular foods and the processes used
3   Lack of low-cost laboratory methods to measure and to discriminate the bacteria in simple foods, mixed foods, precooked and frozen foods, and even dried foods.

The issues that must be faced in setting bacterial limits in foods are analyzed in Ref. 8-10.

The hesitancy on bacteriological tests and standards for foods other than milk does not exist for other tests.   Chemical tests and limits are applied by the Food and Drug Administration, state, and large municipal agencies for all sorts of additives and residues.   These tests use the most recent and sophisticated procedures, which redefine and lower the numerical value of "none shall be detectable."   The last is a favorite phrase of regulation writers.   It defines some number between zero and the skill of the analyst.   It gives consumers the warm glow of security and administrative heads a momentary aura of achievement.   The haggling resumes when a new level of sensitivity is reached by improved analysis. Physical tests are used to determine watering, correct weight and volumes, color, excesses of filth and fillers and foreign matter, excesses of imperfections in fruits and vegetables, drained weight, firmness, viscosity, spreading characteristics, size, shape, consistency, and turbidity. The subjective responses of odor, taste, and sight are termed *organoleptic tests.* These measure flavor, texture, and appearance.

CHANGES AND DEVELOPMENTS TO COME

The driving forces which will intensify changes and developments in food technology, and hence in food protection, are the same three that have liberated man to this time from depending on what he could gather, grow, catch, or kill within a few days of eating it. These are:

1 A growing population which in past millennia migrated to uninhabited regions of unfamiliar climates and used new land and water as an added food source;

2 The concentration of people in urban life patterns in which most individuals are totally incapable of gathering, growing, catching, or hunting their food while at the same time conforming to the urban pattern;

3 The demand of people, including the world's most miserable and apathetic, to be able to feed themselves and their children better both in quantity and quality and with nutritional balance.

The "green revolution" is being hailed as an easy answer to these three forces. The hail and hurrah are based on new record yields from "miracle rice" both where it was developed in the Philippines and where it is in use in other Southeast Asian countries, and on the increased wheat yields in Turkey from introducing carefully selected strains from the United States. All wish the green revolution well.

Such agricultural production triumphs will demand more immediate use of advanced food technology, including food protection, not less. The more rapid plant use of soil nutrients will require the replacement by chemical fertilizers. This was a precondition of the use of high-yield wheat in Turkey. The fertilizer will also feed more weeds, with a demand for weedicide use. The luxuriant stands of rice and wheat will be a splendid maternity ward for insects, old and new, and possible plant diseases unknown in the area until the crowded soil provided a lush environment. The high yields will require more and longer storage, and will require longer hauls to the markets. Storage and transport require a lot of the armamentarium of food technology and protection, including pesticide and antioxidant use. The greater its success, the more widespread will be the green revolution's requirement for the use of agricultural chemicals.   With the extended use, the issue of chemical residues in foods will have to be faced more widely and more realistically.

The requirements of food quantity and quality produced in high yields, with minimum labor time in the advanced countries, and with maximum keeping time will be very strong pressures for the adoption of two techniques already at the laboratory stage.   The first is the use of plant growth regulators on the food crops, not merely as weedicides as at present.   A. J. Vlitos states the readiness in Ref. 8-4 (pp. 89–126).   The second is the use of antibiotics to control microorganisms on meat and poultry.   Using much of his own work, H. H. Weiser states the experimental results of such antibiotic use in Ref. 8-11 (pp. 267–283).   The Food and Drug Administration has backtracked on antibiotics in the rinse and cooling waters on the assembly-line dressing of poultry, and for dips of poultry prior to wrapping.   After several years of use, approval was rescinded in 1967 without new evidence of risk or injury.   The behavior of micro-organisms in frozen foods is not well defined.   The freeze-dry process produces a dried product, not a frozen one.   The fate of microorganisms in that process in its present applications has not been examined extensively.   Freeze-drying will be applied to more foods and food mixes.   The microbiology of the process must be better known. More information on the behavior of bactericidal and bacteriostatic agents in frozen foods and in freeze-dried foods is needed.

Storage and transport of foods in the United States and other well-developed countries can continue satisfactorily with present dependence on refrigeration, and for a few high-priced perishables, on airfreight.   Refrigeration and airfreight are already combined in Styrofoam containers shaped to jet-airfreighter fuselage dimen-sions.   These "igloos" are chilled by liquid-nitrogen cooling units, or less satis-factorily by plug-in electromechanical refrigerating units.   The only restraint in these developments is competitive costs.   For the developing countries, refrigeration is still a luxury in the reach of no more than 10 to 20 percent of a country's population. Refrigeration is not applied to more than a third of the foods which would have a longer time in storage and transport, and less spoilage loss, if it were.   The use of antibiotics and chemical bacteriostatic agents and gamma irradiation must be pursued for these people.   The gamma irradiators are independent of large electrical power sources.   Portable units are already in test use.   Their movement to central points, in step with the harvesting times and places, would greatly cut present losses in storage and transport.   Their use to disinfest grain would alone be worth a great amount of effort.   The Food and Drug Administration approves that use.

Canada and the U.S.S.R. each have a facility for irradiating potatoes on a large scale.   The U.S.S.R. has officially cleared more irradiated foods than any other country—potatoes, grain, dried fruits, dry food concentrates, fresh fruits, and vege-tables.   Additionally, the U.S.S.R. approves "experimental lots" of partially pro-cessed meats, partially processed poultry, kitchen-ready meat products, and onions.

Purposes, doses, and dates of approval are given in Ref. 8-7 (pp. 43 and 657).   The Atomic Energy Commission supports studies in Israel, Iceland, Argentina, India, Pakistan, Venezuela, and Chile by loans of irradiator units for use on fish, wheat, potatoes, citrus fruits, fresh fruits, and vegetables.   France, as is her custom between invasions, is going it alone with installations at Cadrache, Lyon, and Saclay.

The rate of these changes, so dependent on better information on the human physiological effects from chemical residues, is in turn dependent on developing or doing at least three things.   The first is better toxicological methods to assess the effects of chemical residues in foods.   There is something out of scale between human eating patterns and feeding caged experimental animals a test diet for 2 years, in which the test food makes up 35 percent of the dry weight of the animal's total food intake. The second is more epidemiological studies on the behavior of toxicants in human beings.   This is extremely difficult.   The development of techniques and the collection of data by sampling and analyzing blood, fatty tissues, and urine, and by autopsies and organ analysis must be accelerated.   The third is the development of techniques for more comprehensive and extensive prospective studies of new chemicals before these are carried to large-scale manufacture and use.   Such studies must include the fate in the free environment, and some thought of effects on the ecosystems which make man's present way of life what it is.   At least the questions, Do we need to apply this new compound for this purpose at all? and Is there an alternate? would be asked. These three fine, high-sounding proposals are part of the whole effort to clean our dirty environment.   These will require a mobilization of talent and an expenditure of materials that no nation has yet made to better life on earth.

AN APPRAISAL OF FOOD PROTECTION

On the First Level and the Prevention of Disease

The most visible accomplishment of food protection for disease prevention is the roll-back of milk-borne diseases in the United States and countries of northwest Europe. The components of milk sanitation have been applied to public eating establishments in the United States with zeal and a large time commitment.   That effort has produced cleaner premises, cleaner utensils, equipment, food, and waitresses.   Without any clear baseline of how much food-borne disease dirty restaurants were producing, the disease reduction cannot be documented.   A series of specific techniques for the control of cream-filled pastries, control of shellfish, accurate heat treatment of canned food and of shelled eggs heading for the freezer have reduced food-borne outbreaks of staphylococci food poisoning, typhoid fever, and botulism, and of salmonellosis from frozen eggs. Therefore, the rationale and the methods are judged to be sound. Administrative and management questions particularly for local health department food activities are: How much staff time must be committed to a particular phase to hold the benefits? Are there alternative management mechanisms that can deliver an equal return? Are the priorities in use the best ranking?

Poisonings by single acute doses in food still happen from time to time. Cadmium poisoning by ingestion of high concentrations in citrus juices, synthetic and natural, from cadmium-plated containers has been mentioned. Berton Roueché's *Eleven Blue Men* reports what happens when sodium nitrite is put in salt shakers for customer use *ad libidum*, rather than just in meat products to brighten their red. The records of the Philadelphia Health Department have the results of very heavy nitrite sprinkling on spoiling fish to get these from the distributor through a chain of supermarkets before the fish became stinking rotten. Control of such events depends on knowledge, labeling, distinctive dye additives, limiting the use of certain toxic compounds at the point of manufacture or of processing, prohibition of poison-container reuse, and rules on cargo storage. As such events are rare, control is satisfactory, although not optimal.

Poisoning—actual, alleged, or potential—by the cumulative responses to small ingestions over months, years, or a lifetime is truly a dilemma. The nature of the toxicological issues have already been stated. It is difficult but possible to set control limits on any poisons for which there is a specific pathology, such as lead, arsenic, selenium, and aniline. On such poisons, either control is satisfactory, man is tougher than supposed, or medical detection and diagnosis scores misses, for the records show neither cases nor deaths by ingestion in food or water. The lead poisoning in children is from sucking, gnawing, chewing, or swallowing lead-painted objects and surfaces, and parts of these. The lead does not enter with these children's food supply.

The controversy, confusion, and growing dissatisfaction with our present control approaches to low-level ingestions of natural and man-made chemicals has come up in trying to cope with the risk of nonspecific pathology or with the risk of possible pathology. Cancer is largely nonspecific on cause and entry of the etiological agent, until in a particular case the site and the exposure history give some basis for likely cause. Accumulations of DDT and DDE in fatty tissue are possible pathology. Nothing medically identifiable has happened yet in man. The only epidemiological evidence of pathology from prolonged ingestion of low levels of suspect materials in the diet is the high prevalence of stomach cancer in Iceland. Niels Dungal found stomach cancer among 35 to 45 percent of all malignant tumors in Iceland, higher amounts of carcinogens in farm-smoked foods than in commercially smoked ones. High prevalence of stomach cancer is recorded in Japan and Chile without explanation. If epidemiological evidence has not triggered the hunt for carcinogens in our food, what has?

The Delaney clause has been stated earlier in this chapter.   The Food and Drug Administration has responded to a most difficult task with a conservative scientific concept and with a pitifully small scientific staff to determine facts either through its own efforts or through contracts and grants.   As petitions on particular substances and uses have come to it, the Administration must use and interpret someone else's facts.   Its decisions are bound by an extremely explicit statement of law.   It must deal with an emotionally charged disease issue with consequent political sensitivity. The Food and Drug Administration has yet, over 12 years after being given the responsibility, to be given the resources to undertake a systematic study of food additives, or even to evaluate by its own study, the methods of doing such work.

These circumstances have left the regulatory agency, petitioners, independent scientists, and the people vulnerable to alarmists and cranks, all too often abetted by the mass media.   The Food and Drug Administration has taken rather defensive positions.   Among these are:

1 A feeding test must contain 35 percent by dry weight of the total diet of the food under test.
2 It is not enough to prove a food substance is not hazardous; it must be proved safe.
3 A feeding test must be carried on for 2 years.
4 Any reaction product that is a consequence of a process must be regarded as an additive and subject to test.
5 An approval may be rescinded at any time by the Administration when new evidence appears or its further review of an approved petition raises doubts that the safety has been proved.

The conflicting views that these positions produce is revealed in the testimony before the Joint Atomic Energy Committee of Congress (Ref. 8-7).

No one can validate the hypothesis of the Delaney clause.   That hypothesis is that any substances that cause any cancer in any animal at any dose administered by any means for any length of time is not safe to be added to any food of man in any amount whatsoever.   One example which casts doubt on it is tannic acid.   It is barred as a food additive, as it has been shown to be carcinogenic in test animals. Tannic acid is a natural component of tea.   In that form it does not come under the Delaney clause.   Tea drinking has neither been banned nor discouraged.   There has been no epidemiological evidence that tea drinkers have a higher prevalence of cancer or any other disease.   A law and an administrative process which becomes overly restrictive puts in jeopardy the very benefits for which they were set up.   A satisfactory rationale for dealing with lifelong and generation-after-generation-long exposure to low-level concentrations of man-made toxicants will be developed from ecological and epidemiological information. Experimental animal toxicology is a necessary starting point. It must be recognized that it is a starting point which is not likely to provide information final for man or biological systems generally.

On the Second Level—Comfort, Convenience, and Esthetics

Food protection has delivered the goods. Cleanliness, freedom from filth, and attractiveness first urged by health and food control people have become a competitive selling point. So has the cleanliness and attractiveness of eating places. Some visitors from overseas believe this to be an American obsession. If so, it has a one-sidedness to it, for the patrons as a group do not exhibit either responsibility or inclination to do their part to maintain cleanliness and tidiness. Being automobile-borne seems to confer particular liberties to leave the picnic areas a mess, drive-in areas a sea of tossed-out single-service paper and plastic, and the roadsides littered with beer cans and soft-drink bottles.

On the Third Level—Safeguarding the Ecological Balances

Food protection or the lack of it contributes only indirectly to ecological balances. Use of the persistent pesticides for food protection is a very small part of the total use. However, the use of such pesticides in producing our food is sizable despite the much larger amounts used on cotton crops and for the control of forest pests like the spruce budworm and the fire ant. Food production per se is quite another story, as man's rising number takes new land for food growing, discards the worked-out land, over-fishes, overhunts, and overgrazes. Forests are burned to clear land for crops without a thought of the wildlife. Water is diverted for irrigation. Areas are flooded to impound water for irrigation. Man has never let conservation interests stand in the way of getting food. He is not likely to do so in the future. At best, he will accept the better of two alternatives to manage his use of land and water resources, so that there is something left after he has got his food. He can be made to heed the warning not to hunt and fish a species to extinction. Food protection is directed toward making better use of our foods and conserving food resources. To that extent it is a positive force for managing ecological balances.

In a 1969 report, Indicative World Plan, the United Nations Food and Agriculture Organization projects a population increase in the developing countries from 1.5 billion in 1965 to 2.5 billion in 1983. China with three-quarters of a billion people is not included. The organization estimates that the population increase demands a food supply increase of 3.9 percent a year. In these countries the annual food production increase had been 2.7 percent a year from 1955 to 1965. The gap is evident and threatening to social stability. In the part which it plays in meeting the gap, food protection must be a positive force to speed production, to extend storage and transportation, to reduce losses to insects and rodents, to curb spoilage, and to minimize contamination of all sorts. Those responsible for food protection will be overrun if their policies and actions are negative, delaying, and arbitrary. When it comes to a bitter test and choice of survival, food protection that has an overly restrictive approach will be an early casualty.

REFERENCES

8-1 SARTWELL, PHILLIP E. (ed.): "Maxcy–Rosenau Preventive Medicine and Public Health," 9th ed., Appleton Century Crofts, New York, 1965.

8-2 United Nations Joint FAO-WHO Expert Committee on Milk Hygiene: Third Report, *WHO, Tech. Rep. Ser.* 453, 1970.

8-3 Toxicants Naturally Occurring in Foods, *NAS-NRC Publ.* 1354, 1967.

8-4 AYRES, J. C., A. A. KRAFT, H. E. SNYDER, and H. W. WALKER (eds.): "Chemical and Biological Hazards in Food," Iowa State University Press, Ames, 1962.

8-5 POTTER, NORMAN H.: "Food Science," Avi Publishing Co., Inc., Westport, Conn., 1968.

8-6 Milk Hygiene, *WHO, Monogr. Ser.* 48, 1962.

8-7 Joint Committee on Atomic Energy: *Status of the Food Irradiation Program*, 90th Cong., 1968.

8-8 NIVEN, W. W.: "Industrial Detergency," Reinhold Publishing Corporation, New York, 1955.

8-9 SAWYER, CLAIR N., and PERRY L. MCCARTY: "Chemistry for Sanitary Engineers," McGraw-Hill Book Company, New York, 1967.

8-10 The Evaluation of Public Health Hazards from the Microbiological Contamination of Foods, *NAS-NRC, Publ.* 1195, 1964.

8-11 WEISER, H. H.: "Practical Food Microbiology and Technology," Avi Publishing Co., Inc., Westport, Conn., 1962.

9

IONIZING RADIATION AND ITS CONTROL

The control of ionizing radiation is the tour de force of the management of a class of environmental contaminants and of the exposure of people to external and internal risks from radiation sources and radioactive elements. This form of energy is the most fascinating and fantastic that man has yet harnessed for his use. It was identified in the form of x-rays by Wilhelm C. Röntgen on January 4, 1896, and from radium by Antoine H. Becquerel in November 1896. Forty-nine years later it was an incidental energy release of a devastating bomb that made radioactivity a vocabulary item of all speaking people. Their comprehension of the phenomena may yet be limited and may be erroneous in the scale of relative risks and benefits. A sufficient number of people have a sufficient amount of knowledge to deter politicians and war makers from recklessly deploying weapons which release ionizing radiation and, even, from testing the weapons in the open atmosphere. The destructive capacity of nuclear weapons from the heat and air pressure generated by the detonation has deterred their use by the conventional routes of military decisions on tactics. But even in those considerations, the radiation releases and effects have sobered all but the most maniacal. Why has the management of ionizing radiation been a tour de force, while easily controllable chemicals continue to cause occupational diseases, and the understanding of the effects of food additives remains vague and emotional?

There are seven identifiable reasons why the control of ionizing radiation has been extremely effective and successful.

1 Overt injury was immediately recognized.   In the very month that Röntgen announced the discovery of x-rays, E. H. Grubbe, working in Chicago with Crookes tubes to fluoresce chemicals, saw the back of his hand reddening, swelling, and becoming very sensitive.   The skin cracked, ulcerated, and scarred.   X-rays were tried on a variety of human ailments in the 10 to 15 years after Röntgen's discovery.   Cancers, skin abnormalities, and rheumatic joints were the targets for treatment.   Paradoxically, the rays also produced the first two.   By 1911, O. Hesse of Germany had 94 case histories of tumors from x-rays.   Fifty of these were among physicians using x-rays on their patients.   By 1901 Becquerel had chest burns under the vest pocket in which he had carried a radium source, and M. Curie had hand burns.   The delayed effects required time to be recognized. Skin malignancies appeared in physicians 10 to 25 years after their last use of x-rays for fluoroscopic examination.   By 1922 more than 100 radiologists had died of occupationally induced cancers.   These occurrences among knowledgeable people were warnings that were heeded.

2 By the nature of the early sources, the limited application, and the cost of the sources, particularly radium, the use of, and exposure to, ionizing radiation was restricted to a very few people.   Most of these were professionals with a modicum of understanding of the danger.   Between World Wars I and II the use of radium for self-luminous instrument dials and for the radiography of large castings such as ship propellors required a few skilled and semiskilled people to work with radioactivity.   In the case of the dial painters, mouth tipping of brushes carried radium into the body with disastrous cancers and radium poisoning the consequence.   The decision of the United States in 1941 to attempt to build an atomic fission bomb changed the numbers of workers handling radioactive materials from a few to many.

3 Ionizing radiation signals its presence by an energy transfer and an ionizing event which makes its detection and measurement by electronic devices and radiation-sensitive media relatively certain and simple.   These physical methods are much more sensitive than chemical and biological methods for detecting toxicants and pathogens.   The very same energy behavior which makes these radiations useful and injurious also makes these detectable and measurable in very minute quantities.   In milk ^{90}Sr can be detected at 10 picocuries per liter (pCi/l).   That is a radioactivity equal to 3.55×10^{-16} g of ^{90}Sr in a liter of milk.   No chemical or biological contaminant of milk can be detected at such remarkably low concentrations.

4 Radioactive elements follow the same biological and chemical pathways as the stable, nonradioactive forms of the same element. Additionally, radioactive forms behave chemically similarly to the elements in the same group on the periodic table of the elements. This follows, as orbital electron structures of radioactive elements are not different. It is the number of neutrons in the nucleus which makes an atom radioactive. Thus, chemical and, in part, biological behavior of a radionuclide can be predicted and explained to a practical degree.

5 When the Manhattan District project was organized in 1942 to build atomic bombs, a large-scale chemical and metallurgical operation began. Protection against ionizing radiation from sources of unprecedented magnitude and of unknown characteristics was an operational necessity. The mismanagement of these radioactive materials not only endangered people, but equipment, buildings, and land. The risks and consequences of mishandling are a couple of magnitudes greater than for most toxic, flammable, and explosive materials.

6 Nuclear energy and its product, radionuclides, have been nearly a government monopoly in the United States and entirely so in the United Kingdom, France, U.S.S.R., China, Canada, and India, because of military security requirements and because of the tremendous capital investment to develop the technology. Therefore, radioactivity from ^{235}U and ^{239}Pu production and use has been tightly regulated by governments. As regulation has been gradually and partially relaxed in the United States, the United Kingdom, and Canada, there has been time to build protection and safety into nuclear energy and man-made radionuclide use to a degree unprecedented by any other chemical, biological, or physical technology. In the United States since 1948, health physics has extended beyond the Atomic Energy Commission's fences and has stimulated the development of radiation protection with concern for all radiation sources in general use.

7 Public fear of ionizing radiation, which many cannot dissociate from the single-bomb demolitions of Hiroshima and Nagasaki, has made control not only acceptable but demanded as a condition for the presence of radiation sources in the community. When rational and emotional influences enter decisions and actions, paradoxes appear. Communities bitterly fight the location of a nuclear energy installation, while oblivious to community traffic and fire hazards, and may concurrently create flood and mudslide risks in unplanned land use.

THE ORIGIN OF IONIZING RADIATIONS

The emissions, which ionize when absorbed by matter, radiate from changes in orbital electrons of an atom or from the nucleus of an atom. These are energy releases from a system which is stabilizing. The state of imbalance or of excitation results from one of four occurrences.

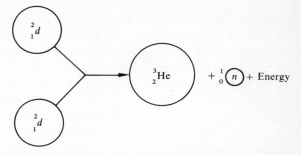

Two deuterium nuclei are fused to form a $^3_2$He atom
with a release of one neutron and energy.

FIGURE 9-1
Fusion of deuterium.   [*Source*: "*Atomic Fundamentals*," *DASA, Field Command
Sandia Base, Albuquerque, N. Mex.*, 1963, p. 13.]

1 The nucleus of an atom of a particular element has an excess, or deficiency, of
one or more neutrons above, or below, the stable neutron-proton ratio for that
element.   The excess neutron state occurs in nature, as in radium and polonium,
or may be induced by neutron bombardment and capture, as in controlled
reactors and in uncontrolled nuclear weapon reactions.

2 Electromechanical devices accelerate electrons or other atomic particles with
collisions and capture which produce excitation.   The x-ray machine is the most
common of these devices.

3 Nuclear reactors produce a controlled chain reaction of neutron release and
capture in a mass of ^{235}U.   In the splitting of each ^{235}U nucleus, a variety of
ionizing emissions are released from the fission and from the new nuclei formed
by the fission.

4 Fusion of elements of very low mass numbers, such as hydrogen, deuterium, and
tritium, produces fast neutrons which in turn produce other radiations.   Fusion
goes on in our sun and other stars, and in thermonuclear bombs.   Experiments
to produce and sustain controlled fusion continue in the United States at Oak
Ridge, Princeton, and the Lawrence Radiation Laboratory, and in England, in
West Germany, and in the U.S.S.R.   See Fig. 9-1.

Radioactive Nuclei

Excepting hydrogen, the nuclei of the elements are made up of protons and neutrons
and an energy state which holds these together.   The sum of the number of protons p
and of neutrons n is the *atomic mass number*, that is, ^{40}Ca (calcium) has $20p + 20n$.
The number of protons is the *atomic number* and is also the number of orbital electrons

in the un-ionized state, that is, the atomic number of Ca is 20. Calcium has 20 protons and 20 orbital electrons. Note that the n/p ratio of ^{40}Ca is 1. This condition of equal numbers of n and p holds for the stable elements from ^{4}He to ^{40}Ca, moving up the periodic table from helium to calcium with increasing atomic mass. Elements with a mass above 40 have more neutrons than protons in their most usual mass, and in their stable isotopes. Iron, ^{56}Fe, has $26p$ and $30n$, and a ratio of $n/p = 1.15$. Silver, ^{107}Ag, has $47p$ and $60n$ for $n/p = 1.27$. Lead, ^{208}Pb, has $82p$ and $126n$ for $n/p = 1.53$. Bismuth, ^{209}Bi, has $83p$ and $126n$ for $n/p = 1.52$. The increasing number of neutrons to protons in the heavier elements indicates that these neutrons are needed to form a stable nucleus. Above ^{209}Bi all elements in natural state are radioactive despite continued rises in n/p ratios. Uranium, ^{238}U, has $92p$ and $146n$ for $n/p = 1.59$. All 11 of the man-made transuranic elements have large n/p ratios, and all are radioactive. Californium, ^{251}Cf, has $98p$ and $153n$ for $n/p = 1.56$.

The 81 stable elements from hydrogen to bismuth have 282 isotopes. An isotope has a different number of n than is in the most common number, but always has the same number of protons. Tin has 10 stable isotopes. Of the 282 isotopes, 264 are completely stable, 18 are so weakly radioactive with very long decay times that they are essentially nonradioactive. Seven elements below bismuth have natural radioisotopes of quite long decay times with readily detectable radiations. Five are quite rare elements. One is extremely common and in all of our bodies. It is potassium. Its radioactive form is ^{40}K with $19p$ and $21n$. The stable form, ^{39}K, has $19p$ and $20n$. Another of the seven is platinum 190. These radioactive isotopes were formed with the earth's crust. Their continued existence is due to their initial relative abundance and long decay time. There are some radioactive isotopes which are continuously produced by natural actions and, in turn, decay. Two of interest are tritium, or ^{3}H, and ^{14}C. Both are formed naturally in the upper atmosphere by cosmic radiation interactions. The two are also products of man-made nuclear reactions in reactors and in weapons. In the time scale of nature, only ^{14}C has a half-life of consequence, 5,730 years. That is short compared with ^{40}K, 1.3×10^9 years, ^{138}La (lanthanum) 7×10^{10} years, and ^{209}Bi, 2.7×10^{17} years, among those which were formed with the earth's crust. Tritium has a half-life of 12.3 years.

Up to this point radioactivity has been identified with nuclei with an excess of neutrons above the usual number. That is usually the case. However, among naturally occurring radionuclides, ^{22}Na has one neutron less than normal sodium, and ^{7}Be has two neutrons less than normal Be. A deficiency of neutrons in the nucleus also produces natural radioactivity in some elements. It is a condition of instability. The neutron number is an index of instability, not an explanation. The next step to understanding is F. W. Aston's *packing fraction*, and then the apparent disappearance of minute amounts of mass which provide the energy to hold the repelling positively charged protons in the densely packed nucleus. All the man-made radioisotopes

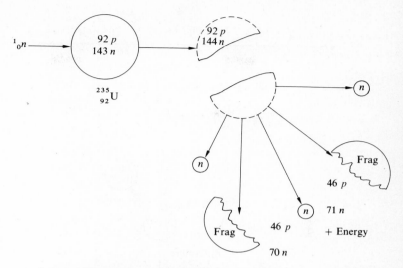

A neutron bombards a nucleus of $^{235}_{92}U$ with its 92 protons and 143 neutrons. The resulting fission produces two nearly equal mass fragments, nuclei with 46 protons and 70 or 71 neutrons. Three free neutrons are released.

FIGURE 9-2
Fission of uranium 235. [*Source*: "*Atomic Fundamentals*," *DASA, Field Command Sandia Base, Albuquerque, N. Mex.*, 1963, p. 12.]

produced in reactors by neutron bombardment have nuclei with an excess of neutrons over the stable state. Thus ^{90}Sr compared with ^{87}Sr, ^{131}I with ^{127}I, ^{137}Cs with ^{133}Cs, and ^{143}Ce with ^{140}Ce are examples of radioactive forms which are significant environmental contaminants from weapon testing, and potentially so from spent reactor-fuel elements and discarded radionuclides.

In a uranium-fueled reactor and in a uranium fission bomb, ^{235}U is the fissionable atom. Its state of instability is such that the penetration of a neutron splits the nucleus, see Fig. 9-2. Quite a mix of radioactive elements result. These are at present largely a nuisance. The valuable products are the energy produced by the small loss of mass and the extra neutrons released in the nuclear fission. The sum of the masses of the fission nuclei is less than the ^{235}U. In accord with Einstein's equation $E = mc^2$, the energy released equals the mass difference, the loss, multiplied by the speed of light squared. In a ^{235}U or ^{239}Pu bomb the fission of 56 g of material in the supercritical mass produces the explosive equivalent of 1,000 tons of TNT. In a proper detonation, this power is generated and released in an extremely rapid sequence of events. The expansion of the fireball blast is 50 percent; 35 percent is heat, radiated from the fireball; and 15 percent is ionizing radiation. Prompt gamma rays and

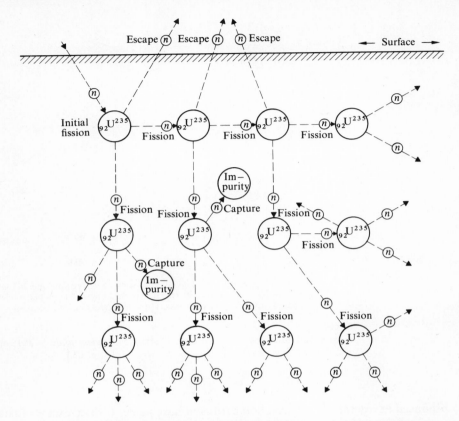

Few impurities reduce the number of neutrons lost by capture. Close spacing of the $_{92}U^{235}$ atoms reduces escape. Two neutrons per fission cause more fissions, and the neutron population increases rapidly. The fission fragments have been omitted from the drawing for clarity.

FIGURE 9-3
A multiplying chain reaction.   [*Source*: "*Atomic Fundamentals*," *DASA, Field Command Sandia Base, Albuquerque, N. Mex.*, 1963, *p.* 18.]

neutrons are one-third of the radiation, produced in a few seconds.   Two-thirds of the radiation comes from decaying fission products from the original nuclei and from whatever elemental bits of anything were in the detonation and became activated by absorbing neutrons.

The phenomenon which produces the chain reaction is that the first neutron to split the ^{235}U nucleus releases several neutrons in that fission.   If enough ^{235}U is in the configuration and held together long enough in a bomb, enough of these neutrons penetrate other ^{235}U nuclei to continue the fission and the energy release.   That is the chain reaction in the critical mass.   It is a big event in a hurry, as each 235 g of ^{235}U contains 6×10^{23} fissionable nuclei; see Fig. 9-3.   In a reactor, the rate of fission and of neutron generation is controlled.   Most of the neutrons are absorbed, wasted as it were, by the control rods and moderators.   Cadmium and boron are efficient absorbers.   Purified graphite and heavy water are moderators, slowing down neutrons from the fast class to the thermal class.   In a reactor the useful energy forms are heat, controlled neutrons, and radiation.   The heat can be converted to electricity by a heat transfer system and generators.   The controlled neutrons can produce desired radio-nuclides, and transuranic elements.   The capture of neutrons is the basis for producing ^{239}Pu from ^{238}U and for breeder reactors, which produce fissionable elemental forms faster than the initial fissile charge is fissioned and spent.

Radiation-producing Machines

Whenever electrons or other elemental particles are hurled about, their collisions with matter will produce ionizing radiations.   Electrons are most commonly accelerated about under high-voltage conditions.   Their encounters with orbital electrons produce x-rays.   The encounters may be in well-designed machines and properly controlled as in x-ray devices in the hands of knowledgeable operators, or these may be unrecog-nized, unwanted, and unheeded as in color TV sets, around Klystron vacuum tubes, and electron microscopes.   Unheeded at least until there is damage, detection, and corrective action.   William Crookes started the game in the nineteenth century by causing a stream of electrons to flow from a negative plate, the cathode, to a positive plate, the anode, in an evacuated glass tube, see Fig. 9-4.   That simple arrangement produces the phenomenon which makes neon and other gas-discharge tubes glow, fluorescent lamps to produce light, Lee de Forests' audion vacuum tube to amplify and separate the audio frequency from the carrier radio frequency, the "boob tube" to make pictures in our living rooms, and William D. Coolidge's tube to emit x-rays. Crookes lived to see most of this, as his life spanned 1832 to 1919.   His device provided J. J. Thomson with the means to discover the electron and to prove that electricity is a stream of these.   It was the device which led Röntgen to state that some invisible ray which could pass through opaque material was coming out of his Crookes tube, to be called x-rays until Röntgen found out more.   By 1913, Coolidge mobilized his own brain power and the electrical and metallurgical skills of the General Electric Lab-oratories to invent and produce the Coolidge x-ray tube, a configuration very much like that in Fig. 9-4.   With refinements to permit higher voltages and better cooling of the anode, there are about 200,000 such tubes in use in the healing arts in the United States.

Collisions involve a variety of energies.   A car collision produces noise, heat, crunched metal, broken glass, broken bones, and sometimes, sparks.   Electron

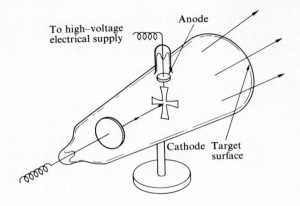

(a) Crookes tube with cold cathode.

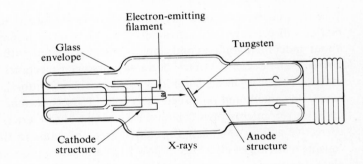

(b) Coolidge X-ray with heated cathode.

FIGURE 9-4
Schematics of Crookes tube and Coolidge x-ray tube.   [*Source*: *Hanson Blatz,*
"*Introduction to Radiological Health,*" *pp. 26–27, McGraw-Hill Book Company,*
1964.]

collisions and near hits produce x-rays, heat, visible light, and ultraviolet radiation.   In
the same way, accelerating other particles such as protons, neutrons, electron-stripped
helium atoms, by such electromagnetic machines as Van de Graaff generators, cyclo-
trons, betatrons, synchrotrons, linear accelerators, and bevatrons, produces a variety
of physical energy releases.   Some are the wanted output.   Some are nuisance energy
exacerbations.   All are dangerous.   We are now past the point in time when these
machines were in use only in the laboratory of experimental physicists, who accepted
some risks for their science and their career advancement.   Betatrons are frequent in
large hospital radiology departments.   Coolidge would be pleased with the voltage

range of x-ray therapy machines at the finger tips of physicians and technicians. Color TV sets boost electrons through the set's tubes at voltages not much below those used to generate diagnostic x-rays.   The TV mechanic or partially "savvy" set owner can jack up the voltage with the turn of a screwdriver to improve the picture.   Booting electrons about ends in collisions somewhere; x-rays result.   If these are not absorbed by shields and barriers, human tissue in the path absorbs the rays and becomes ionized. X-rays penetrate dogs and cats, too, so veterinarians have x-ray machines.   Flaws in welded seams and metallic castings show up under x-ray and gamma rays.   Therefore, industrial radiography is a part of quality control.   The miles of pipelines laid in the United States are radiographed under x-ray or gamma rays from ^{60}Co sources.   Grade school and high school science students generate the emissions in their laboratory exercises.   Some ingeniously step up the voltage on their cold cathode tubes, occasionally unaware that x-rays, which they cannot detect but which they do absorb, are coming off with the ultraviolet they are using to produce fluorescence.

THE EMISSIONS

In the first 10 years of this century, Ernest Rutherford observed the behavior of emissions from uranium salts as these passed through magnetic fields.   One stream bent one way.   Rutherford called it *alpha*.   Another bent in the opposite direction and was labeled *beta*.   By 1914 Rutherford had identified alpha as a helium atom stripped of its electrons, a bare nucleus of two protons and two neutrons.   In the nuclear cosmos, alpha is a massive particle, readily stopped by a few sheets of paper, but ionizing matter strongly in its short path seeking to fill its electron vacancies.   Beta turned out to be a wildly energetic electron with moderate penetrating and ionizing power.   Gamma came on the scene as emission energy.   Its behavior came under further close scrutiny.   Gamma is an electromagnetic energy release shorter in wavelength and higher in frequency than x-rays.   It is emitted from the excited nucleus of radioactive elements in the process of nuclear changes.   The emission of gamma rays releases the excitation energy.   The nucleus is then said to be in its *ground state*.

Table 9-1 summarizes the character of alpha, beta, and gamma.   It is the fruition of a tremendous amount of toil and thought.   It is the key to comprehending radioactivity and radiation protection.   Figure 9-5 shows the nuclear change when an alpha particle is emitted.   Note the reduction of mass number by 4, and the proton number by 2.   A helium nucleus has left to seek electrons and become an inert helium atom.   The depleted nucleus has a new chemical identity as another element. The alchemist's dream, and sometimes fraud, is realized.   Figure 9-6 shows the mechanism of beta emission and its actuality as thorium 234 radiates to become protactinium 234 with one more proton, hence an atomic number of 91.   A neutron converts to a proton, releasing an energetic electron as beta emission. A careful energy analysis of a large number of betas from the same element requires the existence and release of another nuclear bit called the *neutrino*. As it has no charge and negligible mass, the neutrino has been hard to validate by direct observations. Beta emission is 1 neutron in nucleus → 1 proton in nucleus + beta ejected + neutrino ejected.

The nucleus of many beta emitters is in a very temporary state of excitation which results in an immediate gamma emission. The radionuclide of mercury, $^{203}_{80}Hg$, emits a beta and produces a thallium nucleus with an excitation energy, $^{203}_{81}Tl$. The excited thallium nucleus emits a gamma quantum with an energy of 0.279 megaelectronvolt (MeV). A widely used radionuclide ^{131}I follows the pattern of beta-gamma emission with two betas of differing energy and subsequent gamma releases to reach the ground state of ^{131}Xe (xenon). The thallium and xenon exist as soon as the beta emits. These are momentarily excited nuclei which then emit gamma rays.

The decay of radium, Ra, to radon, Rn, has energy from a mass loss, which illustrates the mass-to-energy conversion of nuclear events in which the sum of the reactants is more than the sum of the products. The (unified) atomic mass unit (u) is an arbitrary ratio with carbon, with the original assumed base of 12.00000. The arithmetic of $^{226}_{88}Ra$ to $^{222}_{86}Rn$ is:

Mass of Ra	226.10309 u
Mass of Rn	222.09397 u
Mass of alpha	4.00388 u
Mass of Rn + alpha	226.09785 u
Mass of difference from Ra	0.00524 u

Expressed as energy, the mass difference equals 4.88 MeV, as 1 u is equivalent to 931 MeV. The 4.88 MeV is nearly the energy of an alpha particle ejected by a radium

Table 9-1 CHARACTERISTICS OF THE PRINCIPAL EMISSIONS FROM THE RADIOACTIVE NUCLEUS

Type of radiation	Symbol	Composition	Effect of emission	
			Atomic no.	Atomic wt.
Alpha particle	$_2\alpha^4$	2 protons 2 neutrons	Decrease 2	Decrease 4
Beta particle	$_{-1}e^0$ or $_{-1}\beta^0$	High-speed electron	Gain 1	No change
Gamma ray	$_0\gamma^0$	Form of electromagnetic energy similar to x-ray	No change	No change

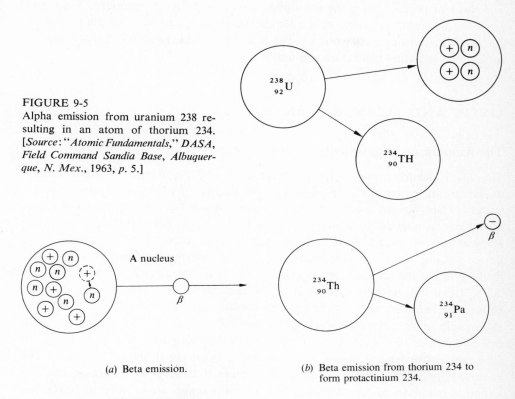

FIGURE 9-5
Alpha emission from uranium 238 resulting in an atom of thorium 234. [Source: "Atomic Fundamentals," DASA, Field Command Sandia Base, Albuquerque, N. Mex., 1963, p. 5.]

A nucleus

(a) Beta emission.

(b) Beta emission from thorium 234 to form protactinium 234.

FIGURE 9-6
The mechanism of beta emission and the change of thorium 234 to protactinium 234 by beta emission.   [Source: "Atomic Fundamentals," DASA, Field Command Sandia Base, Albuquerque, N. Mex., 1963, pp. 6–7.]

nucleus.   The actual value is closer to 4.80 MeV, with the difference in the recoil of the massive Rn nucleus.   It is like the movement of the *Queen Elizabeth II* as a sailor pushes a landing launch from her side.   There are four other nuclear transformations which occur in certain radioactive events:

1   Positron emission, a positively charged beta
2   Electron capture, in which an orbital electron enters the nucleus
3   Internal conversion, in which excess energy in the nucleus moves to an orbital electron that is then ejected from the atom
4   Isomeric transition, in which an excited nucleus releases gamma energy after some considerable lapse of time.

The three of principle concern are alpha, beta, and gamma emissions. These and x-ray are the principal cause of the ionization of tissue, animal and plant, and all inanimate matter upon absorption. The biological effects of such ionization are the reason that radiation protection is a health matter.

UNITS AND MEASUREMENTS

The Amount of Radioactivity—The Curie

The curie is the unit of radioactivity. It is the rate of decay in terms of disintegrations of the radium nuclei in 1 gram of radium per second. In 1911, Rutherford and his student, Hans Geiger, used a counting device to detect the ionizing events in a gas-filled glass cylinder as alpha emissions passed through the gas. They recorded emissions at the rate of 3.57×10^{10} alpha emissions per second from 1 g of Ra. The device became the Geiger counter. The number was later refined to 3.70×10^{10} disintegrations per second. An amount of any radioactive material which produces 3.7×10^{10} disintegrations a second is 1 Ci of radioactivity. It is a very large amount of activity, hence fractions of the unit are needed. These are millicurie (mCi), one-thousandth or 10^{-3} Ci; microcurie (μCi), one-millionth or 10^{-6} Ci; nanocurie (nCi), one-billionth or 10^{-9} Ci; picocurie (pCi), one-trillionth or 10^{-12} Ci. The quantities of a radioactive nuclide in use by a research scientist are in the mCi ranges. The radioactivity of ^{90}Sr in a liter of milk ranges from 10 to 30 pCi. In heavily shielded gamma-irradiation devices, the inventory of ^{60}Co ranges from 5,000 to 50,000 Ci. Until man-made radionuclides came from nuclear reactors in the late 1940s, the world's inventory of Ra was about 5,000 Ci. A useful conversion factor is 2.22 disintegrations per minute, equal to 1 pCi. That is the magnitude of radioactivity which is found in samples of food, air, and water in the free environment. The quantities of radioactivity inhaled or ingested in air, water, and food and excreted in urine and feces are stated in pCi or μCi. The amounts that are deposited for varying lengths, of time in the body, in bone, or in critical organs such as lungs, spleen, liver, or thyroid are stated in pCi or μCi.

Units for Exposure, Absorbed Dose, and Biological Effect

The effect of all radioactive materials and radiation machines is to emit energy forms which transfer energy to the material that absorbs it by ionizing the chemical substances or elements it encounters. The energy is electrical or electromagnetic. The source of the radiation may be external to the body, as a rod of ^{60}Co in an irradiator or an x-ray machine. It may be internal as ^{90}Sr in our bones or ^{131}I taken for a

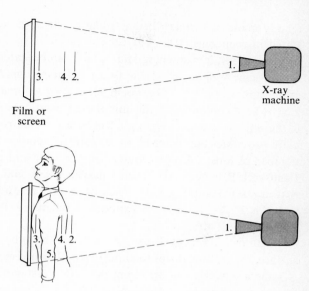

FIGURE 9-7
Points of measurement of x-ray through the human body from tube to film.
(*Source*:   *D. H. Wilhoit, University of North Carolina, Environmental Sciences and Engineering Publ. 202, Chapel Hill, N.C., 1968.*)

diagnosis of thyroid function.   A human being who has had no contact with man-isolated or man-made radioisotopes or elements still has at least one radioisotope in his body, ^{40}K.   Potassium 40 is a part of this planet and moves along with all other forms of K.   Dose estimates from ^{40}K and other natural sources will be found in Table 9-2.   One who has never been near an x-ray tube or any other man-made source of radiation is exposed to natural radiation throughout life from cosmic and terrestial sources, including the rock and mineral materials used for buildings.   All this makes up natural background.   The process of human biology evolved with a basic component of ionizing radiation present.

Figure 9-7 poses the issue of measuring external radiation, its absorption in the human body, and the biological effect on the human tissue.   Consider measurements at points 1 through 5, a little of their meaning, and the units used.   Measurement 1 is of the primary beam from the x-ray tube at its exit point.   It is not the full output from the tube.   Some of the output scatters all about the target.   Some low-energy *bremsstrahlung* x-ray is filtered at the beam port, as it is useless in making the picture, fuzzes the image, and needlessly doses the patient.   Some is added at measurement 1 from scatter bouncing from the tube enclosure, from the walls of the room, and even back from the patient and film holder.   Point 1 is as near a measurement as can be readily made of primary beam strength.   It is the exposure in air.   Its intensity is stated in roentgens (R).   The tube's rate of output is in roentgen per minute.   In physical terms, it is an energy flux which can be stated as the charge of ions produced in a specific weight or volume of air.   The recognized definition is of little help to initial understanding.   One roentgen of x or gamma radiation produces a charge of 2.58×10^{-4} coulomb (C), the unit of electrostatic charge, in 1 kg of air.   The roentgen is the unit to express ionizing effect in air.   One roentgen produces 2.08×10^9 ion pairs per cubic centimeter of air at standard temperature and pressure, an impressive number of ions.   A good ionization chamber and reader such as the Victoreen or Landsverk R-meter makes such a measurement, and every other actual measurement that can be made in Fig. 9-7.   Assume that the reading at 1, which is 4 in from the tube target, is 30 R.   Such an air exposure is the output from an x-ray tube at a voltage of 75 kV for 100 mA/s at 4 in.

At measurement 2, say, 25 in from the tube target and at the patient's skin surface, the reading drops to about 1 R.   The inverse-square law is at work, and there is some attenuation in air along the added distance.   The roentgen still is the unit, as the measurement is the ionizing power in air.   At measurement 3, beyond the patient's body and at the film, there is another air-exposure reading.   Say it is 0.75 R. There are two things that need to be known and expressed in Fig. 9-7.   There is some value for the path from 2 to 3, designated as measurement 4 in the figure, which is the radiation absorbed by the patient.   It is the radiation absorbed dose.   The unit is an acronym of those three words, *radiation absorbed dose*, the rad.   As radiation damage depends on the energy absorbed and is proportional to the concentration of the energy in tissue, absorbed dose is expressed in ergs, an energy unit, per gram; 100 ergs/g is a radiation absorbed dose of 1 rad.   It is an arbitrary unit accepted after conflicting results from attempts to agree on the number of ergs delivered to tissue by an exposure of 1 R measured in air.   The calculated and reported values ranged from 83 to 97 ergs/g, depending on what assumptions on tissue composition were used.   Bone increases the value 3.5 to 4 times for low-energy rays.   The value for an estimate of the energy absorbed in the body, measurement 4 in Fig. 9-7, is expressed in rads.

A conversion from roentgens to rads can be calculated.   Two things must be known.   The energy of the incident radiation and the mass absorption coefficient of the absorbing material.   Figure 9-8 shows how 1 R in air uniformly produces 0.88 rad for rays from 0.01 to 10 MeV energies.   Water absorption is quite close to 1.   That means that the absorption of 1 R, measured in air, produces 1 rad (100 ergs/g) in water.   Soft tissue has a high water content.   It is made up of elements with atomic weights close to that of H_2O, which is 18.   There are C at 12, O at 16, N at 14, and H at the low of 1.   So it is close to H_2O.   Therefore, 1 R into soft tissue produces approximately 1 rad.   Note that bone with its denser mineral composition produces much higher absorption at energies below 0.2 MeV.   Bone has a higher mass absorp-

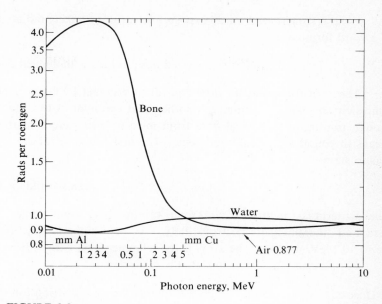

FIGURE 9-8
The rads produced in air, water, and bone on exposure in roentgens. (*Source*: *H. Johns, " The Physics of Radiology," Charles C Thomas, Springfield, Ill.,* 1961.)

tion coefficient.   This indicates the intracacies which escalate as attempts are made to translate air exposure measurements in roentgen to absorbed dose in rads.   Consider the differences between a whole-body exposure to a high-energy gamma and the exposure of the lower spine and pelvic region to a moderate-energy x-ray.

The last and most difficult step is to quantitate the biological effect of the absorbed radiation.   This is diagrammed in Fig. 9-7 as measurement 5.   The means of expressing this measurement continues to undergo efforts to refine it.   In the process, it has become more complex with the same unknown factors still unknown, but at least delineated.   The objective is to state the relative biological effective dose (RBE dose), or in more recent terminology, the dose equivalent (DE).   Why such a measurement? A radiation worker in a year or a lifetime handles alpha, beta, and gamma sources. He works around high-voltage apparatus emitting x-rays.   He is in the presence of neutron fluxes around reactors.   Some denominator must be used to state his total absorbed dose and to estimate the biological effect of the exposures he has accepted. The exposure of all people is becoming more varied as radioisotopes are increasingly used in medical diagnosis, and high-activity sources are used in therapy.

What is sought for a mixed exposure to various ionizing radiations can be stated in a word formula

Dose equivalent = absorbed dose in rads × biological factors

The need for a unit for dose equivalent was met by coining the *rem*, roentgen equivalent in man (or mammal), another neat acronym, with a double meaning, as though translating biological data from mice to men were a matter of what "m" means to you at a particular moment.   The first round to fill out the word formula was to state

rems = rads × RBE

The last term is a multiplier, with some appropriately round values.   For x, gamma, beta, and other energetic electrons, RBE = 1.   For alpha, fast neturons, and protons up to 10 MeV, use 10.   The x-ray is the reference level with RBE = 1.

A refinement has been to state the relation as

Dose equivalent = absorbed dose × quality factor × distribution factor

or

DE, in rems = rads × QF × DF

The QF is a numerical value from 1 to 20, dependent on the density of ionization produced along a radiation's path in an absorbing material.   The physical term for this density along a path is *linear energy transfer* (LET).   A useful analogy is to visual- ize applying an equal force to the skin surface of your forearm with a sharply pointed pencil.   Concentrate all of the force at a single contact point.   You well may puncture the skin.   That is the behavior of an alpha particle.   All its energy is delivered in a very short path.   A high QF of about 10 is appropriate.   Apply the same force as the pencil point travels along 6 to 8 in of skin surface—a very light contact.   The same energy is transferred along a lengthy path.   That is the behavior of an x- or gamma ray, leaving a long path of few ions as it penetrates readily.   A QF of 1 or 2 is appropriate. Values of RBE and QF are of the same magnitude.   Quality factor values can be stated more precisely if there is enough known about the type of emission and its energy and the tissue composition.   For example, a low-energy alpha produces 7,600 ion pairs in a single micron of path.   A gamma from ^{60}Co produces only about 10 ion pairs in the same distance.   However, the gamma continues moving at the speed of light, gradually attenuating its energy long after the alpha has been stopped. The alpha has collected its two electrons and is a neutral atom of helium.   Its energy transfer has been completed.

The DF is best understood for ingested or inhaled radionuclides already within the body.   The radionuclides are not uniformly distributed even within a single organ such as ^{131}I in the thyroid.   The DF is also used to cover the differences in the essential need of the tissue receiving the radiation to the function of a major organ or the whole being.   The DF is an attempt to express relative damage to tissue and the importance of the damage.   Some radiation protection specialists have used DF to mean *damage factor* or *relative damage factor*.   The International Commision on Radiation Units, recommends the words *distribution factor*.   For radionuclides in the body which emit alpha or beta, a DF value of 5 is used.   If the radionuclide is one of a decay series which starts with radium, use DF = 1.   The distribution of the radionuclides from the series will be determined by where the [226]Ra "parked" at the start and where it moves, if at all.

Radium is the material on which human observations of an epidemiological sort have been made.   From such data a safe permissible body burden of 0.1 μg or 0.1 μCi of Ra has been set.   That amount of Ra produces a DE of 0.56 rems/week.   Furthermore, that Ra burden of 0.1 μCi is the basis for permissible body burdens of all other radionuclides.   These are estimated by applying all reliable information on the physical, chemical, and biological characteristics of other radionuclides in comparisons and analogies with Ra.   This introduction to ionizing radiation protection units and what these seek to measure can be supplemented by studying D. J. Rees' chapter, Radiation Dosimetry (Ref. 9-1), and the International Commission on Radiation Units Report 10a, Radiation Quantities and Units.   The latter is published in the United States as the *National Bureau of Standards Handbook* 84, 1962.   The Commission's Report 10a pleads twice in its text that the use of each special unit should be restricted to one quantity:

The *roentgen*   Solely for exposure measured in air
The *rad*   Solely for absorbed dose in the material receiving the radiation
The *curie*   Solely for activity of a radionuclide

To these three, the rem is added as a measure of dose equivalent for equating biological effects from all forms of ionizing radiations from all sources.   The purpose is to sum the cumulative record of dose exposure, the success of radiation protection for an individual, and a unit for that protection.   Less certainly the cumulative dose exposure provides a basis for judging whether delayed biological impairment, such as leukemia late in life, can be ascribed wholly or in part to absorbed radiation.   The nature of the units and the means of measuring these are least well grounded in the biology and chemistry of radiation effects in man.   This makes such judgments most difficult in assessing human experiences.   This makes their use in legal proceedings that adjudicate radiation injury claims a trying affair for all parties, particularly the conscientious expert witness (Ref. 9-2).

BIOLOGICAL DAMAGE FROM THE IONIZATION OF TISSUE

Before stating the nature of biological damage, Tables 9-2 to 9-4 are presented to provide some reference points on the sources of man's exposure to ionizing radiation and the magnitude of the tissue dose effect he is getting. Note the dose units and time periods carefully in making comparisons among these data as well as those from other sources. Table 9-2 reminds us that man has evolved in an ionizing radiation environment which has been giving him from 125 to 150 mrems/year throughout his existence. This is the range of dose effect from natural background to the gonads, and bone materials. About 80 percent of this is from external sources. Twenty percent is from radionuclides that are inhaled and ingested, with a fraction retained. All the radionuclides listed in Table 9-2 have very long half-lives. The issue is how much are man-made sources adding to this and what are the consequences. As a working value, authorities have been loath to sanction more than an amount equal to natural background, except for medical treatment of an individual. Table 9-3 shows that on the average the world stayed within those bounds for the 8 years 1954 to 1961, but not with a large margin to spare. The data are the cumulative values for the 8 years. The annual average for the world's people is 30 mrems from diagnostic medical x-ray, 5 from medical treatment, and about 2 for occupational exposure with gonadal dose as the index (Ref. 9-3, p. 418). Using a bone-marrow dose index raises the diagnostic x-ray dose to the range of 50 to 100 mrems. The three relevant facts are:

Table 9-2 NATURAL SOURCES OF IONIZING RADIATION AND THE TISSUE DOSE EFFECT PRODUCED FROM EXTERNAL AND INTERNAL SOURCES*

Source of irradiation	Dose rates, mrems/year		
	Gonad	Haversian canal	Bone marrow
External irradiation:			
Cosmic rays (including neutrons)	50	50	50
Terrestrial radiation (including air)	50	50	50
Internal irradiation:			
^{40}K	20	15	15
^{226}Ra and decay products (35% equilibrium)	0.5	5.4	0.6
^{228}Ra and decay products (equilibrium)	0.8	8.6	1.0
^{210}Pb and decay products† (50% equilibrium)	0.3	3.6	0.4
^{14}C	0.7	1.6	1.6
^{222}Rn (absorbed into bloodstream)	3	3	3
Total	125	137	122

* UN, 1962.
† ^{210}Pb in excess of that expected from ^{226}Ra and decay products in 35% equilibrium.

1 Medical sources add from 15 to 20 times that from occupational sources.

2 Diagnostic procedures add 6 times that of therapeutic ones, as many more people are "rayed" for diagnosis than treatment.

3 Such data are directed to mankind's plight, not the individual's, so all estimated radiation is apportioned to all.

Table 9-4 is a rather detailed look at the dose effect values on the people of the United States, where an advanced technology has 200,000 x-ray machines in the reach of its physicians and dentists, and where about 100,000 men and women are in the nuclear energy industries.   The bone-marrow dose from diagnostic radiography is already equal to the natural background contribution.   The gonadal dose from the same source is a bit below one-half of the background dose effect, 62 mrems/year versus 125 mrems/year.   Weapon fallout contribution is small by comparison, and the occupational dose effect is tiny.   But these two are so because of control and restraint, which have not been notable qualities of the use of x-rays in United States practice of medicine.

Some Facts and Hypotheses on Mechanisms of Biological Damage

When a bit of ionizing radiation hits tissue, only a few molecules are initially involved in the energy transfer.   These are ionized or excited.   For man 400 rads of gamma is the LD_{50} in 30 days.   It is calculated that in absorbing that 400 rads only about 1 atom of tissue substance in 10 million atoms is affected by the initial ionization or associated excitation.   For a 70-kg man (154 lb) this is about 5×10^{20} injured cells among 5×10^{27} in the body.   The number of injured cells seems large, but the fraction is

Table 9-3   EIGHT-YEAR CUMULATIVE TISSUE DOSE EFFECT TO THE WORLD'S PEOPLE FROM NATURAL, MEDICAL-USE, AND FALLOUT SOURCES

	Total dose delivered, mrems, for 8 years		
Source of exposure	Gonads	Bone	Bone marrow
Natural	1,000	1,040	1,000
Medical and occupational	300	?	400–800
Fallout:			
All but ^{14}C	41	128	84
^{14}C	70	116	70
Total fallout	111	244	154

SOURCE: Ref. 9-3.

exceedingly small.   Yet there is death in 30 days for 50 percent of the cases.   How is this possible?

Those initial events are the direct actions producing dissociations of atoms. When this happens to DNA molecules, which are in all germinal and somatic cells, the original genetic pattern cannot be transmitted to the next generation of cells. What is transmitted are point mutations.   The damaged gene burden is then continuously transmitted.   Another effect of these direct hits is chromosome aberrations, actual morphological breaks in the structure carrying the genes.   These do relink and appear to repair.   There may be illegitimate relinkage and unequal distributions in repaired chromosomes.   Such daughter cells usually die.   Point mutations and chromosome aberrations impair somatic cell reproduction, which injures the irradiated man, and are carried in injured germ cells that he or she uses to transmit their hereditary factors to their children.   The frequency of such germ cell injury and the probability of an impaired child is small for any individual.   The transmitted defect is most rarely gross deformity.   H. J. Muller states the defects are subtle, such as a slightly diminished intelligence, or a high blood pressure which comes on earlier in life.   The stake is the lowering of man's total hereditary quality.   The detriment is directly proportional to the amount of radiation absorbed by man as a total population. These events are direct actions of a radiation emission acting on the protein and nucleic acid molecules in the cell.   These are specific hits.   There are also indirect actions due to chemical changes among the compounds surrounding the specific targets.   As the

Table 9-4   AVERAGE ANNUAL TISSUE DOSE EFFECT TO PERSONS LIVING IN UNITED STATES FROM MEDICAL EXPOSURE, WEAPONS FALLOUT, OCCUPATIONAL SOURCES, AND OTHER USES

Source	mrems/year
Medical exposure:	
Gonad dose from diagnosis, 1964	55
Gonad dose from therapeutic use, 1964	7
Bone-marrow dose from diagnosis, 1964	125
Thyroid dose from diagnosis (mostly dental), 1964	1,000
Weapons-fallout dose, 1966	3
Occupational exposure:	
Nuclear-energy industry, gonad dose, 1966	0.2
All other occupational exposure, gonad dose, 1966	0.4
Other man-made sources (watches, television, shoe-fitting machines, radioisotope applications, etc.), gonad dose, 1966	0.1

SOURCE: *Senate Hearings on Radiation Control for Health and Safety*, pt. 1, 90th Cong, 1967, p. 48.

body is about 70 percent water, the ionizing effect of radiation on HOH is most disturbing.

The normal ionization of water is $HOH \rightleftharpoons H^+ + OH^-$. Under radiation, pure water produces a bizarre assortment of ions and free radicals, that is, neutral molecular fractions without a charge. In the following series, note the charges carefully.

1 Under ionizing radiation $HOH \rightarrow HOH^+ + e^-$, an electron freed.
2 The unstable, charged water molecule $HOH^+ \rightarrow H^+ + OH^0$, a free radical.
3 The free electron combines, $HOH + e^- \rightarrow HOH^-$.
4 The charged molecule immediately separates, $HOH^- \rightarrow H^0 + OH^-$.

The H^0 and OH^0 are free radicals. These and the strange forms in the equations *1* through *4* last about 1 μs. Here are some results:

1 $OH^0 + OH^0 \rightarrow H_2O_2$, hydrogen peroxide, a strong oxidizing agent that is still found in some home medicine cabinets as a disinfectant.
2 $H^0 + H^0 \rightarrow H_2$, a hydrogen gas molecule.
3 If dissolved oxygen is in the tissue, $H^0 + O_2 \rightarrow HO_2$, a hydroperoxyl radical, which in turn combines with free-radical hydrogen.
4 $H^0 + HO_2 \rightarrow H_2O_2$ to form more hydrogen peroxide.

This chemical chaos occurs in irradiated cells in the presence of a variety of carbohydrates, proteins, and traces of metallic forms. The radical OH^0 reacts in steps to form hydroperoxides of the general formula RO_2H. The R, as usual in organic chemistry, is any alkyl group. Some of the combinations in the cell are protective, as the exotic intruders are engaged before strongly influencing cell chemistry. Things that do occur are:

1 Detachment of amine groups from amino acids
2 Removal of carboxyl groups from organic acids
3 Oxidizing sulfhydro, SH compounds
4 Decomposing simple sugars such as glucose

One thing emerges from these cellular reactions to ionizing radiation. It was stated by a United Nations special committee on the effects of atomic radiation in 1958 and repeated by the 1962 committee (Ref. 9-3) in these words: "Biological effects will follow irradiation, however small its amount." Every added bit of radiobiological information has supported that observation. This fact is expressed in two concepts. There is no threshold for a biological effect from any absorbed dose of radiation. Figure 9-9 compares the threshold dose-response curve which fits toxic chemicals and physical energy exposures, such as noise, ultraviolet, and microwave energies, with the no-threshold dose response which fits ionizing radiation. The second concept follows

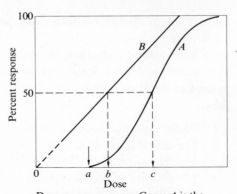

Dose-response curves. Curve *A* is the characteristic shape for a biological effect that exhibits a threshold dose—point *a*. The spread of the curve, from the threshold at *a* until the 100% response is thought to be due to "biological variability" around the mean dose, point *c*, which is called the 50% dose. Curve *B* represents a nonthreshold or linear response; point *b* represents the 50% dose for the nonthreshold biological effect.

FIGURE 9-9
Threshold and nonthreshold dose-response curves. (*Source: H. Cember, "Introduction to Health Physics," Pergamon Press, Elmsford, N.Y., 1969.*)

from the first. If there is damage from any and all ionizing radiation which the body absorbs, there must be a benefit resulting from the acceptance of the dose. Ionizing radiation is the environmental agent which puts the risk-benefit choice most clearly and to a remarkable degree measurably. The pious proclamations that human health is paramount is laid to rest. If that were the case, all man-made and man-manipulated sources of ionizing radiation would be set aside forthwith. Every use produces some release. Every release that is absorbed has a biological effect.

Acute Radiation Effects

A single exposure that results in from 10 to 1,000 or more rems of radiation absorbed by the whole or nearly whole body is an acute exposure and quite immediate effects appear. The scale and nature of these are stated in Table 9-5. The effects described are largely those on the blood system and the gastrointestinal tract. Under doses of 2,000 rads or more, the central nervous system caves in with unconsciousness in a few minutes and death in a day or two. At the low end of the dose scale, the blood-forming system shows the first effects. The outward signs are nausea and vomiting, malaise and fatigue within a few hours of a dose of 200 rems. Within the blood, elements are lost. The bone marrow is first a jellied mass and under doses of 400 rems disappears

altogether.   Some people make a recovery even from so severe an effect with a regeneration of bone marrow.   In severe exposure the white blood cell count plunges
from a norm of 7,000/mm^3 to 2,000 or less.   The person is stripped of normal defenses
against bacterial infections.   Lymphocytes make up about 25 percent of the white
blood cells.   Death is rather certain when the lymphocyte count drops under 500/mm^3
in a day or two of exposure, although men have hung on for a month or two with
rigorous medical support.   In these dose ranges, hair is lost during the second and
third weeks.   At the upper range shown in Table 9-5, gastrointestinal effects are added.
The intestinal lining is stripped off.   The nausea, vomiting, and diarrhea are extreme.
At a dose of 1,000 rads, death in a week or two is likely.   It is a death devoid of heroic
attributes and unlikely to appeal even to war lovers.   Temporary sterility occurs after
single exposures of men to 30 R and of women to 300 R, reflecting the tissue protection
of the ovaries compared with the vulnerable position of the testes.   A 400 to 600 R
exposure of the testes produces permanent sterility.   The roentgen unit is used as these
are reported as air or body-surface exposure measurements.

Delayed Effects

These effects result from external exposure over extended time periods, from the extended inhalation or ingestion (or both) of small amounts of radioactive materials, or
from a single or several large ingestions or inhalations.   From such large intakes,
the radionuclides are deposited in some critical organ or tissue and irradiate that tissue

Table 9-5   PROBABLE EFFECTS OF ACUTE WHOLE-BODY RADIATION DOSES

Acute dose, rems	Probable clinical effect
0–25	No observable effects.
25–100	Slight blood changes, but no other observable effects.
100–200	Vomiting in 5–50% within 3 h, with fatigue and loss of appetite; moderate blood changes; except for the blood-forming system, recovery will occur in all cases within a few weeks.
200–600	For doses of 300 rems and more, all exposed individuals will exhibit vomiting within 2 h or less; severe blood changes, accompanied by hemorrhage and infection; loss of hair after 2 weeks for doses over 300 rems; recovery in 20–100% within 1 month to a year.
600–1,000	Vomiting within 1 h, severe blood changes, hemorrhage, infection, and loss of hair; 80–100% of exposed individuals will succumb within 2 months; those who survive will be convalescent over a long period.

SOURCE: S. Glasstone and A. Sesonske, "Nuclear Reactor Engineering," D. Van Nostrand Company, Inc.,
Princeton, N.J., 1963.

continuously until radioactive decay and biological elimination removes the source of radiation. Radiological half-life is the time required for the curie level of any radionuclide to decay to 50 percent of its level from any time zero. The biological half-life is the time for a radionuclide entering the body to be reduced to 50 percent of its initial curie level at time zero by biological actions culminating as urinating, defecating, and exhaling. The combined actions take place in a time that is always shorter than the radiological half-life. That time is called the *effective half-life*. It is the important time for controlling patient damage, particularly if biological elimination can be made more rapid. An example is the possible use of chelating agents to keep ^{90}Sr from depositing in the bone, so that the ^{90}Sr stays in the body fluids for a better chance of elimination in urine and sweat. An example of effective half-life is ^{131}I. The radiological half-life is 8 days. The biological half-life is 180 days. The effective half-life is 7.7 days. Using the same time unit throughout, this value is from the formula:

$$\text{Effective half-life} = \frac{\text{rad. half-life} \times \text{biol. half-life}}{\text{rad. half-life} + \text{biol. half-life}}$$

Thus

$$\text{Effective half-life } ^{131}\text{I} = \frac{8 \times 180}{8 + 180} = \frac{1,440}{188} = 7.7$$

The derivation of the formula is given by Cember (Ref. 9-4, p. 166). It is based on two simultaneous actions, each following its first-order reaction. If one must ingest a radionuclide, choose one with a short radiological half-life and short biological half-life. ^{24}Na is a good choice. Its radiological half-life is 15 hours. It is readily eliminated in urine.

A concept for the control of the amounts of radionuclides that are inhaled, ingested, or absorbed and subsequently deposited in the body is that there is a quantity above which disabling injury within a life-time is likely. That quantity is the *maximum permissible body burden* (MPBB). When the physiological behavior of a radionuclide is known, the MPBB is defined for one or more specific organs of the body. When one organ is clearly a point of concentration of a radionuclide and vulnerable to the emissions, that organ is the *critical organ*. The thyroid is the critical organ for the radionuclides of iodine. The bone is the critical organ for radium, strontium, thorium, and plutonium. The MPBB is the total radioactivity of a specific radionuclide which may safely be in the critical organ of man or in his total body at any time. The value for ^{226}Ra is 0.1 μg in the bones in equilibrium with its daughter products. That body burden is calculated to deliver a dose of 0.56 rem/week. The completeness of information on the behavior of radionuclides deposited in the human body, in its several organs, and the certainty of the critical organ is quite variable for the number of different radionuclides that enter our bodies. The effective half-life is important in evaluating the hazard.   Other factors are the type of emissions, their energies, and the nature of the decay products.   Maximum permissible body burden is a fascinatingly complex interaction of biological, chemical, and physical processes of a radioactive nucleus which has entered a life system.   The best judgments on MPBB have been prepared by the International Commission on Radiological Protection and in the United States by the National Council on Radiation Protection and Measurement. Both publish lengthy tables of MPBB values.   Cember (Ref. 9-4, p. 204–218) gives the steps in calculations of MPBB values and provides abbreviated tables of the principal ones.

The delayed effects of radiation overexposure are (*1*) cancer, (*2*) leukemia, (*3*) life-span shortening, and (*4*) cataracts.

1   Cancers induced by ionizing radiation are most frequent in the skin, the bone, and the thyroid gland.   The development is delayed from 5 to 20 years.   The progress of skin cancers spans several years.   The widely known bone cancer among some 800 radium dial painters in New Jersey in the 1920s has provided valuable information.   Survivors continue under study.   Their ingestions by oral brush pointing and from contaminated fingers were radium and mesothorium.   About 50 developed bone cancer and aplastic anemia.   Lung cancer from the inhalation of the radioactive gas radon and particulates is supported by ancient lore and modern epidemiological studies.   The decay of radon, a gas, produces nongaseous radioactive daughters which continue to ionize the lung cells close to the site of deposition.   The principal daughters, ^{218}Po and ^{214}Po, are very short-lived emitters of high-energy alphas.   Epidemiological studies in the United States support the strong correlation between lung cancer in uranium miners and the cumulative exposure to radon daughters.   To 1965, the evidence was that those with 5 or more years of underground work had a tenfold increase in respiratory-system cancers.[1]

2   Leukemia is a cancer of the blood-forming tissue with an excessive production of white blood cells and often a concurrent severe shortage of hemoglobin.   It is the malignancy most likely to develop from overexposure of the whole body to ionizing radiation.   In-utero x-raying causes a 40 percent higher leukemia mortality.   In British medical practice, patients seeking relief from the racking pain of spinal arthritis, ankylosing spondylitis, accept the risk of a threefold chance of leukemia.   In the Japan bombings of 1945, of the 60,000 people who received some radiation exposure, 7,000 survived after major symptoms of acute radiation exposure.   To 1958 the Atomic Bomb Casualty Commission had 209 leukemia deaths among those irradiated by the Nagasaki and Hiroshima fission bomb drops

---

[1] J. K. Wagoner et al., *New Engl. J. Med.*, **273**:181 (1965).

in 1945.   That is several times the total number to be expected in the total life span of the group, according to Japan's actuarial experience of leukemia.

3   Life-span shortening as an effect of ionizing radiation is well established for experimental exposures of animals.   It is supported by epidemiological evidence among radiologists in the United States, but not among radiologists in Great Britain.   Work by R. Seltzer and P. E. Sartwell showed life shortening among radiologists to hold in comparison with internists and ear, nose, and throat specialists.   The difference grows smaller in recent time periods.   These data make up Table 9-6.   No satisfactory biological mechanisms for the premature death of man and animals have been validated.

4   Cataracts require comment as this impairment of vision illustrates the universalities and the enigmas of radiation injury.   The injury occurs in man and animals. It is not caused exclusively by ionizing radiation.   The site of damage is extremely specific.   Growing cells in the lens which take the hit develop abnormal lens fibers slowly.   The opacity which eventually shows may appear several years after exposure.   It will be indistinguishable from cataracts produced by other agents or causes.   The damaging exposure can be a single acute event or an extended series of low-level exposures.   Certainly in animals, the young are more sensitive than the old.   The sources of exposure can be accelerators, criticality accidents, nuclear weapons detonations, or emitters of x, gamma, and beta.   There are some 200 cases from x and gamma exposure and an uncertain number from neutron exposure around accelerators.   The Hiroshima-Nagasaki survivors showed 10 cataract cases in 8,000 examined 11 years after the bombings.   Among 425 Nagasaki survivors who were from 1,400 to 1,800 m from the hypocenter, 47 percent had lens opacities which had not developed to cataracts by 1956.

Table 9-6   MEDIAN AGE AT DEATH OF RADIOLOGISTS, INTERNISTS, AND EAR-NOSE-THROAT SPECIALISTS IN THE UNITED STATES IN THREE TIME PERIODS, 1935-1944, 1945-1954, 1955-1958

Medical specialty	Median age at death during		
	1935-1944	1945-1954	1955-1958
Radiologists	71.4	72.0	73.5
Internists	73.4	74.8	76.0
Ear-nose-throat	76.2	76.0	76.4

SOURCE: R. Seltzer and P. E. Sartwell, JAMA, 190:1064 (1964) and R. Seltzer and P. E. Sartwell, Am. J. Epidemiol., 81:2 (1965).

LIMITS ON EXPOSURE AND ON DOSE
SET BY VOLUNTARY AND OFFICIAL GROUPS

The array of documents stating limits, guides, and standards to radiation exposure, radiation dose, and radioactivity concentrations in food, air, and water is not quite so formidable when it is recognized that the committees, commisioners, and councils preparing these have a great overlap in their composition and that each depends on very similar, if not the same, information for their decisions.   Furthermore, the endless tables are assemblies of the same basic numerical values.   In 1928 the Second International Congress of Radiology designated an international x-ray and radium protection commission to state safe practices of medical radiology to protect the physicians and the patients.   In 1930 the commission's name became the International Commission on Radiological Protection.   From it, a number of organizations have proliferated, voluntary and official, at the international, national, state or provincial, and local levels.   In using any statement on standards and limits on radiation, three things which you must have well in mind are the population and conditions of exposure for which you have concern, and the suitability of the standards you are examining for those conditions.

What Population Groups and Circumstances Are Covered?

Two population groups are now recognized and given distinct treatment.   The first group consists of those occupationally engaged in work requiring ionizing radiation use and hence accept some exposure.   This group is under surveillance and control. It is adult.   It is in the prime of physiological and emotional life.   It is knowledgeable of its work and its risks.   Its exposure at work is somewhere between 35 and 50 hours out of 168 hours in each week and not likely more than 50 weeks of a year's 52.   Work cycles have intervals of radiation exposure which may be above background, but not continuously pushed to prescribed limits.   Only accidents and emergencies demand commitments to clearly hazardous exposures, indeed, to sacrificial exposures during rescue work.

The whole population, which embraces all mankind, is the second group. Limits set for all of us have the objective of protecting the species against the deterioration of its genetic quality by man's uncontrolled use of ionizing radiation.   The 1966 recommendations in the International Commission on Radiological Protection Report 9 provide a limit for:

1 A dose effect for occupational workers that averages 5 rems/year to the gonads or total body for the working years, with detailed limits for each quarter year, for single years to a maximum of 12 rems, and for specific body parts and organs

  2 A dose effect for the whole population that is one-tenth of that for occupational workers, 0.5 rems/year to the gonads or total body

The Commission's 1966 report discontinued previous special population groupings with different limits for workers in the vicinity of controlled areas, or near-neighbors living adjacent to major nuclear energy installations such as Oak Ridge, Tennessee, or Harwell, England.   Such groupings will be found in earlier publications of the Commission's, and in those of other agencies, and in reports of professional committees, some as yet unchanged.   Note that the 0.5 rems/year is four- to fivefold natural background.   An ad hoc committee of the National Council on Radiation Protection and Measurement of the United States recommended in 1959 that the whole-population dose effect be held to 0.1 rems/year.[1]   One of that committee's leading members, K. Z. Morgan, holds to the prudence of the 0.1 rems/year level, reminding us that the limit is the sum of internal and external dose and that it is in addition to what man receives from medical and background sources.

What Conditions of Exposure and Dose Effect Do the Limits Cover?

Are the limit statements addressed to external exposure, to intakes in air, food, and water, or to dose effect on total body, gonads, specific body parts such as hands, or to specific organs such as the thyroid?   Careful reading of table captions and footnotes is required.   External dose will be in roentgens.   Absorbed dose should be in rads. Intake limits will be in some fraction of a curie per unit of volume or weight, as quantities of radioactivity are the issue.   Dose effect is in rems or in mrems.   That unit should not be used for any other purpose.   Unfortunately, there are instruments which are held in the air and have dials which read in rems.   There are film badge reports which obviously could only have received air exposures that majestically and authoritatively state the rems of the wearer.   That implies that the dose effect on the wearer is known.

Do You Understand the Intent of the Limit Terminology?

Is your understanding of the terms *maximum permissible dose* (MPD), *maximum permissible concentration* (MPC), and *radiation protection guide* (RPG) that which the authors had in mind?   For a discussion of these terms and their intent, see Ref. 9-5 (pp. 501–508).   Chapter 14 of Ref. 9-5 on Maximum Permissible Exposure Levels— External and Internal, by Dr. K. Z. Morgan is a comprehensive and thoughtful statement on what we are seeking to do when we undertake to assign a number to a judgment of risk versus benefit.   His thinking has useful meaning for all the magic numbers

[1] *Science*, **131**:482 (1960).

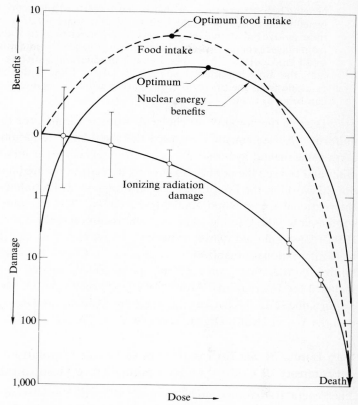

FIGURE 9-10
Schematic of balancing of benefits and damage with dose.   (*Source*: *K. Z. Morgan and J. E. Turner, "Principles of Radiation Protection," p.* 507, *John Wiley & Sons, Inc., New York, 1967.*)

by which we seek to direct the management of the quality of our environment.   Whatever the label, MPD, MPC, RPG, the men of good will and of professional competence who assume the responsibility for stating a number, all seek a value at the inflection points designated by Dr. Morgan as "optima," or a lower value, in Fig. 9-10.   Here are his words on it.

Ideally, the health physicist who sets the exposure limits would like to balance the risks against the benefits as shown in Fig. 14-1.   [See Fig. 9-10.]   Here it is assumed that all doses from ionizing radiation are harmful to man, and at high doses the magnitude of the damage to the individual becomes more certain, that is, the probable errors are smaller, and eventually the damage approaches negative infinity or death.   On the other hand, the curve of nuclear energy benefits has a maximum.   At low doses, the benefits become negative (or damaging) because of the deprivation of nuclear energy benefits and at high doses the benefits again become negative (or damaging) because of the excessive radiation damage that is uncompensated by benefits.   The curve of benefits from nuclear energy is similar to the curve of benefits from intake of food, except that a small intake of food probably does not produce a negative benefit (or damage).   Perhaps the most important responsibility of the FRC is the balancing of the benefits resulting from the proper use of ionizing radiation against the hazard and damage it can bring to man.

Despite the nonuniform choice of words on limits, the radiation units used are uniform.   All statements have used the same basic radiation units even though it takes some mental gymnastics to shift from picocurie per liter to microcurie per milliliter and to keep the negative exponents in focus.   We are on uniform units throughout the world as the First International Congress on Radiology in 1925 organized the International Commission Radiological Units.   The international and the national commissions, the Atomic Energy Commission, and the Federal Radiation Council (FRC) have followed its recommendations on units and use them.   Fortunately, so have international organizations related to the United Nations, which have responsibilities for radiation protection in aspects directly related to their missions.   These included the International Atomic Energy Agency (IAEA), Vienna; the International Labor Office (ILO), Geneva; the Food and Agriculture Organization (FAO), Rome; and the World Health Organization (WHO), Geneva.

Can Limits Be Set for the Intakes of Whole Populations, and Can an Intensity of Control be Recommended to Hold to the Limits?

The Federal Radiation Council has made affirmative answers to that two-part question. As their answers have a direct bearing on the amounts of radioactive material released to the free environment and the amounts we can accept in our intakes of air, food, and water, the approaches used and the recommendations made require analysis.   Federal Radiation Council statements on radiation protection issues have two forms:

1   A memorandum for the President of the United States, which is quite concise. Upon his approval, it is published in the *Federal Register* and is applicable to all federal agencies.
2   There is a staff report which provides the background of technical data and the rationale used to prepare the memorandum.

The questions raised in this section were answered in a Council memorandum for the President which was approved by President John F. Kennedy and printed in the *Federal Register* of September 26, 1961, and in Staff Report 2 of September 1961 (Ref. 9-6).   The objective of the Federal Radiation Council's work is the protection of all people by a policy of continued assessment of radiation use for assured and necessary benefits with the minimum of necessary risk.   It provides the President of the United States with a policy on radiation protection for the nation.

Federal Radiation Council Report 2, 1961, covers four matters.

1 Recommendations on dose effect limits for public exposure to specific selected body organs and the use of a "suitable" sample of the public. These recommendations are compatible with its first report on whole-body and 30-year gonadal limits. This is its *Radiation Protection Guide* for public exposure.

2 Recommendations on how the guide can be translated into three ranges of total daily intakes for the whole population, and intensities of control fitted to each of the ranges.

3 Recommendations of specific ranges for four of the most significant radioactive isotopes which are in the free environment and, therefore, in our air, food, and water. These are ^{226}Ra, ^{131}I, ^{90}Sr, and ^{89}Sr. The Radiation Protection Guide's values for these are in Table 9-7.

4 Recommendations on graded scales of action to be taken in accord with the environmental concentrations observed for the four radionuclides.

The graded scale of action, Table 9-8, recommends the intensity of control fitted to the three groupings of average daily intakes over a period of a year for a large collection of people. The wording for the first two ranges is moderate. Routine actions are sustained and gradually escalated as highs persist. The origin and derivation of the numerical value of the upper boundary of range 2 makes the recommended actions comprehensible and expeditious. It is not a number which is intended to trigger the panic button automatically. It is a point at which the risk is rising, and at

Table 9-7   THE RANGES OF TRANSIENT RATES OF DAILY INTAKE OF ^{226}Ra, ^{131}I, ^{90}Sr, AND ^{89}Sr IN A SUITABLE SAMPLE OF THE EXPOSED POPULATION FOR APPLYING THE GRADED SCALE OF ACTIONS RECOMMENDED BY THE FEDERAL RADIATION COUNCIL OF THE UNITED STATES

Radionuclides	Intakes, pCi/day		
	Range 1	Range 2	Range 3
^{226}Ra	0–2	2–20	20–200
^{131}I*	0–10	10–100	100–1,000
^{90}Sr	0–20	20–200	200–2,000
^{89}Sr	0–200	200–2,000	2,000–20,000

* In the case of ^{131}I, the suitable sample would include only small children. For adults, the values in the Radiation Protection Guide for the thyroid would not be exceeded by rates of intake higher by a factor of 10 than those applicable to small children.

SOURCE: FRC Memo for the President, Sept. 13, 1961.

which a close look at the happening, the trend of it, the benefit from the usage that produces it is required.   The causes for reaching that level must receive a timely and calm study.   Recall that this deals with radioactivity in the general environment reaching all people in their air, food, and water.   It is not the occupational setting of a research laboratory, a power reactor, or a radioactive pharmaceutical prescription laboratory.

At the end of 1969, the ^{131}I in the general environment illustrates the control requirements.   In the fluid milk supply in the United States the ^{131}I has been below levels detectable by routine sampling and analytical methods.   The number of analyses of milk samples for ^{131}I should be very few, enough to keep the sampling, analytical, and reporting network viable.   There must be alert response to any events which we know release ^{131}I to the atmosphere, an accident such as at Windscale, the United Kingdom reactor fire, or a leakage from a peaceful-use detonation test, or the news that the " Kingdom of Oceania has entered the Nuclear Weapons Club by the first bang of Operation Mollusk of their test series, Clambake."   Testing milk intensifies in frequency and geographic coverage in accord with air-surveillance results, meteorology, and whatever intelligence can be gleaned about the event.   It will also intensify if the few samples being run begin to show detectable amounts of ^{131}I, which would raise the question of why, what is going on in nuclear materials used to cause rising releases to the free environment.   In practice the ^{131}I would show in air samples before it would show in milk.   Therefore, increases in air sample reports would step up milk analyses.   This is moving from range 1 to range 2 action.   Continued rises into range 3 intakes require action that is beyond sampling and analysis.   Certainly the search for and pinpointing of sources and causes is necessary, along with verification of control at known sources.   The network of response expands and intensifies in accord with findings of rising risks.   Milk cows in fallout areas can be taken off grass and fed stored ensilage and hay.   It is not necessary to sewer all the milk in

Table 9-8   THE GRADED SCALE OF ACTION FOR RANGES OF DAILY INTAKES OF RADIOISOTOPES RECOMMENDED BY THE FEDERAL RADIATION COUNCIL OF THE UNITED STATES

Ranges of transient rates of daily intake	Graded scale of action
Range 1	Periodic confirmatory surveillance as necessary
Range 2	Quantitative surveillance and routine control
Range 3	Evaluation and application of additional control measures as necessary

SOURCE: FRC Memo for the President, Sept. 13, 1961.

sight or to wreck milk transport vehicles in outrage and panic at the first report of a rise in ^{131}I above range 2.   There is time for calm, measured, and deliberate response by intensifying surveillance and control.

RADIATION PROTECTION—PRINCIPLES AND TECHNIQUES

Protection against external radiation can be provided by three means:

1 Manage the distance between the source and the man, as each doubling of the distance reduces external exposure by one-fourth.
2 Manage the chronological length and spacing of the exposure, as the dose at the skin is a linear multiple of time exposed and dose rate.
3 Place barriers between the source and the man so that he is shielded by the material's absorbing the energy of the radiated emissions.

The control of radioactive materials which can enter the body and then produce internal exposure can be achieved by one or more of the following:

1 Contain or capture (or both) the radioactive gas, particulate, or large solids so that none gets into the air or water, or is left exposed for contact.
2 If any gaseous particulate or coarse solids get into the air or water at the point of use or processing, clean that air and water before these leave the use and process area.
3 If after treatment of the waste stream any residual fractions must be discharged into the air or into water, or be disposed of in solid form, use dilution, control the discharge, and trace the dispersal of the residuals.
4 Use isotopic dilution to limit the absorption of the radioactive isotope by all forms of life subsequently using that element.   Nonradioactive carbon burned during the incineration of an animal that had ^{14}C in its body for tracer studies results in diluting the release of $^{14}CO_2$ with stable CO_2 formed simultaneously. The method spreads the burden.
5 Prevent inhalation, ingestion, and skin absorption of radioactive materials by protective devices used by workers.
6 Protect the whole population by regulatory surveillance of the free environment to limit the intakes in air, food, and water.

There are five precepts of radiation protection that apply to all situations of use and exposure:

1 The use of radioactive materials and of radiation sources is regulated so that where there is no benefit from that use, nonradioactive materials and methods are satisfactorily substituted.

2 Persons using radiation sources are well trained and cognizant of the dangers to themselves and others and, in the case of health service uses, the danger to the patients.

3 Equipment required in radiation use is fitted to the job, functioning correctly, maintained, and checked for its performance.

4 The inventory of radioactive materials is current and accurate from receipt to final disposition, and the use of radiation machines is recorded.

5 The design, construction, and installation of machines and devices producing ionizing radiation are controlled so that unnecessary emissions are at a minimum and properly absorbed or attenuated during the intended use of the machines and devices.

The principles and techniques of achieving all these control objectives share many methods used in industrial hygiene, air pollution control, water treatment, and even food protection.   The distinctive differences are:

1 Radiation protection must deal with very small quantities.   As an example, chemical contaminants of water are in milligrams per liter, while radioactive ones are in picocuries per liter; that is 10^{-3} g versus 10^{-12} g if Ra is the radioactive contaminant.   This is a factor of 1 billion.

2 Radioactivity gives off an ionizing emission, an electromagnetic signal, which can be detected by very sensitive instruments.   This can be shown by turning on any Geiger-Müller counter anywhere on earth and picking up background radiation of 10 to 50 counts/min.

3 Radioactivity cannot be neutralized or cancelled out.   Nor can there be immunization against its effects.   It must be confined, captured, or, in sparing quantities, diluted and dispersed in our environment.

Initial Precepts on Radiation Use and for Radiation Users—Five Questions

Is the use necessary? must be asked about all radiation use, extant and proposed. When this question was put to the users of fluoroscopic x-ray shoe-fitting machines, which were common in local retail shoe stores, the answer was, No.   It was a sales gimmick.   Experienced salesmen did not depend on it or need it.   Unlamented, it has left the shoe sales scene in the United States.   Should there be radioactivity in children's toys?   Should automobile instrument dials be radio-luminescent by tritium as in the case of Army tanks?   If so, what about the residual radioactivity, however small, in the 8 million cars that go to junk each year?   All but a few cherished antique cars go to junk in 4 to 10 years.   Tritium, ^3H, has a half-life of 12 years.

There are already more than necessary residuals of radioactivity in military surplus stores, unlabeled and unrecognized. The question of benefit versus risk must be asked in each use of an ionizing radiation emitter.

Does the person who is using an ionizing radiation-emitting material or machine know what he or she is managing? Perhaps that should be the first question. The answer for users of licensed radioisotopes from the Atomic Energy Commission is quite good. Somewhere in the chain of control the instruction of such users must be verified. The answer is not good for those handling x-ray machines in industrial and health service use. There is too much button pushing by unsupervised, poorly instructed, and transiently engaged workers. A large collection of them are in our hospitals. The private practitioners of medicine without specialization in radiology are another large group using x-ray imprudently (Ref. 9-7).

The testimony of Hanson Blatz of the New York City Health Department and of K. Z. Morgan at the U.S. Senate hearings in 1967 is illuminating and disturbing (Ref. 9-8).

Does the design, construction, and installation of radiation emitting devices control and minimize the exposure of the users, of those nearby, of those in adjacent rooms? If the beam is directed at human beings, does the design and use of equipment limit the exposure to that required to produce the beneficial information? Devices utilizing Atomic Energy Commission licensed radioisotopes are well controlled and subject to inspection. Devices generating x-rays and radium sources have been decidedly lacking such control in the recent past and are only beginning to receive the attention that is commensurate with the risks and hazards of poor design, inattentive construction, and careless installation. X-ray tube enclosures that have sufficient shielding and are free of gaping leaks are now on the market after years of production of inadequate units. X-ray units have been installed in apartment and office buildings without a thought about the direction of the primary beam, about backscatter or about the attenuation provided by existing walls, floors, and ceilings. The work of local and state health departments is correcting gross defects and gaining correct practices in new installations. In industrial radiography, fixed units can be managed by structural safeguards. Portable units are most difficult to control with dependence resting on the operators' skill and concern in making his setups. The question must be answered for all uses, from a student laboratory's use of a Crookes tube or a few microcuries of ^{60}Co to use of nuclear reactors and accelerators.

Is the equipment, including protective devices, maintained so that it functions as designed and built? Is it calibrated and checked so that electrical outputs and radiation emissions are as designed and specified? These corollary questions to those on initial design and assembly apply equally to the instruments the maintenance man and the radiation protection officer carry and use for their work. No dial reading can be accepted at its face value without an independent check with calibrated sources and instruments.   Instruments should be calibrated at intervals of three months to a year by a professional person.

Is there an accounting of radioactive materials and of the use of radiation-generating machines?   Despite stringent requirements on inventories, Atomic Energy Commission inspectors encounter unrecorded transfers of radioisotopes by licensed users, usually within the same institution.   Radium losses are not rare in the light of its cost and the professionals who handle it.   Hanson Blatz reported nine losses of a total of 432 mg of Ra in New York City through carelessness by physicians in 1963 through 1965.   A warning of radium-use license suspension, provided in New York City procedures, reduced the loss in the following 2 years to one of 3 mg.   There has been no satisfactory single answer to recording radiation emitter use.   For large installations requiring high operational costs and skilled persons there are complete logs of their use.   These are for accelerators, reactors, high-voltage and high-curie therapy, and industrial radiography units.   It is burdensomely impractical to require such logs on every x-ray unit and every radioisotope use.

Illustrations of Protection Against Internal Radiation

Internal radiation results from breathing in, drinking up, eating up, or absorbing through the skin radioactivity in gaseous, dissolved, or particulate form, which then "parks" in specific or generalized sites in the body for periods of a few hours to life's remaining time. The preventive techniques apply that are used against toxicants in industrial hygiene and against biological pathogens in food protection and in hospital and nursing-home sanitation.   Adaptation and improvements of these techniques are used in the work environment.   Examples are:

1   Confine, contain, and capture radioactive releases and spills with local exhaust ventilation and with high-efficiency cleaners in the line; use removable blotting-paper covers on bench tops; use strippable paints on walls and ceilings; use full enclosures such as glove boxes and "hot cells."

2   Segregate and collect air- and waterborne radioactive wastes for high-efficiency removal before discharge.   Airborne ^{131}I is removed on banks of activated carbon filters before the collected air is discharged.   Radioactive forms of the noble gases, argon, krypton, and xenon, must be stored for decay.   Airborne particulates are caught on ultrafilters and electrostatic precipitators.   Low concentrations of radionuclides in water are removed on ion-exchange beds.   Waterborne ^{32}P, ^{90}Sr, and ^{137}Cs are precipitated in water treatment units quite similar to conventional mixing, flocculating, and settling basins.   Coagulants are carefully chosen and applied in high doses to achieve 95 to 98 percent removals.   The settled sludges must be buried.   These treatment methods work for intermediate-level wastes for which the radioactivity concentrations are in one or two digits

of millicuries per liter.   Wastes are grouped in levels given in Table 9-9.   Low-level concentration can be stated in one or two digits of microcuries per liter. High-level concentrations can be stated in one or two digits of curies per liter.

3   The assimilative capacity of the air and of water is used for the direct discharge of low-level wastes and of intermediate-level wastes after treatment.   Limits for disposal are prescribed for specific radionuclides by the Atomic Energy Commission in Code of Federal Regulations, Title 10, Part 20.   These are approximately one-tenth of the values recommended by National Council on Radiation Protection for 168 h/week in the drinking water of radiation workers. The correct apportioning of these discharges to fit the hydrology, meteorology, and ecology of the receiving environment requires in-depth knowledge of the behavior of radionuclides in a free environment, conscientious and concerned management, and vigilant monitoring by regulatory agencies.

To date in the United States, there have been few major nuclear energy installations, with all under government contract such as the Argonne, Brookhaven, and Oak Ridge National Laboratories, and the vast production facilities at Savannah River, Paducah, Kentucky, and the Hanford Works at Richland, Washington.   Control of discharges from these installations have met the requirements.   Very large nuclear reactors for power generation, however, are increasing in number.   This increase in reactors requires an extension of surveillance and monitoring of the same caliber as developed for the major sites.   There are continuous low-level discharges from nuclear power stations to the local air, water, and ground.   A valuable fund of information on how these contaminants behave in the open environment has been developed by lengthy studies at the Oak Ridge, Hanford, and Savannah River sites in the United States, at Chalk River in Canada, and at Windscale in the United Kingdom.   The U.S.S.R. has contributed useful data at international conferences on its procedures and experiences, although not usually pinpointed and detailed.

Table 9-9   THREE LEVELS OF RADIOACTIVE WASTE LIQUORS DEFINED BY DECONTAMINATION OR DILUTION FACTORS REQUIRED BEFORE DISCHARGE

Waste	Decontamination or dilution factor required before discharge	Examples of usual waste liquors source
Low level	1,000	Nuclear-reactor process water
Intermediate level	1,000–100,000	Radioisotope preparation laboratory
High level	Over 100,000	Fuel-element reprocessing plant

The needs to be met are:

1   Competent coverage of the increase from a few sites in the United States to over 100.
2   The sorting out of jurisdictions, as power companies already respond to several federal and state agencies.
3   The resolution of what number and types of samples and analyses are useful and meaningful.
4   The concomitant control of wastes from the fuel-fabricating and spent-fuel reprocessing plants, where high-level wastes result, and of the transportation of high curie quantities of radioactive materials in new and spent fuel elements.

All this requires a continuing assessment of the assimilative capacity of the whole environment and control adjustments to hold the balances. As for our management of the whole environmental quality, neither reckless, panicky diatribes, nor feckless, delayed, or short-sightedly rigid regulatory action contribute to the needed deliberated decisions for the beneficial use of our environment.

The toughest and least satisfying control of radioactive wastes has been the handling of high-level liquids from fuel-element reprocessing. The cladding of stainless steel and Zircaloy, a zircon-steel alloy, must be stripped from the radioactive materials within the fuel element by strong acids. The mixture is processed to recover the " unburned " uranium, the fissionable plutonium that has been produced in the fuel element, and at least in part, the fission products that are abundant, long-lived, and recoverable. These include ^{90}Sr, ^{137}Cs, ^{144}Ce, and a few other rare element radioisotopes. What remains is a nasty acid mix with unrecovered fission products and traces of unrecovered uranium and plutonium of 5 to 10 Ci/gal. All are still very active. The mix has the amusing acronymic label *purex waste* (plutonium-uranium extract waste). In the United States, this is being stored in underground tanks at Savannah River, Hanford, the National Reactor Testing Station at Idaho Falls, and in much smaller volumes at Oak Ridge. The fuel-element reprocessing plant in New York, the first in wholly private management, is storing its high-level waste on site. The curie quantities are staggering, the heat generated by the decay is considerable, and the corrosiveness of the wastes formidable.

A reactor which has operated for 6 months with a thermal output of 500 MW has a fission-product inventory of about 400 MCi, measured 1 day after shutdown. Such a reactor is capable of generating 150 to 170 MW of electricity, enough for the per capita needs of about 150,000 people. But it is only one-tenth of the capacity of some in design and construction and about one-fifth to one-sixth of several already operating. That initial radioactivity is equivalent to the activity of 400 tons of Ra. Most of the activity is short-lived isotopes, for in 1 week the level is 80 MCi, in 1 month 8 MCi. From there on decay is slowed, as the long-lived nuclides remain. This is the material that ends presently in steel storage tanks, underground, surrounded by concrete vaults, with steel catch pans below the tanks to intercept leakage, with piping systems to manage temperature and vapor-condensate cycles, with off-gas vents, and with extensive monitoring facilities for expected and unexpected releases and leaks. Ten years ago, there was already 50 Mgal of high-level wastes in underground storage tanks at Hanford, Washington, largely from plutonium production.   Some of these tanks stay at a boil from their decay heat and will continue so for 100 years.   Projecting waste volume and curies from estimated power reactor capacity to 1990, almost 20 years hence, shows that the United States will have over 10 GCi of fission products in storage in a volume of over 100 Mgal.   That is an activity of 100 Ci/gal.   Changes in reactor technology will reduce these estimates, but not substantially or rapidly, as existing plants will operate for their capitalized lives.   The economic use of alternative methods of managing high-level wastes is still in development.   Laboratory batches and modest pilot plant runs have been demonstrated in the United States, the United Kingdom, and France by which the high-level material is brought to a solidified, non-leachable mass in such forms as glass, ceramics, and sinters.   This, too, would have to be stored, but in smaller volumes and without liquid leakage risk.   Burial in deep salt formations is most promising.   These approaches must continue, as the commitment to centuries of storage of millions of curies in corrosive liquids is not a fitting or acceptable end to the elegant and sophisticated technology of controlled nuclear fission.

The inevitability of uncontrolled discharges finding their way back to man has been marked by radioactive fallout from weapons testing appearing in man, most accurately determined by ^{90}Sr in our bones.   No living creature with an internal or external bony structure, from mollusks to man, has been spared the added risk, however small, of a new body burden of radioactive strontium and its daughter ^{90}Yt, a radionuclide of yttrium.   These follow the chemical and biological pathways of calcium.   Table 9-10 shows the ^{90}Sr content of milk and of young bone in picocuries of

Table 9-10 ^{90}Sr IN MILK AND IN BONE OF YOUNG CHILDREN IN NEW YORK CITY IN PICOCURIES PER GRAM OF CALCIUM

Year	Milk	Year	Milk	Bone	Year	Milk	Bone
1954	1.4	1958	7.6	2.1	1964	23.2	6.2
1955	2.7	1959	11.0	2.7	1965	19.0	6.0
1956	3.9	1960	8.0	2.4	1966	12.0	5.6
1957	4.5	1961	6.1	3.1	1967	10.0	4.9
		1962	12.1	3.3	1968	9.0	3.5
		1963	25.6	5.6			

^{90}Sr per gram of Ca in New York City.   Note the milk response to weapons tests which increased up to 1959.   In that year there was a mutually voluntary "moratorium" of tests by the United States and the U.S.S.R.   Tests resumed in 1962 and concentrations in milk rose immediately.   The rise was sustained until the formal treaty banned air tests in 1963.   Concentrations in bone rose steadily during the period of bone record, 1958 to 1964, excepting the slight dip in 1960.   These have declined since 1964.

Illustrations of Protection Against External Radiation

External radiation risks for radiation workers are inherent in the use of radiation in hospitals, laboratories, any radiographic work, reactors, accelerators, and radioisotope processing and use.   The protective procedures are three straightforward measures:

1   Increase the distance between source and the worker and those around him. Cember (Ref. 9-4, p. 281) gives an example of a 100-mCi source of ^{60}Co, which would expose a worker to 1,490 mR/h at 1 ft.   Equipping him with remote-handling tongs 8.65 ft long reduced his exposure to 20 mR/h.   That's not an exposure recommended for a whole workday or week.   It can be accepted for the few minutes required to place the source for a radiograph exposure.

2   Regulate the time for which workers are in high-radiation fields so that their cumulative exposure for a week, for 13 weeks, for a year, and for their work-lives does not exceed the occupational exposures recommended by international and national radiation protection commissions for whole-body, body parts, and gonad exposure.   The elemental number is 5 rem/year in each year beyond age 18.   The time restriction is that not more than 3 of the 5 rem can be received in any single 13-week period of the year.   Furthermore, for women in their reproductive years the 3 rem is reduced to 1.3 rem.   This value holds any fetus she may carry to 1 rem in the first 2 months of term, possibly an unacknowledged pregnancy to that point, and to 1 added rem in the remaining 7 months of pregnancy ahead.

3   Shielding is elementary in principle and instinctive as a response to a barrage of external assault.   In practice, the factors which must be known or estimated are the types of radiations, their energies, and the stopping power of the shielding materials.   There are resultant actions of the absorption of the primary radiation, as there are secondary radiations emitted in particular interactions. There is scatter prior to hitting the absorber barrier and from hitting it.   The fundamental behavior of radiation attenuation conforms to a first-order equation.   A fixed fraction of incident radiation is absorbed for each unit of thickness of a particular material.   The fixed fraction is stated as an exponential fraction, e^{-ut}, with u the attenuation constant, and t the thickness.   A shield may be ordinary structural materials, a stack of lead bricks at the face of a laboratory hood, lead sheathing on the walls and ceiling of an industrial radiography room, a barytic concrete mix containing barium sulfate poured around a power-reactor core, or a transparent-plastic window in a glove box if the emission is solely alpha and low-energy beta.   For methods of calculations for shielding, see Ref. 9-4, p. 285.

In power-reactor construction, shielding and containment vessel are distinct structures and for different purposes.   The shielding is around the core and likely to be below ground level.   The containment vessel on pressurized-water reactors is the usually photographed, large domed cylinder on reactor sites that is built about and above the core.   The purpose of the containment vessel is to hold the released gases, vapors, and particulates so that there is no escape of radioactivity in case of an excursion.   There is structural strength to contain the type of steam or chemical explosion that can happen in a reactor.   As reactor configurations of fissionable materials cannot produce a nuclear detonation, such forces are not used in calculating shielding and containment.

INSTRUMENTAL MEASUREMENT

The radiation protection practitioner, whether called health physicist, radiological health specialist, or radiation safety officer, and whether a highly educated professional or a well-trained technician, has a dazzling array of instruments for measuring ionizing radiation.   These are quite expensive, to the dismay of budget officers.   These also provide remarkably misleading information when used for tasks and in situations for which they were not intended or when not calibrated.   The instruments are exquisitely sensitive and equipped with electrical circuits which can express an initial event by sound, light, needle swings, and amazingly rapid counters.   It's royal fun to have clicks, chirps, flashes, and warning blares at the touch of one or several knobs identified in obscure symbols to further humble the uninitiated.   Some carry beguiling names, as *Cutie Pie* and *Juno* of World War II security origin, and *Sparrow* for its bird sound. A few markers can be blazed to transverse this lovely forest of instrumental technology. Table 9-11 is the master guide, modified from a table in Cember (Ref. 9-4, p. 229).   The table groups instruments by the initial effect of ionizing radiation into four physical or chemical responses, states the class of instruments for the four effect groups, and cites commercial examples for each class by common or trade name.

Electrical-effect Instruments

The first three classes of instruments in Table 9-11 function by radiation emission that creates an ion pair in a low-pressure gas mixture in a chamber across which a voltage is impressed either from batteries or from a plug-in ac line which has been rectified to dc.   The creation of the ion pair in the existing preset circuit causes a disruption by an ion current, a flow of electrons which have been freed by the ionizing event.   For each 34.5 eV (a minute amount of energy) absorbed by the gas molecules from the radiation entering the gaseous mix, one pair of ions form—a negative and a positive one.   Numbers increase, of course, as the radiation energy rises.   One roentgen of radiation produces 1.6×10^{12} ion pairs in a gram of air.   There is no shortage of ions at such an exposure.   The voltage across the chamber collects the ions, anions to the anode chamber walls and cations to the cathode axial wire in the chamber.   Figure 9-11 diagrams a simple ion chamber device.   The collected ions produce a reading on the current meter.   The reading is translated on the dial as roentgens of ionizing radiation in air, by previous calibration and the designer's ingenuity.

By carefully regulating the voltage across the detection chamber and by carefully designed, built, and calibrated equipment. the basic circuit shown in Fig. 9-11 will provide three different types of instrumental responses.   These are the three groupings in Table 9-11 for electrical effects.   At low voltages, the response is that of ionization chambers.   At higher voltages, the response is that of proportional counters.   At

Table 9-11   TYPES OF INSTRUMENTS FOR MEASURING IONIZING RADIATION, GROUPED BY EFFECT BY WHICH THESE OPERATE, AND EXAMPLES OF EACH GROUP

Effect	Type of instrument	Example by common or commercial name
Electrical	Ionization chamber	Pocket chambers and dosimeters; survey meters, Cutie Pie, Juno, Samson
	Proportional counter	Internal gas-flow, proportional counter
	Geiger counter	Geiger-Müller tubes and counters, survey and laboratory types
Chemical	Film	Personal film badges with selective filters
	Chemical dosimeters	Solution vials, treated plastics, activated glass
Light	Scintillation counters	Sodium iodide crystals for gamma spectrometry on environmental samples and whole-body counting
		Liquid scintillation for low-level beta counting and low whole-body gamma counting
Thermoluminescence	Thermolumiscent dosimeters	TLDs of lithium and calcium fluoride Ruby crystals

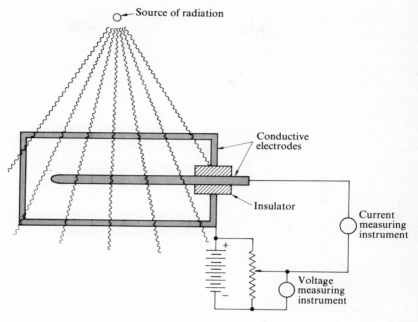

FIGURE 9-11
Schematic of ionization chamber circuit. (*Source: Hanson Blatz, " Introduction to Radiological Health," p.* 130, *McGraw-Hill Book Company, 1964.)*

still higher voltages, the response is that of the Geiger counter. The ionization chamber type of instrument is made in a variety of forms for measuring personnel exposure and for detecting and measuring environmental sources and contamination. The proportional counter type of instrument is well adapted to laboratory counting of environmental samples of air, water, and food. Careful preparation of the samples frequently includes complex chemical separations and concentration to get countable amounts. The behavior of the basic ionization chamber permits alpha response to be separated from the combined response to alpha and beta. Therefore, the proportional counter can be used to distinguish between the alpha-emitter and beta-emitter content of the material being counted. The Geiger counter is made in many configurations with a wide range of cost and price. The advice of an experienced person is most desirable so that the proper type of instrument is in use for the exposure situation at hand. Radiation protection requires more than the muscle power to turn on a switch on a yellow, gray, or black box.

Measurement by Chemical Effect

It takes a second thought to accept the film emulsion response to ionizing radiation as a chemical effect.   As in all photochemical reactions, whether visible-light photography or the smog formation over Los Angeles, electromagnetic energy is absorbed by atoms and molecules.   The absorption alters elemental and molecular groupings to produce, in the case of film, visible changes.   The most common is the darkening of silver-coated cellulose acetate film in black and white and x-ray pictures.   As alpha, beta, gamma, and x-ray energy absorption ionizes and produces molecular changes, film emulsion responds to these emissions.   The most widely used detector, and if properly used, measure of exposure in air, is the film badge.   The Atomic Energy Commission's requirement of "badging" its employees and its contractor employees extended to licensed radionuclide users.   In due course, the vogue spread to x-ray users, just as "hard hats" spread from the World War II shipyards to general construction jobs. Badge wearing does convey a poorly grounded sense of being protected.   At best it is a rough approximation of exposure measured in air.   A combination of metal filters in the badge holder provides some basis for distinguishing among beta, gamma, x-ray, and neutron exposures.   Some of the sources of poor and misleading results from film badges are:

1 Poor choice of emulsion for the intended use.
2 Poor choice of filters in the badge holder.
3 Ignorance of the energy dependence of emulsion response, particularly the poor response of conventional film to the energies of diagnostic x-ray.   Errors of 90 percent low occur; that is, the badge report is only 10 percent of the actual air exposure.
4 Badge orientation to the emission must be at 90° for full response, with low readings proportionate to deviations from the 90° incident angle.
5 Sloppy development methods lacking temperature control, agitation, and developer concentration control.
6 Poor reading of developed film density.
7 Stereotyped reporting and interpretations of readings without the necessary information about the sources and conditions of exposure.

A number of chemical compounds change color when there are radiation-induced ionic changes.   Some are in solutions, as the change of ferrous sulfate to ferric sulfate, or cerric sulfate to cerrous sulfate.   Some are in plastic films, blocks, or slices.   Some are not color changes, but optical changes in glass strips and chips with new optical properties or photoluminescence induced by radiation.   High-radiation fields produce these chemical effects.   Therefore, these are not useful for human protection.   They are useful for measuring dose in such applications as the extemely high radiation doses required in food irradiation.   Doses to foods are planned and controlled by dosimeters showing chemical colorimetric responses.

Measurement by Light Generation

Another credit to Rutherford is his detection of alpha emissions with his naked eye by having a zinc sulfide crystal in their path.   The alpha energy converts to a flicker of light as it is absorbed by the zinc sulfide.   In less than 50 years, a series of photo-electronic events have replaced the human eye for measuring low-energy beta and all sorts of gamma emissions.   Three components are required.

1 The phosphor which converts an ionizing radiation event to a flash of light.
2 One or more photomultiplier tubes which convert the light flash to electrons and then multiply each tenfold through seven to nine stages for a total multiplication of 10^7 to 10^9.
3 A series of amplifiers and discriminators that produce the sort-out and readout of the electrons which are produced by the photomultiplier tubes and arrive as pulses.   For gamma the formidable assembly of electronic gear makes up a multichannel analyzer with readout by such devices as oscilloscopes, automatic typewriters, tape punch-out, and automatic graphic plotters.

Scintillation techniques are used for gamma measurement in environmental samples, with thallium-activated sodium iodide crystals as the phosphor scintillator. Whole-body counters measure gamma emitters in the body, either by one or more TlNaI, or less successfully by xylene-toluene liquid, scintillators in an annular tank around the body.   In studies of biochemistry using beta emitters like ^{32}P or ^{14}C as tracers in living systems, samples are dissolved or suspended in liquid scintillators such as terphenyl and counted in the sample tube in low-beta counting equipment.   Other phosphor scintillators are organic crystals of anthracene and stilbene, terphenyl dissolved and cast in solid polystyrene, and xenon gas.

Measurement by Thermoluminescence

Thermoluminescent dosimetry (TLD) is the most recent means of radiation measurement to move from research study to field practice.   Crystals of calcium fluoride or lithium fluoride containing manganese impurities store the absorbed energy of gamma, x, beta, electron, and proton radiations.   When the capsule of crystals is heated, the stored energy is released as visible light directly proportional to the absorbed radiation. Readout is by a photomultiplier tube and a digital voltmeter.   The heating "wipes out" the absorbed energy, which makes the dosimeter ready for reuse.   Calibration of the thermoluminescent dosimeter to exactly the same quantities and types of radiation as are being observed is the basis for interpreting the readout, displayed as *glow curves*. Calcium fluoride is the more sensitive of the fluorides in wide use. Lithium fluoride, LiF, has the advantages of being almost energy-independent for gamma emissions with energies of from 100 KeV to 1.3 MeV, and of being closely equivalent to soft tissue in its absorption of radiations. This is not happenstance. It results from effective atomic numbers of the two being close to one another with soft tissue at 7.4 and LiF phosphor at 8.1. Thermoluminescent dosimeters have a wide range of usefulness from 10 mrads to 100,000 rads. They are available through commercial channels in the United States in the same way as film badge services. They can be used in place of film badges in some exposure situations and can supplement film badges.

CHANGES AND DEVELOPMENTS

Radiation protection and the three things on which it is dependent, radiation effects information, formulation of standards and limits, and measurement methods, must respond to the increased usage of ionizing radiation sources. The three uses that are accelerating in the United States are nuclear-fueled electricity generation, medical use of radioisotopes, and use of x-ray in health services. Like patterns are evident in other countries. Ionizing radiation sources for testing in manufacturing and construction are increasing. Sources are entering our homes as high-voltage equipment such as color TV receivers, which bash electrons about to produce x-rays in collisions, planned or unplanned. Finally, there are two collections of people who as they age, will test the validity of our knowledge, assumptions, and practice of radiation protection. These are the radiation workers and those born since July 16, 1945, the day of the Alamogordo test bomb. They have developed and lived in an environment in which the ionizing radiation factor is a bit larger and definitely longer than other people before them have experienced. The exceptions are the quite small numbers of professional and occupational specialists such as radiologists, industrial radiographers, radium handlers, and miners in radioactive rock formations. Continued careful account must be kept of those who have survived the high-level radiation of the two bombs used in Japan, of the high fallout on the Marshall Islands and on the Japanese fishing boat *Lucky Dragon* in 1954, and of radiation accidents.

From 1945 to 1965, there have been, in the world, 14 occupational accidents that produced high doses of radiation and acute effects which N. Wald records as valuable sources of human data. In the 14 accidents, 57 people suffered injury. These are tabulated with specific references in Ref. 9-5 (p. 452). There were 267 people on the Marshall Islands and 23 on the *Lucky Dragon* who were caught in the unpredicted fallout pattern from a United States bomb test in the Pacific in 1954.   The uranium miners on the Colorado plateau are a unique group under close medical surveillance. Epidemiological study of the consequences of their inhalation of radon and its daughters is vital to the protection of all miners working in radioactive rock, and of limited use for extension to all people.

Biological Effects

Efforts to resolve reparable and nonreparable cellular damage from radiation are being strengthened by the momentum of molecular and cellular biology.   The significance of chromosome aberrations and the relation of those caused by ionizing radiation to those from other causes requires painfully long and exacting planned epidemiological studies.   Automated cytogenetic and automated blood culture techniques can be used for such work.   The benefits from such work concern not only radiation, but alleged risks from low-level chemical environmental contaminants, side effects from drugs taken for treatment and for " kicks," food-production residues, and occupational exposures.   To measure provoked chromosomal aberrations requires the base line of the usual range of aberrations in a less disturbed population.   This, along with the cycles of change of elemental physiological indices such as blood chemistry, blood pressure, renal function, has scarcely been observed for accurate mapping.

Limits, Standards, Guidelines, and Criteria

No substantial change in the recommendations of the International Commission on Radiological Protection and the National Council on Radiation Protection is likely for the intended applications and stated purposes and circumstances.   Changes will result if there is firm and confirmed evidence of human injury or of ecological damage to plant or animal systems, marine, terrestrial, or aerial.   No other environmental contaminant from man is monitored as accurately and as frequently as radioactive discharges to air, water, and land, and with as continuous observation of biological markers such as trees, plants, rodents, shellfish, and finfish.   The international and national radiation protection committees have been hesitant to make recommendations directed to general population exposures.   These highly responsible groups must recognize the presence of ionizing radiation sources in our homes in electromechanical devices and in radioactive seeds implanted in family members on long-term therapy. No alarmist view is intended, and indeed the therapists are sensitive to the risk of the implant patient's being a radiation source to those near him.   It is in part for this reason that ^{125}I, which decays without a gamma emission, is used in place of ^{131}I, which has eight gamma emissions in its decay scheme with enough energy and tissue penetration to emerge from the body of the patient.   Professional health physicists, who have given major attention to in-house matters, are recognizing their responsibilities for contributing to public protection and public understanding.   The two protection commissions always responded to the needs of their peers.   Under public law 90-602 of the United States, the Secretary of the Department of Health, Education, and Welfare must regulate radiations from electronic products.   The first standards were issued in 1970 as governmental regulations.   The value of having professional societies and groups pooling their experience in promulgating standards has been demonstrated in water and wastewater management and industrial hygiene.

Protection in Health Services Use

Three things will continue in the control of x-ray use in health serivces.

1 Technological changes are at hand.   Automatic collimators are sufficiently developed to be applied widely.   Automated control of film development is ready.   Standardization of film identifications will result from the extensive work on commercial film characteristics by Drs. Russell Morgan and Lloyd Bates of The Johns Hopkins University.

2 The licensing of x-ray technicians will become widespread, and consequently their training more formalized and improved.

3 More governmental regulation is coming.   In states where registration of x-ray equipment is voluntary, it tends to become mandatory.   In states where compliance starts as a voluntary response, it gains the force of law.

The acceleration of hospital use of radioisotopes for diagnosis and therapy and of high-voltage x-ray, ^{60}Co sources, and betatrons is imposing an added task of preparing people to use and manage these effectively and safely.   This preparation requirement exists at the highest professional levels, technician levels, and among radiation protection people.   The most difficult technical matters are those of dosimetry.   How must the source be controlled to get these very powerful radiations at the points in the human body where they are most beneficial with the least damage to surrounding cells?   The patient must be protected so that he receives the maximum benefit at the minimum risk.   The staff must be protected, mindful that young females in their first reproductive chances are numerous in hospital employment.

Nuclear-fueled Power Generators

The issues of this complex technology have already been cited.   The Atomic Energy Commission and the power companies continue to face public suspicion and misunderstanding, which surfaces when new stations are being sited.   They are going through public hearings on safety.   Their new stations are going on the line.   The credibility of the two groups is widely discounted among some people, some organized as conservationists, or as antibomb, or as nearby property owners. The reasons for the difficulties are:

1 The statements come from two publicly authorized monopolies and hence are regarded as lacking competitive views.

2 The Atomic Energy Commission is placed by law in the conflicting roles of judge, jury, and attorneys for plaintiff and defendant in several uses of nuclear energy. For power generation, the Commission is the promoter, the entrepreneur to the extent of providing the nuclear fuel, the controller of design criteria, the licenser, and the regulator of operation.

3 The simplest of issues become confused and obfuscated when charges and refutation fail to distinguish among such matters as (a) low-level discharges and criticality risks, and the proposed means of managing each; (b) the makeup of a nuclear reactor, and how it differs from a bomb and thus cannot become a bomb; (c) attributing uniquely to nuclear-fueled plants things which are common with fossil-fueled plants, such as the discharge of condenser cooling water, the esthetics of the layout of buildings, stacks, and transmission towers, and the acquisition of transmission-line right-of-way.

The Atomic Energy Commission made a formal agreement to have the Bureau of Radiological Health of the Public Health Service, Department of Health, Education, and Welfare report on the needs and proposals on low-level discharges from nuclear-fueled generating stations from site selection to operation, on the environmental surveillance plan, on the plan for radiological assistance from public and private sources in emergencies, and on the potential dose to the population during the " most credible " accident. The reports were the *Public Health Evaluation* of the proposed plans and procedures. The procedure has the virtue of coming from a third party whose sole concern is public health and safety. The function has now been transferred to the Environmental Protection Agency, and this provides a means to broaden the agreement to other environmental impacts. An extension of the use of third parties which are highly qualified, which have the people's interest and confidence, and which do not have conflicting objectives in the nuclear power projects will be necessary to reduce the abrasive encounters experienced in communities where reactors are sited and operated. Clear divisions and assignments of what are and are not radiation and of other environmental matters will have to be made among the federal and state agencies.

Controversies on nuclear-fueled generating stations are not confined to the United States. Japan's plans to meet soaring power demands by nuclear stations run into heavy public opposition, with the Hiroshima and Nagasaki bombings adding to the fear. The United Kingdom, similarly confined to small island geography, has its difficulties, further complicated by the National Coal Board's demand that its mines be kept in production.   The people's suspicions in Spain as an aftermath of the United States bomber crash in which nuclear weapons fell at Palomores without detonating but causing some surface contamination, have dampened the interest of the government of Spain in nuclear reactor projects.

Environmental Surveillance

The very coining of these two words was to describe the response of the U.S. Public Health Service in the 1950s to the Atomic Energy Commission's request to take them "off the hook" of public disbelief on its weapons-test fallout information.   Testing on the desert north of Las Vegas, Nevada, and on the Pacific atolls was distributing radioactivity to every chemical system on the earth.   Russian testing was increasing and adding to it.   The United Kingdom shot off a few, too.   The Atomic Energy Commission's reports of off-site fallout were simply not accepted by the American people as objective or from a group that had a well-rooted concern for public health and safety.   Environmental surveillance came into being to measure and track weapons-testing fallout off-site, meaning beyond the Commission's security fences and boundaries.   Sampling, analytical, and instrumental techniques were developed.   Surveillance networks were set up to cover the nation's milk, food, water, and air supply for radioactivity measurement.   The sample taking and collection is not much more sophisticated than in the 1950s.   The analysis and data processing are.   In state health department laboratories and in the regional radiological laboratories—at Montgomery, Alabama; Las Vegas, Nevada; and Winchester, Massachusetts—detection, counting, and plotting gear, with the use of the latest methods, some developed in-house, give the readout on the raw samples.   Statistical methods are used to minimize the number of samples analyzed.   Computers are used to sort out the myriad of numbers.

The surveillance network must be kept sharp for three reasons:

1   Surveillance continues to supply information on the radioactivity already loose and circulating.   The behavior of the world's present burden is not so well known as to permit forgetting it like so many loads of rubbish in the town dump.
2   International harmony or mutual fear is not so certain that more weapons testing in air is precluded.   Two nuclear nations, France and China, test when they will—as neither have signed the nuclear test ban treaty.
3   Peacetime use of nuclear materials adds to the total environmental load in circulation.   We must know where it is and how it is behaving.

Disposal of Wastes

Radioactive waste is inherently hazardous and stays so for many half-lives, with at least a few radionuclides with half-lives longer than all man's recorded time on earth.   Whatever the option, dilute and disperse, delay and decay, or concentrate and confine, radioactive wastes and related procedures must be monitored. The control methods merely move the contaminant from one medium to another, from the airstream to the filter material, from the liquid stream to the settled sludge, from the collection container to the burial ground. It still must be watched. Improvements in treatment technology will continue. For a price, removals will be made more efficient in cleaning air and liquid waste streams. Further automation of such processes is certain. Coagulant aids, new exchange and adsorption media, and improved filter materials for air and water are coming into use. The regulatory headache rests in the increase in use of nuclear materials and the disposal of the consequent wastes. The number of users and nations engaged in controlling substantial amounts has been relatively small. Much of the material has been in direct government use and at least easily pinpointed. Peaceful use requires transfers to private users across many jurisdictional lines.

Aside from the need for enduring records and markers and for reasonably uniform measures for control and regulation, inevitable pieces of the environment will reach an assimilative limit for a particular waste or mix of these. It may be a stretch of stream, a reach of an estuary, a meteorological zone, or an expanse of land. Administrative and legal mechanisms for coping with analogous matters of nonradioactive contaminants and pollution have been poor, cumbersome, and slow to respond to gross conditions. Put globally and internationally, agreement on the issue will be most difficult to reach. The International Atomic Energy Agency directs much of its efforts to waste matters. Conferences, exchange of personnel, and publications are the means for communicating and for reaching for understanding. In the United States there is scarcely agreement among the federal agencies which have the final say on some matters; the state versus federal questions are just arising as states assert their power and responsibilities on such matters as reactor siting, effluent concentrations to air and water, and the use of salt deposits for solidified high-level waste entombment.

APPRAISAL

The opening statement of this chapter stands. The countryside is not strewn with bodies broken by radiation damage. That is more than we can say for our management of our cherished automobiles. Hospital beds and dayrooms are not filled by physiological and psychological wrecks induced by radiation. That is more than we can say for our handling of our cherished social beverage, alcohol, in various beguiling forms and the more recent indulgences in habituating drugs. Despite the vulnerable position that has been ascribed to the AEC in this chapter, the AEC and its predecessor the Manhatten District project have an exemplary record not only for the low occurrence of radiation injuries, but for all injuries and for the health services it provides for its employees and for its contractors. Its radiation record is more creditable than that of physicians, a profession dedicated to human health repair, if not protection.   In their use of the magic of ionizing radiation, the physicians have not spared themselves.   But they have learned to accept protection for themselves.   The benefits of radiation protection to radiologists is in Table 9-12.   Radiologists have cut their leukemic liability from 10 times that of all other physicians to $3\frac{1}{2}$ times.   Considering the bad prognosis for leukemia, the differential is worth continued effort to sharpen radiation protection consciousness among radiologists and among their staffs, for whom there are no reports on leukemia.

There are data on the integrated working-life doses of all 5,145 employees of the Oak Ridge National Laboratory to March 1966.   Some have been at work on the site since 1943.   Of the 5,145 employees, 4,425, or 86 percent, have received a total working-life dose of less than 5 rems, the annual acceptable dose for radiation workers.   Of the 700 over 5 rems, only 127 have received more than 20 rems; and 18, more than 50 rems, the acceptable total for 10 working years.   The two largest single doses at Oak Ridge laboratory have been 63 rems to a person mistakenly entering an area of highly radioactive material, and 13 rems to a person entering a hot cell to check an agitator that was mixing radioactive chemicals.   Despite lapses, it is an impressive record of effective radiation protection.   Not every major nuclear energy center has been that successful, as some require more hazardous manipulation of critical assemblies of fissionable materials.

One criticality accident was at the Y-12 plant in Oak Ridge in 1958.   This installation is operationally separate from the Oak Ridge National Laboratory, although

Table 9-12   THE RATIO OF INCIDENCE OF LEUKEMIA AMONG RADIOLOGISTS AND ALL OTHER PHYSICIANS IN THE UNITED STATES FOR THREE INTERVALS, POINTING TO THE BENEFIT OF INCREASED RADIATION PROTECTION

	The ratio of leukemia among	
Interval	Radiologists	All other physicians
1929–1943	10.3	1
1944–1948	6.7	1
1952–1955	3.6	1

SOURCE: "Effects of Ionizing Radiation on the Human Hemapoietic System" Publ. 875. Committee on Pathologic Effects of Atomic Radiation, NAS/NRC, Washington, D.C. 1961.

under the same management, the Union Carbide Corporation, Nuclear Division. During a uranium salvage operation $2\frac{1}{2}$ kg of ^{235}U were inadvertently drained into a standard 55-gal drum. The ^{235}U became critical in about 50 liters of initial solution and continued so for 20 min until a continued waterflow terminated the reaction. In that time 1.3×10^{18} fissions occurred. Eight men, one within 6 ft of the drum, received dose equivalents of 461 to 28.8 rems before an automatic alarm alerted them to evacuate. That action saved their lives and spared them from any permanent disabilities.

Records of the world to 1967 show eight deaths in reactor and criticality accidents. There have been seven deaths in the United States, three at Los Alamos, three at Idaho Falls, and one in Rhode Island, and one death in Yugoslavia. Thirty-eight others survived reactor and criticality accidents from 1945 to 1965, with recorded doses of from 20 to 550 rads, including two Russians who took 450 and 300 rads in 1954 (Ref. 9-5). For the year 1960, Merril Eisenbud shows the dose in rems to 82,197 workers of the Atomic Energy Commission and its contractors to be 0 to 1 for 77,522, 1 to 5 for 4,629, 5 to 10 for 41, 10 to 15 for 2, and over 15 for 3. He cautions (Ref. 9-9):

> There remains the important question of the frequency with which injuries can be expected to occur because of delayed effects of repeated small doses of radiation. To date there have been no known injuries of this kind in the atomic energy industry, an observation that must be tempered by acknowledging the long latent period associated with chronic radiation injury and the fact that the industry is only a little more than two decades old.

In addition to the reactor and criticality accidents and the heavy fallout on the natives and Americans on the Marshall Islands and on the Japanese fishermen, there have been 15 serious exposures from handling radionuclides in AEC or contractor installations or among licensed users. These occurred from 1948 to 1962 and exposed 26 identified people. In these 15 serious exposures, there were no deaths, 2 permanent partial disabilities. The injury to 8 of the 26 identified people was localized skin burns from beta emissions (Ref. 9-5, pp. 47–48). Clearly, no one is immune from the concatenation of behavioral and environmental conditions which produce accidents. Two lessons from nuclear accidents have been that panicky actions happen before informed authority applies the radiation emergency plan and that dose investigation is very frustrating.

There has been an emphasis on safety in the nuclear energy industry since the design, construction, and start of the reactor pile under the stands at Stagg Field, University of Chicago, on December 2, 1942, under the direction of Enrico Fermi. At the start-up, Fermi had two backup men behind the one who was ready to shut down the reactor by normal means. One man had a hatchet in hand ready to cut a rope which held up the first control rod. Another man had a hammer at the side of a bottle of boric acid ready to douse the pile with the strong neutron absorber. Commissioner James Ramey, of the Atomic Energy Commission, calls those the days of the "hatchet and the hammer." All who deal with nuclear energy must have the double backup of "hammer and hatchet" in their thinking and action. Dating the nuclear energy industry from 1942, radiation protection has four accomplishments:

1 Protection began with use, being built into operations.
2 Instrumental and analytical development kept pace with use and perceived risks.
3 Environmental surveillance, tracking discharges in air, water, and the ground, were started early. This coverage extended to food, plant, and animal cycles. Important parts of surveillance were made the independent responsibility of other federal, state, and local agencies to assure third-party objectivity.
4 Surveillance data and the need to interpret these spur a continued and comprehensive study of the fate of radioactive contaminants along environmental pathways. This information confers the power to predict. He who can predict can control.

REFERENCES

9-1 REES, D. J.: "Health Physics—Principles of Radiation Protection," Butterworth & Co., Ltd., London, 1967.
9-2 WILLHOIT, D. W.: "Radiation Quantities and Units and the Significance of Recorded Measurement," University of North Carolina Department of Environmental Sciences and Engineering, Chapel Hill, 1968.
9-3 United Nations Scientific Committee: Effects of Atomic Radiation, UN 17th Sess. Suppl. 16 (A/5216), 1962.
9-4 CEMBER, HERMAN: "Introduction to Health Physics," Pergamon Press, New York, 1969.
9-5 MORGAN, K. Z., and J. E. TURNER (eds.): "Principles of Radiation Protection," John Wiley & Sons, Inc., New York, 1967.
9-6 Background Material for the Development of Radiation Protection Standards, *Fed. Radiat. Counc.*, *Rep.* 2, Reprinted by U.S. Public Health Serv., 1961.
9-7 Population Exposure to X-rays, U.S., 1964, *U.S. Public Health Serv.*, 1966.
9-8 *United States Senate Hearings, Radiation Control for Health and Safety Act of 1967*, 90th Cong., 1968.
9-9 EISENBUD, MERRIL: "Environmental Radioactivity," McGraw-Hill Book Company, New York, 1963.

10

ELECTROMAGNETIC ENERGY IN THE RANGE OF ULTRA VIOLET, VISIBLE LIGHT, LASER, THE RADIO FREQUENCIES, AND MICROWAVE

The electromagnetic energy spectrum is a resource just as certainly as land, air, and water are. It is a peculiar one, as the question is not so much one of our using what nature provides in the form of electromagnetic energy as one of what forms man creates and how he manages his energy creation. These forms can be defined in the physical characteristics of frequency, wavelength, and energy. In what sense is the electromagnetic energy spectrum a resource? It is a continuous spectrum of wavelengths. Man has various devices for generating electromagnetic energy at specific wavelengths. He imparts a certain energy to it and then sends it somewhere. It may be only a short few inches confined in a microwave oven. It may be literally broadcast, cast abroad, without the slightest notion of where it will be received and converted to radio speaker sound or a TV screen picture. There is a limit to how all this electromagnetic energy can be emitted without interfering with someone else who is emitting his form of energy at the same or a near wavelength or at an uncontrolled, unspecified, and undirected energy. There is interference of the function of an electronic device by the stray pickup of electromagnetic energy from a known or unknown source. An example is the airport radar disturbance of an electronic heart pacer on a person in an airplane or in a ground crew in a radar field. Warnings on highway construction sites to turn off two-way radios (so as not to detonate explosives) and on airplanes to turn off pocket radios (as these interfere with radio navigation equipment) bring the point to your daily experience and observation.   Less evident is the growing complexity of allocating the frequencies of the electromagnetic energy spectrum for radio and TV uses among civilian and military, public and private, national and international, profit and nonprofit, and educational and entertainment uses.   There are agreements and systems of wavelength allocations within countries and internationally.   The demand for use has outstripped capacities originally thought adequate.   The most critical overloads of assigned frequencies are those used for mobile two-way radio; police and fire service, marine service, citizen-band business service, and air traffic service. All but one of these directly involve public safety.   The development of car control on multilane throughways, of bus dispatching by phone-radio, and of document transmission is limited by present allocations.

The technical complexities of these issues and paths to solutions are in Ref. 10-1. That joint committee report, "Spectrum Engineering—The Key to Progress" has a section on side effects and a lucid charting of these by frequency.   *Side effects* is the committee's term for biological effects.   There is a potpourri of observations of effects. These are responses, not necessarily impairments or injuries.   They include such things as caged chickens involuntarily extending wings and legs when in a radar beam, changes in the brainstem potentials in cats by pulse-modulated electromagnetic energy at the UHF of 1 GHz (1×10^9 cycles/s), pearl-chain reactions in bacteria in the radio and TV frequencies, buzzing and knocking sounds in the head under radiation at TV frequencies, a 200 percent increase in gladiola growth and insect kills at international and citizen's band radio frequencies.   Eye damage and internal tissue heating occur in man and mammals across the radio, TV, and radar frequencies.   The latter effect is the basis for medical diathermy.   There have been isolated cases of eye cataracts in patients unknowingly or carelessly exposed during diathermy.

Two things must be emphasized.

1   The physical parameters of the radiations causing many reported biological observations are often not precise and lack the information important to the physicists.   The biologists often have not had the collaboration of physicists to be aware of standing waves, interference patterns, and reflection phenomena.   In some cases frequency and energy measurements have not been well instrumented. In exchange, the physicists have their share of gaps and ignorance of biology. The need for joint work was very evident in a research symposium on microwaves at the Medical College of Virginia in September, 1969 (Ref. 10-14).

2   The effects that have been observed are moderate.   Eye cataract is the most serious.   The reported cases have come from severe, overt, and usually repeated exposures to radar with the eyes close to the source.   Exposure to the energy forms discussed in this chapter carry nothing like the biological effects of standing

in a medical x-ray beam. With all of us continuously in an electromagnetic energy field usually of very low energy, if the biological effects were serious or common, there would be epidemiological evidence of impairment. Such impairment would be observed first in those exposed at work.

The diversity of terms and units used to describe electromagnetic energy causes confusion and uncertainty for those not experienced with the parlance used by those who deal only with particular segments. The radio or TV station's frequency is given in kilohertz if it is broadcast AM (amplitude modulated), in megahertz if it is broadcast FM (frequency modulated), and in megahertz if it is TV broadcast. All stations state their irradiated power in watts. Many of us are aware that most radio tuning dials are in kilohertz for AM and megahertz for FM. These are three- or four-digit numbers for AM, 550 to 1,700 kHz; and in two- or three-digit numbers for FM, 88 to 108 MHz. Television set designers saved us that bother by identifying a sending station's frequency by channel number, adding recently the mild mystery of UHF to the original VHF ranges. Appendix 2 fixes these in the total spectrum. Figure 10-1 shows their positions in the radio frequencies. International public broadcasting is identified by wavelengths in meters, such as the 18-m band. Compared with AM radio at 550 kHz (or kc/s) with a wavelength of 550 m, the international station at an 18-m wavelength is short. At 18 m the station has a frequency of 16.7 MHz. Remember that throughout the spectrum the product of frequency in hertz (cycles per second) and the wavelength in centimeters equals 3×10^{10} cm/s, the speed of light. In this chapter frequencies will always be in hertz (Hz) even at the cost of using the powers of 10. The prefixes kilo, 10^3; mega, 10^6; giga, 10^9 are used in covering the ranges of the radio frequencies, including microwave.

ULTRAVIOLET

In 1801, J. W. Ritter observed a blackening of silver chloride by the sun's energy beyond the visible violet range. Man had recognized ultraviolet radiation. He had and has been exposed to it throughout his existence, as the sun is the principal source of it. In 1899, N. R. Finsen showed that sunburn was caused by the ultraviolet in sunlight. An effective proponent of UV for therapy, Finsen was awarded a Nobel prize in 1903. His name is a unit of measurement for UV, the Finsen unit. The definition of a Finsen unit illustrates the necessity of identifying wavelength, or frequency, and energy in any electromagnetic energy component. One Finsen unit is a radiant flux of 10 microwatts (100 ergs) per square centimeter per second of homogeneous radiation of a wavelength of 2967 angstrom units (Å). One Å equals 1×10^{-10} m or 1×10^{-8} cm. Therefore, a 2967-Å emission equals 2.967×10^5 cm and has a frequency of 10^{15} Hz.

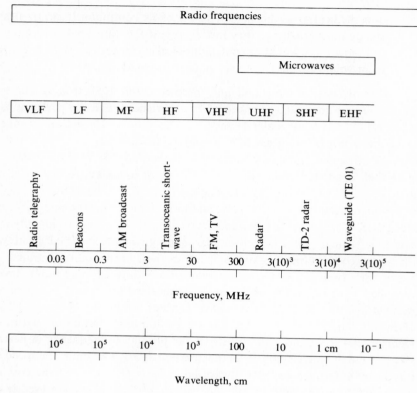

FIGURE 10-1
The electromagnetic energy spectrum from infrared to radio. (*Source: Redrawn from W. W. Mumford, Ref. 10-12, p. 427.*)

The characteristics and effects of UV are usually divided into three ranges, extreme UV, far UV, and near UV. The degrees are in distance from the visible range as wavelength shortens. These are significant observations:

1 In the extreme UV of 7.5×10^{16} to 1.5×10^{15} Hz (40 to 2000 Å), the UV effects at 3×10^{16} Hz (100 Å) are ionizing emissions.
2 The specificity of effects are dependent on frequency (wavelength) with marked changes in the peaks of effects for small shifts in frequency. This is important in selecting, ordering, or using UV lamps. The emission spectrum of a lamp must be fitted to its application.
3 Ultraviolet effects have stages specific to frequencies or wavelengths as indicated in the entry in Appendix 2 on skin reddening and subsequent tanning and pig-

ment darkening.   This occurs at 8.9 to 8.6 × 10^{14} Hz (3400 to 3500) Å.   This is in the near UV range of 1 × 10^{15} to 7.5 × 10^{14} Hz (3000 to 4000 Å).

4   Ultraviolet is an energy form which drives photochemical reaction.   Among these are ozone and the Los Angeles type of smog formation, photosynthesis, and vitamin D synthesis from ergosterol.   The range for these reactions is the far UV from 1.5 to 1.0 × 10^{15} Hz (2000 to 3000 Å).   It is the range of germicidal action, which peaks at 2650 Å.

5   The biological effects are not serious impairments, with the exception of skin cancer, as UV is fully absorbed in the skin.   The cancer from the sun's radiation develops after years of continued exposure.   It appears solely in whites and is markedly associated with the sunny climates.   Eye injuries including arc welders' flash burn and snow blindness are severe temporary discomforts.   There have been cases of permanent blindness from arc flash exposure.   A blistering sunburn is painful but recovery is complete.   These effects are all at the long-wavelength end of far UV range with flash burn at 2880 Å, skin cancers at peaking range of 2900 to 3200 Å, and the peak of skin reddening at 2970 Å.   This is at the edge of the near range.

6   *Black light* is in the near UV range, close to the visible range.   Lamp sources for it are in frequencies of 9.4 × 10^{14} to 8.0 × 10^{14} Hz (3200 to 3800 Å).   The human eye sees no light from the source in these ranges.   The photons in the UV range are absorbed by many fluorescent materials.   The absorbing atoms release that energy in the visible range, 7.5 × 10^{14} to 4.5 × 10^{14} Hz (4000 to 7000 Å, or 400 to 700 nm).   Many minerals fluoresce naturally and many man-made dyes and compounded pigments do so.   The reaction under UV provides identification on demand and is the basis for a variety of detection, inspection, and identification uses of UV.   The eerie to brilliant visible light emission is a spectacular event capturing visual attention.   This is its appeal for advertising displays and show lighting.

The widest use and widest variety of UV lamp applications are in the black light range.   It is fortunate that there is no recognized biological effect from the exposure to this range of UV except impaired vision from prolonged looking directly at the source or at strong reflections.   When such exposure is necessary, protective goggles that completely absorb the UV at 8.25 × 10^{14} Hz (3660 Å) and 90 percent of the UV at 7.25 × 10^{14} Hz (4055 Å) must be worn.   For seeing, such goggles should transmit at least 85 percent of the visible blue-green range of 5.8 × 10^{14} to 5.2 × 10^{14} Hz (5200 to 5800 Å, or 520 to 580 nm).   Reference 10-3 provides comprehensive information, except on goggle protection.   Lamp types, characteristics, and advantages are tabulated in detail.

In comparison with these biological impairments, UV stands as a significant form of energy to synthesize organic compounds on the primitive earth (Ref. 10-2, pp.

174–175).   The UV component of solar energy is important in photosynthesis, the source of all our stored energy on earth.   Photosynthesis not only provides all the earth's green life, it utilizes carbon dioxide and releases oxygen.   Its past productivity of plant and animal tissue is the basis for all our fossil fuels—coal, oil, and gas.

THE VISIBLE RANGE

The physiological and psycholgical responses of reasonably well-managed visible light are wholly beneficial.   There are a few good practices that must be followed to prevent undesirable effects.   There is no evidence that normal use of natural or artificial lighting is adverse to health, eye comfort, and easy seeing.   The issues are those of proper control of light suited to the visual task.

Good lighting will be defined in units peculiar to artificial illumination and in the intensities recommended for particular visual tasks.   These will be more meaningful if you consider your own experiences in seeing under what you intuitively recognize as satisfactory lighting.

1   High intensities facilitate seeing fine work whether in print or in manipulating small parts.   Compare the work in an iron foundry with that at the watchmaker's bench.

2   Satisfactory lighting reduces obscure ocular symptoms.   Subjectively, this is readily accepted by those who have put in a long day of demanding visual work at the drafting table under poor lighting compared with good lighting, with the illumination differences being those of intensity and the minimum of annoying reflections.

3   Older people realize that they can see things more easily, including newsprint, if the lighting is good.   High incident lighting appears to increase the contrast so long as glare is not a product.   The demands for extremes of ocular accommodation are lessened.   Similarly, at an inspection station on a conveyor belt of production items, the benefits of good lighting are observed both in efficiency of detecting defective items and in how the worker feels about that job at the end of a full working day.

4   Good lighting promotes cleanliness if by no more than revealing the accumulated filth and litter, and by making the cleaning job easier and more rewarding to see. A casual look at public toilet rooms and public corridors will support this.

5   There are psychological and behavioristic responses to lighting.   In most manifestations these are products of our color perception and our color associations. The cones in the fovea of the retina of the eye are highly sensitive to the energy differences of visible light that are color differences (see Fig. 10-12).   That rad-

iant energy is transformed to chemical energy in the cones and conveyed to our brain by the optic nerve.   The brain's interpretation of the stimuli received produces the mental concept of color.   Color associations are similar among many cultures in our world.   Reds, oranges, and yellows are stimulating, gay, exciting.   These predominate in festive occasions of holidays and dance ceremonies. Blues, violets, and purples are solemn and associated with the subdued passions of sorrow, mourning, and profound respect.   The greens are cooling and calming. Theater, opera, musicals, and shows make skillful use of these associations to produce a mood or effect.   A wholly unsubtle attempt to use illumination to modify human behavior is lighting for security against the crimes of robbery, assault, rape, arson, and bombing and for accident prevention at road intersections, along streets and highways, on stairways, walks, and construction projects. Documented or not, campus areas, parks, public buildings, and areas of recorded repeated crimes are being lighted to much higher intensities to prevent crime. Specific data on the value of lighting to prevent accidents are not offered.   It does appear that lighting sufficient to improve seeing in high-risk areas and situations would result in individual responses to an imminent accident speedily enough to prevent the occurrence.   Street and highway intersection lighting to high intensities is being tried in the United States.   The lighting on motor vehicles of United States specifications is patently inadequate, as the beam does not reach to the stopping distance of the vehicle at 60 mi/h.   Glare from on-coming vehicles is an obvious limitation on what a vehicle lamp can project.

6   Natural light has bactericidal power primarily due to the UV component.   The desiccation of organisms deposited or in suspension by the heat effect of natural light contributes to the kill.   Laboratory data support these contentions.   Epidemiological data are not in common coin.   This bacterial kill is of value in our total environmental effort to hold down the transmission of communicable diseases.

Figure 10-2 from Ref. 10-5 is a general graphic scaling of the benefits of higher-intensity lighting to accomplish a visual task.   The resultant benefits are graphed as increases in accuracy, speed of seeing, sensitivity to contrast, visual acuity, and ocular motor accommodation reserve.   Note that a factor of 10 applies to intensity required for like increases between light tasks and dark tasks.   The curves display data from observations on seeing responses of many volunteer subjects in diverse seeing situations.

Illumination Characteristics and Their Measurement

White light is an unequally distributed mix of visible frequencies from 7.9×10^{14} Hz (380 nm) through 3.85×10^{14} Hz (780 nm).   There is a segment of UV and infrared, above and below the visible range in the white light.   Table 10-1 states the physical

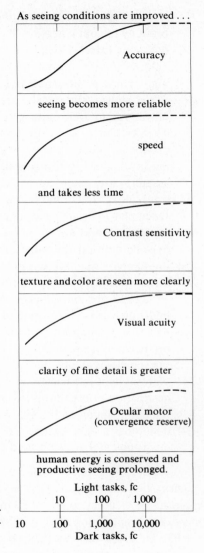

FIGURE 10-2
The benefits of good lighting in accomplishing the visual task. (*Source*: *Redrawn from Ref*. 10-5, *p*. 5.)

parameters.   This was the visible spectrum which Newton discovered when he passed white light through a prism.   The short-wavelength violets and blues bend more than the longer-wavelength oranges and reds, which produces the rainbow band.   The sequence in Table 10-1 is from high frequencies to low and from short wavelength to long. The numbers for the color bands in the table are approximate, as there is a continuous gradation.   Some data sources end the red band at 3.95×10^{14} Hz (760 nm).   Indeed, when it comes to seeing, there is little help to the human eye outside the range 7.5×10^{14} Hz (400 nm) to 6.3×10^{14} Hz (700 nm).   Note that the color bands are not uniform in width.   Blue and yellow have quite narrow ranges.

Table 10-1 introduces color definition by the temperature of a blackbody radiator.   The colloquialisms "red hot" and "white hot" are physical realities.   These are the absolute temperatures in kelvins at which a perfect blackbody radiator will display that color, (0 K equals $-273°C$).   Color temperatures can in actuality be a characteristic of incandescent materials.   General-purpose tungsten filament incandescent lamps have color temperatures in the range of 2600 to 3000 K.   Studio flood lamps have filament temperatures of 3100 to 3400 K, close to the melting point of tungsten, 3500 K.   Color temperature is used to specify the degree of whiteness and spectral composition of sources of illumination.   The degree of whiteness can be stated in *apparent color temperatures*, although the sources are not incandescent materials and hence not at such temperatures.   Such designations are imprinted on various types of fluorescent tubes.

Units of Measurement

Once upon a time the units of lighting were based on an international standard candle of prescribed composition not very different dimensionally from a common kitchen candle.   The unit of luminous intensity is now the *candela*.   It is one-sixtieth of the

Table 10-1   THE VISIBLE RANGE DEFINED AS COLOR, FREQUENCY, WAVELENGTH, AND COLOR TEMPERATURE

Color	Frequency, Hz $\times 10^{14}$	Wavelength, nm*	Color temperature, K
Violet	7.9–6.65	380–450	
Blue	6.65–6.15	450–490	Pale blue 8000 K
Green	6.15–5.35	490–560	White 5000 K
Yellow	5.35–5.18	560–580	3000 K
Orange	5.18–5.0	580–600	
Red	5.0–3.85	600–780	800 K

* One nanometer (nm) equals 1×10^{-9} m and is equivalent to 1 millimicron.

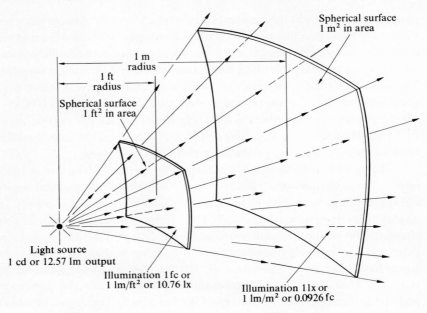

FIGURE 10-3
A schematic of lighting units, the canedla, the footcandle, and the lumen. (*Source*: *Ref.* 10-6, *p.* 5.)

intensity of a square centimeter of the surface of a blackbody radiator at the temperature of molten platinum, 2047 K. Of course, if you want a luminous source equal to 1 or more candelas (cd), you purchase a carefully made and precisely calibrated incandescent lamp and control the applied voltage. Two practical sets of units immediately emerge from the candela. These and their relations are displayed in Fig. 10-3. The candela, still pictured as a candle in Fig. 10-3, puts out a luminous flux. The intensity of light from that flux at a distance of 1 ft is 1 footcandle (fc). The "quantity," or perhaps better, the luminous power of a source which uniformly lights 1 ft^2 of surface to an intensity of 1 fc is 1 lumen. Figure 10-3 shows a 1 ft^2 segment of sphere of a radius of 1 ft, illuminated to an intensity of 1 fc and therefore receiving 1 lumen. As that sphere has a total of 12.47 ft^2, the 1 cd at its center has a luminous power output of 12.47 lumens. For metric use, the process is related to a 1-m distance and results in 1 lux of intensity, equal to 0.0926 fc, as the inverse-square law applies. The luminous power is not changed, but it is distributed uniformly across a square meter. We specify footcandles as the desired intensity at the point of the visual task. Lighting design is the process of having the number of lamps and their distribution of light so that their output in lumens delivers the specified number of footcandles at the point

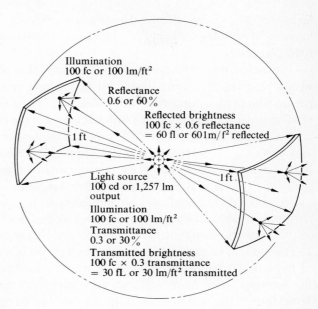

Illumination
100 fc or 100 lm/ft²

Reflectance
0.6 or 60%

Reflected brightness
100 fc × 0.6 reflectance
= 60 fl or 60 lm/f² reflected

1 ft

Light source
100 cd or 1,257 lm
output

1 ft

Illumination
100 fc or 100 lm/ft²

Transmittance
0.3 or 30%

Transmitted brightness
100 fc × 0.3 transmittance
= 30 fL or 30 lm/ft² transmitted

FIGURE 10-4
A schematic of lighting terms, reflectance, reflected brightness, transmittance, and transmitted brightness. (*Source*: *Ref.* 10-6, *p.* 5.)

required and specified.   We order footcandles at the visual task surface and purchase lumens at the lamp.

There is a very large spread between those two numbers due to three things:

1 The inverse-square law applies.
2 Reflectance is considerably less than 100 percent and hence a loss in reflected brightness.
3 Transmittance is usually considerably less than 100 percent.

All this arises from the fact that we see brightness, not the light beam itself.   We see what is reflected or emitted by a luminous surface.   In lighting terms, this is brightness and is expressed in footlamberts or in candelas per square inch or any area unit. Therefore, we perceive or see footlamberts, the light emitted or reflected.   A surface which emits or reflects light perfectly at the rate of one lumen (lm) per square foot of area has a brightness of 1 footlambert (fL) viewed from any direction.   The unit is named for Johann Heinrich Lambert, a German scientist of the eighteenth century. Figure 10-4 shows the relations of reflection, transmission, and adsorption.   Note that a 100-cd source puts 100 lm/ft² on the surfaces at a radius of 1 ft and provides 100 fc. The surfaces in Fig. 10-4 have reflectance factors of 60 percent and transmittance factors of 30 percent.   Thus, the reflected brightness is 60 fL.   Of the initial 100 lumens, 10 have been absorbed.   Therefore, the absorbtion factor of these surfaces is 10 percent.

A major limiting behavior of brightness is that of having too much of it in the wrong place at the wrong time.   Misplaced or ill-timed brightness is glare to the person who finds it interfering with his seeing.   The glare of the high-beam headlights of an approaching car interferes with the seeing of the driver of the second car, indeed can be dangerously blinding.   The driver of the first car has the benefit of the bright-ness of his high-beam lights.   He sees better,   When he switches to the low beam, the illuminated path before him is shortened, narrowed, and diverted from the center of the road.   The second driver is grateful for less glare.   Uncontrolled sources of trans-mitted and reflected brightness are difficult to manage to the satisfaction of all in both natural and artificial illumination design and practice.

Measures of brightness enter in another matter vital to efficient and easy seeing. It is the ratio of brightness between the center point of visual task upon which the fovea of the retina is being focused and the large visual field within the eye's view, called the *surround*.   The fovea subtends an angle of not more than 2° encompassing the visual task.   The *near surround* is the zone subtended by an angle of about 60° covered by the peripheral retina of the eye.   Whatever is in view beyond is defined as the *re-mote surround*.   The physiology and optics of the process of seeing are intricate.   It is recognized that optimum conditions prevail when the brightness ratios between the visual task and the surround are 1:1.   This is achieved in uniform daylight and nearly so with luminous panel lighting, which has high and uniform brightness at the trans-mitting surface.   Satisfactory conditions prevail when the brightness ratio of the visual task to the near surround is 3 or 4:1.   Figure 10-5 diagrams the relations.   Slightly different terms and values are used, as these were the choices of M. Luckiesh, a fore-most investigator on the subject, at the time he set down his ideas.

Most of the brightness we see is reflected light.   Reflectance is expressed as a percentage of incident light.   Figure 10-6 shows a simple method of approximating reflectance with an inexpensive light meter, and then an example of the arithmetic of its determination from observations.   Figure 10-7 shows three types of reflection, diffuse, spread, and glossy, and gives examples of surfaces which produce them.   These occur from all surfaces.   Reflection makes seeing a fact, as our eyes see things because of reflected light or recognizable differences of brightness, shadow, and color.   Color is our response to selective absorption and reflection.   Fresh grass is green, as it reflects light in the frequency of 6.65 to 5.3×10^{14} Hz (490 to 560 nm).   All other inci-dent ranges of energy are absorbed by the grass, including those which energize photo-synthesis.   The management of reflectance and its undesirable manifestation as glare is a necessity in lighting design and practice.   It is paramount in the selection of mat-erials and shapes of luminaires.   A luminaire is that part of a lighting fixture that

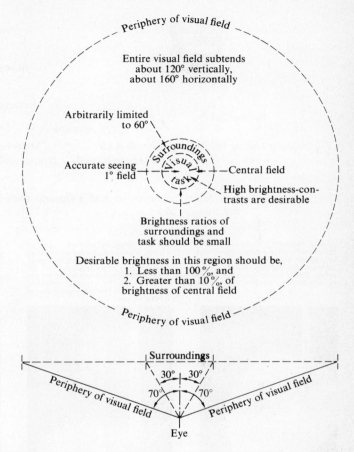

FIGURE 10-5
A diagram of the visual field of the human eye, showing the areas of vision and desirable brightness ratios. (*Source: M. Luckiesh, "Light, Vision and Seeing," Van Nostrand Reinhold Company, New York.*)

transmits, reflects, or absorbs the lumen output of the lamp housed in the fixture. The specifications of the luminaire manufacturer must be known and used well to get efficiency from the electricity consumed to light the lamp.   Reflectance is determined by the finish of a surface, its texture, and its color.   Composition enters in the case of paints containing high-reflectance particulates in their pigment.   Lighting manuals and handbooks provide reflectance data on usual surfaces and finishes.   Paints vary from a 75 to 90 percent reflectance from flat matte whites to 10 to 15 percent for the reds.   The use of reflectorizing paints for road striping and traffic signs for easier night seeing and consequently for safety are familiar.

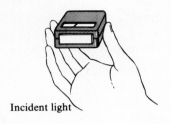

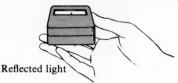

Cell 2″–3″ from wall (no shadow)

Reflected light

Incident light

Example

Meter reading with base against wall = 65   Meter reading with cell facing wall = 40

Reflectance of wall: $= \frac{40}{65} = 60\%$ (approx.)

FIGURE 10-6
Reflectance measurements with a General Electric 213 light meter. (*Source: Ref.* 10-6, *p.* 20.)

Diffuse reflecting surfaces, such as matte paint, fresh white plaster, blotting paper, and magnesium carbonate produce no bright mirror image spots. These surfaces appear almost equally bright from all angles of view.

Spread reflecting surfaces, such as etched aluminum, spread the light so the source is not definitely mirrored. The diffusion is incomplete, and the surface brightness varies with the viewing angle. This type of reflecting surface is useful for wiping out source irregularities.

Glossy diffusing surfaces, such as glossy paint, glossy paper and porcelain enamel show a combination of diffuse and specular reflection. The glossy finish produces a small specular component at the angle of reflection.

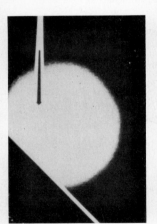

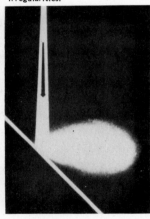

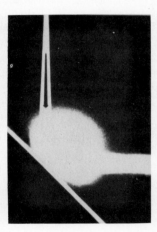

FIGURE 10-7
Three types of reflecting surfaces. (*Source: Ref.* 10-6, *p.* 19.)

The Control of Lighting and Lighting Standards

There are four elements of lighting that are controllable in artificial illumination design and practice: footcandles, brightness ratios, color, and glare.

Footcandles The number of footcandles provided at the visual task and the surroundings are readily and economically a matter of choice. The development of inexpensive

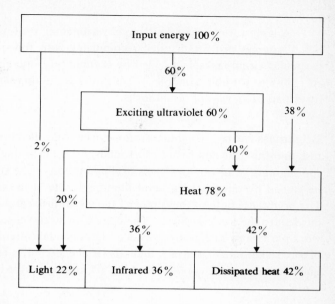

FIGURE 10-8
The energy distribution in a typical cool white fluorescent lamp. (*Source*: *Ref.* 10-7, *p*. 18.)

and durable lamps, the availability of low-cost electricity, and the acceptance and expectation of good lighting have permitted a steady rise in footcandle recommendations for specific tasks and for general lighting during the last 50 years. Classroom lighting of 10 to 15 fc was considered satisfactory in the 1930s. Today, levels of 100 fc are common, and 200 not unusual. Precision assembly areas as in electronic component plants go to 500 fc.

The two cardinal characteristics of a lamp are its lumen output per watt and its heat output which must be dissipated. The visible light output of a fluorescent lamp totals a still disappointing 22 percent of the input energy. The balance, heat, is that dissipated at the lamp and luminaire, 42 percent, and that transmitted as infrared, 36 percent. The lumen output per watt of such a 40-W fluorescent is from 75 to 80 lumens. The lamp puts out a total of 3,000 to 3,200 lumens. Figure 10-8 diagrams this energy distribution. A comparable lumen output from an incandescent tungsten filament lamp is 2,700 lumens from a 150-W lamp. That is 18 lm/W. In such a lamp the energy output is about 10 percent as visible light, 70 percent as infrared, and 20 percent as internal heating of gases which cool the tungsten filament and of the lamp materials. Whether from fluorescent lamps or incandescent ones, the heat loads from artificial illumination of buildings is an energy that can be utilized in cold seasons and that must be included in computing cooling system capacities for summer air tempering.

A large variety of tables from governmental, professional society, and manufacturers' sources provide detailed recommendations for specific footcandle values for particular visual tasks subdivided by occupations, operations, and locations.   Reference 10-5 is a usable example.   Table 10-2 is an alternate guide to footcandle levels for broad categories of visual tasks.

Brightness ratios   Brightness ratios can be controlled between the center of the visual task and the near and remote surrounds.   The attachment of many to high-intensity spot lighting results in low levels of illumination of the surrounds.   Better seeing can be gained by raising the general illumination level to reach lower brightness ratios. The brightness ratio at the center of the visual task rarely depends on the footcandles incident to the work surface.   These are usually sufficient.   It is the reflectance of the work pieces and background surfaces that demands attention.   The texture and finish of the background surfaces frequently can be altered to reduce reflectance with consequent increase of the contrast between workpiece and the background surface.

Color   Color is a manageable component of lighting as we well recognize from our continuous response to our visible surroundings.   Three examples of light and color manipulations are (*1*) show effects on stage, screen, and TV tube; (*2*) interior decoration use to express the desires of owners, occupants, or decorators; and (*3*) color coding for safety and hazard identification, which is a productive supplement to industrial lighting practice and is worldwide in traffic designations of go, slow down, and stop.

Table 10-2   FOOTCANDLES RECOMMENDED FOR FIVE CLASSES OF VISUAL TASKS, EXAMPLES OF THESE, AND THE BRIGHTNESS EMITTED IN FOOTLAMBERTS AT A 60 PERCENT REFLECTANCE

Class of visual task	Examples of such work	Range, fc	Range, fL
Most difficult	Precision instrument making, jewelry making	700 and up	420 and up
Very difficult	Fine benchwork and machining, sewing in low-contrast colors	200–700	120–420
Difficult	Drafting, proofreading, classroom, and office	70–200	42–120
Ordinary	Rough benchwork and machining, medium assembly, and inspection	30–70	18–42
Easy	Rough manufacturing processes, as in clay, concrete, and steel products	Below 30	Below 18

Glare Glare has already been identified as misplaced brightness. Motor vehicle drivers and riders recognize that by day and by night. It holds for many sources, low sun positions at dawn and dusk, high-beam headlights by night, and reflections from wet or ice-glazed roads. These are examples of direct glare. A less evident form of glare is from the bright sources in the peripheral visual field. The eye responds to such sources by increasing and decreasing the iris opening. The iris adjustment may not be advantageous to the visual task in the central visual field. That results in continuing changes in iris opening. The eye has three accommodations to reach optimum seeing: iris opening, focus, and convergence. When these are continuously responding to change without reaching a fairly stable state fitted to the task and the lighting, the ineffectual adjustments produce the conditions of eye strain. The form of glare that is most likely to produce that response is veiling glare. It is the excessive brightness reflected from the background of the visual task. The most common experience of veiling glare is in the reflections from glossy finished paper. The ubiquitous and variable sources of glare make its control difficult. Management of the color and texture of reflecting surfaces that come in the anticipated light paths is the most productive approach. Careful placement of luminaires in relation to the surfaces and position of the visual task reduces the risk of veiling glare.

The Management of Daylight

Daylight illumination of the interiors of our homes and workplaces has been in the hands of architects and builders with surprisingly little help or concern of others, except occasionally troublesome clients. Before energy sources for lighting and heating became unlimited, at least to the wealthy, architects had to compromise interior illumination from natural light with heat losses and, in some seasons and latitudes, heat loads through the light openings. When that compromise was not imposed, magnificent use of natural light testifies to the ingenuity of architects and builders. The medieval cathedrals of Western Europe, the edifices of Central India of which the Taj Mahal is best known, and the temples of Southeast Asia are wonders of natural light use and control.

In the western temperate zones, building designers with an armamentarium of thermal control and artificial lighting, of special-purpose glass, and of window structural materials are working in both extremes of windowless buildings and all glass-faced buildings. A balance is surely in the offing. John Marston Fitch, Professor of Architecture of Columbia University, put it this way:[1]

> For most purposes, however, the windowless building seems not only impracticable but also undesirable. Apart from the question of cost (involving the expense of the lighting system and the cooling needed to remove the waste heat it produces), people do not

[1] J. M. Fitch, "The Control of the Luminous Environment," *Sci. Am.*, **219**(3):192

relish being cooped up in a windowless building. Human vision and well-being apparently suffer when vision is restricted to the shallow frame of man-made perspectives and is denied the deep views of nature. That eye wants variety in the optical conditions and freedom for occasional idle scanning of a visual field broader than the work at hand. In the home and at work people hunger for view windows, if only to "see what the weather is like outside."

Some rules on windows for natural lighting of a room have evolved. Some are in building codes. Most were in school sanitation guides and standards of the 1930s, receiving avid attention particularly for rural schools before the electric line came down the road.

1 A window area to floor area ratio of 1:4 is optimal.
2 The window height should be one-half the room depth for satisfactory distribution.
3 The top of the window should be as close to the ceiling as possible.
4 Ceilings should have white matte finishes for high reflectance. The wall areas between windows should be in light finishes to diminish contrast between windows and wall areas.
5 The windows should have from one-half to one-third of their area present a "sky picture." That is, the viewer should be able to see a piece of sky. In an effort to produce that, generally unsuccessfully, building codes in large cities required minimal distances between walls with windows and setbacks in multistoried buildings. The setbacks were also intended to admit direct sunlight to street levels for part of a day.

All these desirable features of fenestration arise from the very rapid decrease in light intensity as measurements are taken from a window sill into the depth of a room. In direct sunlight, sill readings with the sun overhead will range from 6,000 to 10,000 fc. At the far corner from that window the readings will be from 30 to 50 fc. Factories, shops, arcades, and occasional hotel lobbies and stairwells are illuminated by skylights and sawtooth roof construction. An initial architectural decision which is an important factor in natural-light use is the orientation of the building and the choice of which walls should have windows and which should be windowless. Because of the wide swing of apparent sun position from the winter to summer solstices in the temperate zones, a wholly satisfactory choice is not achieved. The choice is easier in the equatorial zones, as the apparent sun position varies very little.

Building orientation and window position are supplemented by light control devices. These include shades, venetian blinds, exaggerated overhangs, fixed and movable vertical sun deflectors, awnings, prismatic glass, and glass blocks with selective transmittance and diffusion. One development of recent years is tinted glass carefully fabricated for selective transmittance and reflectance. Some tints and their transmittance are bronze, 51 percent; neutral gray, 42 percent; and blue-green, 75 percent. Glass that absorbs infrared is in commercial production to reduce interior heat loads. So is one-way mirror glass with a thin layer of metal on the inside.   This allows privacy through all-glass walls as one can see out but not in.   Drapes, shades, and blinds are not needed.   The entrance of infrared is reduced.   A most startling product of glass technology is photochromic glass.   This glass darkens under the incidence of ultra-violet, blocking high-intensity sunlight.   As the ultraviolet intensity diminishes, the glass proportionately regains transmittance.   It is practical to hold a nearly steady level of sunlight intensity through photochromic glass.

Fitch, already cited above, closed his article this way:[1]

> It is apparent that the nature of the luminous environment exerts profound physiological, psychological, social and economic effects of life in our urban culture.   So far neither the effects nor the possible means of ameliorating them have been adequately analyzed.   Obviously the establishment of a harmonious relation between man and his new environment of artificial illumination calls for cooperative studies by physical and biological scientists, engineers and architects.

LASER, COHERENT LIGHT

In 1917 Albert Einstein stated the basis for the laser phenomenon.   In 1960 T. H. Maiman built and operated a ruby-crystal device that emitted coherent light at a frequency of 4.35×10^{14} Hz (694.3 nm in wavelength).   Einstein's postulate was fulfilled.   Since Maiman's first device, a growing family of laser devices has flooded the scientific scene. These have found amazingly rapid utilization ranging from aligning a subway tunnel under the San Francisco Bay to virtually bloodless liver surgery at a medical sciences center in Cincinnati.   The predicted major use as a communications carrier is yet to come. Its fantastic use in holography which projects a three-dimensional image from a plane hologram, produced by laser light and projected by it, is a fact which challenges the adage "Seeing is believing."   Laser is an acronym of *light amplification by stimulated emission of radiation*.   That radiation is a photon, a quantum of electromagnetic energy. The first laser photons were in the visible range, but their range has already been extended, commercially into the infrared, and experimentally into the ultraviolet.   Although the observed injury from laser energy absorption in man has been limited to eye and skin burns, the wide use of laser devices in teaching, research, and industrial laboratories and in a variety of practical applications requires the management of their output (Ref. 10-8).

[1] Ibid.

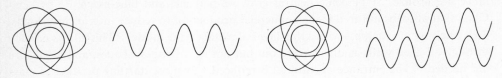

FIGURE 10-9
Photon multiplication by stimulated emission.   (*Source*: *Ref*. 10-8, *p*. 9.)

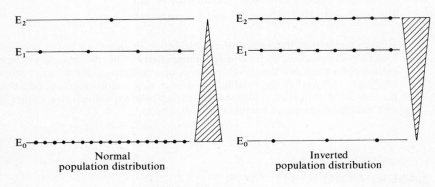

FIGURE 10-10
Illustration of population inversion.   (*Source*: *Ref*. 10-8, *p*. 12.)

The Production and Characteristics of Laser Energy

Einstein said that if a photon released by an excited atom interacted with a similarly excited atom, that second atom would release a second photon identical in frequency, energy, direction, and phase.   Furthermore, the first photon would continue on its way unchanged.   One has produced two.   The two can replicate the action if similarly excited atoms are encountered.   Figure 10-9 diagrams the events.   In a laser device, mirrors or prisms at the ends of the unit send the identical photons back and forth along the path until a cascade of photons pass through one of the reflectors which is less perfect in reflectance.

In order to produce laser energy from a medium, say, a ruby crystal, a very large number of its atoms must be in an excited state.   That is, the electrons of the atoms are at an energy level above their ground state designated as E_0.   Normally, only a few atoms will have their electrons at excited states, designated as E_1 and E_2.   The necessity is to invert that distribution among a population of atoms.   Figure 10-10 shows the normal population distribution and the inverted population distribution, or population inversion.   Excitation is achieved by "showering" the laser medium with

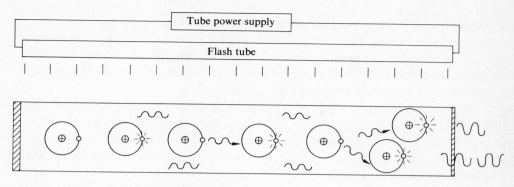

FIGURE 10-11
Schematic of a laser-energy-generating device.   (*Source*: *Ref.* 10-10, *p.* 4.)

an energy which is readily absorbed by the medium's atoms and raises its electrons to excited states such as E_1 or E_2.   In the case of a ruby crystal, a xenon flash lamp directs its output of 5.52×10^{14} Hz (or 545.1-nm wavelength) to raise the electrons of the chromium in the aluminum oxide structure of the ruby to an E_2 excited state.   Figure 10-11 is a schematic of a laser generator.

A laser device has three components.

1 The medium in which the population inversion of millions of excited-state electrons will be created.   In a ruby crystal these are in the chromium atoms which are the impurities in the aluminum oxide and which give the ruby its characteristic color.

2 A source of energy external to the medium which will "pump" in the energy. On absorption of that energy the electrons of the absorbing atoms go into their excited state.   The source is called the *pump* in laser devices.   For a ruby laser, the pump is a xenon flash lamp.   It is similar to a xenon strobe light used in photography, with higher outputs.   It is mounted along or around the ruby.

3 A space in which the photon production is controlled to produce the necessary photon cascade is the third component.   It is called the optical cavity.   For a ruby laser, it is the rod of ruby itself with its ends polished and silvered.   One end is less silvered.

The laser energy leaves the optical cavity through that end.   It is a beam of coherent light at 4.35×10^{14} Hz and wavelength of 694.3 nm.   It can be focused, refracted, and reflected.   It is a brilliant red.   It carries a high energy of visible light which diverges very little along great straight-line distances.   For example, a ruby laser beam in use to align the San Francisco Bay subway tunnel is 2 in wide at the source and diverges to 9 in at the receiving camera $1\frac{1}{2}$ mi away.   Its energy is manifest as heat in the absorbing bodies.   Thus, it can be used to burn holes of exact dimensions, as in diamonds for wiredrawing dies.   It can burn precise patterns on metal-foil-covered surfaces, as in cutting and shaping electronic circuit boards.   It can "weld" detached retinas back in place, but it can also burn healthy retinas of the eyes of unsuspecting people who look at the direct beam or high reflection of it.

      There are three major types of laser media, solid state, gas, and liquid.   The ruby crystal is the solid state in widest use.   Gaseous laser media include a mix of 90 percent helium and 10 percent neon; carbon dioxide, which emits infrared; argon; and krypton.   The liquids are organic dyes which emit coherent light of specific frequency and wavelength, depending on the dye and its concentration.   A fourth type of laser medium is a sandwich of two layers of semiconductor materials.   These have high efficiency and small size.   Gaseous media are pumped by electrical discharge through the gas, which produces electron collisions.   The liquid media are pumped by a laser beam from a solid-state laser.   The photon cascade is produced in the optical cavities with sets of mirrors or prisms to direct beam propagation.   The beam delivered is usually continuous for low-power beams, and pulsed for high-power beams.   Short, powerful pulses can be produced by the technique of Q-switching.   The Q-switch interrupts and delays the photon cascade in the optical cavity until a very high level of population inversion is reached.   Then all these excited electrons join to produce a short and powerful pulse of laser energy.   These techniques result in pulsed laser devices in distinction to continuous-wave lasers, denoted as CW lasers.

The Properties of Laser Energy and Their Application

Four properties of laser energy make it unique, useful, and dangerous.   These properties are:

1 Divergence is very slight compared with a usual noncoherent light beam.   As a result the energy of a laser beam is not markedly dissipated as it travels.   A helium-neon laser device produces a beam with divergence of 1.5 to 4 minutes of arc. This property is used in range finding and in plane surveying.

2 Laser media output is very nearly monochromatic.   A ruby laser's output is at 4.35×10^{14} Hz (694.3 nm) in the red spectrum.   Related to its monochromaticity is laser energy's behavior in an interferometer.   This permits measuring and controlling distances in such diverse operations as metalworking and earth moving.   It allows precise measurement of earth settlement, building sway, and bridge movements.

3 Laser energy is spatially coherent in frequency, phase, amplitude, and direction. This means that all points in all three dimensions remain equidistant as the wave propagates.   Coherent light can be focused into a very narrow beam.   Its

energy can be transmitted to an absorbing body with precise control of the locus. High-energy density levels can be applied to very small areas.   This makes laser energy useful in piercing and cutting materials, in welding minute electronic components, doing attachment surgery, and removing tatoos from human skin.

4   Despite cumbersome and unfamiliar units, the intensity of laser energy can be appreciated when compared with the emission from our sun.

The sun at its surface: 7×10^3 W/(cm^2)(sr)(μm)
Laser energy now produced : 1×10^{10} W/(cm^2)(sr)(μm)

That is an intensity difference of 1.4×10^6 times, nearly 1.5 million times.

The units used describe the intensity of pulsed bursts.   Laser devices and their outputs are rated in joules (J) for their energy, and in watts or joules per second for their power.   A device emitting 10 J of laser energy in 1 s is a 10-W laser.   If 10 J were released as a pulse that lasted 0.01 s, the source would be a 1,000-W laser device. It is these levels of energy and power and the ease of focusing them that make piercing, cutting, and welding of very hard materials a rapid task for laser energy.   The absorbed energy is transformed to heat in the material receiving the laser beam.   Power density is expressed in watts per square centimeter.

The Biological Effects of Laser Energy Absorption

The primary mechanism of laser energy absorbtion is heating, a thermal effect.   This is linear.   It is the consequence which is best documented in animals and man.   There is an array of secondary and even tertiary events that is not well defined due to the wide variations in the energy received and the absorbtion mechanisms of the live tissue. These effects are not proportional to the energy absorbed and are therefore grouped as nonlinear.   These are mechanical, including impulse and recoil in the target tissue; pressure effects from thermal expansion of heated tissue and tissue water and from shock waves; and three which appear to be unusual and minimal: ionization effects, the formation of free radicals, and the generation of harmonics of the absorbed energy wavelengths (Ref. 10-9).

The critical organs of experimental animals and men for laser absorption are the eye and skin.   As skin injury is usually immediately evident, repairs itself readily, or can be remedied by grafts, the eye is the organ of principal concern.   The eye is a remarkable optical system with a variable lens opening controlled by the pupil dilation or contraction, a variable focal length by eyeball axial length change, and a specialized set of receptors in the retina and its central structure, the fovea.   It has a protective cover transparent to visible light, the cornea.   Figure 10-12 provides an orientation to the elements of the anatomy of the eye.   The questions that must be answered are:

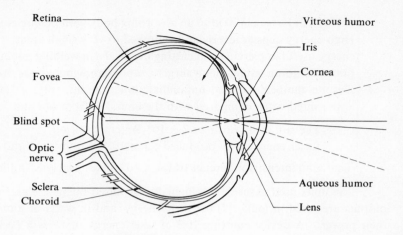

FIGURE 10-12
Schematic of the human eye.   (*Source*: *Ref.* 10-8, *p.* 29.)

1   What energies are absorbed?
2   Where in the eye are these absorbed?
3   What is the effect of the heating of that part of the eye?
4   Are there any subsequent events which are injurious?
5   Is the event a single acute effect with or without repair?.   Are there delayed effects?
6   Are there cumulative effects after repeated repairable effects?   Are there cumulative effects from absorptions which do not produce clinically observable damage shortly after the identified exposure?

Within a year of Maiman's invention of the ruby laser device in 1960, Solon, Aronson, and Gould wrote on the ocular hazards of laser energy.[1]   As the ruby laser was the first and is the most widely used, the most extensive observations on eye injury are on laser energy at 4.35×10^{14} Hz (694.3 nm).   There have been major exposures and a few serious eye injuries.   The retina is the critical part of the eye for laser energy in the near ultraviolet, visible, and near infrared ranges.   These ranges are transmitted through the human ocular media with an 80 percent transmission in the range of 500 to 950 nm.   Light at 694.3 nm at axial incidence has at least 94 percent transmission to the retina.   Three eye conditions affect the probability of retinal damage by laser in transmissible ranges.

[1] L. R. Solon, R. Aronson, and G. Gould, Physiological Implications of Laser Beams, *Science*, **134**:1506 (1961).

1 The pupil size determines how much light enters the eyes.   Wide open for dark seeing, say, a 7-mm diameter, is the worst condition.   Closed down to 2 mm as in daylight, the pupil contraction restricts laser light entry.

2 The degree of pigmentation of the retina and choroid determines absorption. More pigmentation results in more absorption and more injury.   There are wide variations in the pigmentation of these structures among individuals and within areas in the eyes of each of us.

3 The size of the image focused on the retina determines the area of the absorption of the incident energy.   A greater image size results in a greater absorbing area with consequently less energy transfer per unit area and less damage.   Time of exposure and the rate of retinal temperature rise and of heat dissipation are conditions of exposure and absorption which affect the risk of damage.   These in turn are determined by the beam energy, beam power density, and whether the beam is pulsed or continuous.

The present accepted hypothesis for the effects of ruby-laser damage to the retina is that the melanin in the pigmented epithelium of the retina absorbs most of the energy.   The heating of tissue changes the proteins by denaturing and coagulation. Further heating vaporizes the tissue water and may produce steam which disrupts the tissue.   At the threshold for a retinal burn in rabbit eyes, sufficient to cause slight coagulation, temperature rises of 12 to 20°C above the normal of 39°C have been reported (Ref. 10-9, pp. 2).

In 1971 the American Conference of Governmental Industrial Hygienists published five values for certain stated wavelengths and operational modes of laser energy. These cover Q-switched and non-Q-switched pulsed laser energy at 694.3 nm in energy density at the cornea, continuous-wave laser energy from 400 to 750 nm in power density at the cornea, and pulsed and continuous-wave laser energies in the visible, near infrared, and infrared wavelengths for skin protection.   The values are maxima, or *ceiling values*, and apply to the occupational setting.   The numerical values are not stated here, as these should be read in the context of Ref. 10-11 (pp. 62–64).

The biological consequences of skin exposure are much less than for ocular exposure.   The greater the degree of pigmentation, presence of hair, and the hair color, the greater the risk of skin injury.   Thick keratinized surfaces are protective.   The consequences of skin absorption range from immediate mild reddening and loss of sensitivity to the touch which lasts 4 to 5 days, to superficial charring, crusting, and even ulceration.   The effects of repeated, chronic exposures are not yet established beyond cases of hypersensitive individuals.   The laser energy levels that may injure the skin exceed the corneal-surface threshold levels for the eye by 100,000 to 1 million times. Skin exposure effects are confined to the surface layers, as absorption is complete and penetration very slight.

Safe Practices for Laser Use

1 Avoid looking at the primary beam or strong reflections of it, and do not align the beam by eye.

2 Work in high illumination levels to keep the pupil of the eye contracted.

3 Safety goggles are specific for particular wavelengths. Use those that correspond to the beam wavelength generated.

4 Target backgrounds and test patches must be of low reflectance and fire-resistant.

5 There are electric shock, electric fire, and x-ray risks at the high voltages required for many units.

Special precautions are required in using high-powered, pulsed lasers, CO_2 infra-red-generating lasers, and CO_2 N_2 gas lasers in which UV is generated in the optical cavity by the electron-discharge gas encounters. The use of lasers out of doors requires clear paths, free of pedestrians, vehicular, and airborne traffic. Even rain, snow, dust, and fog make the operation risky for others. There must be vigilant control of the curious and of horseplay by the operators and their fellow workers. The risk of injury to domestic animals, pets, and wildlife requires attention.

THE RADIO FREQUENCIES AND MICROWAVE

Table 10-3 and Fig. 10-1 provide a closer look at this most useful segment of the elec-tromagnetic energy spectrum. The table comprises all frequencies less than infrared and correspondingly wavelengths longer than infrared. Note that in microwave oven range, the wavelengths are from 10 to 100 cm. In the AM radio broadcast range the wavelengths are from 10,000 to 100,000 cm (or 100 to 1,000 m). Short-wave radio falls in wavelengths of from 1,000 to 10,000 cm (or 10 to 100 m). In Fig. 10-1, it is clear that the term microwave is applied to the three highest frequency ranges of the radio frequencies, the ultrahigh, superhigh, and extrahigh frequencies. This is a range of from 3×10^7 Hz (30 MHz) to 3×10^{11} Hz (300 GHz). Microwave in usual military and civilian use is in a slightly narrower range, 50 MHz to 10 GHz. The range of photon energies in electronvolts corresponding to the last two frequencies are 2×10^{-7} to 4×10^{-5} eV. These are very small values compared with 1.24 eV for red visible light. The wavelengths for the frequency range cited is from 6 m to 3 cm. These lengths have a bearing on microwave behavior when a human body is in the beam. The low energies of the photons account for failure of microwave and radio frequencies to produce ionization in the absorbent materials. Hence, these are identi-fied as nonionizing radiations.

The primary effect of absorbing nonionizing radiations is heating. That, of course, is the basis of microwave ovens in manufacturing operations, in commercial food processing, as warmers in food-vending machine lines, and for kitchen cooking. The interaction of microwaves and of material in their path depends on the conductivity of the material. A nearly perfect conductor, such as any metal, reflects microwave energy completely. That is the basis for radar detection and tracking. A perfect insulator provides no absorption mechanism and only some reflection at its surfaces; therefore, there is transmission. Biological tissue interacts in an intermediate way; there is some surface reflection, some absorption, and some transmission. The thickness of the tissue largely determines the proportions reflected, absorbed, and transmitted. The depth of penetration depends on frequency; penetration decreases as frequency increases. Depth of penetration is about 2 cm at 300 MHz, about 5 mm at 3 GHz, and less than 1 mm at 30 GHz.

The power of microwave is expressed as power density in an appropriate fraction of a watt per square centimeter. The measurement is meaningful at a point some distance from the source, termed the *far field*. In the far field the power level follows the inverse-square law, and the radiation pattern has sinusoidal properties in time and locally in space. Close to the microwave generator, there are complex patterns dependent on the source and its surroundings. This is called the *near field*. There is no adequate instrumentation for measuring power densities in the near field. Presently, assessing exposures close to the high-powered radar generators and antennas, such as those which produce very directive beams for military use, is complex. Military and support personnel have been exposed to high near-field strengths inadvertently through failure to follow prescribed operating procedures. Some precautionary measures have been difficult to observe in the close quarters aboard radar picket planes

Table 10-3 THE EIGHT REGIONS OF RADIO FREQUENCIES IN DECADES OF WAVELENGTH IN CENTIMETERS, IN FREQUENCY UNITS, AND BY SOME ASSIGNED USES

Designation	Wavelength by decades, cm	Frequencies, multiples of Hz	Some assigned uses
Very low frequencies	10^7–10^6	3–30 kHz	Radio telegraphy
Low frequencies	10^6–10^5	30–300 kHz	Radio beacons
Medium frequencies	10^5–10^4	300 kHz–3 MHz	AM broadcast
High frequencies	10^4–10^3	3–30 MHz	Transoceanic short-wave
Very high frequencies	10^3–10^2	30–300 MHz	FM radio and TV
Ultrahigh frequencies	10^2–10	300 MHz–3 GHz	Microwave ovens, radar, and some diathermy
Superhigh frequencies	10–1	3–30 GHz	TD2 radar, microwave communications relay
Extrahigh frequencies	1–0.1	30–300 GHz	Wave guide, TE 0.1

and ships, particularly immediately after the installation of new high-powered or additional units. Except for direct exposures during generator-tube repair, near-field strengths in civilian applications are controlled by enclosures, positioning in space, and delineating nonentry zones.

In the near field, which is up to 100 m in front of the antenna in certain military radar units, the average power density remains quite constant with distance and the wavefront has extreme field curvature and power density variation. In the area beyond this, the far field, the wavefront is planar and average power density decreases with the inverse of the distance squared. In microwave communication the far-field power densities are in the order of microwatts per square centimeter. In radar detection and tracking the emitted beam in the far field is in the order of milliwatts per square centimeter, and the reflected beam in the order of microwatts per square centimeter. In ovens, microwave is a power delivery system. Therefore, within the oven cavity the power density is in the order of watts per square centimeter. Otherwise, that round of beef would not be cooked so grandly. The magnetron tubes of home ovens deliver about 800 W of microwave power. However, outside the oven, with door closures and seals and with interlocks and power controls functioning as designed and built, the levels within 2 or 3 cm of the door-cavity seal will not exceed 1 mW/cm^2. Home microwave ovens are entirely safe, provided operating procedures are followed, interlocks and safety devices are not compromised, and the door seal is kept clean and to tolerances prescribed by the manufacturers (Refs. 10-12, 10-13).

The Biological Effects of the Upper Frequencies

As Jacques A. d'Arsonval recognized tissue heating at 100 kHz in 1890, and as patients were given "long-wave diathermy" at 1 to 3 MHz by 1900, the thermal energy transfer in tissue from the radio frequencies has not been news. The Federal Communications Commission assigns six specific frequencies for medical diathermy, 13.56, 27.12, 40.68, 915, 2,450, 5,850 MHz, and 18 GHz. Note in Table 10-3 that these lie in frequencies from high to superhigh. The 915 and 2,450 MHz are the frequencies used for home microwave ovens. The questions on biological effects of microwave energies are:

1 How much heating is there in predictable human exposure?
2 What tissues or organs are critical?
3 What has been the evidence of injury to date?
4 Are there tissue responses other than heating?

Heating effect   The heating effect of absorbed microwaves has been measured in doll phantoms and calculated by Lawrence D. Sher and associates at the University of Pennsylvania (Ref. 10-13, pp. 441–453). Considering absorption variations of fat and

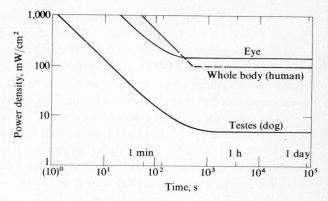

FIGURE 10-13
Estimated threshold levels for three sensitive structures versus time and power
density of microwaves, in milliwatts per square centimeter. (*Source: T. S. Ely
et al., Res. Rep. Proj. NM*001 56.13.02; *March* 21, 1957, *Nav. Med. Res. Inst.,
Bethesda, Md.*)

muscle, of angles of incidence, and of frequency, it was concluded that absorption is
somewhat less than 100 percent. Using the U.S. Armed Forces' level of 10 mW/cm²
as safe and 1 m² as a man's exposed unilateral body area, the absorbed power is 100 W.
This is comparable to our bodies' basic metabolic rate of 70 to 80 W.   Adding moderate activity to the basic metabolic rate produces about 300 W; 1 W equals 0.86 kcal/h.
As we know from diathermy, the microwave frequencies do penetrate and do produce
heating deeper in the body's tissue and organs to some degree.   Heat exchange mechanisms are not effective for deep heating.   Anesthetized rabbits exposed for 30 min to
microwave at 2,500 MHz, a 12-cm wavelength, showed temperature rises of more than
40°C in their small intestines, although rectal temperatures rose less than 1°C.   Rats,
rabbits, and tranquilized dogs exposed to power densities of not more than 100 mW/
cm², ten times the Armed Forces safe level, died of induced fevers.   No animal survived exposures that raised the body temperature to 44°C, 112°F.   A continued exposure to 25 mW/cm² maintained a body temperature increase of 1°C (Ref. 10-12, pp.
434, 435).

Critical tissues and organs   The issue of critical organs other than the whole body
has centered on the eye, with cataracts as the consequence, and on the testes, with
infertility as the consequence.   Figure 10-13 (Ref. 10-12, p. 435) summarizes the estimates of T. S. Ely and a team of investigators at the U.S. Naval Medical Research
Institute, Bethesda, Maryland, the estimates being based on animal exposures and three
terminal temperature points in the structures.   The tolerable terminal temperatures

were taken to be 39.0°C (102.2°F) for the whole body, 45.0°C (113.0°F) for the eye, and 37.0°C (98.6°F) for the testes. As indicated in Fig. 10-13, the power densities to maintain these temperatures are 100 mW/cm^2 for the whole body, 155 for the eye, and only 5 for the testes. The basis for the testicular temperature level is that undescended testicles which are at the body temperature of 37.0°C (98.6°F) are sterile. The power density of 5 mW/cm^2 is one-half of the U.S. Armed Forces safe level.

The first experimental evidence on cataracts resulted from exposure of rabbit eyes in 1949. The eye of the rabbit is well suited for study, as it is close to the human eye in size and structure. More recent information reported by S. Michaelson, H. D. Baillie, and R. L. Carpenter substantiate the earlier findings with some refinements of data from animal experiments (Ref. 10-14, pp. 41–46, 64, and 80). Microwave radiation has specific effects on the lens capsule. There are increases in capsule permeability, thermal coagulation of lens protein, reductions in ascorbic acid level, and inhibition of DNA and cell synthesis in the lens epithelium. There are increases in interocular temperatures up to the range of 45 to 55°C. Without a direct blood vascular connection, the eye cannot dissipate heat readily. Lens opacities following single exposures of experimental animals appear after a 1- to 7-day latent period. Cumulative effects are recognized when a single damaging event includes protein denaturation. Lesser injury is believed reversible by repair processes provided there are not repeat exposures before repair is complete. There has been animal confirmation of testicular temperature rises and reduced sperm production. But mating of mice and of rats and reproduction of dogs and of guinea pigs was not affected.

Evidence of injury The evidence of human injury, at least in the United States, has been confined to cataracts and lens opacities. The number has been remarkably small. To September 1969, M. M. Zaret found 44 reported cases of microwave cataracts, of which his own work accounted for 42. All were among young men without predisposing factors for cataracts. All had worked with high-powered radar systems and had had repeated exposures to power densities far exceeding 10 mW/cm^2 (Ref. 10-14, p. 82). Zaret has additionally reported a number of radar workers who have lens opacities revealed by meticulous examination and against a record of previous eye characteristics. In addition to Zaret's work, N. Telles found three published reports assessing possible effects of microwaves on radar workers. These covered fewer than 400 exposed individuals with less than 3 years in radar work (Ref. 10-14, p. 254). Controlled clinical and epidemiological studies of microwave workers simply have not been undertaken despite many such workers in military, governmental organizations, and governmental contractors.

Nonthermal effects The literature on biological effects of microwave energy absorption is rife with discussions on thermal and nonthermal effects. S. Michaelson reviewed such alleged effects as embryonic development differences, alterations in protein activities, behavior changes of amino acids in the liver and testes, genetic modifications, central nervous system and cardiovascular system changes and pearl-chain formation of tissue particulates.   He includes a quote from an extensive critical review: "However, a review of the literature, which claims the existence of such [nonthermal] effects, fails to be quantitatively convincing." (Ref. 10-14, p. 49.)   The physical basis for non-thermal effects is the concept of field-induced force effects.   The force of the electrical field effects real or induced charges in the absorbing material and affects the dielectric properties of the material.

Control of Microwave and Management of Microwave Workers

Protection depends upon the following:

1 The initial design and construction of the entire microwave unit determines its safety in use for its expected life.   This holds particularly for microwave ovens in general consumer use.   Control and safety depend on the integrity of the design, durability of all parts, quality of assembly, and ease of keeping filth from surfaces whose effective performance requires cleanliness.

2 Maintenance of the equipment in proper working order and wholly as designed and built.   Locking out safety switches, bypassing interlocks, and altering opening seals and shields is certain to risk exposure for the users.

3 Defining safe zones, using "in-service" signals, and limiting access to authorized personnel are standard operating procedures in radar installations.

4 Reflective barriers providing partial body shielding are of limited usefulness. Head surrounds of copper wire mesh are in test as eye protection.   Use and acceptance of such devices require persistent training and discipline.

The management of microwave personnel for health protection rests upon:

1 The worker's understanding of microwave behavior and its hazards.   Initial and repeated instruction is needed to gain such understanding.   The needs and means to accomplish this among home appliance repairmen working on microwave ovens in the Los Angeles area have been reported by J. C. Rogers and P. I. Gill (Ref. 10-15).

2 A preassignment eye examination for any lens opacities is necessary for the protection of all parties, employee, employer, insurance carriers, and any other third-party interests.   A detailed record of that examination and subsequent ones provides a baseline for the early observation of changes.

3 Supervision for compliance with operating procedures which incorporate safe practices must be part of the overall work plan.   Proper maintenance of all equipment is a component of safety. Periodic monitoring by skilled persons with well-calibrated instruments suited to the exposures reinforces the work forces' will to do their jobs without foolish breaches of built-in safety devices and established procedures.

The protection levels in use in the United States in 1972 cover occupational exposure and the performance tests on microwave cooking ovens at the factory for leakage. Both use the average power density values under far-field conditions. The occupational level is 10 mW/cm^2, and it is used by the Armed Forces and corporations such as General Electric, Raytheon, and the Bell Telephone System. The value is stated as a safe level for work-period exposure. The American Conference of Governmental Industrial Hygienists uses the same level for a control guide for continuous 8-hour workday exposure. Reference 10-11 (p. 65) provides the conference's full statement covering other levels and shorter time periods. Effective October 6, 1971, microwave commercial and home cooking ovens offered for sale in the United States meet a prior-to-sale performance test which limits emissions to 1 mW/cm^2. Furthermore, the ovens must meet an emitted-radiation level of not more than 5 mW/cm^2 throughout the useful life of the equipment.

POSSIBLE CHANGES AND DEVELOPMENTS IN THE USE OF CERTAIN SEGMENTS OF THE ELECTROMAGNETIC ENERGY SPECTRUM

No large increase in ultraviolet light use is indicated. Display lighting and spectacular show use is likely to continue as at present. Despite an energetic effort to control hospital-acquired infections, it does not appear that ultraviolet germicidal lamps are an important means of protection in the hospital setting. More elemental methods of disinfection, cleaning, and sanitary measures are producing more consistent results. Ultraviolet use for revealing invisible identification marks is expected to increase. Such use is readily managed, as low intensities on small areas is all that is required. The consequences of overexposure are directly evident as skin reddening and eye discomfort. Therefore, the warnings of misuse and failure to use protection should be sufficiently early to avoid repeated discomfort.

Artificial lighting will continue to be used more generously with higher intensities accepted and expected. This will surely lead to more careful designing and installation. Five elements are identified as requiring integration for a satisfactory lighting system: visual factors, thermal balances, noise effects from poor ballasts in fluorescent lamps, spacing and positioning of luminaires to get efficiency and to minimize glare, and esthetically pleasing responses. There is concern for people's response to spending long periods during daylight hours in windowless rooms and work areas. Extended investigations of such environments in schools, offices, and factories would be necessary to determine if there are unfavorable physiological or psychological responses.

Coherent-light generators, lasers, are certain to increase in number, in power, and in variety of applications. Their place in surgery is already assured as bleeding during cutting major organs is exceedingly small without recognized disadvantages in healing or of wound infection. The major predicted application of laser energy is as a communications carrier. Without neglecting other developments, the large communication companies of the United States are working on laser carriers for transmission of what are initially voice or sound inputs.

In the radio frequencies, microwave for heating and more specifically for cooking is most certain to have a great increase. In the United States, at the end of 1970 there were 120,000 microwave cookers in use. Only 40 percent of these were home units. The remainder were in institutions, restaurants, and on vending machine lines. Sales at the rate of 80,000 a year were expected to accelerate, so that by 1976, microwave ovens would account for 25 percent of the oven market. This would require sales of 1.8 million a year. With the oven manufacturers reconciled to the national performance standard, design and construction to meet it are underway.

Reference 10-16 presents extensive information on microwave heating in industrial processing in the United States in 1970. Examples are, in food processing: drying potato chips, precooking poultry and bacon, heat input required in freeze drying, and doughnut cooking; in the forest products industry: drying hard woods, veneers, and paper; and in other applications: sealing certain plastics, curing concrete, permanent-pressing fabrics, and drying leather, grain, film, and match heads. Speed, precision of control, and lower overall costs are causing, and will continue to cause, adoption of microwave heating.

Electromagnetic compatibility is one facet of conservation and control of that peculiar resource, the electromagnetic spectrum. One example which has been recognized for some 10 years by a few authorities confronting the problem is the sensitivity of certain types of cardiac pacemakers to electromagnetic radiations from external sources. These include electrosurgical and diathermy devices in hospitals, and close proximity to radar and communications systems. There have been isolated instances of interference from an electric shaver, from spark coils, and from gasoline engine ignition systems. With an estimated 50,000 patients wearing pacemakers in the United States, work is underway on the effect of microwave ovens on the demand type of pacemakers (Ref. 10-17). Under some conditions of leakage and of close proximity, microwave ovens do interfere with the normal outputs of demand pacemakers. Redesigning pacemakers to provide shielding against various sources of interferences is underway. Indeed, some pacemakers already have a high degree of shielding. On removal from the interfering field, the pacemaker resumes its normal performance.

The problem is not at all unmanageable. It may be a foretaste of others to come as further utilization of electromagnetic energy in various forms and for diverse purposes continues.

AN APPRAISAL OF MAN'S MANAGEMENT OF CERTAIN SEGMENTS OF THE ELECTROMAGNETIC ENERGY SPECTRUM

Man's utilization of ultraviolet, visible light, coherent light, and the radio frequencies, including microwave energies, has been remarkably free of grave or widespread injury to himself or to other forms of life. Certainly, more people are self-inflicted by sunburn from excessive exposure to the ultraviolet of the sun in a single summer than have been afflicted by overexposure to man-made sources of ultraviolet since their invention. Perhaps it is more to the credit of good fortune than great wisdom that these forms of electromagnetic energy have such a favorable health record. Other than for visible light and the radio communication frequencies, the number of people exposed to these forms has been quite few and usually in an occupational setting. Microwave in the home kitchen and public vending-machine line is a change in that pattern. However, there is clear evidence that microwaves from ovens at the point of manufacture are in good control. Furthermore, the injuries from these forms of electromagnetic energy that have been recognized to date have been specific, confined to rather severe exposures of a few, and nonfatal and remediable. These can be prevented with our present knowledge of source control and personal protective action. Compared with burns from fossil-fueled heat sources at work, at home, and at play, and compared with burns and fatal shocks from electricity, the toll from the energies under discussion has been exceedingly small. It can, of course, be said that artificial lighting has made man much more of a nocturnal animal with such unfortunate results as more exposure to accident hazards and risks of being a victim of night crime and of compromising social situations. Better light sources and fuller understanding of the benefits of good lighting are changing many badly illuminated workplaces, including office and commercial areas.

The second level of man's comfort and convenience can only be regarded as having been augmented by the use of the electromagnetic energies being considered. These range from the personal choice of lying under an ultraviolet lamp in midwinter, to seek solace from an aching muscle under medical diathermy. Of course, the largest convenience benefit is that of electric lighting. It is so taken for granted in the Western countries that it is a matter of complete astonishment to visit towns of considerable size in other countries of the world where electric lights are still to come or, more commonly, where electricity is supplied only from twilight to midnight or 11 o'clock.

On the level of ecological balances, there has been no evidence of disturbances from the electromagnetic energy sources under discussion. Neither animal nor plant life has undergone changes due to man-made ultraviolet, visible light, or the radio frequencies. Man has manipulated plant and animal behavior and growth rhythms by exposure to ultraviolet and visible light. He accelerates plant growth by artificial light. He puts egg-laying chickens on forced feeding to increase egg production by lengthening the chicken's day by artificial lighting. Phototropic insects and animals are led into traps, and glare-blinded animals are killed in their confusion on roadways. There is clear evidence that microwave fields produce escape reactions in a variety of birds. Chickens and pigeons show immobilization and initiation of collapse or of flight. Seagulls tend to initiate flight. Birds in flight take avoiding action when they encounter a microwave field. These reactions have been studied, with their possible usefulness for clearing airfield flight paths of birds hazardous to aircraft by collision or by being drawn into jet-engine intakes (Ref. 10-14, p. 185). A remarkably fortuitous event is that not man, nor other animal forms, nor plants have shown any observable damaging physiological response to the communication frequencies of 3 kHz to nearly 300 MHz. The energies, the wavelengths, and the power densities usually in use may account for this lack of observed unfavorable response. There have been observations that in proximity to the antenna structures of very high-powered naval radio transmitters there are electric field strengths that may be injurious to man (Ref. 10-14, p. 222). There have also been reports of individuals who convert radio frequencies directly to audio responses in their brains without the usual receiver apparatus (Ref. 10-14, p. 260). One explanation has been the particular array of metal fillings in their teeth or metal pins in repaired joints. At any rate, these bits of evidence suggest that electromagnetic fields of various sorts may produce some kind of interaction in biological systems. As man's use of these energies continues to increase and as power levels rise, watchfulness will be in order not only for effects on man but on life around him.

REFERENCES

10-1   Spectrum Engineering—The Key to Progress, IEEE and EIA, Jt. Tech. Advis. Comm., 1968.

10-2   HANDLER, PHILIP (ed.): "Biology and the Future of Man," Oxford University Press, New York, 1970.

10-3   Black Light, *Gen. Electr. Large Lamp Dep., Tech. Publ.* 125, Nela Park, Cleveland, Ohio, 1969.

10-4   Light and Color, *Gen. Electr. Large Lamp Dep., Tech. Publ.* 119, Nela Park, Cleveland, Ohio, 1968.

10-5   Footcandles in Modern Lighting, *Gen. Electr. Large Lamp Dep.*, *Tech. Publ.* 128, Nela Park, Cleveland, Ohio, 1969.

10-6   Light Measurement and Control, *Gen. Electr. Large Lamp Dep.*, *Tech. Publ.* 118, Nela Park, Cleveland, Ohio, 1965.

10-7   Fluorescent Lamps, *Gen. Electr. Large Lamp Dep.*, *Tech. Publ.* 111, Nela Park, Cleveland, Ohio, 1970.

10-8   VAN PELT, W. F., H. F. STEWART, R. W. PETERSON, A. M. ROBERTS, and J. K. WORST: Laser Fundamentals and Experiments, *Bur. Radiol. Health*, SWRHL 70-1, 1970.

10-9   Biological Aspects of Laser Radiation, *Bur. Radiol. Health, U.S. Public Health Serv., Publ.*, 1969.

10-10   Laser Safety Standards Announced, *Safety Standards*, **17**(6):1–5 and 12 (November–December 1968).

10-11   Threshold Limit Values of Airborne Contaminants and Physical Agents—1971, *Am. Conf. Gov. Ind. Hyg.*, 1971.

10-12   MUMFORD, W. W.: Some Technical Aspects of Microwave Hazards, *Proc. IRE*, **49**:427–448 (February 1961).

10-13   SHER, LAWRENCE D.: Interaction of Microwave and RF Energy on Biological Material, *Bur. Radiol. Health, Div. Electron. Prods.*, 70-26, 1970, pp. 431–464.

10-14   CLEARY, STEPHEN F. (ed.): "Biological and Health Implications of Microwave Radiation," *Bur. Radiol. Health*, 1970.

10-15   ROGERS, JACK C., and PHILIP I. GILL: A Survey of Microwave Oven Repair Procedures in the Los Angeles Metropolitan Area, paper at *APHA Annu. Meet., Houston, Texas*, 1970.

10-16   Survey of Selected Industrial Applications of Microwave Energy, *Bur. Radiol. Health, Div. Electron. Prods.*, 70-10, 1970.

10-17   RUGGERA, PAUL S., and ROBERT L. ELDER, "Electromagnetic Radiation Interference with Cardiac Pacemakers," *Bur. Radiol. Health, Div. Electron. Prods.*, 1971.

11

THE ENERGIES OF HEAT AND SOUND

HEAT AND MAN

The Mechanisms of Heat Transfer

The heat transfer processes are conduction, convection, radiation, and evaporation. In maintaining his heat balance, man has a minimal dependence on, or use for, conduction, as it depends on direct contact. To be sure, there is conduction while walking barefooted on hot sand or on a cold tile floor. Convection is a special case of heat conduction to a fluid and the movement of that fluid, as a warm air current, or cold water current, to facilitate heat transfer. Air movement is a very significant factor in cooling or heating man. A part of that is heat transfer by convection. Radiation is the transfer of heat as electromagnetic energy in the infrared range, 7.5×10^{14} to 1.5×10^{12} Hz (0.7 to 200 μm). The earth and human body radiate principally at 3×10^{13} Hz (10 μm). In most situations evaporation is the major means of cooling for man as the air temperature rises above 28.6°C (75°F). Relative humidity is a paramount factor in the success of evaporative cooling. The inhibiting effect of high relative humidity on evaporative cooling is recognized in the summer euphemism, "It's not the heat, it's the humidity that's killing me." The effectiveness of evaporative cooling is due to the transfer of 580 cal to each gram of water that is energized from the liquid to the vapor state at body temperature.

The heat exchange between the human body and the environment results from a balance of five rates:

1 The rate of body heat production q_M, the metabolic heat which is determined by activity. Typical q_M rates are shown in Table 11-1 in both British thermal units (Btu) per hour and kilocalories per hour; 1 Btu equals 0.2520 kcal.

2 The rate of convective transfer q_C, which may be plus if the surrounding air blanket is warmer than the body, or minus if it is lower. Note that in home heating by warm air systems, the air temperature is not actually warming the body. It is damping down the rate of loss by convection, usually augmented by various layers of clothing.

3 The rate of radiation q_R, which is a gain if there are radiant sources in direct line of transmission that are at a higher temperature than the body. This is the warming experience before an open fire, a steam-heated radiator, or an electric heater. The q_R will be minus when the surroundings are below body temperature. This is the experience in standing in a cold walled cave or basement. The radiant flux is from the mass at the higher temperature to that at the lower

Table 11-1 ESTIMATES OF BODY HEAT PRODUCTION FOR VARIOUS TYPES OF ACTIVITY

Kind of work	Activity	q_m,* Btu/h	kcal/h
Light work	Sleeping	250	62.5
	Sitting quietly	400	100
	Sitting, moderate arm and trunk movements (e.g., desk work, typing)	450–550	112.5–137.5
	Sitting, moderate arm and leg movements (e.g., playing organ, driving car in traffic)	550–650	137.5–162.5
	Standing, light work at machine or bench, mostly arms	550–650	137.5–162.5
Moderate work	Sitting, heavy arm and leg movements	650–800	162.5–200
	Standing, light work at machine or bench, some walking about	650–750	162.5–187.5
	Standing, moderate work at machine or bench, some walking about	750–1000	187.5–250
	Walking about, with moderate lifting or pushing	1000–4000	250–350
Heavy work	Intermittent heavy lifting, pushing or pulling (e.g., pick and shovel work)	1500–2000	375–500
	Hardest sustained work	2000–2400	500–600

* Values apply for a 154-lb man and do not include rest pauses.
SOURCE: Ref. 11-1, p. 119.

temperature.   This is in accord with Clausius' second law of thermodynamics. Rooms heated to about 21°C (70°F) by radiant panels, floors, or ceilings frequently bring occupant complaints.   They do not have a sense of warming as the radiant flux is low.

4   The term q_E is the rate of evaporative cooling.   It is always a loss in heat regulation of the human body.   The environmental determinant of this rate is the amount of water vapor already in the air relative to the amount that the air can hold at that dry-bulb air temperature, the saturation value.   The body's evaporative cooling devices are the sweat glands secreting body fluid to the skin surfaces.   When these skin surfaces are uncovered and when the relative humidity of the air is low, evaporation of sweat proceeds efficiently and immediately.   It will not be so in a high-humidity, high-temperature air such as in a tropical rain forest.   Any air movement helps, as it sweeps away the saturated air layer close to the skin to bring in less-humid air.   At a 100 percent relative humidity in still air at body temperature, evaporative cooling is at a standstill.

5   The final item is q_S, the rate of change of heat stored in the body.   This is reflected in body temperature readings, oral or rectal.   The body is not much of a heat sink, plus or minus.   There can be limited short withdrawals at low-temperature exposure, but soon there is a shutdown of the blood circulatory transfer rate.   The body sacrifices its extremities and exposed surfaces to freezing.   The body's capacity for storage of metabolic heat or of excess heat received is quite limited.   Any condition which does not permit loss of all metabolic heat results in storage and an immediate body temperature rise.   A few individuals can continue to work with body temperature rises above 39°C (102°F) to nearly 40°C (104°F), but most people drop sharply in productivity or just drop.

The relation of the five rates is stated by

$$q_M = \pm q_C \pm q_R - q_E \pm q_S$$

with the units either British thermal units per hour or kilocalories per hour.   Table 11-1 shows q_M values for different levels of human activity.   Figure 11-1 shows the responses of the five rates of heat exchange as the dry-bulb air temperature rises from 10°C (50°F) to 43°C (110°F) at a relative humidity of 45 percent.   The data are for clothed subjects seated at rest.   Note that q_S rises above the zero line at the point at which total heat loss drops below heat production.   Above 37°C (98.6°F) at a relative humidity of 45 percent, the body depends solely on evaporation to maintain a thermal balance.

Dropping the q notation, using only the subscript capital letters, and doing an algebraic transposition, the relation among the five heat rates can be expressed to show that the body maintains thermal equilibrium when $S = 0$.   Thus from

$$M \pm C \pm R - E = \pm S$$

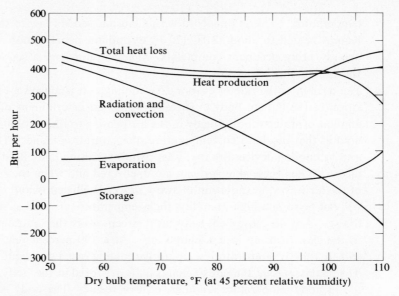

FIGURE 11-1
Rates of body heat production and of exchanges with the environment for healthy, young, clothed men seated at rest.   [*Source: Ref.* 11-1, *p.* 114.]

there is equilibrium at

$$M \pm C \pm R - E = 0$$

This formula was first suggested by C. E. A. Winslow and associates in 1936.[1]   It continues to be the basis for all analyses of the body's heat exchange response to external thermal stresses.

The Physiological Effects of Heat Stress

Hooke's law of the mechanics of materials is that within the elastic limit, the strain, deformation, or other change is proportional to stress, the load.   All is well, and all the structural members bearing the load return to normal shape when the stress is removed.   When the stress produces a strain beyond the elastic limit, deformation is permanent and well may tear the member asunder in complete failure.   Heat stress on man follows Hooke's law with three evident, measurable strains:

1   Increased sweat loss.
2   Increased heart rates.   See Fig. 11-2.

[1] C. E. A. Winslow, L. P. Herrington, and A. P. Gagge, *Amer. J. Physiol.*, **116**:641 (1936).

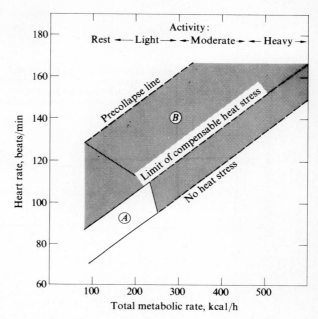

FIGURE 11-2
Effect of heat stress on heart rate at different levels of energy expenditure.
[*Source*: *Ref.* 11-2, *p.* 15.]

3 Increased heat storage causing rises in deep body temperature reflected in rises
in rectal temperature.   See Fig. 11-3.

When these strains exceed the elastic limit, each in turn results in the acute failure sig-
naled by:

1 Heat cramps
2 Heat prostration or exhaustion
3 Heat stroke or sun stroke

At the maximum body heat production given in Table 11-1, 600 kcal/h (or 2400
Btu/h) in an external temperature about equal to body temperature, a man can hold
his thermal equilibrium by producing and evaporating 1 liter of sweat per hour.   That
is a high rate of sweat loss and cannot be sustained for a whole working day.   Recorded
values do not exceed 12 liters in 24 hours.   The limitation is not the performance of
the sweat glands but the strain on the water and salt balance of the body (Ref. 11-2,
p. 19).

In Fig. 11-2, note the ranges of heart beat from a low of under 70 beats per minute at " no heat stress " to over 160 at the "limit of compensable heat stress " and a heat

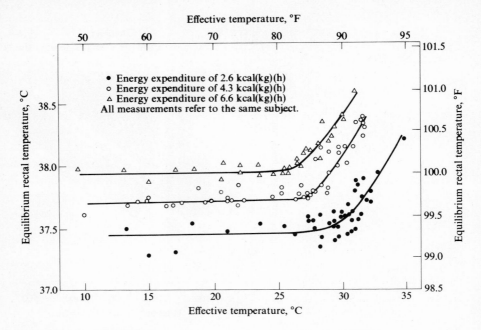

FIGURE 11-3
Equilibrium rectal temperatures at different rates of working at various effective temperatures. [*Source*: *A. R. Lind, J. Appl. Physiol.*, **18**:51 (1963), *WHO dwg.* 81667.]

production rate of 600 kcal/h (2400 Btu/h.) In the figure, *A* denotes a man doing steady, light work with a heartbeat of 100 per minute. Neither acute nor cumulative effects of heat stress will be felt by a healthy individual. The *B* denotes a man at moderate work in the heat with a heart beat of 142 per minute. It is tolerable for a fit young man for several minutes. Longer work periods will produce severe strain likely to produce acute failure. Short work periods must be alternated with recovery periods (Ref. 11-2, pp. 15–16). Laboratory studies suggest 100 heartbeats per minute as an allowable maximum during heat stress. That number is not applicable to a work setting without considering age, sex, health status, nutrition, and the intake of fluids and salt. The general level of sodium chloride with the daily diet in many countries appears to support the production of 5 liters of sweat per 8-hour shift in acclimatized men (Ref. 11-2, p. 19).

In making comparisons with other data, note that in Fig. 11-3 the work rate is in kilocalories per kilogram of body weight per hour. Using 70 kg (154 lb) as an average European, perhaps low for a United States male and surely high for an average adult male of most countries of Asia and Latin America, the work rates are 180, 300,

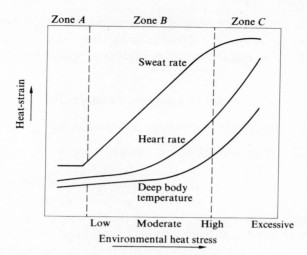

Zone *A*: No heat stress.
Zone *B*: Zone of increasing heat stress where sweat loss increases rapidly and nearly linearly
but through a large part of the zone, body temperature is not greatly affected. Strain
in terms of heart rate increases exponentially. Sweat loss is a good physiological
indicator of the heat strain experienced.
Zone *C*: Zone of increasing heat stress where sweat loss approaches or reaches its maximum
and can no longer be used as an index of stress or strain. Heart rate and body temperature
now rise rapidly and are the best physiological measures of the strain experienced.

FIGURE 11-4
Changes in sweat loss rate, heartbeat rate, and deep body temperature with
increasing environmental heat stress.   [*Source*: *Ref*. 11-2, *p*. 22.]

and 460 kcal/h (or 720, 1200, and 1840 Btu/h).   At the highest work rate, the break
point in rectal temperature equilibrium is at an effective temperature of 25°C (80°F);
for the intermediate rate, at 27°C (85°F) and for the lowest work rate, at 30°C (92°F).
These effective temperature values, which will be defined, can be simulated by a dry-
bulb air temperature of the same number at a relative humidity of 100 percent in still air.
    The data in Fig. 11-3 are all on the same subject.   Nevertheless, these are indic-
ative of the behavior of the body's heat exchange mechanisms.   As external exchange
by convection, radiation, and evaporation is slowed, the rising rectal temperature signals that thermal equilibrium is being lost.   Figure 11-4 summarizes the three elemental physiological responses, or heat strains, as the external heat stress rises from nil to
excessive through the ranges of low, moderate, and high.   Note the linear rise in rate
of sweat loss in zone *B*, that of increasing heat stress.   This observation has made the
rate of sweat loss an attractive physiological indicator of heat strain.   In zone *C* with
heat stress rising from high to excessive, the sweat rate levels off.   It would no longer
be a useful predictor.   Heartbeat rate and deep body temperature readily measured

by rectal temperature are in exponential rise from moderate heat stress at mid-range of zone *B* to excessive in zone *C*. These indicators are considered the best measures of heat strain in these ranges of heat stress (Ref. 11-2, p. 22).

Measurements of the Thermal Environment and Predictions of Heat Stress

Four physical measurements of the thermal environment are:

1 The dry-bulb temperature (DBT) is familiar to all, either in the Fahrenheit or Celsius (Centigrade) scale.

2 The wet-bulb temperature (WBT) introduces the rate of cooling by evaporation. A thermometer bulb is enclosed in a thin cloth sack which is kept wet. Uniform air movement is maintained by whirling the thermometer or by a mechanically blown current around the bulb. To the extent that evaporation takes place, the reading of the WBT is lower than the DBT reading. At vapor saturation in the air, there is no evaporative cooling. The WBT and DBT will be the same. The relative humidity is 100 percent.

3 The black-globe temperature (BGT) provides an index of radiant heating. A thermometer bulb is enclosed in a copper sphere about 4 in in diameter, usually painted a matte black. Infrared is well absorbed by the surrounding globe so that the thermometer gives a measure of the radiant temperature.

4 Air velocity strongly influences evaporative cooling and has some effect on convective transfer. It must be known to predict heat stress.

Combinations of the four measurements produce useful information on thermal stress and lead to predictions of that stress and of the resultant strain. Three of the combinations useful for defining comfort in heated and cooled spaces are illustrated. Three others which are useful to predict heat stress in hot work places are noted.

1 With the use of a table, nomograph, chart, or formula, readings of the DBT and WBT taken simultaneously yield the relative humidity expressed in percent. This is the weight of water vapor that is in the air at that DBT as a percentage of the weight of water vapor at saturation in the air at the same DBT. Figure 11-5 provides much more information, but it also gives relative humidities for observed DBT and WBT. At DBT 80°F and WBT 70°F, the relative humidity is just over 60 percent. A psychrometer is a pair of thermometers, one wet bulb and one dry bulb, mounted side by side with a means for uniform air flow across the wet bulb. The simplest form is the sling psychrometer. The two thermometers are mounted in an open frame which is rotated by hand with a peripheral speed of about 15 ft/s. That is a comfortable slinging motion of a frame about 1 ft long. The wet-bulb reading of itself is quite informative. In a report in

1904 on the health of Cornish tin miners, the Scottish physiologist and proponent of mine safety, John Scott Haldane, advised the Secretary of State for Health that in hot, humid mines whenever the WBT was higher than 85°F, the miners would be in increasing distress and could not maintain high rates of production.

2 The further information that Fig. 11-5 provides for known DBT and WBT is a subjective value called the *effective temperature*. This is an empirical index that has been in development and use in the United States for nearly 50 years. Trained subjects, young, healthy, white American men and women, many of them college students, responded, in test rooms, to varied combinations of DBT and WBT, and subsequently to air velocities, in a seven-point psychophysiological scale from cold, − 3, thru neutral, 0, to hot, + 3. Figure 11-5 plots data for clothed, sedentary subjects in essentially still air, having linear velocities of 15 to 25 fpm (feet per minute). A velocity of 50 fpm is a barely perceptible air movement. An approximate but satisfactory conversion to metric units is 1 m/s equals 200 fpm, more exactly, 196.8 fpm. The bell-shaped curve in the upper quadrant of Fig. 11-5 is the percentage distribution of subjects reporting themselves as comfortable at the corresponding diagonals for effective temperatures of 64° to 78°F. Each effective temperature diagonal is plotted as a continuing series of DBT and WBT readings with these two values also providing the relative humidity percentages plotted as another set of diagonals.

Effective temperature values are for use in comfort heating and cooling for sedentary activities. These are not for the high ranges of hot work spaces. At a latitude of 42°N, an effective temperature of 67 to 68°F (19.5 to 20°C) is satisfactory for winter in normal indoor clothes. In winter relative humidities above 30 percent are difficult to hold and result in condensation on windows; therefore a DBT of 73°F (22.8°C) would be needed. At a relative humidity as low as 10 percent, a DBT of 77°F (25°C) would be needed to reach an effective temperature of 68°F (20°C). A chart correcting for air velocities from 100 to 700 fpm with DBT and WBT readings from 30 to 120°F (−1 to 48.9°C) for sedentary and light work activities is available (Ref. 11-1, p. 117).

3 Figure 11-6 shows a nomograph in metric units, which includes air velocities. It allows use of the BGT readings and therefore takes radiant heat sources into account. It is for men working stripped to the waist. It provides a corrected effective temperature (CET) value. The readings are considered satisfactory for mild heat stress under intermediate humidity levels. It is not suggested for use in relative humidities less than 40 percent. There has not been a satisfactory means to take differing rates of work into account in using the CET chart. There has been enough experience to make clear that widely differing climates which may have the same CET reading do not produce the same heat strains of rectal temperature and heartbeat increases. The CETs of high DBT values with high

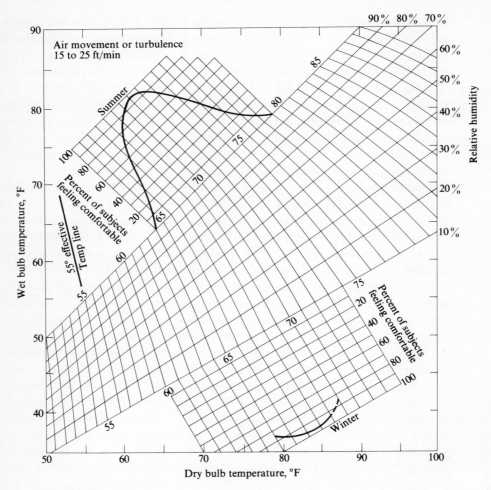

FIGURE 11-5

An effective temperature chart for air velocities of 15 to 25 ft/min. [*Source*: *Ref*. 11-1, *p*. 122.]

air velocities tend to exaggerate the heat stress. The CETs of high DBT and WBT values at low air velocities tend to underestimate the heat stress (Ref. 11-2, pp. 23–25).

To meet the demands for predicting conditions of hot work areas, formulas have been devised. Among these are the predicted 4-hour sweat rate (P4SR). By a nomogram the heat stress from sweat loss can be predicted for young, fit, acclimatized

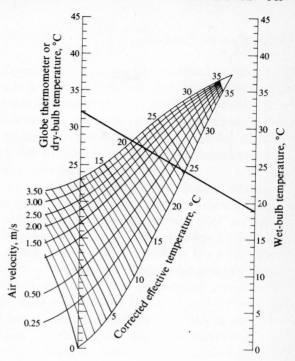

FIGURE 11-6
Corrected effective temperature chart in metric units for varying air velocities. [*Source*: *F.V. Lavenne, Rev. Inst. Hyg. Mines*, **29**(1):3 (1965), *WHO dwg.* 81 556.]

European men.   The knowns must include DBT, WBT, BGT, air velocity, clothing worn, and the rate of work.   Another formula is the H. S. Belding and T. F. Hatch heat stress index (HSI).   Values for R, C, and E of the basic formula

$$M \pm R \pm C - E = 0$$

at thermal equilibrium, are modified by a series of coefficients dependent on actual observations of BGT, DBT, air speed, and the vapor pressure in air.   A third formula, B. Givoni's index of thermal stress (ITS) is a mathematical model relating the sweat rate required to hold the thermal equilibrium, expressed by the basic thermal equilibrium equation.   Six coefficients are used to account for clothing, reflected radiation, and the man's position relative to the sun.   The DBT, air velocity, and vapor pressure in the air must be known.   In a conclusion on the P4SR, HSI, and ITS, the report of a WHO scientific group (Ref. 11-2, p. 29) states:

> All the indices of heat stress described above, as well as a number of others not considered, are regarded as having proved useful within specified limits.   In the long run, the thermal balance approach appears likely to have the widest applicability, because it is aimed at the development of a rational index, based on the physics of heat transfer. However, the important problem of relating the values to actual physiological strains, such as elevation of heart rate and body temperature, is still largely unsolved.

What Can Be Controlled?

For comfort heating and cooling of homes, public places and sedentary workplaces, such as offices and light assembly plants and also buses, cars, airplanes, trains, and passenger boats, control of the thermal environment is gained by regulating the DBT and relative humidity and by providing a moderate air movement of about 50 to 75 fpm (0.25 to 0.4 m/s). Existing effective temperature data is sufficiently satisfactory to define the requirements. These are then modified by the occupants to suit their activities, clothing habits, and in some instances cultural patterns and personal whims. Figure 11-7 makes clear that very small air volumes are required to replace the oxygen used in human respiration, about 1 cubic foot of air per minute per person, and about four times that rate to maintain carbon dioxide concentrations under 5,000 ppm by volume (0.5 percent). The requirements, as shown by curves C and D, for removing body odors and holding thermal comfort during moderate activity are considerably higher and dependent on the air space per person. These purposes of dilution ventilation during human occupancy were characterized by Professor F. S. Lee in a report on New York State school ventilation in 1923. He stated, "The problems of ventilation are physical, not chemical; cutaneous, not respiratory."

For the control of physiological distress and acute failure in hot work, the means of control are not as certain owing to human variation not only between ethnic groups, but within groups, and within the same individual. Nevertheless, a lot of practical preventive measures can be applied without delaying corrective measures because complete physiological data are not at hand for each ethnic cultural group for each climatic situation in each industry. There has been more than a bit of delaying action with "lack of complete data" as the excuse as industrialization and mechanization of agriculture move into the humid tropical and hot arid regions of the world. The plea of "we don't know enough" is not heard in providing comfort cooling in luxury hotels, bars, embassies, corporate offices, and the homes of the wealthy. Environmental measures that can be applied are:

1   Lower the relative humidity to improve evaporative cooling in hot areas. Isolate the hottest processes to minimum volumes and space to hold down the costs of dehumidification.
2   Provide the maximum of air movement by natural and mechanical ventilation. Natural ventilation can be improved by building orientation and construction of wall and roof openings to utilize prevailing winds. The day is past when the architecture of Birmingham factories has to be replicated in Bombay. Mechanically moved air should be directed to the hot work spots to cool the man.
3   Provide simple radiant-reflecting shields of aluminum between the man and the high-radiant source. Very few hot metallurgical operations require constant

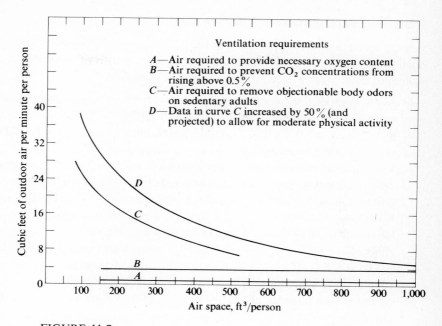

FIGURE 11-7

Ventilation requirements of spaces for human occupancy. [*Source*: " *Industrial Ventilation*," 11*th ed., sec.* 3, *p.* 3-1, *Am. Conf. Gov. Ind. Hyg., Lansing, Mich.,* 1970.]

attention. Shields with sight slots provide protection when the man is not directly manipulating the hot material.

Brief mention is in order on personal measures to minimize heat strain in man: Selection and acclimatization of individuals are practical measures at the time of hiring and training. C. H. Wyndham reports on procedures used in recruiting and preparing Bantu men for work in the hot South African gold mines (Ref. 11-4, pp. 177–203). There is no doubt of considerable variation in susceptibility to heat stress within a group having apparently like characteristics. Some sort-out can be made.

The provision of ample, accessible, high-quality water, of salt, and of rest intervals will help to keep heat strain within bounds. The promotion of good habits of personal hygiene and the provision of facilities to practice these during work hours are needed. Good nutrition, regular sleep patterns, moderate use of alcohol, cleanliness of body, clothing, and surroundings, and recreation contribute to the physical and mental well-being which makes severe heat stress endurable.

The Stresses and Strains of Extreme Cold

Military operations and exploration in the polar regions and high altitudes have provided ample and at times painful experiences on the strains of exposure to severe and prolonged cold. Four specific pathologies are identified:

1 Acute transient inflammation with considerable pain to exposed skin occurs when the skin temperature drops to 59°F (15°C). Numbness sets in at a skin temperature of 50°F (10°C). Under these conditions the peripheral circulatory system is alternately dilating and constricting.

2 Trench, or immersion, foot results from having cold and wet feet for several hours near the freezing point, as in the winter trench warfare of World War I. Blood and lymph ooze into the tissues of the exposed foot. Gangrene is the end point.

3 Frostbite occurs when the skin and tissue freeze. Freezing can begin at a tissue temperature of 28°F (−2°C), but lower ranges are more likely to produce the effect, 23 to 14°F (−5 to −10°C). Still lower temperatures of skin and tissue, +5 to −4°F (−15 to −20°C), cause necrosis and gangrene in as little as 10 to 15 min. Frostbite must be treated immediately to save the tissue. Rewarming by immersion in water at exactly 107.6°F (42°C) is recommended. Better yet, prevent it.

4 General body cooling, or hypothermia, causes blood at lower-than-normal temperature to be circulated to the heart and brain. At a rectal temperature of 92°F (33.3°C), brain function impairment begins. At 88°F (31.0°C), consciousness begins to slip away. At 80°F (26.7°C), coma is likely and cardiac performance is seriously disturbed. At a body temperature of 77°F (25°C), death is likely and is virtually certain at 70°F (21°C). Any extended immersion in water below 68°F (20°C) cools the body faster than any capacity to produce metabolic heat. Unless there is rescue, death is increasingly certain at lower temperatures. Survival times for water immersion are up to 8 hours at 62°F (16.7°C); 2 to 5 hours at 60°F (15°C); and about 1 hour at 40°F (5°C) (Ref. 11-5, p. 726).

In the cold air exposure, the DBT and wind velocity are dominant in determining tolerances. Values have been set for still-air temperatures for inactive subjects without special clothes or other protection. Tolerance, exposure times, and temperatures are 6 hours at −10°F (−23.3°C); 1½ hours at −40°F (−40°C); and 25 min at −70°F (− 56.7°C). Nude exposure is tolerable for only 8 hours at 40°F (7.6°C), which shows man's dependence on his clothing and shelter to hold his thermal equilibrium (Ref. 11-5, p. 725). Douglas H. K. Lee discusses three cold indices, including his own, and states that these are no more satisfactory than analogous attempts for hot environments. (Ref. 11-6, pp. 29–31). A concise and practical guide on analysis, measurement, and management of temperature extremes in the occupational setting with emphasis on environmental engineering is *Heating and Cooling for Man in Industry* (Ref. 11-7).

SOUND, THE UNWANTED FORM—NOISE

The opening sentence of the foreword by the editors of *Noise as a Public Health Hazard* (Ref. 11-8) is: " Noise—in the sense of ' unwanted sound '—has been a problem since Eve first poked Adam in the remaining ribs and told him to stop snoring." Characterizing noise as unwanted sound, as in Eve's case, means that it is defined subjectively. Noise is an objectionable sound. It is in the wrong place at the wrong time. It is told that Britishers living near the combat airfields of World War II blessed the roar of the nightly takeoffs to subdue the Nazi and gave thanks for each return, however faltering the engine sounds might be. With World War II ended, it was not long before nearby residents complained of the noise of night training flights. Just as glare is misplaced brightness, noise is misplaced sound. Furthermore, there are some disagreeable effects on hearing thresholds, speech intelligibility, and physiological states. Some of these effects are well documented by medical facts correlated with environmental measures. To that extent, the effects are not subjective but a normal response of a large portion of exposed people, with immediate recognition that a small portion are very sensitive to noise and another portion are able or willing to endure it.

The Nature of Sound, Units for It, and Its Measurement

Sound is a mechanical energy from a vibrating surface, transmitted by a cyclic series of compressions and rarefactions of the molecules of the material through which it passes. In a pure tone, the wave pattern of the alternating positive and negative sound pressure is an ideal sinusoidal form with fixed wavelength, frequency, and amplitude. As our experience indicates, sound is transmitted through gases including air, liquids, and solids. Only a vacuum, in which there are no molecules to compress and decompress, alternately, fails to transmit mechanical energy as sound. The speed of transmission is a function of the transmitting medium and its temperature. The speed in air is 340 m/s at 20°C (1,125 fps at 68°F). The speed of sound is proportional to the absolute temperature of air. In water, it is 1,470 m/s (4,860 fps). In steel, it is 5,000 m/s (16,500 fps). As in the case of light, all frequencies travel at the same speed. Frequencies are now expressed in hertz, equal to cycles per second. The audible range for an exceptionally good human ear is 35 to 20,000 Hz. A more limited range of 80 to 15,000 Hz is considered normal for young adults who have had no hearing losses or ear abnormalities. Even that range is wider than that in which most of us in adult years can hear. For the testing of hearing, the standard procedure is to use eight frequencies, 250, 500, 1,000, 2,000, 3,000, 4,000, 6,000, and 8,000 Hz.

A vibrating source producing sound has some total power expressed in watts and designated W. In free space that power is transmitted omnidirectionally in a spherical form. The intensity I is the power per unit area of the spherical boundary. Intensity

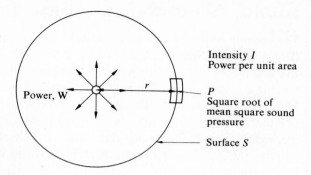

FIGURE 11-8
Relations of a sound source with a power of W (watts) to intensity I, and root-mean-square sound pressure. [*Source*: *Ref.* 11-9, *p.* N2-3.]

decreases inversely with the square of the radius r of the sphere.   Intensity is not readily measured directly.   Instruments have been devised to measure the effective sound pressure.   As sound pressure is alternately rising to a maximum pressure of compression and dropping to a minimum pressure of rarefaction, the square root of the mean-square sound pressure P_{rms} must be used.   The P_{rms} equals $0.707P_{max}$.   Derivations and calculations are given in Ref. 11-9 (pp. N2-3, N2-4).   Figure 11-8 diagrams the relations.

These values do not provide a practical unit for sound or noise measurement for two reasons.

1   There is a tremendous range of sound power and sound pressures produced. Expressed in microbars, one-millionth of 1 atmosphere of pressure, the range is from 0.0002 microbar (μbar), the minimum sound pressure a healthy young human ear can detect, to 10,000 μbars for peak noises within 100 ft from large jet and rocket propulsion devices.   In units of physics, 1 μbar equals 1 dyne/cm^2.

2   Our ears do not respond linearly to increases in sound pressure.   The nonlinear response is essentially logarithmic, as are our other sensory responses to odors, pressures, and weight differences.   This nonlinear response pattern is described by the Weber-Fechner law.

The needs are met by a term, *sound pressure level* (SPL), expressed as a logarithmic ratio to a reference level and stated in a dimensionless unit of power, the decibel (dB).   The reference level is 0.0002 μbar, the threshold of human hearing.   The expression looks formidable, but has the advantage of resulting in values of two and three integers for the SPL we experience in our increasingly noisy environment. The expression is

$$SPL = 20 \log \frac{P}{P_0} \quad dB$$

with P_0 equal to 0.0002 μbar.

Table 11-2 orients you to the decibel scale of SPL by giving examples of recognized noise levels, the sound pressure in microbars, and the SPL in decibels. Here are some examples of the arithmetic of the decibel SPL scale:

$$dB = 20 \log \frac{P}{P_{\text{ref}}},$$

where $P_{\text{ref}} = 0.0002$ μbar threshold for human ear response.

At $P = 0.0002$,

$$dB = 20 \log \frac{0.0002}{0.0002} = 20 \log 1 = 20(0) = 0$$

At $P = 0.2$,

$$dB = 20 \log \frac{0.2}{0.0002} = 20 \log 1,000 = 20(3) = 60$$

Table 11-2 THE DECIBEL SCALE OF SPL, WITH SOUND
PRESSURES IN MICROBARS, AND RECOGNIZED
SOURCES OF NOISE IN OUR DAILY EXPERIENCES

Sound pressure, μbar	SPL, dB/0.0002 μbar	Example
0.0002	0	Threshold of hearing
0.00063	10	
0.002	20	Studio for sound pictures
0.0063	30	Studio for speech broadcasting
0.02	40	Very quiet room
0.063	50	Residence
0.2	60	Conventional speech
0.63	70	Street traffic at 100 ft
1.0	74	Passing automobile at 20 ft
2.0	80	Light trucks at 20 ft
6.3	90	Subway at 20 ft
20	100	Looms in textile mill
63	110	Loud motorcycle at 20 ft
200	120	Peak level from rock and roll band
2,000	140	Jet plane on the ground at 20 ft

At $P = 20$,

$$dB = 20 \log \frac{20}{0.0002} = 20 \log 100,000 = 20(5) = 100$$

At $P = 20,000$,

$$dB = 20 \log \frac{20,000}{0.0002} = \log 100,000,000 = 20(8) = 160$$

The unit decibel is not uniquely reserved to describe the power of sound and noise. It will be encountered in other uses in electronic technology. As the SPL-decibel scale is logarithmic, decibel values are not additive. For example, an SPL of 74 dB from one source superimposed on one of 75 dB does not result in 149 dB. An SPL of 77.6 dB results. To determine the total effect, it is necessary to convert decibel readings to intensity ratios, add the intensity ratios, then reconvert the new sum back to a decibel value. Reference 11-9 (p. N2-5) details an example and more conveniently provides Table 11-3 for determining the cumulative decibel values of two or more known observations on individual sources. The value in the difference column in Table 11-3 is always added to the highest of the two decibel values being handled.

Very few sounds or noises are in a single frequency or pure tone. The human ear is not uniformly sensitive to all frequencies nor does it perceive noise equally across the frequency spectrum. For audiometry some scheme of frequencies had to be

Table 11-3   DETERMINING THE CUMU-
LATIVE DECIBEL SPL WHEN
THE DIFFERENCES
BETWEEN TWO OR MORE
LEVELS ARE KNOWN

Difference between levels, dB	No. of dB to be added to higher level
0	3.0
1	2.6
2	2.1
3	1.8
4	1.5
5	1.2
6	1.0
7	0.8
8	0.6
10	0.4
12	0.3
14	0.2
16	0.1

SOURCE: Ref. 11-9, p. N2-6.

agreed upon.   The use of three expressions of physical auditory stimuli, expressed in units unique to these, requires an analysis of the frequencies of the noise.   These are the loudness level in phons, the loudness in sons, and noisiness in noys or as the *perceived noise* level in decibels (PNdB).   Therefore, the frequency of sound is assigned an octave band distribution.   An octave is any frequency range with an upper value twice that of the lower.   Until 1960 the frequency limits generally used were 75 to 150 Hz, 150 to 300 Hz, and on to 4,800 to 9,600 Hz.   Since then by international agreement among workers in acoustics, the frequencies given in Table 11-4 have been in use. Each octave band is specified by the center frequency, which is the geometric mean of the high and low cutoff frequencies of a particular band.   Note that 125 Hz is not the arithmetic mean of 90 and 180.   It is the square root of their product.   Instruments for analyzing sounds by frequencies are called *octave-band sound analyzers*.   There are full-octave and divided-octave analyzers.   The usual division of an octave band is in thirds so that a high-quality analyzer produces readings on 24 one-third octave bands. There are two types of analyzers, a constant-bandwidth analyzer and a constant percentage bandwidth analyzer.   To interpret and to attempt to compare readings from the types of sound analyzers available, it is necessary to know what type was in use. W. Rudnose's excellent statement, Primer on Methods and Scales of Noise Measurement is recommended for those venturing to measure the noisy environment (Ref. 11-8, pp. 18–34).

Table 11-4   FREQUENCIES FOR ACOUSTIC MEASUREMENTS SHOWING THE GEOMETRIC-CENTER FREQUENCIES AND THE LIMITS OF THE OCTAVE FILTER PASSBANDS

Center frequencies, Hz	Limits of band, Hz
63	45–90
125	90–180
250	180–355
500	355–710
1,000	710–1,400
2,000	1,400–2,800
4,000	2,800–5,600
8,000	5,600–11,200

SOURCE: Ref. 11-10, p. 47.

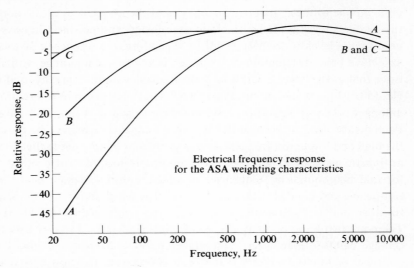

FIGURE 11-9
Frequency response curves of A, B, and C weighted networks on SPL meters. (*Source*: *A. P. G. Peterson and E. E. Gross, Jr., " Handbook of Noise Measurement," 5th ed., p. 8, General Radio Co., West Concord, Mass., 1963.*)

Before reaching the sophistication of a sound analyzer, field measurements are made with a sound-level meter. By a microphone, battery-powered amplifier, and meter scaled in decibels, SPLs are read. There is no separation into octave bands. There is a separation by means of electrical circuits known as *weighting networks*. These three networks, A, B, and C, have distinct responses to different frequencies. They simulate the characteristics of the sensitivity of the human ear for different frequencies. The ear has less sensitivity to frequencies below 400 Hz and above 10,000 Hz at low sound intensities. As can be seen in Figure 11-9, curve A is less responsive below 400 Hz than B or C is. The A weighted network is intended for use at low SPL, 55 dB or less. At high sound levels, human response shows less difference with frequency. The B network, used least in practice, is flatter than the A weighting. It is intended for SPLs from 55 to 85 dB. The C response is quite flat from 40 to 6,000 Hz. It is used for SPLs above 85 dB. It comes closest to indicating actual SPLs, as SPL is based on a flat response. When readings are not on the C network, the sound pressure should be recorded with the network letter as a suffix, as 50 dBA or 60 dBB. In the United States since 1969, the decibel A value has taken on added interest as permissible noise exposures of the Department of Labor are stated in exposure time in hours per day and decibel *A* sound level with the meter set for slow response (refer to Table 11-5).

Sound-level meters and sound analyzers are designed to measure steady noises with few interruptions.   Impulse noises, as from a drop-hammer forge or a gun, require a different arrangement of the instrumental elements of microphone, amplifier, and read-out.   The requirements depend on the frequency and the rise time to peak pressure of the impulse sound.   Readout is usually by an oscillograph, as dial indicators are too slow and easily misread.   Sonic boom from high-speed aircraft poses another measurement situation, as there is a time pattern described by a stretched out N with a compression peak and a rarefaction peak.   What must be determined is the peak-to-peak pressure difference.   Meaningful noise measurement requires the proper instrumentation in correct calibration in the hands of a skilled person (Refs. 11-8, pp. 18–28, and 11-10, pp. 40–51).

Effects of Noise

Information on effects of noise is best for hearing loss due to noise at work.   Other effects of occupational noise, except speech intelligibility interferences, are less certain. These are changes in psychological and physiological states, including annoyance and sleep interruptions.   The last two are the principal complaints against community and aircraft noise.   Property damage by actual vibrational or boom destruction and by depreciation because noise paths and patterns impinge on the property is known, and is to some degree measurable and predictable.   Effects on animals seem to have been studied very little.   These effects are of concern for wildlife around airports and along highways, and for fish and wildlife in the pathways of sonic boom.   In the first instances habitats may be lost, but the creatures have a chance to migrate and to reestablish beyond the reach of the noise.   If there are bad immediate effects on those in the sonic boom paths, there is no escape time.   Noise effects are examined as hearing changes and losses, interference with speech communication, annoyance and sleep interruption, other physiological and psychological responses, and the impairment of property values.

Two baselines are needed to evaluate hearing changes and losses ascribed to noise exposure.   These are provided in Fig. 11-10 and 11-11.   The first is the curve of auditory sensitivity.   It indicates that very much higher SPLs are needed for hearing at frequencies below 400 and above 8,000 Hz.   The human ear is most sensitive in the frequencies needed for hearing speech largely from 500 to 4,000 Hz.   It is a marvelous product of evolution.   Indeed, ears or hearing mechanisms of all animals are remarkable.   A splendid account of these developments is in Ref. 11-11 (pp. 38–75).   The second set of base lines, Fig. 11-11, shows the hearing-loss levels that come with age, presbycusis.   For speech communications, the severe losses illustrated in the

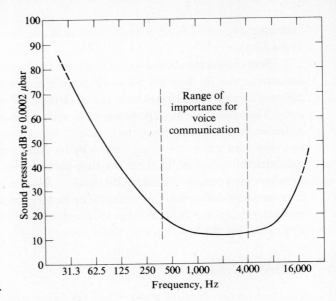

FIGURE 11-10
Curve of auditory sensitivity.

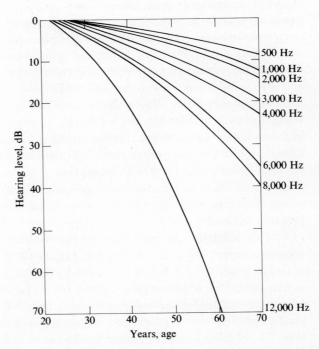

FIGURE 11-11
The relation between age and hearing level. [*Source*: *R. Hinchcliffe, The Pattern of the Threshold of Perception for Hearing and Other Special Senses as a Function of Age, Gerontologia,* **2**:311 (1958).]

frequency curves of 12,000, 8,000, and 6,000 Hz are not of consequence, as these are above the speech frequencies.   The importance of data on presbycusis in medical-legal evidences on losses ascribed to occupational exposure is evident.   This holds particularly in United States workmen's compensation procedures, in which the awards are scaled to the extent of disability.

There are two types of hearing changes caused by noise exposure.   Temporary threshold shift (TTS) is the lessened ability to hear weak auditory signals, from which there is recovery in a matter of hours and at most in 2 to 4 weeks.   Noise-induced permanent threshold shift (NIPTS) is a loss from which there is no recovery.   The relations between the two are not clear.   It cannot be assumed that the second is an extension of the first in terms of changes in the auditory response system (Ref. 11-8, p. 40).   For both conditions higher SPLs for long time periods increase severity.   By its nature TTS has been easier to study.   Some things that are known about TTS is that it increases linearly with the average noise level, from about 80 dB up to 130 dB.   It is proportional to the fraction of time that the noise is present; therefore steady noise is the major offender.   Noise with its maximum energy in the low frequencies produces less TTS than that at high frequencies.   The locus in the ear structure of physiological impairment associated with TTS is specific, the hair cells of the cochlea.   There is no treatment specific or palliative.   The remedy is removal from the noise to allow recovery.   Recovery is exponential, with the greater regains in the periods immediately after removal.   For those with losses less than 40 dB, complete recovery within 16 hours is usual (Ref. 11-8, pp. 41, 42).

From extended observations several things can be said about NIPTS, a form of deafness (Ref. 11-8, pp. 44–47).

1   Exposures of 8 h/day for several years, to SPLs above 105 dBA are sure to produce NIPTS in a normal unprotected ear.

2   The first and most severe NIPTS is at frequencies in the neighborhood of 4,000 Hz.   The ear transmits sound to the brain best at frequencies between 1,000 and 4,000 Hz.   In this range more energy reaches the cochlea.

3   If there is going to be partial recovery of the loss, that is, if part of the loss is TTS, almost all such recovery will occur in 2 weeks.   There will be some added recovery in a month.   Single event injury, as a gun shot near the ear, may show recovery up to 2 months.

4   Noise-induced permanent threshold shift is not progressive after the person is removed from the noise.   Neither is a noise-damaged ear more susceptible to further injury than a normal ear.

5   Regular exposure to moderate noise does not make the ear more resistant to occasional exposures to high-intensity noise.   The ear does not toughen.

6   Susceptible individuals cannot be identified before they suffer hearing losses. Monitoring audiometry detects early NIPTS before it becomes severe.

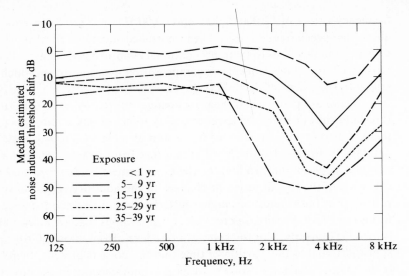

FIGURE 11-12
Median noise-induced hearing changes for jute weavers as a function of years of
exposure.   [*Source*: *W. Taylor et al., Study of Noise and Hearing in Jute Weaving,
J. Accoust. Soc. Am.,* **38**:113 (1965).]

7   After onset, further NIPTS cannot be avoided except by reducing the noise exposure.   There is no way to restore loss from NIPTS.

8   In the occupational setting, NIPTS will appear in almost all men exposed 8 h/day
to broadband noise above 105 dBA.   It will appear in about 50 percent of those
exposed similarly to a level of 95 dBA.   It will not appear in anyone at a level
below 80 dBA.

Figure 11-12 shows the characteristics of noise-induced hearing losses among
workers in noisy operations.   The maximum losses at 4,000 Hz and the increases with
time of exposure are usual.   Extensive and detailed data of a like sort for a variety of
manufacturing operations in the federal prison industries were gathered by audiomet-
ric and environmental observations from 1953 to 1959.   The operations produced
overall noise levels of from 75 to 110 dB.   Shifts in hearing level correlated well with
duration and severity of exposure.   It was greatest among the four noisiest operations
in furniture making, the weave rooms of a cotton and a woolen mill, and the twist
room of the cotton mill.   The findings supported the damage-risk criteria that had
been proposed up to that time for exposure to continuous spectrum noise (Ref. 11-12).

Interference with speech communication by noise impedes our activities and
understanding of one another at work, in the home, and in the general social scene.

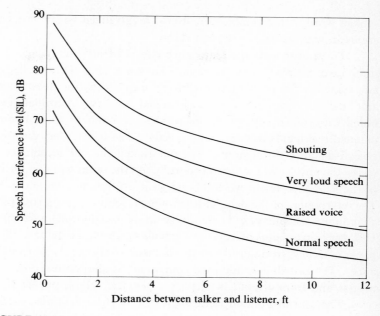

FIGURE 11-13
Transmission distances at four voice levels in the face of SILs of 40 to 90 dB.
[*Source*: "*Bioastronautics Data Book*," *NASA*, *SP*-3006, *p*. 301, 1964.]

With the increase of the speed and power of machines in manufacture, construction, office work, on the highways, and in the home, the interference noise has become all pervasive. Those responsible for the success of electronic communication have given much effort to defining the speech interference level (SIL). It is the average SPL of noise in decibels in the three octave bands, 600 to 1,200 Hz, 1,200 to 2,400 Hz, and 2,400 to 4,800 Hz. These are the frequencies which carry a large part of our spoken words in the range of maximum auditory sensitivity. When the SIL is over 75 dB, a loud voice is needed to get the word more than 1 ft and telephone use is impossible. When the SIL is between 65 and 75 dB, a raised voice can pass the word about 2 ft. A loud voice would move it 4 ft, and a shout 8 ft. Telephone conversation is difficult at the 65 to 75 dB SIL. Things get better at the 55 to 65 dB SIL, with telephone conversation unimpaired. An SIL of 55 dB is tolerable in open office areas. A 45-dB SIL or lower is desirable for private offices and conference and class rooms. Figure 11-13 diagrams the transmission distance at four voice levels in the face of SILs of 40 to 90 dB. The real remedy is to quiet down the space in which interference is happening. There has been some use of sound-powered amplifiers used at close range. Amplifier systems such as hearing aids are of no use, as the SIL is amplified along with the spoken word.   In some bad situations, prearranged vocabularies and sign language are used, with writing as the last resort.

To venture into the annoyance effects of noise is to encounter the subjective response of people to noise head-on.   Facts are few.   Those collected by the question-aire route are fraught with many biases, imposed by the questioners, the questioned, and finally the interpreter of the assembled answers.   A brilliant example is the Okla-homa City, Oklahoma, study on resident reaction to sonic boom from a series of planned overflights at supersonic speeds.   The questioners did their best to hold an objective stance throughout.   The questioned showed acceptance at the start of the series, the posture of the "good sport."   As the series wore on, their sportsman's view of the field experiment wore off and their attitude became increasingly antagonistic. The interpreters of the data, at least in press releases, saw a rosy picture in the data of community acceptance of being shook-up six to eight times a day by sonic boom.   The U.S. Air Force claims officers see a greenish picture, the shade of the reverse side of our paper currency, paid out to satisfy, claims or to silence the raucous but spurious claim-ants.   The British have reported community studies on responses to noise of multiple origins and from aircraft in airport zones (Ref. 11-10, pp. 99–107 and 206–234).

The central London noise survey of 1963 by field measurement supported the opinion surveys against street traffic noise.   It predominated in 84 percent of 400 locations at which noise analyses were made.   In the remaining 16 percent of the locations, the predominant noises were industrial, 7 percent, railway, 4 percent; building operations, 4 percent; and unclassified, 1 percent.   The traffic noise reached 90 dBA, with diesel trucks the main source, followed by buses, and occasional motorcycles and sports cars.   This 1963 survey was away from airport areas.   These received separate attention.

At London's Heathrow Airport the nearly 200,000 aircraft movements per year in 1965 is expected to reach nearly 350,000 by 1975.   The 1975 projected traffic requires nearly 1,000 landings and takeoffs per day.   Small wonder that the planners for second airports for large cities encounter firm and furious resistance from public and private sources whenever a proposed site is revealed.   The resident and property owner ob-jections are to the noise, the annoyance, and the limitations on property use these impose.   The Heathrow study of 1961, the start of the jet engine era, presaged what has come.   Nearly 2,000 of the 1,400,000 residents within 10 mi of Heathrow were interviewed in depth, while on-the-ground noise from aircraft was measured at 85 locations.   Figure 11-14 gives a statistical summation of the annoyance rating— from 1 equals "little annoyed" to 4 equals "very much annoyed"—of the PNdB (Perceived Noise in Decibels), and of three groupings of the number of overflights per day.   Note that the latter numbers are rather few compared with what must now pre-vail in some sections of the Heathrow area.   The figure is nevertheless much like Leo

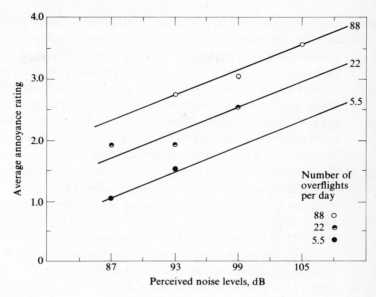

FIGURE 11-14
Relation between average annoyance and perceived noise levels from jet aircraft.
(*Source*:   *Ref.* 11-10, *p.* 225; *original from Committee on the Problem of Noise,*
1963, London.)

L. Beranek's graphic composite of four studies (Ref. 11-8, p. 260).   Beranek uses a
descriptive annoyance scale from "noticeable" to "unbearable," a range of 20 to 40
overflights a day, and an outdoor PNdB of 80 to 130.

Beyond hearing loss and annoyance, what other noise effects have been considered?   Four items are found in research reports on noise effects.   There is not clear
agreement on any of these.   The reason is that there is a large network of an individual's
whole personality, environmental adaptation, and value set involved in his real or
imagined reaction to noise.

1   Disruption of sleep and rest is a common and accepted product of noise, particularly loud unexpected noise.   At the other end of the scale is the drip, drip of
the faucet and the second undropped shoe.   There is the case of the window-air-
conditioner noise in the bedroom being welcome to mask more distant noise
sources.   People accommodate to noise.   Disruption results when an added or
new noise penetrates the accommodation level.

2   Changes in work capacity or performance due to noise or its reduction has not
been demonstrated in field studies, with one exception.   That exception is for
tasks requiring vigilance in monitoring instrument control panels.   Under noisy

conditions there is a loss of attentive response.   The importance of this mounts as more tasks require responding to signals from automated systems.   The results of some field studies have been in doubt or subsequently disproved because of lack of control group observations.   Efficiency in complex tasks may be reduced initially by noise, but the loss is regained with exposure time and practice. There are favorable responses in morale, motivation, and attitude in worker groups when management shows concern for them.   This response to noise reduction rather than the noise change itself may produce improved outputs. Because such factors enter, it has not been possible to determine cause-effect relations between noise reductions and such measureables as accident rates, absenteeism, and turnover (Ref. 11-9, p. N4-11).

3   There have not been any disease symptoms or physiological impairment attributable to noise other than hearing loss.   There are responses such as pupil dilation, reduced blood flow to the skin owing to vasoconstriction, and temporary increase in blood pressure (Ref. 11-8, pp. 89–91).   In part, these responses are in keeping with elemental alert and defense reactions to danger signals.

4   With physical signs of noise stress difficult to assess and very much in doubt, the much less measurable and indefinite mental signs or even behavioral signs of noise stress are wholly uncertain.   W. Burns cites a U.S. Navy study among jet aircraft carrier crews to determine if noise increased the probability of signs of nervous conditions to which a man might be predisposed.   No evidence to support the hypothesis was obtained (Ref. 11-8, pp. 113–114).

The hard facts readily available on the costs of property damage from noise is limited to the special case of sonic boom damage from U.S. Air Force supersonic flights over the continental United States.   The Air Force procedures and experiences on sonic boom claims for the fiscal years, July 1 through June 30, 1956 through 1968, are summarized by W. F. McCormack (Ref. 11-8, pp. 270–277).   The number of claims rose from 36 in 1956 to a peak of 9,574 in 1965, the year of the Oklahoma City test flights.   The total claims for the 12 years were 38, 483, for $22,209,000.   Of these about one-third were approved in whole or in part for a total of about $1.5 million. The damages adjudicated were rather minor, covering broken or cracked glass, damage to plaster, and fallen objects.   The Oklahoma City sonic-boom-effect tests required 1,253 supersonic flights in the first 6 months of 1964.   The tests produced 4,901 claims for an average of $93 per claim, predominantly for glass and secondarily for plaster damage.   Human injury from sonic boom is very infrequent and limited to being cut by glass or struck by falling objects.   Domestic animal injury is also rare.   No effects have been found on productivity of female animals or the hatchability of eggs. Any damage to egg shells is minimal.   A high percentage of animal claims are for injury resulting from startle and occasionally panic among confined animals.

Acceptable Noise-Level Risks

The goal of studies of human effects from noise and of existing environmental noise levels is to determine a set of values which most people can accept, tolerate, or withstand with some identifiable risk of impairment, speech interference, or annoyance. There has been agreement in the United States for such levels in the occupational setting. Table 11-5 states permissible noise exposure in the SPL-dBA for time periods of 8 to $\frac{1}{4}$ h/working day, or less. The noise exposure range is from 90 dBA for 8 hours to a maximum of 115 dBA for 15 min or less in an 8-hour working day. When occupational noise remains below these levels, nearly all workers may be repeatedly exposed to such noise without impairing their ability to hear and understand normal speech. Hearing impairment has been medically defined as an average hearing threshold level in excess of 25 dB at 500, 1,000, and 2,000 Hz. The permissible exposures have been adopted by the American Conference of Governmental Industrial Hygienists, and in 1971 were adopted by the Department of Labor for use under the Occupational Safety and Health Act of 1970.

The noise readings are those observed in using a standard sound-level meter operating on the A weighting network with slow meter response. The exposure to impulsive or impact noises should not exceed 140 dBA peak sound pressure. K. D. Kryter notes that these permissible noise exposures appear to accept the risk of unlimited hearing losses at frequencies above 2,000 Hz, and that the use of the decibel A weighting leads to underestimates of relative damage risks to higher-frequency bands. He

Table 11-5 PERMISSIBLE NOISE EXPOSURES IN OCCUPATIONAL SETTINGS

Duration/day, h	Sound level, dBA
8	90
6	92
4	95
3	97
2	100
$1\frac{1}{2}$	102
1	105
$\frac{1}{2}$	110
$\frac{1}{4}$ or less	115

SOURCE: *Federal Register*, **34**(96), Tuesday, May 20, 1969, Washington, D.C.

suggests the use of a decibel *D* weighting network, as it is more responsive from 2,000 to 10,000 Hz than the *A* weighting network (Ref. 11-13, pp. 159 and 162).   The justification for using the decibel *A* readings is that many industrial noises are low frequency and that hearing losses above 2,000 Hz have not been considered in damage criteria for workmen's compensation in United States procedures.   Meeting the permissible noise exposures will not remedy many speech interference situations.   Shouting would be required at face-to-face range for speech communication in almost all environments just meeting the permissible noise exposures given in Table 11-5.

Defining community noise has moved from the rather crude surveys of the 1920 to 1940 period of isolated measurements and complaint compilations.   Two parameters in use are the noise rating (NR) and the PNdB.   From such measurements, suggested or recommended values for varying community situations are proposed.   A very straightforward example without resort to these special parameters is given in Table 11-6.   It is the result of the deliberations of a group of Swiss experts who were called upon by their government to provide a base for community planning, police action, and court judgments.   The group recognized the compromises between scientific knowledge and the need for practical protective action (Ref. 11-8, p. 101). Note the differentiation among use of areas, for day and night levels, and among background, frequent-peak, and rare-peak noise levels, all on the decibel *A* scale.   The notes below the table define the point of measurement and the terms used.   The British Committee on the Problem of Noise of 1963 recommended noise levels in decibel *A*

Table 11-6   RECOMMENDED NOISE LIMITS IN SWITZERLAND

Area	Background noise		Frequent peaks		Rare peaks	
	Night, dB*A*	Day, dB*A*	Night, dB*A*	Day, dB*A*	Night, dB*A*	Day, dB*A*
Health resort	35	45	45	50	55	55
Quiet residential	45	55	55	65	65	70
Mixed	45	60	55	70	65	75
Commercial	50	60	60	70	65	75
Industrial	55	65	60	75	70	80
Traffic arteries	60	70	70	80	80	90

Measurement with microphone at open window recommended.
 Desirable values 10 dB less, but not more than 30 dB less.
Background noise: mean value (average noise value without peaks).
Frequent peaks: 7–60 peaks/h.
Rare peaks: 1–6 peaks/h.
SOURCE: Ref. 11-8, p. 101.

for the inside of dwellings which should not be exceeded more than 10 percent of the time.   These were grouped for three residential areas and for day and night as follows: country, 40 day, 30 night; suburban, 45 day, 35 night; busy urban, 50 day, 35 night. With a good quality of wall construction, these interior noise levels can be maintained between dwelling units of apartment buildings.   Wall attenuations of 45 and 50 dB can be attained with proper materials and workmanship.   This means a neighbor's 80-dB noise would be contained in his apartment.   European building standards have been more specific in sound transmission requirements than those in use in the United States.

The NR scheme is of British origin.   It has been proposed for adoption by the International Standardization Organization.   Its application requires the use of a family of NR curves in which the decibel intercept at 1,000 Hz is the NR number.   A recorded noise spectrum is given an NR by comparing it with the NR curves.   The NR can be interpreted for particular situations by the use of two tables covering several room occupancy uses and corrections for differing swelling requirements (Ref. 11-10, pp. 115–120).   The NR scheme has a number of applications.   One is to predict community reaction to noise.   Table 11-7 shows five levels of estimated community reaction for five ranges of corrected NR.   Under present traffic patterns and motor vehicle design and condition, very few of our busy metropolitan commercial arteries will escape the last two reaction classifications, threats of community action and vigorous community action.   Readings in five major intersections such as Times Square and Union Square in the Borough of Manhattan ranged from 64 to 76 dB.   As there is habituation to existing noise, the introduction of a new noise, such as the transformer station, poses unpredictable resident responses.   P. N. Borsky points out that very few annoyed people carry their serious complaints through formal official channels.   In British and United States experience that number is from 6 to 10 percent, the tip of an iceberg of the actual number of annoyed citizens (Ref. 11-8, p. 191).

Table 11-7   ESTIMATED COMMUNITY RE-
ACTION AT FIVE RANGES OF
CORRECTED NR

Estimated community reaction	Corrected NR
No observed reaction	Less than 40
Sporadic complaints	40–50
Widespread complaints	45–55
Threats of community action	50–60
Vigorous community action	Above 65

SOURCE: Ref. 11-8, p. 186.

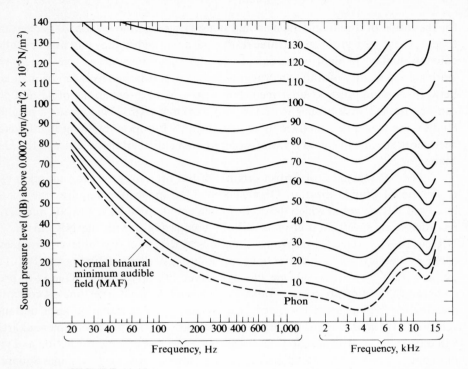

FIGURE 11-15
Equal loudness contours in phons for pure tones. [*Source*: *International Standardization Organization, R*226, 1961.]

Instruments measure the physical characteristics of sound. There is no instrumental measure of loudness, which is our subjective response to the sound energy reaching our ear and brain. To measure or to find an equivalence scale of the sensation of loudness, three terms are in use, the phon, the sone, and the PNdB and an associated unit, the noy.

The phon expresses the loudness level, judged by listeners, hence subjective, to be equivalent in loudness to the SPL in decibels of a simple tone at 1,000 Hz. From compilations of many subjective responses, a graph of equal loudness contours has been constructed. The value in phons can be read for known octave band analyses in decibels. Figure 11-15 shows equal loudness contours in phons of 20 to 15,000 Hz (Ref. 11-10, p. 305).

The sone is a unit of loudness. It is defined as the loudness a listener perceives when hearing a simple tone at 1,000 Hz, 40 dB above threshold, an SPL of 40 dB. That loudness is 1 sone. Other sounds are then judged as twice as loud, 2 sones; as three times as loud, 3 sones, and so on. The loudness of 1 sone, as defined, equals 40

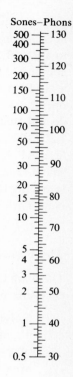

FIGURE 11-16
Nomogram for the conversion of phons
to sones. [*Source: International Standardization Organization, R532,* 1967.]

phons.   For simple tones an average young person will indicate a 10-phon increase in
loudness level for each 10-dB increase in SPL in frequencies from 600 to 2,000 Hz.
Correspondingly, he will rate the sound as twice as loud, that is 2 sones.   The usefulness of all this is the converse.   The acoustic expert uses these responses and units to
analyze complex sounds and to calculate their loudness.   Figure 11-16 is a nomogram
for converting from phons to sones.   For a sample calculation on sones, see Ref. 11-10
(pp. 306–308).

The PNdB has been devised by Karl D. Kryter to cope with the noise annoyance from jet engines.   Due to the high frequencies of jet noise, the overall SPL values
do not correlate with the judgments of noisiness.   Kryter's scale of "equal-annoy-
ance contours" gives more weight to the high frequencies.   The PNdB scale of noisiness is analogous to the sone scale of loudness.   Kryter designates the unit as the noy
with a base of 40 dB above threshold in a bandwidth of one octave rather than the simple tone of 1,000 Hz used for the sone.   W. Burns provides a graph of contours of perceived noisiness in noys as adopted by the International Standardization Organization
in 1966.   The x axis is frequency in hertz.   The y axis is in SPL in decibels.   Burns

gives a sample calculation illustrating how a frequency band analysis of jet aircraft noise is converted to PNdB.   A table or a formula must be used to convert noy values to a PNdB number (Ref. 11-10, pp. 308–312).   The Port Authority of New York has adopted 112 PNdB as the limiting noise from jet aircraft.   The London Heathrow uses a 110 PNdB for day operations and a considerably lower value of 100 PNdB for night operations.   These limits apply to ground-level readings during takeoff, made in residential areas nearest to the runways.   Usually the planes are at an altitude of 600 to 1,200 ft when passing such monitoring points.   Beranek states that perceived noise level in PNdB can be approximated by adding 13 dB to the decibel A reading of a standard sound-level meter.   Such readings are at the maximum intensity of the noise which lasts only for a second (Ref. 11-8, pp. 256–275).   At 112 PNdB, those dwelling near New York airports are far from rural quietude.

The Rationale of Noise Control

There are three elemental approaches to noise control, reduction of vibrating sources, enclosure of the source, and attenuation by absorption after generation and release.

1 Noise is produced by an aerodynamic disturbance such as air moving in a duct, discharging from a pneumatic tool, and being pushed about along the surfaces of speeding cars and trucks, beat about by propellors, or squeezed and thermally expanded through jet engines.   Or noise is generated by the vibration of structures purposefully set in motion, as an internal-combustion engine or the shuttle of a loom.   Noise is also produced by a surface that is vibrating as it is connected to the moving parts of machinery, such as a fan housing or a mounting of a punch press or packaging machine.   Control at the source then depends on altering the aerodynamic characteristics of the vibrating air by dimensional changes, by smoothing its flow to reduce turbulence, and by absorbent materials along its path.   Control of vibrating surfaces requires choices of such alternatives as flexible materials in toto or at joints and mounts to limit vibration, or the use of solid rigid material of such mass that the sound energy cannot vibrate it.   Other alternatives are the use of viscous frictional coatings such as car body undercoatings which resist vibratory motion, or the use of porous materials which absorb the mechanical and sound energy so that the surfaces vibrate very little if at all.   In control at the source, attention is directed to the vibrating components which create the noise.   Efforts by mechanical engineers, who design machinery, to moderate built-in noise have just begun.   Equipment noise specification at the time of purchase is being more widely practiced.   It is more economical to pay more for quieter equipment than to pay to control the noise from it after installation and during use.

2   The escape of noise can be prevented by complete enclosure of the noisemaker. With provision for heat dissipation, motors and production machines can be put on vibration mounts and housed in sound-absorbent materials.   Escape can be somewhat reduced by partial enclosure.   Absorbent baffles at air inlets and outlets can reduce the escape of fan noise.   Mufflers control the escape of exhaust air and gas noise partly by altering the aerodynamics and partly by absorbing existing vibrations.

3   The behavior of noise which has already been generated and which has escaped into a room can be modified.   Acoustic characteristics which influence the behavior of emitted noise in a room are the absorption coefficients of surfaces exposed to the noise; the reverberation time which depends on the noise source and the room; and the transmission losses through the walls, floor, and ceiling. Acoustically, reverberation time of a room is the period required for any sound to decrease by 60 dB after the source is cut off and absorption takes place.   In practice the concern is for the steady state of noise that results from a steady source from which the room continuously absorbs a part of the radiated sound energy.   In this dynamic state, reverberation time is measured to determine the average absorption characteristics of a room.   This technique of control depends on reducing the noise level by improving the absorption characteristics of the room.   Suspended absorbent baffles have been used in the always noisy weave rooms.   Modification of wall and ceiling qualities is the principal procedure, and floors as well where change does not interfere with floor serviceability. Application of this approach is a demanding task for a skilled, experienced acoustic control expert.

The methods of noise control in the United States are well formulated for controlling industrial noise.   The publication of the American Industrial Hygiene Association (Ref. 11-14) sets forth the procedures in principle and practice.   The principles embrace plant planning; substitution of quieter equipment, processes, and materials; reduction at the source and reduction by transmission by air.   Explanation of these tenets and thirty-three plates covering control of typical noisy machines and tools illustrate the practice.   Community noise control has been dependent on zoning of land use and regulatory action on complaints.   With traffic the dominant source of noise, more effective results would come from traffic routing and stricter control of major-artery planning, design, and material selection.   Deflecting embankments and absorbing trees and shrubs are helpful.   Noise transmission within buildings in the United States has worsened with the use of lightweight wall construction and extensive duct work for the widely used forced-air systems for space heating and cooling.   Thin-section floors and ceilings have higher transmission of noise.   The use of thin concrete pourings and precast panels make noise control between dwelling units of apartment buildings and from street and air space above less effective.   Year-around air temper-ing has helped against outside noise by making it unnecessary to open windows for ventilation.

The Society of Automotive Engineers has standardized on a loudness level of 125 sones as a "new-vehicle standard" for trucks.   Under most conditions of use it is doubtful that this will meet the proposed environmental sound level of 88 dBA measured 50 ft from the moving-vehicle source.   Tire noise is a major contributor. New York State has a law limiting truck noise to 88 dBA with 2 dBA as a tolerance. The unresolved tire-noise problem has limited enforcement to speeds less than 35 mi/h! In 2 years, six summonses were issued where traffic exceeds 1,000 trucks per hour (Ref. 11-8, p. 310).   Much remains to develop community demand for traffic noise control that compels action by officials, truckers, and manufacturers.   To the credit of the Society of Automotive Engineers is their development of standards on sound levels for passenger cars, tractors, bulldozers, shovels, cranes, home lawn mowers, and power garden tools.

The issue of aircraft noise is summed up by Leo L. Beranek of Bolt, Beranek and Newman, acoustical consultants, in two statements (Ref. 11-8, pp. 263 and 269).

> The noise that residents of a neighborhood experience from aircraft flyovers may be reduced in varying amounts by a variety of methods:
>
> 1   Reduce the noise power generated by aircraft when the engines are operated at full thrust.
> 2   Require aircraft to reduce thrust and climb at a lower rate when above some minimum safe altitude and when over inhabited areas.
> 3   Turn aircraft away from residential areas during the climb-out phase of takeoff.
> 4   Institute preferential runway systems to direct aircraft away from communities.
> 5   Limit the number of operations and maintenance runups during nighttime hours (e.g., 11 P.M.–7 A.M.).
> 6   Increase the rate of climb or descent upon takeoff or landing.
> 7   Construct runways in directions away from noise-sensitive areas.
> 8   Soundproof and air-condition residences.
>
> In conclusion, I wish to emphasize that aircraft noise will not go away by itself. In the next 10 to 15 years the only possible, significant alleviation of annoyance will be through improved flight procedures and substantial modification of houses to exclude exterior noise.

CHANGES AND DEVELOPMENTS

On Thermal Stress

Thermal stress on workers in the United States will be lessened for three reasons.

1   Enough is known about the physiology of heat strain and its prediction, and enough industrial hygiene methodology is in hand to manage the severe exposures and adverse environments.   Many such situations have remained unrecognized

and neglected because the balance of power among workers, management, and government has left the worker without easy access to remedial action. In some instances, workers have accepted the conditions as "part of the job" and perhaps with some added "hazard pay." Agricultural workers have generally been left without resource, protection, or public concern.

2   These areas of neglect will diminish as the federal Occupational Safety and Health Act of 1970 comes into full effect. As it requires joint state, federal, and employer action, there will be delays, foot dragging, and intentional inequities. In balance is the creation of an institutionalized momentum which will accelerate changes. The benefits will finally trickle down in some diluted form to our most neglected workers, the migrant farm laborers.

3   The continued increase in the use of machines, remote control, and automation in manufacturing, including metallurgic processes, is reducing the exposure of men to hot environments. These changes are characteristic of large operations. There continue to be thousands of small, "job" foundries with unchanged radiant-heat exposures, and hundreds of small textile mills in which the spinning and weave rooms are as hot and humid as a century ago. The percentage of workers forced or willing to accept these conditions for their working lives is going down.

4   There is a factor that is almost certain to be negative in the balance of heat stress and the physiological strain it produces. That is drug abuse in the daily work force.

The knowledge gained and lessons learned from our explorations of the antarctic continent in an intensive and continuous plan for 20 years and from our military operations in the arctic region should serve well in protecting civilian work forces used to exploit oil on the north slope of Alaska on the edge of the arctic seas. Conditions of work and of discipline are likely to vary. The result from neglect of precautions is immediate and may be most severe. In such circumstances, even slow learners accelerate. Russian experiences in the development of northern Siberia should be useful if these are accessible.

The explosive urbanization and rising industrialization of the tropical and subtropical regions are imposing thermal stresses in new forms and in new time schedules on those who leave the rural village agrarian life for the city and whatever work it offers. Compared with the social stresses, thermal stress may be small. It is there though, and it is most evident in manufacturing operations. The agrarian schedule is flexible. It can be fitted to the sun with a predawn start, a midday to midafternoon siesta, and a twilight work resumption. The factory schedule is geared to the capital investment in machinery and plant, and to the order book. There are far too many instances of the plant's architecture and its ventilation, machinery layout, and machinery heat dissipation following the schemes of the temperate zone. Too little thought and capital have been directed to the very different climatic and meterological conditions of the subtropical and tropical regions. It may have been too much to expect of the foreign consulting engineers. It is not too much to expect from the new generation of managers and engineers who have their roots, their practice, and their future in their native lands.

On Noise

In the United States, Japan, and the United Kingdom, community action against more imposed noise from aircraft has and will continue to block the unrestricted use of air space solely for the convenience and requirements of the airborne interests. Four specific examples in 1970 and 1971 actions are:

1 The inability of the Ports Authority of New York to acquire a site for another jet airport in the New York–New Jersey area within a radius of 100 mi. Property owners and communities reject airport operations as incompatible with their expectations of the quality of life.

2 The Los Angeles Airport Commission has resigned itself to issuing revenue bonds that will cost $300 million to purchase all homes, business, and public buildings in a 400-acre area. This will give undisputed air rights of the area to the airport authority and its clients. Houses ranging from $28,000 to $115,000 in value are being sold and moved when possible or demolished. This acquisition has nothing to do with the safety of the airborne passengers. It is to silence complaints and threats of suit from the land-bound neighbors (*New York Times*, July 21 1971).

3 The London airport authority has bowed to community resistance to a new airport near London and settled for a site on the uninhabited Channel coast 80 miles east of London. The Tokyo site for a new 1971 airport also distant from the city is under development and under seige, not by noise-sensitive residents, but by objectors to scenic despoilment for an airport.

4 The Ninety-second Congress of the United States twice voted down further public tax money in the spring of 1971 for the Boeing supersonic transport. Environmental issues of ground-level noise, sonic boom, and stratospheric contamination generated strong public urging for the action. The specter of high cost overruns was also in the minds of congressmen. The risks for very many outweighed the advantages for too few. The prototypes of the Concorde and TU-144 supersonic passenger planes may provide the technology for an environmentally acceptable aircraft. Data on sonic boom over pressures, on civilian reactions, and of predictions of boom paths and composite noise ratings are in Kryter's chapter (pp. 208–227) of Ref. 11-8. Use of the SST in the United

States on medium routes, 1,200 to 1,800 mi, and long routes, 2,000 to 2,400 mi, by 1975 would subject 50 million people to from 10 to 51 booms per day. The booms alone would produce an environment with a composite noise rating of 101 to 115 dB.   Experts offer the opinion that such exposures will result in strong complaints and legal action.

In the United States, public law 91-604, the Clean Air Act of 1970, contained a title IV, Noise Pollution.   It is identified as the Noise Pollution and Abatement Act of 1970.   Under its authority, the administration of the Environmental Protection Agency began a series of public hearings in eight metropolitan centers through the summer and fall of 1971 on the effects of noise, on control technology, on legal and economic aspects, and on research needs.   Systematic coverage of major public noise sources—construction, transportation, agriculture, recreation—urban and domestic will provide a base for further action by federal, state, and local government.   It is a step toward forming public policy on noise.   This legislation and action under it is a move on noise in the public sector comparable to, and in parallel with, that in the occupational setting being made by the Department of Labor in collaboration with state agencies under the federal Occupational Safety and Health Act of 1970.   Under that, the first action on occupational noise has been an extension of the standards that were set for those under the Walsh-Healey Public Contracts Act, to all employers covered by the new act.

APPRAISAL

For the management of the diverse energy forms of heat and sound to safeguard man's health and to provide for his comfort and well-being, the technology is adequate. What lacks is the will to devote capital, public, private, and personal, to apply control methods.   It should be noted that part of that willingness is to accept a higher cost of the products offered on the market.   In the United States, manufacturers and processors delay as long as possible environmental control costs that cannot be passed on to the buyer or that are not paid for by the taxpayers through subsidies, or tax relief by accelerated depreciation, or by reduced evaluation for property tax.   In the United States governmental structure, federal actions applicable across the nation are often favored by management as a last resort in accepting environmental control.   Their feeling is that at least competitors will not gain an advantage by being outside the jurisdiction of effective enforcement.   This explains, in part, the entrance of the federal government into new actions in occupational safety and health and in noise control.

Another price that each of us must be willing to pay in the environmental control of the factors under examination and of all others examined in this book is that of personal restraint and discipline.   This borders on and is in some instances a further surrender of our personal license of unrestrained action.   This price is most evident in terms of restraint in how we dispose of our solid wastes, and how and when we generate sound which is noise to others.   The payment of the price is acceptance of behavior that may not always immediately be fitted to what we judge to be self-esteem and to the expectations of our immediate peers.   Changes in behavior to fit the needs of the general good and our own long-term benefit require maturity.

REFERENCES

11-1   Handbook of Fundamentals, *ASHRAE*, 1967.

11-2   Health Factors Involved in Working under Conditions of Heat Stress, *WHO, Tech. Rep. Ser.* 412, 1969.

11-3   THRELKELD, JAMES L.: "Thermal Environmental Engineering," 2d ed., Prentice-Hall, Inc., Englewood Cliffs, N.J., 1970.

11-4   LEE, DOUGLAS H. K., and D. MINARD (eds.): "Physiology, Environment and Man," Academic Press, Inc., New York, 1970.

11-5   SARTWELL, PHILLIP (ed.): "Maxcy-Rosenau Preventive Medicine and Hygiene," 9th ed., Appleton Century Crofts, New York, 1965.

11-6   LEE, DOUGLAS H. K., Heat and Cold Effects and Their Control, *U.S. Public Health Serv., Monogr.* 72, 1964.

11-7   "Heating and Cooling Man in Industry," *Am. Ind. Hyg. Assoc.*, Westmont, N.J., 1970.

11-8   WARD, W. DIXON, and JAMES E. FRIAKE (eds.): "Noise as a Public Health Hazard," *Am. Speech and Hearing Assoc.*, Washington, D.C., 1969.

11-9   Industrial Noise, *U.S. Public Health Serv., Publ.* 1572, 1967.

11-10   BURNS, WILLIAM: "Noise and Man," J. B. Lippincott Company, Philadelphia, Pa., 1969.

11-11   STEVENS, S. S., and FRED WARSHOFSKY: "Sound and Hearing," *Time Inc.*, New York, 1965.

11-12   Noise and Hearing, *U.S. Public Health Serv., Publ.* 850, 1961.

11-13   KRYTER, KARL D: "The Effects of Noise on Man," Academic Press, Inc., New York, 1970.

11-14   "Industrial Noise Manual," *Am. Ind. Hyg. Assoc.*, Westmont, N.J., 1958.

SELECTED INFECTIOUS DISEASES, THEIR ENVIRONMENTAL AGENTS AND VECTORS, AND COMMENTS ON THEIR EPIDEMIOLOGY AND CONTROL

Disease	Agents and vectors in evident priority	Comments on epidemiology and control
Bacteria:		
Anthrax	Contaminated animal hair, wool, hides; contaminated, undercooked meat; inhalation of airborne spores.	Cases and outbreaks almost wholly from occupational contact with contaminated animal products; total reported cases in U.S., 1945–1951, were 372.
Botulism	A thermolabile toxin produced in nonacid foods under an aerobic packaging; organisms from soil and intestinal tract of animals.	Commercially canned foods not implicated since 1920s in U.S., except for two cases in 1971 from canned potato soup, 1966 outbreak caused by *Type E. Clostridium botulinum* in smoked white fish in vacuum-packed plastic containers.

SELECTED INFECTIOUS DISEASES (Continued)

Disease	Agents and vectors in evident priority	Comments on epidemiology and control
Brucellosis or undulant fever	Contact with infected pigs, cattle, sheep, goats, and horses; use of raw milk and milk products the cause of sporadic cases and outbreaks.	Iowa study by A. V. Hardy, 1930, showed the occupational character of brucellosis; there are economic benefits from control of the disease among animals.
Cholera	Feces of cases or carriers contaminate water, milk, food, and flies; initial wave of epidemic cholera is waterborne.	The Hamburg-Altoona epidemic of 1892 demonstrated the effectiveness of filtration in decontaminating water.
Leptospirosis, Weil's disease or Ft. Bragg fever	Contact with water contaminated by urine of pigs, cattle, dogs, rats, and some wild animals.	Caution in swimming and bathing in farm ponds receiving barn drainage.
Plague, bubonic and sylvatic forms	Organism transmitted by fleas from rats and wild rodents; contaminated vomitus of flea enters skin during biting.	14th century "black death" pandemic, estimated to have killed one-fourth of Europe's people; 1903–1908, sylvatic plague started in U.S. from San Francisco outbreaks of 1900–1907; in 1959, under 300 cases reported in the world.
Rat-bite fever, 2 diseases, Haverhill fever and sodoku	*Streptobacillus moniliformis* or *Spirillum minum* transmitted by bite of infected rat; milk implicated in a few outbreaks	Rat control in slum areas to reduce rat bites of infants.
Salmonellosis	Feces of animals and infected persons contaminate foods; organisms multiply in unrefrigerated foods to deliver massive doses.	Yields to food storage rule, "Keep it cold, keep it hot, or don't keep it."
Shigellosis or bacillary dysentery	Four groups of the dysentery bacillus, *Shigella dysenteriae*, *S. flexneri*, *S. boydii*, and *S. sonnei* leave via feces and return to the mouth directly or via water, food, flies, or fecally soiled objects.	Highest frequency is among low socioeconomic groups in jails, orphanages, and mental hospitals, and among field troops; sanitation in managing feces, food, flies, and water is required.
Staphylococcal food poisoning	A true poisoning by toxin produced by organism during storage above 50°F and below 130°F.	Reheating after improper storage destroys the organsim, but not the thermostable toxin.
Typhoid and paratyphoid fever	Feces and urine of cases and carriers contaminate water, milk, food, and flies.	1849 William Budd deduced the waterborne origin of outbreaks in England; sanitation in managing human excreta, water, food, and flies is required.

SELECTED INFECTIOUS DISEASES (Continued)

Disease	Agents and vectors in evident priority	Comments on epidemiology and control
Viruses:		
Dengue or breakbone fever	Mosquitoes of species *Aedes aegypti*, *Aedes albopictus*, and some *Aedes scutellaris*.	Outbreaks in Caribbean islands, 1963; sporadic cases on U.S. Gulf Coast.
Infectious hepatitis	Outbreaks have been related to contaminated water, milk, and food, including shellfish.	Sewage at intakes of New Delhi, India, water supply produced an estimated 29,300 cases in 1955–1956.
Mosquito-borne viral encephalitides	Virus transfer from wild birds, pigs, and horses by mosquitoes.	Geographical identification of specific viruses producing eastern equine, western equine, Japanese *B*, Murray Valley, and St. Louis encephalitis.
Viral hemorrhagic fevers, mosquito-borne; term *dengue hemorhagic fever* coming into use	Virus may be same as dengue virus, probably from man and *Aedes aegypti* by *Aedes aegypti* bite.	All recognized outbreaks have been in urban areas of the Phillipines, Malaysia, Thailand, South Vietnam, and in localized areas of India; very severe among children in slum and squatter housing; increasing.
Yellow fever	Urban yellow fever from human cases by *Aedes aegypti*; jungle yellow fever from monkeys and marmosets by forest mosquitoes; presence of *Aedes aegypti* in large areas of Africa and Southeast Asia requires vigilance despite absence of yellow fever.	No yellow fever in the Americas since 1942, except for many cases and a few deaths in Trinidad in 1954; Yellow fever has never been present in Asia or the Pacific islands; *Aedes aegypti* eradicated from large areas of Central and South America; reappearance a continuing threat.
Protozoa:		
Amebiasis or amebic dysentery	Hand-to-mouth transfer, contaminated raw vegetables, flies, soiled hands of food handlers, water.	Waterborne epidemic in Chicago, 1933, traced to plumbing defects; 1,409 recorded cases.
Malaria	Three plasmodium types are transmitted from man to man by 1 of about 20 anopheline mosquito species, which are efficient vectors.	1878, C. L. A. Laveran identified plasmodia in patient blood; 1897, R. Ross saw malaria in anophelines after feeding on an infected man; 1904–1914, W. C. Gorgas and J. A. LePrince control malaria and yellow fever in the Panama Canal zone by anti-mosquito measures.

SELECTED INFECTIOUS DISEASES (Continued)

Disease	Agents and vectors in evident priority	Comments on epidemiology and control
Rickettsia: Endemic typhus or murine typhus	Fleas transmit the rickettsiae from rat to rat and from rats to man; organisms in fleas' feces enter through fresh bites and abrasions.	Annual cases in U.S. down from 5,000 in 1945 to under 100; killing rat ectoparasites by DDT dusting of rat runways provides effective control; antirat measures are helpful.
Q fever	Contact with infected ticks, body lice, bandicoots, cattle, sheep, and goats or with their tissue, feces, hair, or hides; transmitted by airborne dust and by raw milk.	Etiological agent discovered in 1937; pasteurization inactivates organism in milk.
Helminths: Ascariasis or round worm	Soil contaminated with feces of infected persons contains embryonated eggs; ingestion of such soil or raw foods after soil contact is the infection route.	Reduction in worm loads among children requires privy use, handwashing, and composting of feces before use as fertilizer.
Hookworm disease	Penetration of skin by larvae developing in soil contaminated by feces of infested persons.	Controllable in rural areas by the use of privies and wearing shoes.
Schistosomiasis or bilharziasis	Eggs of *Schistosoma mansoni* and *japonicum* pass with feces from man and *S. hematobium* with urine to cycle in water through specific snail types, to the cercaria form which penetrates human skin; domestic animals and wild rodents host *S. japonicum*.	An estimated 200 million cases are increasing as more land is irrigated in Asia and Africa; snail kill by Frescon or Bayluscide (Bayer 73) is effective; sanitary disposal of excreta necessary.
Strongyloidiasis	Worm infestation very similar in cycle to hookworm; entry via skin from soil contaminated by feces; dogs are hosts.	Controllable in rural areas by privy use and wearing of shoes; control stray dogs, and treat infected ones.
Taeniasis, beef or pork tapeworm and cysticercosis	Inadequately cooked or raw beef or pork produces infestation with, *Taenia saginata* or *T. solium*, respectively; direct ingestion of eggs of *T. solium* from human feces produces cysticercosis.	Care in feces disposal and use of sewage for pasture irrigation, inspection of cattle and pigs at slaughter, and cooking of garbage before hog feeding are required.
Trichinosis	Pork containing the cysts of *Trichinella spiralis* is main source of human infection; bear, seal, and walrus meat is a source of infection among Eskimo.	Thorough cooking of pork in all forms is a certain protection; cooking garbage at 100°C for 30 min before hog feeding breaks the hog-to-hog cycle.
Trichuriasis or whipworm disease	As for ascariasis.	as for ascariasis.

THE ELECTROMAGNETIC AND SONIC SPECTRUMS IN TERMS AND UNITS USED BY PRACTITIONERS CONCERNED WITH ITS PARTICULAR SEGMENTS

Spectral segment	Frequency, Hz ($=$cycles/s, cps)	Practitioner's usual terms		
		In wavelength	In frequency	In practitioner's parlance
Gamma	3×10^{19} to 3×10^{21}	0.1–0.001 Å (angstrom unit)	Rarely used	0.001 Å $= 1$ x unit
X-ray	3×10^{17} to 3×10^{19}	10–0.1 Å	Not used	Soft, 10–1 Å (or 1–10 keV) Hard, 1–0.1 Å (or 10–250 keV)
Ultraviolet	1.75×10^{14} to 3×10^{17}	4000–10 Å (or 400–1 nanometer, nm) (1 nm $= 1 \times 10^{-9}$ m)	Not used	Near UV, 4000–3000 Å, black light Far UV, 3000–2000 Å germicidal peak, 2537 Å
		10 Å $= 1$ nm (1 nm $= 1$ millimicron)	....	Extreme UV, 2000–40 Å, ionizing UV, 100–40 Å

THE ELECTROMAGNETIC AND SONIC SPECTRUMS (Continued)

Spectral segment	Frequency, Hz (=cycles/s, cps)	Practitioner's usual terms		In practitioner's parlance
		In wavelength	In frequency	
Visible light	4.5×10^{14} to 7.5×10^{14}	720–380 nm	Not used	By colors, red–violet at 720–380 nm
Infrared	7.5×10^{14} to 1.5×10^{12}	0.7–200, μm	Not used	Heating and cooking, 1.5 to 4×10^{14} Hz Radiation from the earth and the human body, 3×10^{13} Hz
Radar	3×10^{10} to 1×10^{9}	0.3–0.01 m	In gigahertz and megahertz (GHz and MHz)	SHF, 0.1–0.01 m UHF, 1–0.1 m Microwave ovens, at 915 or 2,450 MHz
Television	1×10^{7} to 1×10^{9}	10–0.3 m	UHF TV, 1,000–500 MHz (or megacycles) VHF TV, 250–150 MHz (or megacycles) VHF TV, 85–55 MHz (or megacycles)	UHF TV, channels 83–14 at 0.3–0.6 m wavelength VHF TV, channels 13–7 VHF TV, channels 6–2
Radio	3×10^{7} to 3×10^{5}	1,000–10 m	Public broadcasting L (long wave), 150–290 kHz M (medium wave), 515–1,620 kHz S (shortwave), 3–31 MHz	U.S. AM in M band, as 515–1,620 kHz (or kc/s) Europe, M and L bands used Shortwave intl. public radio, set in wavelengths in 7 bands, 12–48 m
Sonic Energy :				
Ultrasonic	3×10^{5} to 1×10^{4}	Not used	100–10 kHz	Ultrasonic cleaning, at 100–10 kHz Electronic induction heating, 100–10 kHz Sonar detection systems, 40–18 kHz
Sonic	20×10^{3} to 20	Not used	20,000–20 Hz (or c/s, cps)	Human voice, 16,000–30 Hz Human ear, 16,000–30 Hz Brain waves, 30–8 Hz ac electricity, 60 Hz
Infrasonic	20–0.01	Not used	20–0.01 Hz	In seismic exploration sonic and infrasonic frequencies, 25–1 Hz are used

Name Index

Abbe, Moigno, 182
Agricola, Georgius, 7
Appert, Nicolas, 391
Ara, F., 331
Aronson, R., 496
Aston, F. W., 422
Ayres, J. C., 417

Baille, H. D., 502
Barber, M. A., 324
Baskaran, T. R., 179
Bates, Lloyd, 466
Baylis, John, 106
Becquerel, Antoine H., 418, 419
Belding, H. S., 519
Beranek, Leo L., 534, 542, 544
Berg, G. G., 138
Berg, Gerald, 53, 62
Besselievre, E. B., 173, 174, 177, 194
Bilharz, Theodor, 350
Birdseye, Clarence, 394
Bjornson, B. F., 358
Black, A. P., 106, 122
Blatz, Hanson, 426, 453, 461
Block, S., 388
Bloodgood, Don, 109

Bolin, B., 277n.
Borden, Gail, 391, 392
Borsky, Paul N., 539
Bramah, Joseph, 186
Brown, J. H., 206n.
Brown, Robert M., 9, 35
Budd, William, 37–40
Burns, William, 541, 548
Buswell, A. C., 183

Caius, John, 37, 38
Caldwell, Elfreda L., 179
Camp, Thomas, 106, 109, 133
Campbell, J. E., 379, 380
Carpenter, R. L., 502
Carroll, Robert E., 42
Carson, Rachel, 10, 357
Cassell, E. J., 42
Cember, Herman, 440, 442, 443, 458, 472
Chang, S. L., 49, 52n.
Charnes, A., 291
Chick, Harriet, 149
Clare, H. C., 158n.
Clark, L. R., 358
Clarke, N. A., 52n.
Cleary, Stephen, 508

Cockburn, W. C., 388
Cohn, M. M., 194
Conley, W. R., 114n.
Cook, K. M., 206n.
Cook, Warren, 220
Coolidge, William C., 425
Cottrell, F. G., 256
Crookes, William, 425
Cumming, Alexander, 186
Curie, Marie S., 419
Cushing, E. J., 358

Dale, Edwin, 18, 35
Daniels, Farrington, 63
Danielson, John D., 276
d'Arsonval, Jacques, 500
Darwin, Charles, 381
Davis, David E., 345
Davis, Kingsley, 2
Densen, Paul, 42, 43
Desrosier, M. W., 399
Dietrich, Berend H., 72–74, 138
Dimitriades, B., 227n.
Douglas, C. G., 204
Dublin, Louis L., 7
Dubos, René, 45
Duprey, Robert L., 268
Dyer, B. R., 179

Ehrlich, Anne H., 34
Ehrlich, Paul R., 34
Einstein, Albert, 422, 491
Eisenbud, Merril, 138, 242, 471, 472
Elder, Robert L., 508
Eliassen, Rolf, 20–22, 97, 109
Ely, T. S., 501
Enslow, Lynn, 106, 115, 116

Fair, Gordon M., 49, 70, 106, 109, 133, 138,
    163, 167
Fermi, Enrico, 471
Ferris, B. G., 61
Finsen, N. R., 475
Fitch, John Marston, 489, 491
Forest, Lee de, 425
Foter, M. J., 401–403
Frear, Donald E. H., 377
Friake, James E., 548
Frost, Wade Hampton, 57, 149
Fruh, E. G., 189
Fuller, George, 106, 109, 112

Gabbai, Albert, 372n.
Gagge, A. P., 512n.
Geiger, Hans, 430
Geir, P. W., 358
Geldreich, E. E., 134
Geyer, John C., 109, 138, 163, 187, 188
Giemsa, G., 324
Gill, P. I., 503, 508
Givoni, B., 519

Glasstone, Samuel, 441
Gloyna, Ernest, 109
Goldsmith, John, 239
Golueke, C. G., 291, 310
Gorgas, William C., 332
Gotaas, H. B., 32, 109, 182, 194
Gould, G., 496
Grafar, M., 329n.
Greenberg, Morris, 334
Gross, E. E., Jr., 528
Gross, Paul M., 17
Grubbe, E. H., 419

Haagen-Smit, A. J., 231, 232, 234
Haggard, Howard, 203, 276
Haldane, J. B. S., 204
Haldane, John Scott, 204, 517
Hamann, C. L., 133
Hammar, B. W., 399
Handler, Philip, 507
Haney, Paul D., 109, 133
Hanks, Thrift G., 284
Hardenbergh, William A., 70, 138
Hardy, A. V., 369
Harrington, Sir John, 186
Hatch, Theodore F., 519
Hayes, Wayland J., 379, 380
Hayne, T. B., 324
Hazen, Allen, 106, 109, 151
Heimann, Harry, 237, 239, 276
Henderson, John M., 72–74, 138
Henderson, Yandall, 203, 276
Herrington, L. P., 512n.
Herschel, William, 60
Hertz, Heinrich Rudolf, 60
Hesse, O., 419
Hill, A. Clyde, 245, 276
Hinchcliffe, R., 530
Hippocrates, 7
Hirst, L. F., 358
Hollister, A. C., 136n.
Hommon, Harry, 147
Howard, L. O., 324
Hudson, H. E., 109
Hughes, R. D., 358
Hull, Thomas G., 334, 358
Hunter, Donald, 276
Hurn, R. W., 231, 263
Huygens, Christiaan, 60
Hyde, Charles Gilman, 106

Iglauer, Edith, 243n.
Isaac, P. C. G., 194
Isaacson, Peter A., 27

Jackson, D. D., 85
Jacobson, Jay S., 245, 276
Jenks, Harry M., 155
Johns, H., 433
Jonge, A. W. R., 324
Jordan, E. O., 149
Junge, C., 29

Kastelic, Joe, 383
Katz, Michael, 57
Katz, W. E., 97, 187, 188
Keeling, J., 227n.
Kehoe, Robert H., 242
Kelleher, R. C., 183
Kennedy, John F., 448
Kensett, Thomas, 391
Knipe, F. W., 324
Kormondy, Edward J., 24, 35
Kraft, A. A., 417
Kruse, C. W., 291
Kryter, Karl D., 537, 541, 546, 548
Kupchik, George J., 294

Lambert, Johann H., 483
Langelier, W. F., 106
Lanoix, J. N., 138, 181, 182, 194
Lavenne, F. V., 519
Lawrence, Carl A., 388
Leal, John L., 115
Lee, David, 184
Lee, Douglas H. K., 522, 548
Lee, F. S., 520
Lehmann, E., 183
Lethen, W. A., 365n.
Leyner, John, 214
Liebman, J. G., 291
Lillie, Robert, 276
Lind, A. R., 514
Lindsay, D. R., 331
Ling, L., 314
Linton, Ron M., 17
Littig, Kent S., 358
Logan, John, 318, 358
Longfellow, Henry Wadsworth, 187
Lotka, A. J., 7
Love, G. J., 8
Luckiesh, M., 484, 485

McArthur, Douglas, 332
McCarty, Perry L., 417
McCormack, William F., 536
MacDonald, George, 354
McFarland, Ross, 14n.
McGauhey, Percy H., 99, 100, 109, 130, 133, 138, 187, 188, 291, 311
Mack, W. N., 51
McKee, J. E., 149n.
McKinney, R. E., 157, 194
McLean, W. A., 366n.
Maiman, T. H., 491, 496
Malek, Emile A., 353, 358
Mallman, W. G., 51
Manson, Sir Patrick, 314
Marais, G. V. R., 186n.
Marengo, U., 331
Marston, B. W., 324
Martin, H., 324
Mason, J. O., 366n.
Maxcy, Kenneth F., 355
Maxwell, James Clark, 60, 63
Melkin, Dorothy, 123n.

Mertens, S., 329n.
Metzler, Dwight F., 99
Michaelson, I., 250
Michaelson, S., 502
Miller, M. M., 138
Mills, E. M., 344
Minard, David, 548
Minette, H. P., 343
Missiorli, Alberto, 331
Moffett, J. W., 115n.
Mood, Eric, 119
Moore, E. W., 83
Morgan, Karl Z., 446, 447, 453, 472
Morgan, Russell, 466
Morris, R. F., 358
Mouras, Louis, 182
Muhlen, P., 324
Muller, Hermann J., 438
Müller, Paul H., 324
Mumford, W. W., 476, 508

Napoleon Bonaparte, 332
Neiburger, M., 248
Newton, Isaac, 60, 481
Niven, W. W., 417
North, Charles, 392, 393

O'Connor, Donald J., 109
Odum, Eugene, 24
Okun, D. A., 109, 133, 138, 163, 188, 190
O'Melia, C. R., 110, 115, 133
Ortelee, M. F., 380

Pampana, Emilio, 339n.
Panum, Peter Ludwig, 37, 38, 40
Parr, L. W., 179
Pasteur, Louis, 349
Peterson, A. P. G., 528
Peterson, R. W., 508
Phelps, E. B., 20n., 57, 106, 132, 147, 148, 167, 194
Planck, Max, 29, 62
Plotkin, Stanley A., 57
Pollitzer, R., 37, 335, 358
Potter, Norman H., 417
Pratt, Harry D., 358

Quon, S. E., 291

Ramazzini, Bernardo, 8
Ramey, James, 471
Rao, T. R., 324
Rees, D. J., 435, 472
Reynolds, R., 194
Riddick, Thomas, 109
Ritter, J. W., 60, 475
Roberts, A. M., 508
Rodie, Edward B., 138
Roentgen, Wilhelm Konrad, 60, 418, 419, 425
Rogers, Jack C., 503, 508

Rogus, C. A., 287
Roosevelt, Theodore, 332
Rosenau, Milton J., 7, 391, 392
Ross, G. Parks, 324
Ross, Sir Ronald, 332
Rossano, A. T., Jr., 260
Roueché, Berton, 34, 37, 38, 63, 235, 276, 414
Ruchoft, C. C., 57
Rudnose, Wayne, 527
Ruggera, Paul S., 508
Russell, Paul F., 324, 332, 358
Rutherford, Ernest, 60, 427, 430, 463
Ryon, Henry, 184

Sartwell, Phillip E., 41, 42, 63, 417, 444, 548
Sawicki, E., 230
Sawyer, Clair N., 417
Scharer, H., 392, 393
Schrader, G., 324
Sedgwick, William, 106
Sekar, C. C., 179
Seltser, Ray, 444
Sesonke, A., 442
Shaw, H., 324
Sher, Lawrence D., 500, 508
Shuval, H., 141n.
Smith, W. W., 8
Snow, John, 37–40
Snow, W. Brewster, 152n.
Snyder, H. E., 417
Solon, L. R., 496
Soper, Fred, 318
Souza, Soares de, 330
Spallanzani, Lazzaro, 39
Spiegelmann, M., 7
Spilhaus, Athelstan, 17
Stern, Arthur C., 276
Stevens, J. F., 332
Stevens, S. S., 548
Stevenson, A. H., 118
Stewart, H. F., 508
Stewart, William, 136, 331
Stokinger, H. L., 137
Stone, Ralph, 291
Streeter, H. W., 20n., 109, 147, 149
Stumm, Werner, 133

Talbot, A. N., 183
Taylor, W., 532
Telles, Norman, 502
Theriault, E. J., 147

Thomas, H. A., Jr., 79, 109
Thomson, J. J., 425
Threlkeld, James L., 548
Tilson, Seymour, 233, 239
Tourin, B., 250
Treybol, R. E., 262
Truitt, M. M., 291
Tukey, John W., 17
Turner, J. E., 447, 472

Underwood, William, 391

Van Dyne, George M., 24, 25, 35
Van Pelt, W. F., 508
Viswathan, R., 134, 138
Vlitos, A. J., 381, 412

Wagner, E. G., 138, 181, 182, 194
Wagoner, J. K., 443n.
Wald, Neil, 464
Walker, H. W., 417
Walker, K. C., 380
Ward, W. Dixon, 548
Warshofsky, Fred, 548
Watt, James, 136, 331
Wayne, L. G., 234
Weiner, D. J., 158
Weir, John M., 331
Weiser, Harry H., 394, 412, 417
Werson, S. S., 291
West, Luther S., 331
Whisman, M., 227n.
White, Gilbert, 138
Willhoit, Donald H., 431, 472
Winslow, C. E. A., 14, 512
Wolf, H. W., 149n.
Wolman, Abel, 66, 79, 106, 109, 115, 116
Woodward, W. L., 137
Woodwell, George M., 26, 27
Worst, J. K., 508
Woytinsky, E. S., 4
Woytinsky, W. S., 4
Wurster, Charles F., 27
Wurtele, M. G., 248
Wyndham, C. H., 521

Zandi, Iraj, 310
Zaret, M. M., 502
Zeidler, Othmar, 324

Subject Index

Page references in *italics* indicate table or figure.

Activated carbon adsorption, 108, *262*, 263
Activated sludge:
  biological makeup, 153
  bulking, 155
  flow diagram of plant using, *154*
Activated sludge treatment:
  compared to package treatment plants, 161–162, *162*
  operating characteristics, *162*
Adiabatic process (*see* Lapse rate)
Agricultural use of water, 127–131
Agricultural wastes (*see* Animal manure)
Air cleaners:
  for gases and vapors, methods and applications, 259–263, *261*, *262*
  for particulates, types and efficiency, *255*, 257, *260*
Air movement, vertical, 32–33, *34*
Air pollutants:
  behavior and fate of, 226–232
  carbon dioxide, 226–227
  carbon monoxide, 226
  control of (*see* Control, of air pollution)
  measurement of, 250–252
    by simple methods, 252
  particulates, 228–231, *231*, *240*

Air pollutants:
  in photochemical reactions, 231–234, *233*
  sulfur dioxide, 226, *240*, 246
Air pollution:
  effects, 234–250
    acute episodes, 235–236, *236*
    on animals and vegetation, 244–247
    on man's health, 234–243
    on materials and property, 248–250, *249*
    on solar radiation, 247–248
    on visibility, 247–248, *248*
    on weather and visibility, 247–248
  estimated emissions, 223–226, *224*, *225*
  from motor vehicles, 224, 226, 231
  from power plants, 224
  primary sources, 223–226
  urban factor in, 238, *238*
  warning signs of 268–269
Air quality:
  criteria in U.S., 269–271, *270–271*
  standards in U.S., 269–271, *270–271*
Air sampling, 208–212
  by extended time collection, 209
  by grab samples, 209
  instruments, 209–212
    cascade impactor, *210*

Air sampling:
  instruments: for dusts and fumes, 209–210,
    210–211
    electrostatic precipitator, *211*
    for gases and vapors, 210–213
    impinger, *211*
  interpretation of results, 212
Air-vapor mixtures, effects on density, 202
Airborne allergens, 198
Airborne biological forms, 197
Airborne pathogenic organisms, 197–198
Aircraft, application of ergonomics to commer-
    cial, 13–14
Aitken nuclei, 248
Alkyl benzyl sulfonates (ABS) and linear akyl
    sulfonates (LAS), 81–83
Amebiasis, 368–369
  Chicago waterborne outbreaks, 48, 369
Amebic dysentery (*see* Amebiasis)
American Iron and Steel Institute (AISI), samp-
    ler, 251–252
Aminotrazole in cranberries, 9
Anaerobic stabilization:
  benthal deposits, *166*, 167
  biochemistry of, 165–166
  gas production, 165–166
  ponds, 166
Anesthetic action, *203*
Animal diseases from livestock water, 128
Animal injury from air pollution, 244–245, *244*
Animal inspection, 385
Animal manure, 305–308
  air pollution from, 307
  bacterial content, 306
  BOD equivalents, 305, 306
  from confinement feeding, 305
  options for handling and treatment,
    307–308, *308*
  pathogenic organisms in, 306
  regulation of cattle feed lots, 305
  water pollution from, 306–307
Antibiotic residues:
  in animal tissues, 385
  in milk, 385
  objections to, in raw milk, 385
Aquatic environment, nutrient balance in,
    124–125
Aquatic environmental requirements:
  of fish, *123*, 124–126
  of water fowl, 124–126
Asphyxiant action, *203*

Bacillary dysentery (*see* Shigellosis)
Bacillus coli (*see* Coliforms)
Bacteria:
  survival of pathogens from feces, 47–48
  survival in a stream, 148–150
  survival of *S. typhosa* in water, 149
Bacterial actions on sewage (*see* Stabilization
    of sewage)
Bactericidal agents:
  chemical and physical, *407*
  iodophors, *407,* 408
  quaternary ammonium, *407,* 408

Bacteriological standards:
  alternates for coliform for swimming pool
    waters, 121
  for foods, 410
  for natural swimming sites, 119, *120*
  for swimming pool waters, 121
Bang's disease (*see* Brucellosis)
Benzo-α-pyrene:
  in smoked fish and meat, 370
  from solid waste burning, 286
  in suspended particulates, 230
Bilharziasis (*see* Schistosomiasis)
Bio-oxidation:
  of industrial wastewaters: by complete
    mixing, 175
    by contact stabilization, 175
    by trickling filters, 175
  two-step process of, 155–156
  of wastewaters, 153–158, *153, 154, 156–157*
Blacklight (*see* Ultraviolet light)
Boat registrations in U.S., 126
BOD (biochemical oxygen demand):
  carbonaceous and nitrification stages,
    161–163, *163*
  load on a stream, 147–148
  means of expressing, 157–158
  monomolecular reaction, 147–148
  reaction constant, k, 148
  Streeter-Phelps formula for, 147–148
  test procedure, 147
Bored hole latrine, 179, *180*
Boron in irrigation water, 129
Botulism (see *Clostridium botulinum*)
Bovine tuberculosis, 365
Brucellosis, 365

Cadmium poisoning from ice-cube trays, 8
Cancer of lung in England and Wales, *41*
Carbon alcohol extract, 83
Carbon chloroform extract, 81–83
Carbon dioxide:
  effect on air temperature, 16, 30
  global increases in, 227–228
Carbon monoxide:
  criteria and standards for ambient air, *270*
  physiological effects of, 203–204
Carbonate cycle, 124, 125
Carboxyhemoglobin, prediction of, 204
Carcinogens:
  in food, 414–416
  in water, 133, 137
Catalytic oxidation, 260
Chemical-biological warfare agents, 199–200
Chemical oxygen demand (COD), 147
Chemical reactions of sewage stabilization (*see*
    Stabilization of sewage)
Chemical residues:
  in foods: control from farm use, 386
    factors influencing toxicity, 374
    requirements for managing, 375–376
    studies required on, 412
    toxicological problems of, 375
  in sewage, 188–189
Chemical toilets for aircraft and boats, 182

Chicago water supply, steps in protection of, 103
Chilean Iodine Educational Bureau, Inc., 122n.
Chinese liver fluke disease (*see* Clonorchiasis)
Chloramines, 116
Chlorinated hydrocarbon pesticides:
  concentration in total diet, *379, 380*
  tolerances in fresh foodstuffs, 378–379, *378*
  toxicity of, 376–378, *376*
Chlorination:
  breakpoint, 116–117
  chemical reactions of, 115–117
  killing efficiency in water, 116, *117*
Chlorine disinfection, 407
Cholera in London, 38, *39*
Chronic bronchitis, 237
Chronic disease and environment, 43
Clarifiers for water treatment, 109
Clonorchiasis, 368
Clostridium botulinum:
  fermentation effect on, 395
  poisoning, *361,* 362
  thermal death curve of, *391*
Clostridium perfringens poisoning, *361,* 362
Coagulation, chemical reaction of, 114–115
Cockroach:
  characteristics, *330*
  disease transmission by, 329–330
COH (coefficient of haze), 252
Coherent light (*see* Laser)
Cold:
  physiological effects, 522
  tolerance temperatures and times, 522
Coliforms:
  bacteriological characteristics, 78
  in human feces, 142
  survival in Ohio River, 149–150, *150*
  in swimming waters, 117–119
  in water, 77–79
Combined sewers, 187–188
Community air pollution, 223–270
Composting:
  of human excreta, 182
  of solid wastes: advantages and disadvantages, 293
    material preparation and handling in, 302–303
    mechanized processes for, 302
    process requirements and results, 299–302
    in U.S. and other countries, 302–303, *303*
Contaminant and pollutant movement from excreta pits, 179–181, *181*
Control:
  of air pollution, 252–271
    alternatives for managing, 253–254, *254*
    appraisal of, 274–275
    changes and developments in, 271–274
    from motor vehicles, 263–267
    by particulate removal, 255–259
    program development for, 252–253
    by removal of gases and vapors, 259–263
  of insects, rodents and snails (*see* Vector control)
  of ionizing radiation, appraisal of, 469–472
Coronary artery disease, 41

Coxsackie virus, 51, 52
Cranberry contamination (*see* Aminotrazole in cranberries)

Dairy farm water quality, 127–128
DDD, residuals in Clear Lake, California, 15
DDE, *379, 380*
DDT:
  in environment, 10, 137, 381
  in estuarine food web, *26*
  in fatty human tissue, *379,* 380–381
  insect resistance to, 15, 323–325
  residuals in Miramachi River, 15
  surveillance and epidemiological needs, 381
Decibel scale for sound pressure level, 524–526, *525*
Delaney clause, 373
  Food and Drug Administration response to, 415–416
  hypothesis of, 415
Delhi, India, infectious hepatitis outbreak, 5, 54, 134–135
  (*See also* Infectious hepatitis)
Deoxygenation and reaeration of a stream, 146–148, *146*
Desalination:
  advantages and disadvantages of, 98
  four processes for, 97
  processes in use for, *98*
Detergent sanitizers, 408
Detergents:
  components and action, 405, *406*
  formulation examples, 406
  trade and common names, *406*
Diethylstilbestrol (DES), 383–384
Disinfectant action on hands, *388*
Disposal of solid wastes, 292–305
  advantages and disadvantages of methods, *239*
  composting (*see* Composting)
  dumping, land and sea, *293,* 295–296
  incineration (*see* Incinerators)
  landfill (*see* Sanitary landfills)
  residues and emissions from, 304
Dissolved oxygen:
  requirements of fish, 146
  saturation values of, *143*
Donora, Pennsylvania, 198, 235, *236,* 271
Drinking water standards:
  for bacteriological quality, 78–79
  for chemical quality, 79–85, *80–82*
  for objectionable chemicals, 81–85, *82*
  for radioactivity, 87–88
  for toxic substances, 79–81, *80*
Dustfall:
  classification guidelines, *229*
  measurement of, 251
  in U.S. cities, 229–230, *230*
  warning levels, 268
Dusts and fumes:
  physical behavior of, 204–207
  physiological behavior of, 207–208
  (*See also* Particulates in air)

ECHO virus, 51, 52
Ecological balances:
    electromagnetic energy and, 507
    factors of concern in, 197
    food protection and, 416–417
    wastewaters and, 193–194
Ecology:
    defined, 24
    and ecosystems, 23–27
Economic costs of air pollution, 250
Effective size, defined, 111
Effective temperature, 517, *518, 519*
Electric power, use in U.S., 18–19
Electrodialysis for desalting water, 97
Electromagnetic energy, 60–63, 473–508
    appraisal of management of, 506–507
    changes and developments in use of, 504–506
    divisions and terms used, 475, *476,* 553–554
    as a resource, 473–474, 505
Electrostatic precipitation, 256, *259*
Emphysema, 238
Energy, electromagnetic: generation of, *62*
    spectrum of, *61*
Entamoeba histolytica:
    cyst resistance to chlorine, 49
    survival in free environment, 48–49, *49*
Enteroviruses, 51–54
    recovery from sewage, 51
    survival in water and wastewater treatment, 52
Environment:
    assimilative capacity of, 19–22
    balance among man, causative agent and, 43–45, *44*
    effects of: on balance of ecosystems and natural resources, 14–17
        on comfort, convenience, efficiency and esthetics, 11–14
        on health, 6–11
Environmental quality report:
    by Gross Committee, 1962, 17, 35
    by Linton Committee, 1967, 17, 35
    by Spilhaus Committee, 1966, 17, 35
    by Tukey Committee, 1965, 17, 35
Epidemiology, 37–45
    of air pollution effects, 235
    defined, 37
    and environment, symposium on, 42
    of occupational diseases, 221–222
    temporal associations in, 42
Equation of continuity, 217
Ergonomics, 13–14
Ergot poisoning at Pont-St.-Espirit, 1951, 371–372
Eutrophication, 125, 189, 194
    of Lake Washington, 15, 189
    prevention, at Lake Tahoe, 189
    of Wisconsin lakes, 15, 189
Evaporative losses during irrigation, 128
Excreta disposal without sewers, 178–186
Eye, the, *496*

Fecal coliform:
    Geldreich method for, 134
    MPN for swimming waters, 118–119

First-order reactions, 58–60
Fish kills in U.S. waters, 170, 307
Fluoridation of drinking water, 84–85, *85, 86*
Fluoride concentrations in water, *86*
Fluorides:
    in air, 244–245
        vegetation damage from, 245, 247
    and tooth quality, 9
    in water, 84–85, *85, 86*
Fluorosis in animals, 244–245
Food additives:
    generally recognized as safe (GRAS), 372–373, *373*
    purposes and examples, 372, *373*
    requirements for control, 373
    tolerances for, *374*
Food adulteration, coverage of legal definition of, 384
Food chain in stream receiving sewage, 146
Food changes, causes of, 388–389
Food handler hygiene:
    handwashing in, 388, *388*
    medical examinations in, 387–388
    requirements for, 387
Food handling:
    bacterial responses to temperature during, *404*
    utensils, washing and sanitizing, 405–409
Food preparation and serving, temperatures to control bacteria, 401–404, *401, 402–403*
Food processing:
    bacterial responses to temperatures of, *404*
    by canning, 391–392
    canning times and temperatures, 391–392
    by dehydration, 390
    equipment washing and sanitizing, 405–409
    fermentation, 395
    freezing, methods and rates, 394–395
    irradiation, 395–398
    sanitary requirements for equipment for, 389–390
Food protection, 359–417
    appraisal of disease prevention by, 413–414
    changes and developments in, 411–412
    cleanliness and esthetics of, 416
    goals of, 360
    in preparation and serving, 400–404
    by processing, 388–399
    requirements for, 400
    tests and inspections for, 409–411
Food protection targets:
    adulteration practices, 384
    pathogenic biological agents: bacterial infections, 364–368
        E. histolytica and *H. nana,* 368–369
        massive bacterial ingestions, 363
        parasitic worms and flukes, 367–368
        rickettsia and viruses, 366–367
        toxin producing bacteria, 361–363
    toxic substances in foods: from additives, 372–373
        from chemical residues, 374–384
        naturally occurring, 370–372
Food storage and transportation:
    keeping time at different temperatures, *399*
    refrigerated airfreight for, 412

Food supply and populations, 416–417
Foodborne disease outbreaks and cases in U.S., 1967–1969, *361*
Fordilla, the, 74
Fosse septique, 183
Freeze drying foods, 390
Frozen foods:
    bacterial behavior in, 399, *400*
    thawing and bacterial counts of, 395, *395*, 399, *400*

Garbage grinding:
    advantages and disadvantages, *293*
    Aurora, Colorado, 296
    feeds sewer rats, 296
    Jasper, Indiana, 288, 296
    sewage treatment loads from, 296–297
Grade A Pasteurized Milk Ordinance, 410
Gross national product, growth in U.S., 18
Ground water recharge, 100
Growth regulators, 381–384

Hardness in water, 84, 93
Health effects:
    of asbestos in air, 243
    of beryllium in air, 242–243
    of carbon monoxide and carboxy hemoglobin, *241, 270*
    of lead in air, 241–242
    of oxidants in air, *242, 270*
    of oxides of nitrogen in air, 242, *271*
    of particulates in air, *240, 270*
    of sulfur dioxide in air, *240, 270*
Hearing:
    auditory sensitivity, 529–531, *530*
    loss with age, 529–531, *530*
    losses among workers, 532, *532*
    permanent loss of, 531–532
    temporary loss of, 531
Heat and man:
    acute failures, 513
    changes and developments, 544–546
    equilibrium formulas, 511–512
    mechanisms of transfer, 509–512
    physiological effects, 512–516, *513, 514, 515*
    predictions of heat stress, 516–519
    production with activity, *510*
    rates of exchange, 510–511, *512*
Herbicides (*see* Weedicides)
High volume sampler, particulate selectivity of, 229
Hookworm, survival in free environment, 49–50, *50*
Housefly and diseases, 330–331
Hydrocarbons in air, criteria and standards for, *270*

Ideal gas law, 202, 216, 224
Incinerators:
    advantages and disadvantages, *293*
    apartment building, 288
    number of municipal, in U.S., 203
    operating problems, 294–295
    operating temperatures, conventional and super-high, 295

Incinerators:
    performance requirements, 294
    residues and emissions from, 304
    siting resistance, 294
Industrial hygiene, 272, 274–275
    (*See also* Occupational diseases)
Industrial hygiene control methods, 213–219
    enclosure and isolation, 214
    personal protection, 215
    process change, 214
    substitution, 213–214, *213*
    ventilation, 215–219
    wet methods, 214
Industrial ventilation:
    contrast between general dilution and local exhaust, *217*
    general dilution formula, 216
    local exhaust, 217–220
        capture velocities required, *219*
        design objectives, 219, *220*
        suction and discharge, *217, 218*
        velocity contours, *218*
Industrial wastewaters, 167–178
    bio-oxidation treatment of, 173–176
    combined treatment, 173, *174*
    conditions for agreement on, 173
    control at point of generation, 171–172
    control and treatment, 171–178
    disposal of solids from, 176
    effects of, *168*, 169–171
    electrodialysis applied to, 177
    injection wells for, 178
    land disposal of, 175–176
    objectionable components in, 167–169, *168*
    on-site treatment, 173–178
    oxidation ponds for, 176
    pretreatment, 172
    reverse osmosis applied to, 177–178
    typical sources, *168*
    unconventional treatment, 176–178
Industrial water, 131–132
    boiler feed requirements, 131, 132
    consumptive use, 131
    quality requirements, 131–132
    requirements for condensing and cooling, 131
    requirements in U.S. in 1980, 131
    use per production unit, 131
Infectious hepatitis:
    Delhi, India, outbreak, 5, 54, 134–135
    virus survival in shellfish, 52
    virus transmission by shellfish, 52, 366
    waterborne outbreaks, 54
Infiltration gallery, 91, *92*
Inorganic nitrogen in source waters and treated sewage, *190*
Insect:
    and animal borne diseases, 314, 327–335, 341–343
    biological transmission, *328*, 330–333
    ecological gaps in control of, 354–355
    endemic murine typhus, *8*, 342
    hemorrhagic fever and encephalitis, 334–335, *335*, 366
    mechanical transmission, 327–330, *328*
    needs and new problems in, 356

Insect:
 and animal borne diseases: plague, 333–334,
  341–342, *342*
  transmission from animal host, *329,*
   333–335, *335*
  vectorial capacity for transmission, 332–333
 and rodent damage, costs of crop and food
  losses, 314, 343–344
Insect control by genetic management, 354
Insecticides, 320–327
 chemical grouping, action and use, *321*
 choices and applications, 325–327
 chronology of development, 1867–1951, *324*
 effects on ecological balances, 357–358
 insect resistance to, 323–325
 for malaria eradication, choices and costs,
  326–327, *326*
 natural products, 320
 pre-use assessment by World Health Organization, 354
 restraints on use, 352–354
 structural formulas of organic types, *322–323*
Intermittent sand filters, 152, *153, 156*
Inversion:
 defined, 31
 ground, 31, *32*
 thermal layer, *32*
Ionizing radiation:
 accidents during occupational exposure, 464
 acute effects, 440–441, *441*
 balancing benefits and damage, 447–448, *447*
 biochemical effects, 439
 biological damage, 419, 436–444
  mechanisms of, 437–440
 changes and developments, 464–469
 control, reasons for effectiveness of, 419–420
 from Crookes tube, 425, *426*
 deaths from, in occupational accidents, 471
 delayed effects, 441–444
  cancer, 443
  cataracts, 444
  leukemia, 443–444
 dose effect from man-made sources, *437, 438*
 dose effect from natural sources, 436–437,
  436
 dose-response curve, 439–440, *440*
 genetic damage, 438
 instrument types and examples, 460–464, *460*
 instrumental measurement, 459–464
 leukemia among radiologists, *470*
 life span shortening, *444*
 limits on exposure and dose, 445–448
 machine produced, 425–427
 origins of, 420–427
 protection, 451–459
  from external exposure, 451, 458–459
  in health services use, 466
  from internal exposure, 451, 454–458
  precepts of, 451–454
 units, 430–435
  for absorbed dose (rad), 432–433, *433*
  for biological effect (rem), *431,* 432–435
  for dose equivalent, 434–435
  for exposure (roentgen), *431,* 432
 working-life doses at Oak Ridge National
  Laboratory, 470

Ionizing radiation:
 from x-ray tube, 425–427, *426*
 (*See also* Radioactivity)
Iron ore, output of world and U.S.,
 1880–1960, *4*
Irradiation of foods:
 applications and effects, *396*
 benefits of, 396–397, *396*
 controversial issues on, 397–398
 dose levels, *396,* 397
 in U.S.S.R. and Canada, 412–413
Irrigation for sewage disposal, 158–160, 308
Irrigation water, 128–131
 degradation of, 130–131
Irritant gas-vapor action, *203*

Jackson turbidity unit, *85*
Junked motor vehicles, 277–278
Jurisdictions, political, number of, in U.S., 19

Lapse rate:
 adiabatic process, 32–33, *34*
 normal environmental, 31, *32*
Laser, defined, 491
Laser energy, 491–498, 505
 biological effects of, 495–497
 eye damage from, 496–497
 production of, 492–494, *492, 493*
 properties and applications of, 494–495
 safe practices for use of, 497–498
Light (*see* Visible light)
Light penetration for aquatic photosynthesis,
 124
Lighting:
 benefits of good, 478–479, *480*
 controllable elements of, 486–489, 505
 glare, 484, 489
 lamps compared, *487*
 management of natural, 489–491
 recommended levels for visual tasks, *488*
 terms defined, 482–486, *482, 483, 486*
 units of measurement, 481–484, *482, 483*
 visual fields, 484, *485*
Livestock:
 injury by air pollution, 244–245, *244*
 water quality for, 128
Lung cancer, 238–239
Lung fluke disease (*see* Paragonimiasis)

Madrid, Spain, water system, 111
Malaria:
 management methods compared, *339*
 in military campaigns, 332
 in Panama Canal construction, 332
Malaria eradication, 318, 336–340, *337*
 appraisal of results and problems of, 355–356
 campaign phases, 336, *337*
 choice and cost of insecticides for, 326–327,
  326
 concept of, 336–337
 defined, 336
 progress and success in, 336–338, *337*
 reintroduction in Ceylon after, 339
 risk of reintroduction after, 338–340

Man, environmental situations of, and air pollution, 197–200
Marinas, 126–127
Mass of dose:
  effect of exposed person on, 55
  effect of exposure conditions on, 55
  quantities injurious, 56–57
Measles on Faroe Islands, 1846, 38
Mercury in the Baltic Sea, 125
Meteorological conditions, impeding air pollutant dispersion, 269
Meteorology, 27–34
Methemoglobinemia:
  from nitrates in baby formulas, 9, 81
  from sodium nitrite in oatmeal, 8
Microwave energy:
  biological effects, 500–503, *501*
  characteristics of, 498–500, *499*
  control of, 503–504
  eye effects of, 502
  fields, near and far, 499–500
  future uses of, 505
  management of workers in, 503
  nonthermal effects of, 502–503
  protection levels for, 504
  thresholds of effects, *501*
Microwave ovens, 500, 505
Migrant farm-workers camps, water use and disease in, 136
Milk:
  bacterial growth in, *399*
  pasteurization, 392–393
    and bovine tuberculosis in children, 365
  phosphatase test, 392
  Q fever and pasteurization of, 393
  quality of raw product, 386–387
Molluscicides, 351, *352*, 357
Monomatic flush toilets, 127, 182
Monomolecular reaction law (*see* First-order reaction)
Motor vehicle exhaust emissions:
  control: modification of gasolines for, 266–267
    by positive crankcase ventilation, *264*
    requirements by model years, 264, *265, 266*
    tests on 1975 model prototypes, 267
  effects of control, 1968, 1970, 1980, 267
  percentage reduction, 1962–1975, *265*
  U.S. standards, 1968–1975, 264–267, *265*
Mouse transmission of disease, 343
Multipurpose water impoundments, 137
Murine typhus fever, cases in U.S., 1932–1957, *8*
  (*See also* Insect, and animal borne diseases)

Natural sites for swimming:
  criteria of: New York City, 119, *120*
    Tennessee Valley Authority, 119, *120*
  sanitary surveys of, 119
Neutron-proton ratios, 422
New Orleans, asthma episodes in, 42
Nitrification of sewage, 162–163
Nitrogen cycle, 125
Noise:
  acceptable risk levels: from aircraft, 541–542

Noise:
  acceptable risk levels: for communities, 538–542, *538, 539*
    at work, 537–538, *537*
  airport, 534–535, *535,* 546–547
  annoyance from, 534–535
    in perceived noise in decibels (PNdB), 541–542
  behavioral effects of, 536
  community studies of, 534
  control: for aircraft, 544
    in communities, 543–544, 547
    in industry, 543, 547
    for trucks, 544
  control approaches, 542–543, 547
  effects of, 529–536
    on animals, 536
    on sleep, 535
    on work performance, 535–536
  impulse, measurement of, 529
  loudness of, 540–542
    level in phons, *540*
    level in sones, 540–542, *541*
  physiological effects of, 536
  property damage from, 536
  speech interference by, 532–534, *533*
  (*See also* Hearing; Sound)
Noy (*see* Noise, annoyance from)
Nuclear fission:
  chain reaction from, 424–425, *424*
  energy from, 423, 425
  nature of, 423–425, *423*
Nuclear fusion, *421*
Nuclear power generators, 466–468
  (*See also* Radioactivity, from nuclear reactors)

Occupational and community exposure to airborne toxicants, comparison of, *199*
Occupational diseases, 200–222
  epidemiological studies by Public Health Service, 221–222
Organic phosphate pesticides:
  tolerances in fresh foodstuffs, 378–379, *378*
  toxicity of, 376–378, *377*
Oxidants in air:
  criteria and standards for, *270*
  health effects, *242*
  vegetation damage from, 246–247
Oxidation ponds:
  for animal manure, 308
  for industrial wastewaters, 176
  for septic tank effluent, 186
Oxides of nitrogen, criteria and standards in ambient air for, *271*
Oxygen demand, biochemical, Phelps-Streeter formula for, 20, 147–148
Oxygen sag curve, 146–147, *146*
Ozone, 232–233, 246, 249
Ozonosphere, *28,* 29

P game, 277
Package sewage treatment plants, 160–163
  basic flow diagram of, *161*

Package sewage treatment plants:
  characteristics of, 160–161
  compared to activated sludge treatment,
    161–162, *162*
PAN (peroxxyacyl nitrate), 234, 246
Paragonimiasis, 368
Paratyphoid fever, 364–365
Particulates in air:
  air cleaners for removal of, 255–256, *256–259*
  criteria and standards for, 270
  equivalent aerodynamic diameters of, *205*
  fate in respiratory system, 206–208
  settling of, 204–206
  size ranges, 205
  specific physiological effects, 207–208
  suspended in urban air, 229–331, *231*
Pathogenic organisms, content of human feces,
  142
Pathogens:
  fate of, 45–54
  survival in free environment, 46–47, *46*
Phelp's rule of expediency, 133
Phon, 540
Phosphate cycle, 125
Phosphates in source waters and treated sewage,
  190
Physiological action of gases and vapors,
  202–204, *203*
Phytotoxins in irrigation waters, 129–130
Pit privies:
  construction campaigns in U.S., Brazil, and
    Thailand, 191
  maintenance and use, 192
  provide hygienic disposal, 139–140, *140*
  reduce worm infestations, 142
  and variants, 179–181, *180–181*
Plague, 333–334, 341–342, *342*
PNdB (*see* Noise, annoyance from)
Poisons in foods, 414–416
Poliomyelitis, waterborne, 51, 54
Population:
  urban growth: environmental consequences
    of, 5
  in India, Pakistan, and U.S., 1900–1960, *5*
  of world, *2, 3*
Population equivalent, 157–158
Potentiation, 57–58
Poza Rica, Mexico, 235, *236, 238*
Public water supply organization, 133

Q fever, 366
Quantum, Planck's equation for, 60

Radar (*see* Microwave energy)
Radiation, distribution of solar, 30
Radio frequencies of electromagnetic energy,
  498, *499*
Radioactive nucleii, 421–425
Radioactivity:
  concentrations in well water, 88
  curie, 430
  emissions, 427–430, *428, 429*
  energy from, 428
  environmental surveillance, 468

Radioactivity:
  levels of, in wastes, 454–455, *455*
  limits on intakes, 448–451, *449, 450*
  maximum permissible body burden of,
    442–443
  from nuclear reactors, 455–457, 459
  precepts on intakes of, 86–87
  in public water supplies, *88*
  of strontium in milk and in children's bones,
    457–458, *457*
  waste disposal, 468–469
  in water, 86–89, *89*
  (*See also* Ionizing radiation)
Radioisotopes (*see* Radionuclides)
Radionuclides:
  chemical behavior of, 87
  in Columbia River, 15
  concentrations permissible in drinking water,
    88–89, *88*
  in environment, 10
  unit of measurement, 87
Rainfall:
  division after precipitation, 93–94, *94*
  in the U.S. (*see* Water resources)
Rats:
  control: by predation and disease, 348–349
    by rat proofing, 346
    by rodenticides, 346–348
  domestic species, 344–345, *344*
  habits, longevity, and reproductivity, *344–345*
Raw-water sources:
  degree of treatment required, 106–107, *107*
  quality standards for, 106–107, *107*
Recreational waters, 117–127
  quality criteria for, 118–119
  man's adverse effects on, 126–127
  for swimming, skiing, and surfing, 117–119
Resources:
  consumption of natural, 2–4
  projection of world use, 2–4
  projections for U.S. to year 2000, *3*
  use of natural, *3*
Respiratory defenses against particulates,
  207–208
Retention containers for excreta, 182
Reverse osmosis for desalting water, 97
Ringlemann chart, 251
Rodenticides:
  anticoagulant, *347*
  choices and procedures, 347–348, *347*
  hazards in use, *347*, 348
  inorganic compounds, 346
  natural alkaloids, 346
  organic compounds, 346
Rodents:
  control methods, 345–349
  diseases from, 341–343
  economic losses from, 343–344
  man and, 340–349
  population estimates and changes, 340–341,
    341
  resistance to anticoagulants, 346
  Salmonella transmission by, 342
Roundworm, survival in free environment,
  49–50, *50*

Salmonella typhosa, survival in free environment, 47–48, *48*
Salmonellas:
  growth on chicken a la king, *403*
  growth and decline in temperatures on steam tables, *402*
  time and temperatures to kill, *401*
Salmonellosis, *361*, 363
Salt concentration in irrigation waters, 128–131
San Luis Drain, 130
Sanitary landfills, 297–301
  advantages and disadvantages, *239*
  decomposition processes in, 299
  equipment for, *300–301*
  leachates and gases from, 304
  methods and procedures, 297, *298–301*
  sites and site use, 297
  water pollution from, 297–299
Sanitary sewers, historical information on, 187
Sanitation of animal quarters, 386
Santee wastewater reclamation project, 53–54
SAR (*see* Sodium absorption ratio)
Schistosomiasis, 348–353
  environmental control points in cycle, 351–353, *352*
  environmental effects on snails and schistosomes, *353*
  environmental requirements for transmission, 351
  transmission cycle and vectors, 349–351, *350*
Secchi disk, 134
Septic tank systems, 182–186
  additive effects on, 185–186
  behavior of, 185–186
  in central Africa, 186
  hygienic disposal by, 139–141, *141*
  Public Health Service studies, 1947–1953, 183–185
  sludge accumulations, 184
  soil absorption lines, *141*, 184–185, *185*
  soil percolation tests, 184–185, *185*
  stabilization ponds and, 186
Sewage, composition of domestic, 142–143, *143*
Sewage treatment, 150–167
  anaerobic processes, 164–167
  bar racks, 152
  bio-oxidation processes, 152–158, *153, 154, 155–156*
  chlorination, *151*, 152
  costs by process and size, *158*
  extended aeration, 160–163
  grit chambers, 152
  by irrigation, 158–160
    in Melbourne, 159
  main stream processes, 151–152, *151*
  primary settling, 151–152, *151*
  removal efficiencies of, *151*
Sewer systems:
  and hygienic control of excreta, 140–141
  and wastewater reclamation, 188
Shigellosis, *361*, 364
Sludge digestion, *164*, 165–167
  time and temperature for, 165, 167
Smog, 232–234
  photochemistry of, 232–234, *233*
Snails (*see* Schistosomiasis)

Sodium absorption ratio, 129, 130
Solid wastes, 277–313
  air pollution from, 286
  bag storage and collection, 288
  clandestine dumps, 286
  collection costs and service, 283
  collection innovations, 291
  collection service and frequency, *290*
  collection and transportation, 290–292
  compaction ratios, 291
  composting of, 299–303
    (*See also* Composting)
  conduit transportation of, 310
  costs, capital and operating, for disposal of, 304–305, *305*
  costs for services in U.S., 282–283
  definition and make-up: ashes, 279–280
    dead animals, 281
    debris, 280
    discards, oversized, 280–281
    garbage, 278–279
    litter, 280
    from manufacturing, 281
    from mines and refining mills, 281–282
    rubbish, 279
    from wastewater treatment plants, 281
  disposal (*see* Disposal of solid wastes)
  disposal Act of 1965, 283
  disposal costs and methods, 283
  disposal options, 278, *293*
  ecological aspects of, 312
  esthetics and resource conservation, 286–288, 31
  fly breeding from, 285
  from food processing plants, 279
  future disposal methods for, 310–311
  health relationships, 283–286, 311–312
  hog feeding on, 292, *293*
  home garbage grinders, 288
    (*See also* Garbage grinding)
  hospital handling, 289
  improvements and developments, 309–311
  incineration (*see* Incinerators)
  landfill (*see* Sanitary landfill)
  management needs, 311
  mosquito breeding from, 285
  quantities in U.S., 282–283, *282, 284–285*
  rail transportation of, 292
  recycling and salvaging, 287–288, *293*, 303–304
  roadside litter costs, 286–287
  salvaging, decline in Europe, 287–288
  source handling and storage, 288–289
  stationary packer units, 289
  storage containers on-site, 289
  transfer stations, 291–292
  water pollution from, 286, 304
Sone, 540–541
Sonic boom, 529, 534, 536, 547–548
Sound:
  frequency spectrum of, 526–527, *527*
  measurement of, 526–529
  nature of, 523–524
  octave band analyzers for, *527*
  power, intensity and pressure, 523–524, *524*
  (*See also* Noise)

Sound level meter, network responses of, *528*
Sound pressure level:
  cumulative values on decibel scale, *526*
  defined and illustrated, 524–526, *525*
  familiar noises as, *525*
Stabilization of sewage:
  aerobic and anaerobic, 143–148, *143, 144*
  biochemical reactions of, 144–146, *146*
Stabilization ponds (*see* Oxidation ponds)
Staphlococcal bacteria:
  growth on chicken à la king, *403*
  growth and decline temperatures on steam
    tables for, *402*
  time and temperatures to kill, *401*
Staphlococcic food poisoning, 361–362
Stratosphere (*see* Ozonosphere)
Streptococcal infections, *361*, 365
Substitutes for toxic substances in occupational
  use, *213*
Suburban development and sanitary services,
  192
Sulfur dioxide:
  in air: criteria and standards for, *270*
    from fossil fuels, 273
  effect on air temperature, 16
Surface water sources:
  advantages and disadvantages of, 95–96
  evaporative losses from, 94
Swimming pool waters, 119–122
  alternates to chlorine for disinfection,
    120–121
  bacteriological quality standard for, 121
  chlorine disinfection of, 121–122
  chlorine residual concentration for, 121
  effects on eyes from, 119
Swimming waters:
  epidemiological study of, 118–119
  findings of Public Health Service studies,
    1948–1949, 118
  human adaptation to, 130
Synergism, 57–58
Systems, environmental: air, *21*
    land, *22*
    water, *20*

Tapeworms, 367, 369
Temperature, global increases in, 228
Temperature tolerances of fish, 122, *123*
Thermal environment:
  cold, stresses and strains from, 522
  control of, 520–521
  measurement by: black-globe temperature,
    516–518
    wet-bulb temperature, 516–517
  measurements of, 516–519
    by effective temperature, 517–518, *518, 519*
  (*See also* Heat and man)
Thermal loads:
  alternates to stream discharge of, 123
  from condenser cooling water, 123
Thermoluminescence, 463
Thermosphere, 27, *28*
Threshold limit values, 208, 212–213, 220–222
  assumptions on exposed person, 221
  epidemiological basis for, 221–222

Threshold limit values:
  information base for, 221–222
  precautions in applying, 222
  types of exposure and response, 221
Total oxidizable carbon (TOC), 147
Toxic gases, vapors, dusts, and fumes:
  chronic effects from cumulative exposures to,
    201
  control of, 213–219
  hygienic standards for, 220–222
  transient effects from short exposures to, *201*
  units for concentrations of, 213
Toxicants:
  in foods: from additives, 372
    high dose-acute effect versus low level-
      delayed effects, 370
    of natural origins, 370–372, *371*
  in natural waters, 125, 137
Transportation accidents, source of air
  contaminants, 198
Trichinosis, *361*, 367–368
Trickling filter bed:
  biological make-up, 153
  flow diagram of plant using, *154*
  rates of application on, 155
  recirculation through, 155
Troposphere, *28*, 29–30
Typhoid fever, *361*, 364–365
  Chicago, 1860–1942, 7
  Massachusetts, 1885–1940, *136*
  Wales and England, 1853, 1866, 37–39, *40*

Ultraviolet light, 475–478
  absorption in ozonosphere, 29
  biological effects, 477
Uniformity coefficient, 111
Urban concentrations in air:
  of carbon dioxide, 227–228
  of carbon monoxide, 227
  of hydrocarbons, nitrogen oxides, and ozone,
    231–232
  of particulates, 228–231
  of sulfur dioxide, 226

Vector control, 314–358
  appraisal of benefits for comfort and con-
    venience, 356–357
  appraisal of disease prevention by, 355–356
  methods defined: naturalistic, 318–319, *319*
    permanent, 317–318
    species eradiation, 318
    temporary, 318
  rationale and requirements for, 316–317
  threats to success, 315–316
Vegetation damage from air pollution, 245–247
Venezulean equine encephalitis (V.E.E.), 200
Ventilation:
  in industrial hygiene: general dilution,
    215–217
    local exhaust, 217–220
  requirements for human occupancy, *521*
Vesicular exanthema (V.E.), 292
Vibrio cholera, survival in free environment,
  47–48, *48*

Virus:
  survival in free environment, 50–54
  transmission by water, 51–54, 134–135
Viruses in swimming waters, 118–119
Visible light, 478–491
  range defined, 479–481, *481*
  (*See also* Lighting)

Wastes, quantities generated in U.S., 19
Wastewater:
  inorganic nitrogen and phosphates in,
    189–190
  reclamation, 99–101, 194
    advantages and disadvantages, 100–101
    at Baltimore, Maryland, 99
    at Chanute, Kansas, 99
    at Golden Gate Park, San Francisco, 99
    Santee project, 53–54, *53*, 99
    at Whittier Narrows, California, 99
  sources, protection and selection of, for
    reclamation, 105
  tertiary treatment of, 189–190, *190*
Water distribution, dual systems for, 133
Water filtration, 111–114
  changes in design rates, 112–113
  by diatomaceous earth, 114
  in London, 1828, 105
  mechanisms of, 112
  by mixed media units, 114, 133
  at Paisley, Scotland, 1802, 105
  polyelectrolyte aids for, 133
  by rapid sand units, 112
  at Richmond, Virginia, 1832, 106
  by slow sand units, 113–114
Water flushed commodes, historical information
  on, 186–187
Water quality:
  biological, 75–79
  chemical, 79–85
  for fish, shellfish, and water fowl, 122–127
  goals of American Water Works Association,
    137–138
  nonpathogenic organisms, 75, *77*
  physical characteristics, 85–86
  radioactivity, 86–89, *89*
Water resources:
  beneficial use defined, 66
  consumptive use defined, 66
  fate of rainfall on the U.S., 66, *67*, 68
  quantities in the world, 65
Water-seal latrine 179, *180*, 191
Water sources, 89–101
  desalted waters, 97–99

Water sources:
  ground water, 90–93
  for Los Angeles, *96*
  protection, 102–105
  quality rating of, *102*
  rainfall, capture of, 89–90
  reclaimed wastewater, 99–101
  surface water, 93–97
Water supply in developing countries:
  benefits of improvements, 74
  cost of improving, 74
  effects of metering, 74
  needs, 71–74, *72*, *73*
  per capita usage, 73–74
  quality, 73
Water supply protection for wells, *91*
Water system leakage and loss, 69–70
Water treatment processes:
  chlorination, 115–117
  coagulation, 114–115
  engineering of, 106–109
  flocculation, 110
  flow diagram of, *108*
  mixing, flash or rapid, 109–110
  sedimentation, 110–111
  for softening hard water, 108
  solids contact, 111, *112*
Water use in U.S.:
  demand: average daily, 70
    maximum daily average, 70, *71*
    maximum hourly average, 70
  domestic use by purpose, *69*
  for fire fighting, 70
  for irrigation, 1900–1975, 68
  1900–1975, trends, *68*
  public supply by use, *69*
  rates of increase of use, 70
  for steam electric power, 68
Waterborne disease outbreaks, 135–136, *136*
Waterborne diseases, 75, *76*
Weedicides:
  toxicity issues on, 381–383
  types, toxicity and uses, *382*
Wells, protection for deep, 102, *103*
Winds:
  Coriolis effect, 30
  effects on air pollutants, 33
  global patterns, 30, *31*

Yellow fever in Philadelphia, 1793, 38

Zones, atmospheric, 27–30, *28*